# TODAY'S
# HERBAL
# HEALTH

# TODAY'S HERBAL HEALTH

## The Essential Reference Guide

Louise Tenney, MH

### Sixth Edition
Revised and Updated

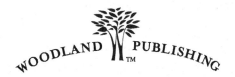

WOODLAND PUBLISHING

For permissions, ordering information, or bulk quantity discounts, please contact: Woodland Publishing, 448 East 800 North, Orem, Utah 84097

Visit our Web site: www.woodlandpublishing.com
Toll-free number: (800) 777-2665

The information in this book is for educational purposes only and is not recommended as a means of diagnosing or treating an illness. All matters concerning physical and mental health should be supervised by a health practitioner knowledgeable in treating that particular condition. Neither the publisher nor the author directly or indirectly dispenses medical advice, nor do they prescribe any remedies or assume any responsibility for those who choose to treat themselves.

Cataloging-in-Publication data available from the Library of Congress.

ISBN 13: 978-58054-416-0
ISBN 10: 1-58054-416-9

Printed in the United States of America

06   07   08   09   10   1   2   3   4   5   6   7   8   9   10

To all those whose lives have been
touched and healed by *Today's Herbal Health*
and the wisdom of nature.

May you be happy
May you be healthy
May you live long

# CONTENTS

## PART 1

### How to Prepare Herbs

## PART 2

### All About Herbs and Natural Healing Agents

## PART 3

### Good Herbs, Good Food, Good Health

## PART 4

### Nutrition, Herbs, and the Human Body

# FOREWORD

FOR MORE THAN TWENTY YEARS, I have watched Louise Tenney write and lecture about something she passionately believes in—the power of herbal medicine. I have to smile when I think about the radical reaction most mainstream practitioners had to her first edition of *Today's Herbal Health*. My, how the tide has turned. Herbal therapies, once referred to as "medieval nonsense," are finally receiving the respect they deserve. Medical practitioners can no longer ignore scores of clinical studies supporting their efficacy. Today, we see herbal supplements routinely sold in pharmacies and grocery stores. And business is booming. Herb sales will reach $2.7 billion in 2006, and according to a new Gallup poll, herb usage among Americans increased by nearly 70 percent. Herbs like St. John's wort and *Ginkgo biloba*, which were relatively obscure twenty years ago, are now considered common household medicines. The idea that for every synthetic drug there is a natural compound that can accomplish a similar effect is rapidly gaining credibility.

Louise Tenney recognized the value of medicinal plants years ago—long before it was the fashionable thing to do. She is one of the most respected herbalist-authors in this country, and for good reason. She not only practices what she preaches but is continually studying to learn more about the disease process and how natural botanicals work to heal the body. Her personal crusade for herbal awareness is centered on the fact that synthetic pharmaceutical drugs only target the symptoms of disease, while plant compounds work to correct the biological malfunctions that caused it in the first place. Always awed by the profound harmony of nature's medicinal formulas, Louise Tenney brings to this book a sense of marvel.

More than two decades ago, her landmark edition of *Today's Herbal Health* boldly set the standard for the rest of us to follow. In this new and completely updated edition, she combines science with personal testimonials to create a reader-friendly herbal guide. Written in a style that has made her one of the most popular American natural health authors, Louise interweaves the common sense application of herbs with holistic protocols. In other words, she advocates treating the body as a whole unit rather than the "in-slices" approach commonly used by most conventional physicians. While she advocates the scientific confirmation of herbal treatments, Louise has always shared less-scientific, yet just as compelling empirical experience. Over the years, some of her views have raised a few eyebrows among conventional practitioners, yet she has never apologized for her belief that when doctors abandoned herbal medicines, they also abandoned centuries of knowledge and, more important, the idea of healing the body as a whole. Vindication in the current widespread acceptance of herbal therapies is now hers.

Easy to read and quantified by years of experience, *Today's Herbal Health* is a book for all people, regardless of their educational background. It discusses which herbs are best for dozens of health problems and cites orthodox treatments as well. In addition, Louise Tenney teaches the reader to look for synergistic herbal combinations that potentiate the medicinal action of single herbs to speed the healing process.

Through her prolific writings on herbal medicine, Louise Tenney has established herself as a foremost expert in her field with a desire to help all people get well. I have seen her in action and consider her both a friend and a mentor. *Today's Herbal Health* takes the guesswork out of the practical application of herbs and comes from the author's profound belief that if you provide the body with what it really needs, it can heal itself. Today, more than ever before, consumers need to get some herbal savvy. I can think of no better place to start than with page one of *Today's Herbal Health*.

RITA ELKINS
AUTHOR OF NUMEROUS
NATURAL HEALTH TITLES

# PREFACE TO THE SIXTH EDITION

When I first wrote *Today's Herbal Health* thirty years ago, I had no idea that it would sell over a million copies, go into six editions, and touch and heal the lives of countless people throughout the world. But much has changed in these thirty years: the advent of genetically modified plants; irradiation of our foods; the increasing use of pesticides, herbicides, antibiotics, and hormones; the near death of the family farm, and the advent of giant factory farms controlled by a handful of agribusiness concerns. Our foods are denatured, toxified, colored, flavored, texturized, saturated with trans fats and sweetened with high-fructose corn syrup. Plus they lack the nutrients and fiber that our bodies really need—and what has this led to—a dramatic increase in the incidence of obesity, diabetes, high cholesterol, high blood pressure, heart disease, strokes, and some cancers.

We've seen dramatic changes in the use of pharmaceuticals since the 1970s. Pharmaceutical companies spend billions of dollars each year advertising drugs for high cholesterol, high blood pressure, diabetes, insomnia, depression, gastroesophageal reflux disease—conditions largely caused by the highly processed, denatured, dead foods that compose the standard American diet (SAD), along with Americans' sedentary lifestyles. Most of these serious health conditions can be prevented, treated, or eliminated with the right herbs, the right foods, and the right lifestyle. So the little book I wrote thirty years ago is needed now more than ever, especially in this revised and expanded edition.

We need to connect with the earth and use plants as Mother Nature intended—for our health and benefit—and we need to avoid as much as possible the unnatural pharmaceuticals and toxic foods that we find everywhere we go. We need to learn from the old traditions and the new research about the healing and sustaining properties of botanicals. Doing anything less can have serious consequences for our health.

Over the years, many people have sent in reviews and letters of thanks for the information on health and healing contained in *Today's Herbal Health*. I'd like to share a few of them with you here:

"I truly feel a new security, peace of mind—excitement—in all that I am doing and in the health of my baby and myself. You are such a healing person, Louise. I can't help but feel blessed in knowing you."

"I don't know what else to say about your research and *Today's Herbal Health*. They have changed my life, and I continue to use your books to educate myself and others."

"I have had so much pleasure and gained so much knowledge from reading your books. Thank you!! Thank you!! They are wonderful."

"You really gave me the incentive to do more and learn more to become a healthier person."

"What an amazing woman! Author and lecturer, in person and on the radio. Louise has done her research and has had lots of experience in her field."

"As I listen to the music of Beethoven and write these lines, I am reminded that music has its innovators and its revolutionaries, like Beethoven , and its great gatherers and synthesizers like Johann Sebastian Bach. Both composers were great, in their own way. So with herbalists. The LaDean Griffins and John Christophers reintroduced the world to herbs and natural health and thereby revolutionized, slowly and surely, the health industry. Others, like Louise Tenney, have synthesized and gathered together the best of all the others into an easy-to-use,

concise, no-nonsense volume that would gladden the hearts of newcomers to herbs. . . . This book is a real winner!"

And finally, Mark Victor Hansen, co-author of the Chicken Soup for the Soul series wrote to me: "You're an inspiration. Thanks for contributing so much."

Thank you all for your kind support of Today's Herbal Health. May it give you the knowledge and tools to find health and healing in your life and in the life of those you love so you can use your energy to make the earth a better, greener, and healthier place for all of us.

# INTRODUCTION

SINCE I WROTE THE FIRST EDITION of *Today's Herbal Health* more than twenty years ago, we have witnessed a remarkable herbal renaissance. Why are so many people turning to herbal remedies? Unquestionably, our disillusionment with the wholesale dispersal of powerful and potentially dangerous drug therapies is part of the reason. Moreover, the surprising popularity of herbal medicines reflects not only the increase of stress on our health, but the consequences of pollution, poor nutrition, and our unfortunate "medicate everything" philosophy. Consequently, many of us have reexamined the value of natural and safe herbal therapies.

In addition, within the past decade, scientific evidence continues to accrue, supporting the notion that herbs are valid medicines and can safely treat the human body. Consider what's happened in this country over the past five years. Herbs like *Gingko biloba* for memory, St. John's wort for depression, and saw palmetto for prostate health are now commonly used. They are even added to mainstream vitamin and mineral formulas, something we would have never seen twenty years ago.

Most people don't know that in the early twentieth century, medical doctors still respected herbology, and as late as 1930, they took herbal courses as part of medical school training. As late as 1960, some herbs were still listed in the *Physician's Desk Reference.* Unfortunately, with the advent of modern pharmaceutical drugs, herbal medicine was abandoned for new, synthetic chemical preparations. What we need to keep in mind is that before the advent of modern pharmaceutical drugs, medicinal compounds consisted of natural substances derived principally from plant life.

Virtually every primitive culture discovered the curative properties of specific plants that grew in their location, and throughout the world, the practice of phytomedicine evolved. Legends and written accounts of herbal treatments are found in hundreds of ancient texts and powerfully attest to their impressive ability to not only ease the symptoms of disease, but to heal the body as well. Herbs listed by Dioscorides in the *Materia Medica* were applied for more than fourteen centuries.

Today, many of the drugs we take are comprised of compounds that have been extracted from botanical sources and synthetically reproduced. It is estimated that 25 percent of all prescription drugs contain compounds that have been derived from plants. For example, aspirin is based on naturally occurring salicin found in white willow bark; Chinese ephedra contains a compound called ephedrine, which is the basis for several over-the-counter decongestants; goldenseal alkaloid compounds have been utilized in many over-the-counter eyedrops; and digitalis, which acts as a powerful heart stimulant, is still extracted from an herb called foxglove.

It must be understood, however, that when we tamper with Mother Nature, we create risks for the human body. When scientists examined plant chemistry, they isolated what they considered the most active compound of a medicinal plant and discarded the rest. In essence, they threw the baby out with the bathwater.

I have learned a powerful lesson from studying herbs over the past twenty years: When you eliminate certain plant ingredients in order to isolate what is considered the active principle of an herb, you can destroy the synergistic or balancing effect of the whole medicinal plant. Simply stated, when nature is tampered with, the natural harmony of plant medicines is disrupted and altered. Granted, synthetic drugs may be more potent, work faster, and can often be administered with great precision. However, the human body has a tendency to identify them as foreign and unnatural substances. As a result, a chain of negative physiological reactions called side effects can occur. Frequently, the body reacts to synthetic and powerful compounds much as it would to poison. Moreover, unlike drugs, herbal medicines not only alleviate the symptoms of disease but actually target the root cause and promote healing, something most drugs can't do.

Unlike the United States, European and Asian countries have continued to study and use herbal preparations. They are leaps and bounds ahead of us when it comes to using herbal medicines. Herbs like milk thistle (silymarin), echinacea, and ginseng are commonly dispensed by reliable medical practitioners who have recognized their therapeutic worth. Hopefully, our physicians will eventually follow suit. Clearly, as scores of clinical studies continually emerge on the efficacy of herbs, medical doctors are starting to pay attention to what we knew all along—that Mother Nature offers us natural compounds capable of safely healing the human body. In addition, I am a strong believer that we can't treat the body in separate parts. In other words, until we address the emotional and spiritual components of disease, we will never really get well.

I have written this herbal reference guide for everyone, from the herbal novice to the most seasoned natural practitioner. It offers what I consider the most important aspects of herbal medicine, including an A-to-Z guide for the herbal treatment of many ailments. In addition, knowing what herbs to take in combination is invaluable.

Today, scientific research supports the ancient idea of herbal "marriages." The notion that combining certain herbs creates a better therapeutic effect can be supported by clinical studies. It's important to remember that the interaction between certain botanicals can be even more important than the individual properties of each contributing herb. Well-designed herbal formulas can exert impressive therapeutic effects on a number of maladies.

# PART 1

# How to Prepare Herbs

# HERBAL PREPARATIONS

THERE ARE A VARIETY OF WAYS to prepare herbs for use. The following section contains descriptions and examples of the most common types of herbal preparations, all of which can be produced in your own home. To determine the best herbal preparation for your situation, you must consider the herb(s) being used and the desired results.

## BOLUS

A bolus is a suppository or internal poultice used in the rectal or vaginal area. It helps draw out toxic poisons and is the carrier for healing agents. A bolus is made by adding powdered herbs to cocoa butter, creating a thick, firm consistency. The mixture is usually placed in the refrigerator to harden and is then brought to room temperature before using. A bolus can be inserted into the rectum to treat hemorrhoids and cysts, or into the vagina to treat infections, irritations, and tumors. The bolus is usually applied at night when the cocoa butter will melt with body heat, thus releasing the herbs. Herbs used in a bolus are usually astringent herbs (such as white oak bark or bayberry bark), demulcent healing herbs (such as comfrey or slippery elm), or antibiotic herbs (such as garlic, chaparral, or goldenseal).

## CAPSULES

Gelatin-coated capsules are a pleasant way of taking herbs, especially when the herbs are bitter-tasting or mucilaginous. Be sure you purchase capsules from a reliable herb company. This ensures the herbs will be prepared, measured, and combined in the right proportion by chemists trained in herbal science. To help with swallowing and dissolving herb capsules, take them with eight ounces of pure water or herbal tea.

## COMPRESS

The effects of an herbal compress are similar to those of an ointment, with the added advantage of therapeutic heat. A compress is basically a soft pad or cloth secured on the body to provide heat, pressure, or medication. It is used when herbs too strong to be taken internally need to be used for healing. Using a compress allows the herbs to be slowly absorbed in small amounts by the body. An herbal compress is used in cases of injury, contusions, and effusions. It is used for superficial ailments including swellings, pains, colds, and flu. A compress always helps to stimulate circulation of blood and lymph in the body.

To prepare a compress, add one or two heaping tablespoons of the herb(s) to one cup of water and bring to a boil. Dip a sterile cotton pad, gauze, or cloth into the strained liquid, drain off any excess, then place the warm compress on the affected area. It is beneficial to cover the compress with a piece of woolen material to hold in the heat. If being used on a small child, the compress should be bandaged into place. After the compress has cooled, replace it with another hot one.

A good example of an herbal compress is one made with ginger. To make a ginger compress, grate two ounces of fresh ginger root and squeeze its juice into a pint of hot water until the water turns yellow. Apply the compress, having hot replacement towels ready as soon as the first one cools. A ginger compress is used to stimulate the circulation of blood and lymph, to relieve colic, to reduce internal inflammation, and to restore warmth to cold joints.

## DECOCTION

To decoct means "to extract the flavor or essence of something by boiling." The term decoction is used to describe the extract obtained after boiling. An herbal decoction is similar to an infusion, but is made from the root and bark of a plant. Decoctions are used when the root or bark is not soluble in cold or hot water, but will often yield its soluble ingredients after simmering in water for five to twenty minutes. A decoction is valuable because it contains an herb's essential mineral salts and alkaloids.

To prepare a decoction, place a teaspoon of the dried herb in an enamel or glass container with one cup of pure water. Instead of steeping the mixture, boil it—five minutes is enough if the material is finely shredded, but if the herb is hard or woody, twenty minutes is necessary to produce a good decoction. It is helpful if the plant is first soaked in cold water and then brought to a boil. Decoctions should always be strained while hot.

## EXTRACTS

An extract is a concentrated form of an herb that is obtained by mixing the herb with an appropriate solvent (such as alcohol and/or water). Herbal extracts are usually made from stimulating herbs, such as cayenne, and antispasmodic herbs, like lobelia. Extracts are rubbed into the skin as a treatment for strained muscles and ligaments, or for the relief of arthritis and other inflammations. (See Appendix for specific formulas.)

Extracts can be made by placing four ounces of dried herbs or eight ounces of fresh, bruised herbs into a jar or bottle with a tight-fitting lid. Add one pint of vinegar, alcohol, or massage oil. With time, the liquid will extract the medicinal properties of the herbs. It takes about four days to get a potent extract if the herbs are powdered, and about fifteen days if the herbs are whole or cut. Your only work is to shake the bottle once or twice daily. If olive or almond oils are used in the extract, a little vitamin E can be added for a preservative. Making an extract with oil is useful if it is to be used for massage purposes. Using alcohol extract (vodka or gin) or rubbing alcohol (for external use only) allows the liquid to evaporate quickly, leaving the herbs on the skin and providing a cooling sensation.

## HYDROTHERAPY: THE HERB BATH

Hydrotherapy, the use of water for treatment of illness, is particularly popular in Europe, where health spas are quite common. But you don't have to go to a spa to enjoy their benefits! You can enjoy an herbal bath in your own home. To make a decoction for a full bath, anywhere from several ounces to a pound of plant parts should be sewn into a linen bag and boiled in a quart or more of water. The water is then added to the bath. You can also put the bag into the bath to extract more of its properties, or you can use it like a washcloth, giving yourself a healthy rubdown. Bathing with herbs accelerates their absorption through the skin. It makes them especially effective for circulation troubles, swelling of broken bones, chilblains, rheumatic diseases, and gout.

## INFUSION

An infusion is an extract made from herbs with medicinal constituents in their flowers, leaves, and stems. It is made by pouring hot liquid over a crude or powdered herb and allowing the mixture to steep, thus extracting the herb's active ingredients. Infusions are prepared like teas, but they are steeped longer and are considerably stronger. This method of preparation minimizes the loss of volatile elements.

The usual ratio used in preparing an infusion is about one-half to one ounce of an herb to one pint of water. Use a glass, enamel, or porcelain pot to steep the herbs for about ten to twenty minutes, then cover with a tight-fitting lid to avoid evaporation.

For general purposes, strain the infusion and drink it lukewarm or cool, but to induce sweating and to break up a cold or cough, drink it hot. Remember that infusions have a short shelf life, so use them soon after you prepare them.

## OILS

When the major properties of an herb are associated with its essential oils, an oil extract will prove a useful way of preparing a concentrate. Herb oils are very useful when ointments or compresses are not practical. Oils are prepared by first macerating and pounding fresh or dried herbs. Olive oil or sesame oil is then added, two ounces of herb to one pint of oil. The mixture should then be allowed to sit in a warm place for about four days before it is used. A quicker method is to gently heat the herbs and oil in a pan for one hour. The oil can then be strained and bottled. Adding a small amount of vitamin E will help preserve the oil. Oil extracts are usually made from aromatic herbs such as eucalyptus, peppermint, spearmint, and spices.

## OINTMENTS

Ointments are used on the skin when the active principles of herbs are needed for extended periods, as in cases of injury, contusion, and effusion. Ointments stay on the skin for an extended time and allow for accelerated healing. To prepare an ointment at home, bring one or two heaping tablespoons of the herb(s) and a good helping of Vaseline to a boil. (There are Vaseline-type products made from natural sources that can be used instead of petroleum products.) The mixture then needs to be stirred and strained. After it has cooled, you can store the ointment in a jar and it will be ready for use when needed.

## POULTICES

An herbal poultice is a soft, moist mass of fresh, ground, or powdered herbs applied hot as a medicament to the body. A poultice is put directly on the skin to relieve inflammation, blood poisoning, venomous bites, eruptions, boils, abscesses, and to promote proper cleansing and healing of the affected area. Many herbs contain ingredients necessary to draw out infections, toxins, and foreign bodies embedded in the skin. Plantain and marshmallow are very good to relieve pain and muscle spasm. Cayenne is added to herbs such as lobelia, valerian, catnip, and echinacea to promote stimulation and cleansing.

To prepare a poultice, moisten herbs with hot water, apple cider vinegar, herbal tea, a liniment, or a tincture. Whatever liquid you use, make sure it is hot. Cleanse the affected area with an antiseptic and then oil the skin before applying the hot poultice. A plaster is similar to a poultice. An effective plaster for drawing out fever can be made by squeezing the water out of tofu and mixing it with pastry flour and about 5 percent fresh ginger root. (See the Appendix for other specific poultices.)

## POWDERS

Powders are simply fresh herbal agents that have been crushed into fine particles. Herbs in powder form can be taken in a capsule, in water, in herb teas, or sprinkled on food. Using powdered herbs is an ideal way to introduce herbs slowly into the diet and become adjusted to a certain dosage. For external use, powdered herbs can be mixed with oil, petroleum jelly, a little water, or aloe vera juice and applied to the skin to treat wounds, inflammation, and contusions.

## SALVES

Herbal salves are similar to ointments. A salve is made by covering fresh or dried herbs with water, bringing the mixture to a boil, and letting it simmer for thirty minutes. The water is then strained off and added to an equal amount of olive oil or safflower oil. Simmer the oil/water mixture until the water has evaporated and only the oil is left. Add enough beeswax to give the mixture a salve-like consistency and pour it into a dark glass jar with a tight lid. If stored well, salves will last up to a year.

## SYRUPS

An herbal syrup is ideal for treating coughs, mucus congestion, bronchial catarrh, and sore throats, because it coats the area and keeps the herbs in direct contact. Syrups are especially good for children and people with sensitive palates. A syrup is made by adding about two ounces of herbs to a quart of water and gently boiling it down to one pint. While still warm, add two ounces of honey and/or glycerin.

Licorice and wild cherry bark are commonly used in syrups as flavors and therapeutic agents. Other herbs used are comfrey, anise seed, fennel, and Irish moss.

## TINCTURES

Tinctures are solutions of concentrated herbal extracts made with alcohol rather than water. They are more highly concentrated than infusions and decoctions, and can be kept for longer periods because alcohol is an excellent preservative. Tinctures are usually made with strong herbs that are not taken as teas. They are also useful for herbs that do not taste good or that need to be taken over an extended period of time. Tinctures are convenient for external application.

A tincture can be made by combining four ounces of powdered or cut herbs with one pint of alcohol such as vodka or brandy. Those who do not drink alcohol can make tinctures using warm (but not boiled) vinegar. Use wine or apple vinegar, but not the white variety. Allow the tincture to steep for two to four weeks, shaking every few days to encourage alcohol absorption of the herbs' medicinal properties. After four weeks, you can strain the herbs out of the liquid, but it is not necessary. Store tinctures in a cool place and keep them out of reach of children.

# HERBAL GLOSSARY

EACH HERB CONTAINS VARIOUS biochemical constituents, including vitamins, minerals, hormones, enzymes, chlorophyll, essential fatty acids, and fiber, which provide the body with what it needs to boost the immune system and aid healing. To make it easier to find the herb needed for a particular problem, the following list categorizes common herbal properties and explains their uses.

## ADAPTOGEN
These herbs have immune-system enhancers that help the body adjust to change, regulate stress, and restore natural immune resistance. Herbs used for this purpose include echinacea, garlic, *Ginkgo biloba*, ginseng, goldenseal, pau d'arco, and suma.

## ALTERATIVE
Alteratives are considered useful in altering body chemistry gradually. Herbs with alterative properties stimulate gradual changes in metabolism and tissue function in acute and chronic conditions and increase overall health, energy, vigor, and strength. Alteratives are similar to tonics, which help the overall system as well as aiding particular organs, tissues, and cells. Alterative herbs include aloe vera, black cohosh, blue cohosh, blue vervain, capsicum, cascara sagrada, chamomile, damiana, dandelion, echinacea, elecampane, fenugreek, garlic, gentian, ginger, *Ginkgo biloba*, goldenseal,

hawthorn, horsetail, milk thistle, red clover, red raspberry, schizandra, suma, yarrow, and yellow dock root.

## ANALGESIC
Analgesic herbs are used to relieve pain without loss of consciousness. Some herbs commonly used as analgesics include feverfew, lobelia, mullein, pau d'arco, skullcap, willow bark, and wood betony.

## ANESTHETIC
Anesthetics are used for their ability to cause physical insensitivity. Examples of herbs with this property are caraway, kava kava, and tea tree.

## ANODYNE
Herbs with this property have the ability to soothe and reduce the intensity of pain. Herbs with this ability include anise, chamomile, cloves, juniper, pleurisy root, and rosemary.

## ANORECTIC
Anorectic herbs help to reduce appetite. Herbs with this asset include chickweed, ephedra, fennel, garcinia, and guarana.

## ANTACID
An antacid is used to neutralize acids in the stomach and intestinal tract. Herbs used for this include

dandelion, fennel, ginger, kelp, Iceland moss, and slippery elm.

## ANTHELMINTIC

Herbs with anthelmintic agents expel or destroy worms in the body. Other similar terms to describe such agents include vermifuge, vermicide, and taeniacide. Herbs with these fighting abilities include black cohosh, blue walnut, gentian, goldenseal, mandrake, prickly ash, pumpkin seed, and senna.

## ANTIASTHMATIC

Antiasthmatics are used to help relieve the symptoms associated with asthma. Some of the antiasthmatic herbs are elecampane, ephedra, gotu kola, lobelia, prickly ash, wild cherry, and yerba santa.

## ANTIBACTERIAL

Antibacterial herbs are those that fight and destroy bacteria and include alfalfa, basil, chamomile, cinnamon, clove, eucalyptus, parsley, peppermint, rhubarb, turmeric, uva ursi, and yucca.

## ANTIBIOTIC

Herbs that work as natural antibiotics help the body's immune system destroy growths of microorganisms. Some herbs commonly used as natural antibiotics include buchu, chaparral, echinacea, garlic, goldenseal, myrrh, red clover, and yellow dock.

## ANTICATARRHAL

These are herbs that help dissolve, eliminate, and prevent the formation of mucus and inflammation of the mucus membrane. Herbs that are considered to be anticatarrhal include comfrey, elecampane, ephedra, fenugreek, licorice, lobelia, marshmallow, mullein, and wild cherry.

## ANTICOAGULANT

Anticoagulant herbs help the body prevent clotting of the blood. Herbs with this constituent include garlic, turmeric, and yellow melilot.

## ANTIEMETIC

Antiemetics prevent vomiting, and herbs with this ability include clove, Iceland moss, raspberry, and spearmint.

## ANTIFUNGAL

Antifungal agents act against and destroy various fungi. Herbs in this category include alfalfa, cinnamon, cloves, garlic, kava kava, kombucha, parsley, St. John's wort, skullcap, thyme, and turmeric.

## ANTIGALACTAGOGUE

Herbs with this property work opposite to herbs with galactagogue properties. Sage and black walnut are examples of herbs in this category.

## ANTIHYDROTIC

Antihydrotics reduce levels of perspiration. Herbs with this ability include astragalus and sage.

## ANTI-INFLAMMATORY

Herbs with this ability reduce inflammation in the body without acting directly on the cause of the inflammation. Herbs in this category include birch, chicory, cranberry, elder flowers, eucalyptus, fennel, feverfew, ginger, licorice, marshmallow, papaya, passion flower, peppermint, pine tree bark, queen of the meadow, rhubarb, rosemary, safflower, turmeric, wild yam, and witch hazel.

## ANTILITHIC

Antilithic herbs work to prevent the formation of stones in the gall bladder and kidneys, as well as aiding the expulsion of those already formed. Antilithics are similar to lithotriptics. Some herbs used for this purpose are buchu leaves, hydrangea, and uva ursi leaves.

## ANTIMICROBIAL

Antimicrobials help the body destroy microbes by affecting their growth and multiplication. Herbs with this ability include fennel, feverfew, myrrh, pau d'arco, rhubarb, tea tree, and uva ursi.

## ANTINEOPLASTIC

Herbs with this quality destroy, inhibit, and prevent tumors. Herbs in this category include aloe vera, black walnut, burdock, cat's claw, chickweed, flaxseed, garlic, hops, horsetail, ho-shou-wu, Irish moss, mistletoe, pau d'arco, periwinkle, pine tree bark, rhubarb, saffron, St. John's wort, slippery elm, and turmeric.

## ANTIOXIDANT

Antioxidant herbs counteract the effects of oxidation on body tissues. Included in this category are barley, bilberry, cat's claw, chaparral, *Ginkgo biloba*, milk thistle, pine tree, rosemary, sage, and turmeric.

## ANTIPERIODIC

This constituent counteracts the effects of periodic (intermittent) diseases, such as malaria. Herbs in this category include angelica, blue vervain, boneset, chinchona, eucalyptus, goldenseal, and willow.

## ANTIPHYLOGISTIC

Antiphylogistic herbs prevent inflammation. Herbs with this ability include chamomile, couch grass, and tormentil.

## ANTIRHEUMATIC

Antirheumatic herbs help to ease and prevent arthritis and rheumatism. Some antirheumatics include alfalfa, buchu, buckthorn, bugleweed, burdock, devil's claw, hydrangea, mandrake, queen of the meadow, and yucca.

## ANTISEPTIC

Antiseptics help to prevent and counteract infection and the formation of pus by inhibiting the growth of infectious organisms. Herbs used are black walnut, chaparral, echinacea, elecampane, garlic, gentian, *Ginkgo biloba*, goldenseal, myrrh, rose hips, tea tree oil, uva ursi, and valerian.

## ANTISPASMODIC

Herbs with this property are used to prevent or counteract spasms. They include black cohosh, blue cohosh, cascara sagrada, catnip, cramp bark, dong quai, gotu kola, hawthorn, juniper berries, kava kava, lobelia, mistletoe, and skullcap.

## ANTITUSSIVE

Herbs with antitussive agents are cough suppressants. Herbs in this category include coltsfoot, comfrey, horehound, mullein, and wild cherry bark.

## ANTIVENOMOUS

Antivenomous agents counteract venom, as from a snakebite. Herbs with this quality include pennyroyal and plantain.

## ANTIVIRAL

Antiviral agents act to destroy viruses in the body. Herbs with antiviral qualities include aloe vera, astragalus, barley, boneset, calendula, echinacea, ho-shou-wu, licorice, maitake, reishi, pau d'arco, red raspberry, and turmeric.

## APHRODISIAC

An aphrodisiac is used to help restore normal sexual potency and function and improve sexual desire. Some herbs used as aphrodisiacs include astragalus, damiana, false unicorn, fenugreek, ginseng, kava kava, and saw palmetto.

## ASTRINGENT

An astringent acts to contract and tighten, similar to styptic. This constricting action can help eliminate secretions and hemorrhaging. Some herbs with astringent actions are amaranth, blackberry root, black walnut, capsicum, elecampane, ephedra, fenugreek, horsetail, hydrangea, mullein, oak bark, queen of the meadow, St. John's wort, slippery elm, and witch hazel.

## BITTER

An agent that acts on the mucous membranes in the mouth to promote appetite and encourage digestion. Herbs in this category include alfalfa, blackberry, blessed thistle, bugleweed, chaparral, chinchona, eyebright, feverfew, gentian, licorice, quassia, watercress, wild cherry, and wild lettuce.

## BLOOD PURIFIER

Agents that clean and remove impurities from the blood, similar to depurative. Examples of blood purifiers include birch, buckthorn, calendula, centaury, couch grass, dandelion, plantain, and watercress.

## CARMINATIVE

Herbs that can help eliminate gas from the stomach and intestine are called carminatives. Some of the herbs commonly used are angelica root, capsicum, caraway seeds, catnip, chamomile flowers, echinacea, fennel, ginger, hops, lemon balm, parsley root, peppermint, saffron, and valerian.

## CHOLAGOGUE

This herb property increases the flow of bile, which aids digestion, as well as acting as a mild laxative. Herbs that are used for this purpose are aloe vera, barberry, culver's root, dandelion, goldenseal, hops, licorice, Oregon grape root, and wild yam.

## DECONGESTANT

An agent that relieves congestion in the upper respiratory tract. Herbs with decongestant properties include ephedra, lobelia, pennyroyal, valerian, and yerba santa.

## DEMULCENT

These herbs work internally to help soothe and protect the mucous membranes in the body. Some herbs with this property are aloe vera, burdock, chickweed, comfrey, echinacea, fenugreek, flaxseed, Irish moss, kelp, licorice, marshmallow, mullein, oatstraw, and psyllium.

## DIAPHORETIC

Diaphoretic herbs help the body produce perspiration to help the skin eliminate toxins, similar to sudorific. Herbs with diaphoretic properties include angelica, blue vervain, boneset, borage, butcher's broom, capsicum, catnip, chamomile, elder flowers, elecampane, ephedra, garlic, hyssop, lemon balm leaves, and yarrow.

## DIGESTIVE

Digestives promote or aid in the digestion process. Such herbs include anise, capsicum, centaury, echinacea, garlic, horseradish, mustard, papaya, safflower, and sage.

## DIURETIC

A diuretic is used to increase the flow of urine to relieve water retention. Some herbs used for this purpose are alfalfa, blue cohosh, buchu leaves, burdock, butcher's broom, damiana, dandelion, devil's claw, false unicorn, fennel, hawthorn, horsetail, hydrangea, juniper berries, lily-of-the-valley, marshmallow, parsley, queen of the meadow, saw palmetto, and uva ursi.

## EMETIC

An emetic is used to induce vomiting. Emetic herbs include bayberry, boneset, buckthorn, culver, false unicorn, lobelia, mandrake, mistletoe, mustard seed, pleurisy, quassia, rue, and senega.

## EMMENAGOGUE

Herbs with emmenagogue properties promote menstrual flow. Some herbs that help with this situation are angelica, aloe vera, black cohosh, blue cohosh, gentian, ginger, goldenseal, horsetail, juniper berries, mistletoe, myrrh, pennyroyal, and saffron.

## EMOLLIENT

This category includes herbs used externally to help soften, soothe, and protect the skin. Some are almond oil, aloe vera, comfrey, fenugreek, flaxseed, Irish moss, linseed oil, marshmallow, olive oil, slippery elm, and wheat germ oil.

## ESTROGENIC

Estrogenic herbs promote or produce estrus. Herbs with estrogenic properties include blue cohosh, dong quai, false unicorn, fennel, and licorice.

## EXPECTORANT

Expectorants help the body expel mucus from the lungs, nose, and throat. Herbs used for this purpose include anise seed, blue cohosh, blue vervain, comfrey root, elder flowers, elecampane root, ephedra, flaxseed, fennel, fenugreek, garlic, horehound, hyssop, Irish moss, licorice, lobelia, marshmallow, mullein leaves, slippery elm, wild cherry bark, and yerba santa leaves.

## FEBRIFUGE

Herbs with this property help reduce fevers, similar to refrigerant and antipyretic. Some febrifuges are bilberry, boneset, borage, buckthorn, catnip, chamomile, elder flowers, fenugreek, garlic, gentian, ginger, hyssop, pleurisy root, sarsaparilla, white willow bark, and wormwood.

## GALACTAGOGUE

Herbs with galactagogue properties stimulate lactation in women. Herbs in this category include anise, basil, blessed thistle, borage, fenugreek, horsetail, and vervain.

## GERMICIDE

Germicides are known for their ability to destroy germs and other microorganisms. Herbs in this category include cloves, eucalyptus, and tea tree.

## HEPATIC

These herbs help to strengthen, tone, and increase bile flow to promote normal liver function. Some herbs with hepatic properties are barberry bark, cascara sagrada, dandelion root, gentian, goldenseal, horseradish, mandrake root, milk thistle, olive oil, Oregon grape, parsley, queen of the meadow, and rhubarb.

## HEMOSTATIC

Hemostatics stop blood flow by acting as antihemorrhagic agents. Herbs in this category include bistort, blackberry, bugleweed, calendula, nettle, periwinkle, shepherd's purse, and witch hazel.

## HYPOTENSIVE

Hypotensive herbs cause low blood pressure, similar to antihypertensives, which are agents that lower blood pressure. Examples of hypotensives include astragalus, barberry, celery, dong quai, kelp, mistletoe, rhubarb, and wood betony.

## IMMUNOSTIMULANT

Immunostimulants enhance or boost the body's natural defense against illness and disease. Herbs with this ability include astragalus, barley, dong quai, kombucha, maitake, queen of the meadow, reishi, and shiitake.

## INSECTICIDE

Insecticides are used to kill insects. An example of an herb with this ability is bayberry.

## LITHOTRIPTIC

These are herbs that help dissolve and eliminate urinary stones from the body. They include buchu leaves, butcher's broom, cascara sagrada, cornsilk, dandelion, devil's claw, horsetail, marshmallow, parsley, queen of the meadow, uva ursi, and white oak bark.

## MUCILANT

Herbs that are considered mucilants have a soothing and demulcent effect. They coat and protect mucous membranes from irritations. Mucilants have a wide variety of applications, including coughs, sore throats, and irritated stomach, bowels, bladder, and kidneys. They can also be used for laxatives, creams, and ointments because of their soothing effects. Mucilant herbs include aloe vera, chickweed, coltsfoot, comfrey, flaxseed, Iceland moss, marshmallow, plantain, psyllium seed, and slippery elm.

## NARCOTIC

Herbs with narcotic agents can be used to soothe intractable pain or to induce anesthesia. Herbs with these agents should be used carefully. They include bugleweed, guarana, and wild lettuce. Herbs that can be used to counteract narcotic effects include alfalfa (for addiction) and marjoram and mustard (for poisoning).

## NEPHRITIC

These herbs are used in healing kidney problems. Herbs with nephritic properties include buchu leaves, couch grass root, goldenseal, horsetail, hydrangea, juniper berries, Oregon grape, and queen of the meadow root.

## NERVINE

Nervine herbs help soothe, calm, and nourish the nervous system. Some of the nervine herbs are black cohosh, blue vervain, boneset, catnip, chamomile, cramp bark, damiana, gotu kola, hops, lady's slipper, lemon balm, lobelia, oatstraw, passion flower, skullcap, valerian root, and wood betony.

## NUTRITIVE

Nutritive agents nourish the body. Herbs with nutritive properties include alfalfa, amaranth, barley, bee pollen, chickweed, comfrey, guarana, Iceland moss, Irish moss, kelp, marshmallow, nettle, oatstraw, papaya, pumpkin, red clover, rose hips, slippery elm, suma, watercress, and yellow dock.

## OXYTOCIC

These are herbs that help stimulate uterine contractions to assist and induce safe labor and delivery. Herbs with oxytocic properties are black cohosh, blue cohosh, pennyroyal, and red raspberry.

## PARASITICIDE

Parasiticidic herbs destroy parasites in the body. Herbs with parasiticidic agents include chaparral, feverfew, figwort, horseradish, mandrake, papaya, parsley, peach, pennyroyal, plantain, pumpkin, rhubarb, sage, thyme, vervain, wild cherry, and wood betony.

## PECTORAL

Pectoral agents give relief and remedy pulmonary and other respiratory conditions. Examples of pectorals are chickweed, coltsfoot, couch grass, hyssop, Iceland moss, and wild cherry.

## PURGATIVE

A cathartic or purgative herb is used for purging and stimulating the action of evacuating the bowels. This action may be mild or strong, depending on the need. Purgatives and cathartics are similar to aperients and laxatives, which are mild purgatives used to relieve constipation. Herbs considered to be purgative include aloe vera, barberry bark, boneset, buckthorn bark, cascara sagrada, elder flowers, goldenseal, mandrake, Oregon grape root, psyllium, rhubarb root, and senna leaves.

## RUBEFACIENT

Herbs with rubefacient properties are reddening agents that help to increase blood flow to the surface of the skin to aid healing in cases such as sprains and muscle soreness. Some herbs used for this purpose include camphor, capsicum, cloves, eucalyptus, garlic, ginger, horseradish, mustard seed, peppermint oil, pine oil, stinging nettle, and thyme oil.

## SEDATIVE

Sedative herbs are used to relieve irritability and promote calm and tranquil feelings. Some are catnip, chamomile, cramp bark, dong quai, hawthorn, hops, kava kava, lady's slipper, lobelia, passion flower, red clover, St. John's wort, schizandra, skullcap, valerian, and wood betony.

## SIALAGOGUE

Herbs with this property help to promote the flow and secretion of saliva to aid in the digestion of starches. Some herbs include bayberry, capsicum, echinacea, gentian, ginger, horseradish, hydrangea, licorice, prickly ash, rhubarb, and yerba santa.

## STIMULANT

These herbs help to increase the function of the body, raise energy levels, heighten circulation, and help eliminate toxins. Herbs with stimulant properties are angelica, boneset, capsicum, damiana, devil's claw, echinacea, elder flowers, elecampane, ephedra, false unicorn, garlic, gentian, ginger, *Ginkgo biloba*, ginseng, ho-shou-wu, milk thistle, prickly ash bark, saffron, sarsaparilla root, and suma.

## STOMACHIC

Stomachics strengthen and tone the stomach. Herbs in the stomachic category include agrimony, anise, barberry, basil, caraway, celery, chinchina, cloves, dandelion, gentian, ginseng, gymnema, hops, horseradish, papaya, peach, pennyroyal, quassia, rhubarb, rose hips, and watercress.

## VASOCONSTRICTOR

Vasoconstricting herbs help to constrict blood vessels and raise blood pressure. Herbs with this property include butcher's broom, ergot, and heather.

## VASODILATOR

Herbs with vasodilating agents expand blood vessels and lower blood pressure. Herbs in this category include feverfew, hawthorn, and ho-shou-wu.

## VULNERARY

Herbs with vulnery properties are used to help promote the healing of wounds, cuts, and abrasions. Some used are aloe vera, black walnut, burdock, capsicum, fenugreek, flaxseed, garlic, gentian, goldenseal, hops, horsetail, mullein, oatstraw, and plantain leaves.

# PART 2

# All About Herbs and Natural Healing Agents

# SINGLE HERBS

## AGRIMONY *(Agrimonia eupatoria)*

*Parts used:* Entire plant
*Properties:* Astringent, diuretic, hepatic, stomachic
*Primary nutrients:* Iron, niacin, vitamins B3 and K

Agrimony is a tall plant that grows two to five feet in height in England and Scotland. It has short branches and pairs of leaves. The flowers are pale lilac with masses of heads blooming in late summer or early autumn, and the stems and leaves have been used to make yellow dye.

Ancient Greeks used this herb for wound and eye healing. In Europe, it was used for wounds, snakebites, warts, and other skin conditions, and Native Americans used agrimony for fevers.

Agrimony strengthens and tones the muscles of the body due to its astringent properties that work to contract and harden tissue. Its astringent properties are also helpful for sore throats and on the skin. Agrimony acts as a diuretic, affecting kidney cells and allowing fluids to pass more readily through the kidneys, as well as aiding liver and gallbladder health. It is used to help acidity and gastric ulcers because it is a safe stomach tonic and helps the assimilation of food. Moreover, the astringent qualities of agrimony help draw thorns and splinters from the skin.

### PRIMARY APPLICATIONS

| | |
|---|---|
| Diarrhea | Gastric disorders |
| Intestinal problems | Jaundice |
| Kidney stones | Liver disorders |

### SECONDARY APPLICATIONS

| | |
|---|---|
| Fevers | Gallbladder problems |
| Hemorrhoids | Rheumatism |
| Skin disorders | Splinters |
| Sprains | Throat, sore |
| Wounds | |

## ALFALFA *(Medicagto sativa)*

*Parts used:* Leaves and flowers
*Properties:* Alterative, antibacterial, antifungal, antirheumatic, bitter, blood purifier, deodorant, diuretic (mild), nutritive
*Primary nutrients:* Essential amino acids, chlorine, chlorophyll, iron, magnesium, phosphorus, potassium, silicon, sodium, vitamins A, B1, B2, B12, E, D, and K

In ancient times, alfalfa was considered a miracle herb. The Arabs called it the "Father of Herbs" (Al-Fal-Fa), and it has been cultivated for more than two thousand years. In 400 BC, the Medes and the Persians invaded Greece and began cultivating alfalfa in that region because of its ability to survive even in harsh climates. The roots of the plant can reach as far as sixty-six feet into the subsoil. Later, the Romans discovered that alfalfa was excellent for their horses, and it was introduced to North America by the Spanish, where it was used to treat arthritis, boils, cancer, scurvy, urinary tract disorders, and bowel problems.

Modern research has documented the health benefits of alfalfa. It is one of the most nutritious foods available. It is considered by herbalists to be beneficial for many problems, and some even recommend it for any ailment because it helps the body assimilate protein, calcium, and other essential nutrients. In addition, alfalfa is used to remove poisons and their effects in the body and is thought to neutralize the acidity of the body and break down carbon dioxide. In fact, alfalfa is often used to treat recuperative cases of narcotic and alcohol addiction and has been found to help build the blood in cases of anemia.

Alfalfa contains antibacterial and antifungal properties that make it a great body cleanser, infection fighter, and natural deodorizer. It has also been used to clean stained teeth. The extracts produce antibacterial activity against gram-positive bacteria specifically.

Alfalfa is known to help with milk production in nursing mothers and to stimulate appetite. It has also been researched and found to help lower cholesterol levels and to neutralize cancer. It has been found to help in healing ulcers and treating arteriosclerosis, pituitary problems, liver toxicity, arthritis, allergies, diabetes, and in strengthening the capillaries and blood vessels. Alfalfa is often used to treat appendicitis, water retention, urinary and bowel problems, muscle spasms, cramps, and digestive problems.

## PRIMARY APPLICATIONS

| | |
|---|---|
| Anemia | Appetite, loss |
| Arthritis | Blood, impurities |
| Diabetes | Hemorrhages |
| Kidney, contaminated | Nausea |
| Pituitary problems | Ulcers, peptic |

## SECONDARY APPLICATIONS

| | |
|---|---|
| Alcoholism | Allergies |
| Appendicitis, chronic | Blood pressure, high |
| Body odor | Bursitis |
| Cancer | Cholesterol, high |
| Cramps, | Gastric disorders |
| muscle and stomach | Gout |
| Intestinal problems | Jaundice |
| Lactation, absent | Muscles, weak |
| Nosebleeds | Teeth, stained |
| Urinary problems | |

# ALOE VERA *(Aloe vera)*

*Parts used:* Leaves
*Properties:* Alterative, antineoplastic, antiviral, cholagogue, demulcent, emmenagogue, emollient, mucilant, purgative, vulnerary
*Primary nutrients:* Calcium, copper, iron, lecithin, magnesium, manganese, niacin, phosphorus, potassium, selenium, sodium, vitamins A, B2, B-complex and C, zinc

Throughout history, there have been few botanicals revered as highly as the succulent leaf of the aloe vera plant. Aloe vera has been used for at least four thousand years for its medicinal value and therapeutic benefits. Today, it is widely used and cultivated in many nations throughout the world.

Aloe vera is a member of the lily family (family Liliaceae), although it looks much like a cactus plant. It is a perennial with yellow flowers. The leaves are tough, stiff, spiny, and triangular, and may grow up to twenty inches long and five inches across. The leaves grow in a rosette of narrow, fleshy leaves with three layers.

Historical records have found evidence of aloe use by many people, including the Egyptians, Greeks, Romans, Hebrews, Chinese, Indians, Algerians, Moroccans, Tunisians, and Arabians. Folklore records many medicinal uses of aloe, and recent research adds validity to the many beneficial uses of the aloe plant.

Aloe vera has traditionally been used to treat wounds, frostbite, burns, radiation burns, and other external pain, as well as aiding digestion and combating constipation, inflammation, ulcers, kidney stones, and tissue damage from X-ray exposure or other radiation. Because it contains enzymes, saponins, hormones, and amino acids that can be absorbed into the skin, aloe vera can be used to prevent scarring, heal minor scars—such as from acne—and promote the growth of living cells. Aloe contains substances called uronic acids that are natural detoxicants and take part in the healing process by stripping toxic materials of their harmful effects.

Aloe vera is probably best known for its external healing and soothing effect on burns, wounds, and rashes. Modern research has found that aloe, when applied externally, can help speed healing and restore skin tissue due to its moisturizing effects. It is easily absorbed into the skin, preventing the air from drying the damaged skin tissue and helping to relieve pain associated with burns and wounds.

Studies illustrate the positive use of aloe juice in the digestive process. Aloe vera has been used to treat stomach disorders, ulcers, colitis, constipation, and other colon-related problems. Aloe can help to soothe, reduce inflammation, and heal the digestive tract. In one study, ulcer patients were completely healed using aloe juice. The researchers compared their findings to commonly used anti-ulcer drugs. The natural aloe juice treatment was just as effective as the drugs, without the chance of toxic side effects.

One of the constituents of aloe gel is acemannan, a complex carbohydrate with immune-stimulating and antiviral properties. Certain lectins found in the aloe gel may help stimulate immune response by increasing the production of lymphocytes that are known to kill bacteria and some tumor cells. The acemannan in aloe has shown antiviral activity against HIV-1. The reproduction of HIV-1 is inhibited using constituents of the aloe plant. It has also been found effective against the spread of some viruses, such as herpes, measles, and rhinotracheitis.

## PRIMARY APPLICATIONS

| | |
|---|---|
| Bites, insect | Body odor |
| Burns/scalds | Gastric disorders |
| Hemorrhoids | Scar tissue |

## SECONDARY APPLICATIONS

| | |
|---|---|
| Abrasions | Acne |
| Anemia | Constipation |
| Heartburn | Poison ivy/oak |
| Psoriasis | Ringworm |
| Sores | Sunburn |

| | |
|---|---|
| Tapeworm | Tuberculosis |
| Wrinkles | Ulcers, legs |
| Ulcers, peptic | |

# AMARANTH *(Amnaranthus spp.)*

*Parts used:* Leaves, seeds, and flowers
*Properties:* Alterative, astringent, demulcent, diuretic, nutritive
*Primary nutrients:* Calcium, iron, l-lysine, niacin, phosphorus, potassium, protein, riboflavin, thiamin, vitamin C

Amaranth is a vitamin-packed herb that was traditionally used by Native Americans in Central and North America as a survival food and has been cultivated for thousands of years in many different cultures because it grows well in most climates and uses minimal water. It contains high amounts of protein and more calcium than milk. It contains the amino acid l-lysine, not often found in plants. The Aztecs used the seeds in their pagan ceremonies. The mature seeds were eaten raw, mixed with cornmeal, or added to soups. The leaves are edible and taste similar to spinach.

Amaranth is often used for gastroenteritis or stomach flu to lessen the irritability of the tissues. A strong decoction of amaranth can be used as an anthelmintic to remove worms and other parasites from the digestive tract. Topical application reduces tissue swelling, so the herb can be used with bandages for medical treatment. It can also help stop excess bleeding caused by sore gums, nosebleeds, and a heavy menses. It is highly digestible and is recommended for infant formulas.

## PRIMARY APPLICATIONS

| | |
|---|---|
| Diarrhea | Dysentery |
| Menstruation, excessive | Nosebleeds |

## SECONDARY APPLICATIONS

| | |
|---|---|
| Canker sores | Gums, bleeding |
| Ulcers, stomach/mouth | Worms |
| Wounds | |

# ANAMU *(Petiveria alliacea)*

*Parts used:* Leaves
*Properties:* Antispasmodic, antipyretic, anticonvulsant, counterirritant, nervine, antirheumatic, anticarcinogenic, emmenagogue, aphrodisiac, abortifacient
*Primary nutrients:* Aluminum, bromine, calcium, cesium, chlorine, cobalt, iron, lanthanum, magnesium, manganese, potassium, rubidium, sodium, zinc

This herb is found growing in Cuba, other Caribbean countries, and Central and South America. Anamu is especially popular in Central and South America. An ethnobotanical survey of the Carib population of Guatemala found that anamu was one of the most frequently used plants in their folk medicine.

The herb has been used for cancer, tumors, osteoarthritis, pain relief, conjunctivitis, prostate hypertrophy, and paralysis. Colombians chew the leaves to ward off dental cavities. The inhaled aroma can treat migraine headaches and sinusitis.

An analysis of anamu extract reveals coumarins, saponins, traces of essential oil, and an antimicrobial compound. The herb also contains oligosulfides that show in vitro activity against bacteria and fungi.

One study examined the effect of anamu tea in fourteen patients with hip and knee osteoarthritis. The patients experienced improvement in pain of motion and pain at night. Research on mouse carcinoma and sea urchin egg development shows evidence that anamu may inhibit tumor growth. In another study, anamu decreased blood sugar concentration by more than 60 percent one hour after oral administration to mice that had been fasting for forty-eight hours. This research shows promise for diabetics. Anamu has strong abortifacient properties, so it should not be used by women who are pregnant or thinking of becoming pregnant.

## PRIMARY APPLICATIONS

| | |
|---|---|
| Bronchitis | Cancer |
| Conjunctivitis | Migraine headaches |
| Osteoarthritis | Pain relief |
| Paralysis | Pneumonia |
| Prostate hypertrophy | Sinusitis |
| Tumors | |

# ANGELICA *(Angelica atropurpurea)*

*Parts used:* Root
*Properties:* Alterative, antiperiodic, blood purifier, carminative, diaphoretic, emmenagogue, stimulant
*Primary nutrients:* Calcium, vitamins E and B12

Angelica was used as a cure for the plague in medieval Europe because of its blood-purifying abilities. Many benefited from its curative powers, at least partly because angelica contains vitamin E and calcium.

Angelica is often used to treat problems of the digestive system, such as poor digestion, heartburn, gas, colic, ulcers, and stomach cramps, by aiding stomach, spleen, and intestinal functions. It is also used for toothaches, wounds, fevers, nervous headaches, backaches, and general weakness. It is used for chronic bronchitis, asthma, lymphatic and prostate disorders, rheumatism, arthritis, and menstrual symptoms.

Modern scientific research has found angelica to help stimulate and strengthen the immune system and relax the nervous system, as well as stimulating the entire body and improving mental well-being. It has also successfully treated those suffering from nervous exhaustion.

## PRIMARY APPLICATIONS

| | |
|---|---|
| Appetite, loss | Blood, impurities |
| Bronchial problems | Colds |
| Colic | Coughs |
| Exhaustion | Gas |
| Heartburn | Rheumatism |

## SECONDARY APPLICATIONS

| | |
|---|---|
| Arthritis | Asthma |
| Backaches | Cramps, menstrual |
| Fevers | Gastric disorders |
| Hemorrhoids | Inflammation |
| Lactation, absent | Liver disorders |
| Lung disorders | Menstrual symptoms |
| Prostate problems | Toothaches |

# ANISE *(Pimpinella anisum)*

*Parts used:* Oil and seeds
*Properties:* Anodyne, anti-inflammatory, antiseptic, antispasmodic, aromatic, carminative, diaphoretic, digestive, diuretic, expectorant, galactagogue, stimulant, stomachic
*Primary nutrients:* B vitamins, calcium, choline, iron, magnesium, potassium

Anise was used in ancient Rome as a flavoring, although it also contains nutrients like calcium and iron. It was added to foods to prevent indigestion when eating large quantities of food and to help with bad breath. Hippocrates recommended anise to relieve coughs and congestion.

Anise is used to help remove excess mucus from the alimentary canal and mucus associated with coughs. It is used to stimulate the appetite, relieve digestive problems, and treat colic pain. Some herbalists recommend anise for stimulating the glands and vital organs such as the heart, liver, lungs, and brain, as well as normalizing estrogen levels.

## PRIMARY APPLICATIONS

| | |
|---|---|
| Colds | Colic |
| Coughs | Gas |
| Indigestion | Lactation, absent |
| Mucus, excessive | Pneumonia |

## SECONDARY APPLICATIONS

| | |
|---|---|
| Appetite, loss | Breath, odor |
| Emphysema | Epilepsy |
| Nausea | Nervous disorders |

# ANTLER (DEER AND ELK)

*Parts used:* Entire antler
*Properties:* Adaptogen, antineoplastic, antispasmodic, aphrodisiac, febrifuge
*Primary nutrients:* Calcium and trace elements

Deer and elk antlers, which are high in calcium, are gathered after they have been dropped and have been used for thousands of years to increase vitality and longevity. A recent study in New Zealand discovered why antlers earned this reputation: It showed that antler consumption improved cell growth and contained antitumor and antiviral properties in the bodies of those who used it.

Traditional Chinese medicine used the powder in combinations for many ailments, such as kidney and stomach problems, as well as for bone strengthening, nourishing the blood, reducing swelling, and increasing sperm production. Russians used antlers for health benefits such as lowering blood pressure, increasing endurance, and healing the body.

The antler is used to maintain vitality and health and is thought to increase energy and strength in those who are in a weakened state. A recent Japanese study found antler improved the function of the immune system. It has been successfully used to strengthen muscle contractions, improve nerve impulses, and help with arthritis. In addition, antler may help with mental and physical stamina, circulation, metabolism, stress, arthritis pain, healing of injuries, inflammation, asthma, constipation, digestion, menstrual and menopausal symptoms, and skin conditions.

Dr. Ivan Kinia found significant benefits from the use of antler in helping athletes with inflammation and helping arthritis sufferers. Athletes given antler have found improvement in performance and have experienced fewer injuries.

## PRIMARY APPLICATIONS

| | |
|---|---|
| Aging | Hormone imbalance |
| Impotence | Infertility |

## SECONDARY APPLICATIONS

| | |
|---|---|
| Anemia | Arthritis |
| Blood pressure, high | Fatigue |
| Fevers | Flu |
| Frigidity | Memory loss |
| Menopausal symptoms | Menstrual symptoms |
| Metabolism, slow | Miscarriage problems |
| Osteomyelitis | Rheumatism |
| Stress | Teeth, weak |

# ASHWAGANDHA
*(Withania somnifera)*

*Parts used:* Root
*Properties:* Adaptogen, amphoteric, aphrodisiac, tonic

A small, woody herb in the nightshade family, ashwagandha is related to tomatoes and peppers. It is the most popular and widely used of the herbs favored by the Ayurvedic healing tradition of India. In English, the herb is sometimes called winter cherry. It grows in areas in Africa, the Mediterranean, and India.

Ashwagandha's properties place it in the same class as ginseng, astragalus, and dong quai. (It is sometimes called Indian ginseng.) The main biochemical components of this herb are steroidal alkaloids and steroidal lactones in a class of constituents called withanolides. These serve as vital hormone precursors, which the body is able to convert into human physiological hormones as needed. If there is too much of a certain hormone, these plant-based hormone precursors occupy the body's hormone receptor sites without converting to human hormones. In this way, they block absorption. Thus ashwagandha can regulate important physiological processes. This herb has been researched in animals to study its effects on immune function, inflammation, and cancer.

Ashwagandha raises metabolism, stimulates digestion, clears mucus, and improves circulation. It has been used for generations to increase vitality, energy, endurance, and stamina; to promote longevity and strengthen the immune system; to counteract anxiety and stress; to boost peace of mind; to reduce inflammation; to treat arthritic and rheumatic conditions; and as an aphrodisiac.

## PRIMARY APPLICATIONS

| | |
|---|---|
| Adrenal exhaustion | Anxiety |
| Arthritis | Cancer |
| Dementia | Eye health |
| Immune dysfunction | Low libido |
| Thyroid health | |

## SECONDARY APPLICATIONS

| | |
|---|---|
| Alcoholism | Alzheimer's disease |
| Anemia | Cough |
| Emaciation | HIV/AIDS |
| Insomnia | Lumbago |
| Memory loss | Mental function |
| Multiple sclerosis | Muscle energy loss |
| Nerve exhaustion | Paralysis |
| Rheumatism | Sexual debility |
| Skin afflictions | Stress |
| Swollen glands | Ulcers |

# ASTRAGALUS
*(Astragali membranaceus)*

*Parts used:* Root
*Properties:* Adaptogen, alterative, antibacterial, antihydrotic, anti-inflammatory, antiviral, aphrodisiac, cardioalterative, diuretic, hypotensive, immunostimulant
*Primary nutrients:* Betaine, B-sitosterol, choline, glucoronic acid, sucrose

Astragalus has been used in traditional Chinese medicine for thousands of years as an energy tonic and to enhance the immune system. It has recently become popular among Western herbalists and is often found in energy drinks along with other herbs.

Because astragalus has a reputation as an immune-system enhancer, it has attracted quite a bit of scientific attention, and subsequent studies seem to support astragalus's reputed abilities. Studies by the American Cancer Society show the positive effects of astragalus on the immune systems of cancer patients tested. Those patients undergoing radiation and chemotherapy recovered faster and lived longer if they took astragalus during treatment. Studies seem to indicate that it increases the production of interferon, which can help the immune system in its function.

Astragalus also has antiviral properties, both preventive and defensive. Studies done in China have found that astragalus can help reduce the duration and incidence of the common cold. In fact, astragalus has been used for many different ailments, including chronic fatigue syndrome, Epstein-Barr, pneumonia, emphysema, chronic infection, immune-related illnesses, digestion, chronic cough, malabsorption syndrome, prolapsed organs, uterine bleeding, chronic nephritis, excessive sweating, edema, abscesses, cysts, and ulcers.

## PRIMARY APPLICATIONS

| | |
|---|---|
| Cancer | Chronic fatigue |
| Colds | Epstein-Barr |
| Gastric disorders | Immune deficiencies |
| Infection | Liver disorders |

## SECONDARY APPLICATIONS

| | |
|---|---|
| Arthritis | Cancer |
| Candidiasis | Diabetes |
| Edema | Flu |
| Kidney, inflammation | Leukemia |
| Stress | Ulcers |

# BACOPA *(Bacopa monniera)*

*Parts used:* Entire plant
*Properties:* Adaptogen, anticonvulsant, antidepressant, antifungal, antimicrobial, antioxidant, sedative
*Primary nutrients:* Alkaloids, saponins, sterols

*Bacopa monniera*, also known as *Bacopa monnieri*, water hyssop, or brahmi, is an Ayurvedic herb. Brahmi is also the Ayurvedic name for gotu kola, so the two are sometimes confused. Bacopa is found in marshy places throughout China, India, Nepal, Sri Lanka, Taiwan, and the southeastern United States.

Studies show that bacopa has antioxidant, anticonvulsant, and antidepressant benefits. It has been used for centuries to relieve epilepsy, boost memory, increase concentration, reduce anxiety, and improve cognitive ability. This herb has also been used as a cardiac remedy, digestive aid, and to improve respiratory function. Recent research results support the traditional Ayurvedic claims and also indicate bacopa may improve intellectual performance in children. It seems only chronic administration is linked to cognitive-enhancing effects in adults.

One study indicated the brain tissue of animals given bacopa showed increased serotonin content compared to a control group, which supports baco-

pa's reputed antidepressant activity. The herb also seems to reduce oxidation of fats in the bloodstream, which is a risk factor for cardiovascular ailments.

Studies of anxiety, epilepsy, bronchitis and asthma, irritable bowel syndrome, and stomach ulcers also support the Ayurvedic history of bacopa use. Animal studies have shown bacopa to have a relaxant effect on chemically induced bronchoconstriction, and research in mice indicated high doses of bacopa extract boosted thyroid hormone.

In vitro and animal studies show bacopa may protect against certain drug side effects, and in vitro studies show bacopa has cytotoxic activity for sarcoma cells. The herb does not have any known side effects.

## PRIMARY APPLICATIONS

| | |
|---|---|
| Anxiety | Asthma |
| Bronchitis | Cardiovascular issues |
| Epilepsy | Irritable bowel (IBS) |
| Memory, poor | Stomach ulcers |

# BANABA *(Laegerstromia speciosa)*

*Parts used:* Leaves
*Properties:* Blood sugar regulator

Also known as crepe myrtle, queen's flower, and pride of India, banaba is a plant found growing in the Philippines, India, and Southeast Asia. In Ayurvedic medicine, the leaves have traditionally been brewed into a tea to treat diabetes and hyperglycemia (high blood sugar). Banaba leaf extract's ability to lower blood sugar is similar to that of insulin. It helps move glucose out of the blood and into body cells. Banaba may be useful for balancing blood sugar, maintaining optimal insulin levels, curbing appetite, controlling food cravings (especially for carbohydrates), and aiding weight loss. Banaba extract has been shown to be safe and effective as a reducer of elevated levels of blood sugar and insulin.

The crucial component in banaba leaf extract is corosolic acid, which helps move glucose into cells. Through this action, banaba helps regulate levels of blood sugar and insulin. Some people find that fluctuations in blood sugar and insulin are connected to food cravings, particularly for refined carbohydrates. By maintaining stable blood sugar and insulin levels, banaba may promote weight loss.

Research has demonstrated banaba's effects on blood sugar and insulin. In isolated cells, corosolic acid is seen to stimulate glucose uptake. Administration of banaba to diabetic mice, rats, and rabbits decreases elevated blood sugar and insulin levels to normal. In people with type II diabetes, banaba extract has been shown to reduce blood sugar levels by 5 percent to 30 percent and to help maintain better control of blood sugar swings. This regulation of blood sugar and insulin is most likely the reason behind banaba's tendency to promote weight loss at an average rate of two to four pounds per month. Modulation of glucose and insulin levels probably lessens total caloric intake to a degree and encourages moderate weight loss.

## PRIMARY APPLICATIONS

| | |
|---|---|
| Appetite control | Blood sugar problems |
| Insulin balance | Weight loss |

# BARBERRY (Berberis vulgaris)

*Parts used:* Bark, root, and berries
*Properties:* Alterative, antibacterial, antineoplastic, antiseptic, aromatic, astringent, blood purifier, cholagogue, diuretic, hepatic, hypotensive, purgative (mild), stomachic
*Primary nutrients:* Iron, magnesium, phosphorus, vitamin C

Barberry has been used for approximately three thousand years in China and India in the treatment of diarrhea and intestinal infections. Native Americans used the barberry plant for treating liver conditions such as jaundice, and ancient Egyptians mixed the berries with fennel seed for protection against the plague. Barberry contains an alkaloid, berberine, which is also found in other medicinal herbs such as goldenseal and Oregon grape, and the therapeutic effects of barberry are attributed to its berberine content.

Studies have found that berberine contains properties effective against a wide variety of bacteria, viruses, and fungi, and that berberine was more effective in treating some bacteria than a strong antibiotic. Other studies have found that barberry can kill microorganisms such as staphylococci, streptococci, salmonella, *Giardia lamblia*, *Escherichia coli*, shigella, and *Candida albicans*. The berberine in barberry has also been found to contain antidiarrheal properties and is recommended to stimulate the immune system.

Barberry's effects include help against cancer, liver problems, kidney problems, coughs, cholera, diarrhea, fever, inflammation, hypertension, and tumors. Barberry is also recommended to increase bile secretions and stimulate the appetite, and it may help in cases of anemia and malnutrition. It stimulates bile production for liver problems and dilates blood vessels to lower blood pressure.

## PRIMARY APPLICATIONS

| | |
|---|---|
| Appetite, loss | Blood, impurities |
| Blood pressure, high | Candidiasis |
| Constipation | Diarrhea |
| Dysentery | Fevers |
| Indigestion | Infections |
| Jaundice | Liver disorders |
| Pyorrhea | Throat, sore |

## SECONDARY APPLICATIONS

| | |
|---|---|
| Anemia | Arthritis |
| Boils | Breath, odor |
| Cholera | Gallstones |
| Heart problems | Heartburn |
| Hemorrhages | Itching |
| Kidney problems | Migraines |
| Rheumatism | Ringworm |
| Skin conditions | |

# BARLEY (Hordeum vulgare)

*Parts used:* Juice, in powder form from young leaves and grass
*Properties:* Adaptogen, alterative, anti-inflammatory, antioxidant, antiviral, blood purifier, demulcent, emollient, immunostimulant, nutritive, stomachic
*Primary nutrients:* Calcium, chlorophyll, iron, live enzymes, magnesium, potassium, protein, superox-

ide dismutase (SOD), vitamins B1, B2, and C with bioflavonoids

Barley was revered by the ancient Egyptians and Greeks and cultivated for its health benefits. Hippocrates wrote of the benefits of gruel made from barley. Settlers in the New World planted barley to sustain health and vitality.

Barley juice contains antiviral properties and helps to strengthen the immune system. It can help cleanse the body on a cellular level, normalize metabolism, and neutralize heavy metals in the body such as mercury. It may benefit the body by lowering cholesterol levels, aiding digestion, and relieving constipation, as well as strengthening the entire body.

One study done in Japan isolated a new antioxidant (2-0-GI) in barley leaves. This was found to be effective in food preservation. The flavonoid 2-0-GI was also found to have anti-inflammatory and antiallergenic activity. Another Japanese study found beneficial results in inhibiting the AIDS virus.

## PRIMARY APPLICATIONS

| | |
|---|---|
| Anemia | Arthritis |
| Blood, impurities | Boils |
| Cancer | Poisoning, metal |

## SECONDARY APPLICATIONS

| | |
|---|---|
| Acne | AIDS/HIV |
| Allergies/hay fever | Bronchitis |
| Candidiasis | Eczema |
| Herpes | Infection |
| Kidney problems | Leprosy |
| Liver disorders | Lung disorders |
| Psoriasis | Skin conditions |
| Syphilis | Tuberculosis |
| Ulcers | |

# BASIL (Ocimum basilcum)

*Parts used:* Leaves
*Properties:* Anthelmintic, antibacterial, antispasmodic, demulcent, diaphoretic, diuretic, febrifuge, galactagogue, stimulant, stomachic
*Primary nutrients:* Calcium, iron, magnesium, phosphorus, vitamins A, D, B2

Basil is a common seasoning found in kitchens around the world and is often used to make pesto and to flavor soups, stews, and other foods. Basil has also long been used throughout the world for medicinal purposes in countries in Asia and Africa, as well as in India, where it was hailed as a sacred herb.

Basil has been used to treat exhaustion and works as a stimulant to promote energy. It has antibacterial properties and may help to draw out poisons from stings and bites.

Not only a flavoring, basil has definite health benefits. One study conducted at the University of Baroda in India found that basil helped to lower fasting blood glucose, cholesterol, and triglyceride levels significantly. It may help non-insulin-dependent diabetics control diabetes. Other research has found basil to be useful for killing intestinal parasites, treating acne, and stimulating the immune system.

## PRIMARY APPLICATIONS

| | |
|---|---|
| Bites, insects/snakes | Colds |
| Headaches | Indigestion |
| Lactation, absent | Whooping cough |

## SECONDARY APPLICATIONS

| | |
|---|---|
| Catarrh, intestinal | Constipation |
| Cramps, stomach | Fevers |
| Flu | Kidney problems |
| Nervous disorders | Respiratory infections |
| Rheumatism | Urinary problems |
| Vomiting | Worms |

# BAYBERRY (Myrica cerifera)

*Parts used:* Root bark and leaves
*Properties:* Alterative, antibacterial, antiseptic, astringent, emetic, febrifuge, insecticide, sialagogue, stimulant
*Primary nutrients:* Calcium, magnesium, manganese, niacin, phosphorus, potassium, silicon, sodium, vitamins B1, B2, C, and zinc

Although bayberry is probably best known for the candle wax made from its fragrant berries, the dried root bark is most often used for its medicinal properties. Bayberry has long been used as a tonic to treat diarrhea and external wounds and as a stimulant, and some Native American tribes used it to reduce fevers.

Bayberry is recommended as a tonic for stimulating the system and increasing immune function, and as a gargle to relieve tonsillitis and sore throat. The astringent value of the plant may work as a wound healer.

## PRIMARY APPLICATIONS

| | |
|---|---|
| Cholera | Colds |
| Congestion | Diarrhea |
| Dysentery | Fevers |
| Flu | Glandular problems |
| Goiters | Hemorrhage, uterine |
| Indigestion | Jaundice |
| Menstruation, excessive | Tuberculosis, primary |

## SECONDARY APPLICATIONS

| | |
|---|---|
| Bleeding | Colitis |
| Gums, bleeding | Liver disorders |
| Mucus, excessive | Scurvy |
| Throat, | Thyroid problems |
| sore and ulcerated | Ulcers |
| Uterus, prolapsed | Veins, varicose |

# BEE POLLEN

*Parts used:* Pollen
*Properties:* Alterative and nutritive
*Primary nutrients:* 21 amino acids, enzymes, essential fatty acids, variable vitamins and minerals (depending on the region)

Bee pollen consists of the fine powder in the male seed of a flower blossom. The bees transport it and mix it with nectar for their own nourishment. The pollen grains are collected and eaten by the bees but also pollinate the flowers. Bee pollen and honey have been recognized since the beginning of time for their healing benefits. Egyptian records dating back thousands of years have references to honey and its healing potential, and marathon runners of ancient Greece recognized the value of bee pollen to increase their strength and endurance. European nations and Asian countries also revered bee pollen for its medicinal value.

Bee pollen is considered a complete food because it contains every chemical substance needed to maintain life, and so it is a great supplement to build the immune system and provide energy to the body. Modern scientific research has found bee pollen to contain properties beneficial to healing, revitalizing, and protecting against radiation therapy. It is a rich source of protein and carbohydrates and can be used as a food supplement or to correct body chemistry and normalize weight.

Scientists at the Institute of Bee Culture in Bures-sur-Yvette near Paris, along with other researchers throughout Europe, studied the effects of honeybee pollen consumption on human beings. The study found exceptional antibiotic properties in the bee pollen. Scientists also found the bee pollen helpful in treating conditions such as chronic fatigue, hay fever and allergies, bronchitis, sinusitis, asthma, colds, balancing the endocrine system, menopausal symptoms, prostate problems such as prostatitis, infertility, indigestion, constipation, colitis, anemia, high blood pressure, premature aging, depression, and hair loss.

It can also help improve concentration and mental function. One study found a group of students' mental performance improved significantly with the addition of bee pollen. It reduces cholesterol and triglyceride levels by preventing plaque buildup in the arteries. Athletes often use this supplement to increase their strength, endurance, and speed.

## PRIMARY APPLICATIONS

| | |
|---|---|
| Aging | Allergies/hay fever |
| Appetite, loss | Endurance, lack of |
| Exhaustion | Fatigue |
| Immune system, weak | Infection |
| Multiple sclerosis | Pregnancy problems |

## SECONDARY APPLICATIONS

| | |
|---|---|
| Asthma | Blood pressure, high |
| Cancer | Depression |
| Hypoglycemia | Indigestion |
| Liver diseases | Prostate disorders |
| Radiation | |

# BILBERRY *(Vaccinium myrtillus)*

*Parts used:* Fruit
*Properties:* Antioxidant, astringent, febrifuge
*Primary nutrients:* Calcium, magnesium, manganese, phosphorus, potassium, selenium, silicon, sodium, vitamins A and C with bioflavonoids, zinc

Bilberry is native to areas of northern Europe, Asia, and the United States. It is a perennial shrub that grows in the sandy areas of the northern United States but is found more often in forest meadows throughout Europe. It has been utilized in Europe to treat fragile blood vessels related to high blood pressure, as well as treating urinary problems, scurvy, diarrhea, and dysentery. Early European apothecaries used the berries mixed with honey to make a syrup as a remedy for diarrhea.

Probably the most common use of bilberry is for eye disorders, because it strengthens the capillaries and small veins surrounding the eyes. Optimal eye health requires the proper amounts of nutrients and oxygen, which bilberry helps to provide. Royal Air Force pilots during World War II ate bilberry jam before night missions to improve their night vision. They swore that it helped them see better and adjust to the darkness more quickly.

Since then, research has been done to support these claims. Bilberry is not only helpful with night vision, but also with day blindness and focusing changes in light. Anthocyanosides found in bilberry are thought responsible for aiding the pigmented epithelium of the retina. Bilberry is also thought to help with glaucoma, eye strain and fatigue, eye irritations, nearsightedness, night blindness, and cataracts.

Bilberry is believed to help improve all capillaries, veins, and arteries, thus improving circulation to the feet, hands, brain, and heart. It also helps with varicose veins, atherosclerosis, and blood clots. It can help to prevent strokes, heart attacks, and blindness. It contains essential antioxidants that are useful in preventing free-radical damage.

Bilberry is used in cases of diarrhea and other intestinal problems. It helps nourish the pancreas in diabetes and aids healing in lung disorders such as chronic coughing, lung ailments, and TB. The extract has been found to kill or inhibit the growth of fungus, yeast, and bacteria, as well as protozoa, such as *Trichomonas vaginalis*.

Bilberry has been used to treat diabetes and blood sugar fluctuations. Oral doses have been given to help with hyperglycemia and diabetes. It appears to have benefits similar to those of insulin with less toxicity.

## PRIMARY APPLICATIONS

| | |
|---|---|
| Blood vessels, weak | Circulation, poor |
| Diabetes | Hands/feet, cold |
| Infection | Night blindness |
| Veins, varicose | |

## SECONDARY APPLICATIONS

| | |
|---|---|
| Diarrhea | Edema |
| Immune deficiencies | Kidney problems |
| Light sensitivity | Raynaud's disease |
| Scurvy | Thyroid problems |
| Water retention | |

# BIRCH *(Betula alba)*

*Parts used:* Bark and leaves
*Properties:* Anthelmintic, anti-inflammatory, antirheumatic, astringent, blood purifier, diaphoretic, diuretic, stimulant
*Primary nutrients:* Calcium, chlorine, copper, fluoride, iron, magnesium, phosphorus, potassium, silicon, sodium, vitamins A, C, E, B1, and B2

Native Americans used birch bark tea to relieve headaches. Some also used tea made from the leaves and bark for fevers and abdominal cramps.

The properties in birch bark help to heal burns and wounds and cleanse the blood. Birch bark also contains a glycoside that decomposes to methyl salicylate, a remedy for rheumatism used in both Canada and the United States. A decoction of birch leaves is recommended for baldness, and it works as a mild sedative for insomnia.

## PRIMARY APPLICATIONS

| | |
|---|---|
| Blood impurities | Eczema |
| Pain | Rheumatism |
| Urinary problems | |

## SECONDARY APPLICATIONS

| | |
|---|---|
| Canker sores | Cholera |
| Diarrhea | Dysentery |
| Edema | Fevers |
| Gout | Gums, bleeding |

# BISTORT *(Polygorium bistorta)*

*Parts used:* Root
*Properties:* Alterative, antiseptic, astringent, diuretic, expectorant, hemostatic
*Primary nutrients:* Vitamins A, B-complex, and C

Bistort is known as one of the strongest astringents in the herbal kingdom. It also contains valuable antiseptic properties to promote healing and prevent infection. Bistort can help stop bleeding both externally and internally. A decoction can be used in mouthwash form to treat gum problems and mouth inflammations.

Bistort is a member of the buckwheat family and can be used as an emergency food. Historically, the root was used in place of flour in times of famine.

## PRIMARY APPLICATIONS

| | |
|---|---|
| Bleeding, external/internal | Breath odor |
| | Cholera |
| Diarrhea | Dysentery |
| Hemorrhoids | |

## SECONDARY APPLICATIONS

| | |
|---|---|
| Canker sores | Diabetes |
| Gastric disorders | Jaundice |
| Measles | Menstruation, irregular |

# BITTER MELON FRUIT
*(Momordica charantia)*

*Parts used:* Fruit, leaves, seeds, seed oil
*Properties:* Abortifacient, antifertility, antimicrobial, hypoglycemic
*Primary nutrients:* Ascorbic acid, glycosides, iron, niacin, riboflavin, sodium, thiamine

Bitter melon, also called bitter gourd, is the fruit of the plant *Momordica charantia*, a climbing vine that originated in Asia, Africa, and Australia and is now grown in warm climates all over the globe. This fruit is among the most bitter of all plant foods. The oblong-shaped bitter melon has a distinctive warty appearance. It is nutritious and can be eaten unripe and green or ripe and yellowish or reddish-orange.

Bitter melon has a history of use in folk medicine all over the world. In the Ayurvedic tradition, it is thought to be a natural insulin and is recommended for diabetics. Bitter melon is also a primary component of the diet in Okinawa, which has the highest percentage of centenarians in the world, the longest healthy life expectancy, and a very low incidence of heart disease. This fruit has been used as a treatment for tumors, asthma, skin infections, gastrointestinal ailments, and high blood pressure. Bitter melon has been a traditional remedy in Africa, China, India, and the southeastern United States.

Bitter melon is being researched as a remedy for diabetes, AIDS, and some kinds of cancer. It can help regulate blood sugar by reducing blood glucose and improving glucose tolerance, but no studies have established a safe and effective dose. The plant's roots and leaf extracts have shown antibiotic properties.

Some studies suggest an element in bitter melon may prevent the HIV virus from infecting human cells, and laboratory research shows one component of the plant may help inhibit the growth of some cancers. In some studies, people taking bitter melon developed headaches. Expectant mothers should not use bitter melon.

## PRIMARY APPLICATIONS

| | |
|---|---|
| Asthma | Cancer |
| Diabetes | Gastrointestinal issues |
| HIV/AIDS | Hypertension |
| Skin infections | Tumors |

# BITTER ORANGE FRUIT
*(Fructus aurantia)*

*Parts used:* Fruit
*Properties:* Antibacterial, antifungal, anti-inflamma-

tory, antispasmodic, cholagogue, demulcent, sedative, tonic, tranquilizer, vascular stimulant
*Primary nutrients:* Flavanones, octopamine, synephrine, tyramine

The bitter orange plant is native to northeastern India and is also grown in southern Europe, southern China, and the United States. The flesh of the orange fruit is bitter and sour.

In traditional Chinese medicine, bitter orange was used as a tonic and a remedy for dyspepsia, to relieve abdominal distension and diarrhea, and for blood in the stool. In Europe, bitter orange flowers and oil have been recommended as a sedative and as a remedy for gastrointestinal ailments, nervous conditions, gout, insomnia, and sore throat. This plant has been used for toxic and anaphylactic shock, cancer, and cardiac conditions. Brazilians have used bitter orange as an anticonvulsant and for anxiety and insomnia.

After ephedra's implication in cardiac events in some consumers, the Food and Drug Administration banned the sale of dietary supplements containing that herb in 2004. Thus many supplement makers have altered their weight-loss products to offer ephedra-free formulas that contain bitter orange extract instead. Because of bitter orange's synephrine content, the safety of these products is being monitored.

Synephrine is an ephedrine-like natural product. There are numerous reports of people having cardiac problems after taking formulas containing bitter orange. Italian scientists discovered that laboratory rats given bitter orange ate less and lost weight but also developed heart abnormalities and died as the dose was increased. The compounds in bitter orange may cause vasoconstriction and increased heart rate and blood pressure.

## PRIMARY APPLICATIONS

| | |
|---|---|
| Anxiety | Cancer |
| Cardiac conditions | Dyspepsia |
| Gastrointestinal issues | Gout |
| Insomnia | Nervous conditions |
| Shock | Sore throat |

# BLACKBERRY *(Rubus fructicosus)*

*Parts used:* Berries, leaves, and root bark
*Properties:* Alterative, astringent, bitter, febrifuge, hemostatic
*Primary nutrients:* Calcium, iron, niacin, riboflavin, thiamine, vitamins A and C

Blackberries are most commonly known for being made into jams and jellies. However, the ancient Greeks and Europeans used blackberry to treat gout, and in Asian countries, the unripe berries were used to treat kidney problems. In the Middle East, the leaves have been used as a remedy for bleeding gums for at least two thousand years, and Native Americans used blackberry root tea to cure dysentery.

The root of the blackberry plant works as an astringent by constricting blood vessels and reducing minor bleeding. Blackberries have also been used to treat diarrhea and as a diuretic. Made into a tea, blackberries can help dry up sinus drainage. An infusion of the unripe berries is recommended for controlling vomiting and loose bowels. External uses also include gargles and eyewashes.

## PRIMARY APPLICATIONS

| | |
|---|---|
| Bleeding | Cholera |
| Congestion | Diarrhea in children |
| Dysentery | Vomiting |

## SECONDARY APPLICATIONS

| | |
|---|---|
| Anemia | Boils |
| Fevers | Genital irritations |
| Gums, bleeding | Menstruation, excessive |
| Mouth irritations | Peristalsis, weak |

# BLACK COHOSH
*(Cimicifuga racemosa)*

*Parts used:* Root
*Properties:* Alterative, antispasmodic, diuretic, emmenagogue, expectorant, nervine, oxytocic
*Primary nutrients:* Calcium, iron, magnesium, manganese, niacin, phosphorus, potassium, selenium, silicon, sodium, sulfur, vitamins A, B1, B2, C, K, F, zinc

Black cohosh was introduced by a Dr. Young in 1831 as a cardiac tonic for a fatty heart, bronchitis, hysteria, and female problems. Native Americans called black cohosh "snakeroot" because of its ability to help with snakebites. The Algonquin Indians also used black cohosh to treat menstrual symptoms, childbirth, and female complaints.

Modern research supports the use of black cohosh for high blood pressure and heart problems because it equalizes circulation, as well as helping with asthma and bronchial complaints. Similarly, its use as an antidote for snakebites and to treat menstrual and menopausal complaints has since been supported by scientific research.

Numerous studies have researched its use for perimenopause and postmenopause and have found it a beneficial alternative to hormone therapy. One study involved 110 menopausal women treated with black cohosh. Symptoms such as depression and hot flashes were reduced significantly. This is thought to be due to the fact that black cohosh reduces the secretion of lutenizing hormone (LH), which is linked to hot flashes, drying and thinning of the vagina, night sweats, and other menopausal symptoms.

Since its first use, black cohosh has been used for many other ailments, including excess mucus, yellow fever, spinal meningitis, nervousness, epilepsy, and hormone imbalance. It is also used to treat all types of inflammation. Research supports its use for nervous conditions, irritability, TB, pleurisy, and tinnitus.

## PRIMARY APPLICATIONS

| | |
|---|---|
| Asthma | Bites, insect/snake |
| Bronchitis | Childbirth pain |
| Diarrhea | Epilepsy |
| Estrogen deficiency | Fevers |
| Hormone imbalance | Hot flashes |
| Inflammation | Lung disorders |
| Malaria | Menopausal symptoms |
| Menstrual symptoms | Spinal meningitis |
| Stings, bee | Tuberculosis |
| Whooping cough | |

## SECONDARY APPLICATIONS

| | |
|---|---|
| Arthritis | Back pain, lower |
| Blood impurities | Blood pressure, high |
| Cholera | Convulsions |
| Coughs | Cramps, uterine |
| Gastric disorders | Headaches |
| Heart problems | Insomnia |
| Kidney problems | Liver disorders |
| Nervous conditions | Neuralgia |
| Pain | Rheumatism |
| Skin conditions | Smallpox |
| Uterine problems | |

# BLACK HAW (*Viburnum prunifolium*)

*Parts used:* Bark
*Properties:* Analgesic and sedative
*Primary nutrients:* Scopoletin

The bark of the black haw shrub was used by Native Americans in tea form to treat menstrual cramps and other gynecological problems. Southern slave owners made female slaves of childbearing years drink black haw bark tea to prevent abortions. Europeans adopted the use of black haw for menstrual pain and miscarriage prevention.

Studies have found black haw to be a beneficial treatment for menstrual cramps. It contains analgesic and uterine-relaxing components and acts as a sedative, which is why it helps with cramping. Black haw is considered an alterative for the uterus. It may also help with asthma. The salicin in black haw is similar to aspirin and is not recommended for use during pregnancy.

## PRIMARY APPLICATIONS

| | |
|---|---|
| Asthma | Childbirth after-pains |
| Contractions, uterine | Menstrual pain |
| Miscarriage tendency | Nervous disorders |

# BLACK WALNUT (*Juglans nigra*)

*Parts used:* Hulls and leaves
*Properties:* Alterative, anthelmintic, antigalactagogue, antineoplastic, antiseptic, astringent, vulnerary
*Primary nutrients:* Calcium, chlorine, iron, magnesium, manganese, niacin, organic iodine, phosphorus, potassium, selenium, silicon, selenium, vitamins A, B1, B2, B6, B15, C, P, and bioflavonoids

Black walnut has been used for centuries in Europe for skin ailments and constipation. Research supports its use for skin problems such as boils, eczema, herpes, and ringworm. Its benefits for the stomach are also well represented. Native Americans used black walnut as a laxative, and during the Civil War, black walnut was used as a remedy for diarrhea and dysentery.

Black walnut has also been used for syphilis, TB, varicose veins, chronic infections of the intestines, and urogenital problems. Herbalists consider black walnut very useful for killing parasites, tapeworms, and ringworm. Black walnut causes oxygenation of the blood, which kills parasites and has been proven through recent research. Also, the brown stain found in the green husk of black walnut contains organic iodine, which has antiseptic and healing properties.

Scientific research has found that black walnut contains astringent properties healing to the skin and mucous membranes of the body, and it can be gargled to clean stains on teeth.

## PRIMARY APPLICATIONS

| | |
|---|---|
| Athlete's foot | Candidiasis |
| Canker sores | Cold sores |
| Dandruff | Fungus |
| Gum disease | Herpes |
| Infection | Malaria |
| Parasites | Rashes |
| Ringworm | Tapeworm |

## SECONDARY APPLICATIONS

| | |
|---|---|
| Abscesses | Acne |
| Asthma | Body odor |
| Boils | Cancer |
| Colitis | Diarrhea |
| Diphtheria | Dysentery |
| Eczema | Eye diseases |
| Fevers | Hemorrhoids |
| Liver disorders | Lupus |
| Poison ivy | Skin diseases |
| Tonsillitis | Tuberculosis, primary |
| Tumors | Ulcers |
| Veins, varicose | Wounds |

# BLESSED THISTLE
*(Cnicus benedictus)*

*Parts used:* Entire herb
*Properties:* Alterative, antibacterial, bitter, blood purifier, diaphoric, emmenagogue, galactagogue
*Primary nutrients:* Calcium, magnesium, niacin, phosphorus, potassium, selenium, sodium, vitamins A, B-complex, and C, zinc

Herbalists have recommended this herb for female problems, headaches, and fevers. The Quinault tribe of Native Americans used the whole plant, steeped, for birth control, while monks in Europe used blessed thistle as a treatment for smallpox.

Traditional uses of blessed thistle include digestive problems, headaches, stomach problems, heart conditions, circulation, liver problems, and internal cancer. It strengthens the heart and lungs, as well as increasing circulation to the brain to improve mental function. Research also suggests its ability to strengthen the stomach, spleen, intestine, liver, and nervous system.

Blessed thistle contains nutrients that help support estrogen and balance other hormones in the body. It is sometimes taken in combination with red raspberry, not only to stimulate milk production for nursing mothers, but also to enrich the milk for newborns.

Modern research has shown that the extract of blessed thistle contains antibacterial and anti-yeast properties that can help with *Candida albicans*. In addition, it is used to reduce fevers in childhood diseases such as chicken pox and measles.

## PRIMARY APPLICATIONS

| | |
|---|---|
| Angina | Blood circulation, poor |
| Cancer | Constipation |
| Fevers | Gallbladder problems |
| Gastric disorders | Headaches |
| Heart problems | Hormone imbalance |
| Lactation, absent | Liver disorders |
| Lung disorders | Memory loss |

## SECONDARY APPLICATIONS

| | |
|---|---|
| Arthritis | Blood impurities |
| Cramps, uterine | Edema |

| | |
|---|---|
| Gas | Jaundice |
| Kidney problems | Respiratory infections |
| Senility | Spleen ailments |
| Vaginal discharge | Worms |

# BLUE COHOSH
*(Caulophyllum thalictrodies)*

*Parts used:* Rhizome
*Properties:* Alterative, anthelmintic, antispasmodic, diuretic, emmenagogue, estrogenic, expectorant, oxytocic
*Primary nutrients:* Calcium, chlorine, iron, magnesium, manganese, niacin, phosphorus, potassium, selenium, silicon, sodium, vitamins A, B1, B2, C, and E, zinc

Blue cohosh, one of the oldest indigenous plants in America, was used by Native Americans to treat rheumatism, colic, cramps, epilepsy, and fevers, as well as aiding childbirth and acting as a contraceptive. The early settlers adopted this herb for both delivery and to help reduce fevers. The dried root was an official herb in the United States Pharmacopoeia from 1882 to 1905, where it was listed for inducing labor and menstruation.

The chemical caulosaponin, found in blue cohosh, is what induces uterine contractions, but it should be used only under medical supervision. In addition, a study published in the *Journal of Reproduction and Fertility* found that blue cohosh inhibited ovulation in animals.

Herbalists have recommended blue cohosh for irregular menstrual cycles, inflammation of the uterus, and to stop false labor pains. It has also been used as an antispasmodic and to relieve muscle cramps. These uses have been validated by scientific studies, especially the herb's estrogenic and antispasmodic properties. Its hormone- and menses-regulating powers work best when blue cohosh is combined with pennyroyal.

Blue cohosh may also help stimulate the immune system. It helps with cases of toxemia and has been found useful in reducing emotional and nervous tension.

## PRIMARY APPLICATIONS

| | |
|---|---|
| Childbirth pain | Cramps |
| Epilepsy | Estrogen deficiency |
| Menstruation, absent | Urinary problems |
| Uterine problems | |

## SECONDARY APPLICATIONS

| | |
|---|---|
| Blood pressure, high | Bronchitis |
| Colic | Convulsions |
| Cystitis | Diabetes |
| Edema | Heart palpitations |
| Mucus, excessive | Neuralgia |
| Spasms | Vaginitis |
| Vaginal discharge/leucorrhea | |
| Whooping cough | |

# BLUE VERVAIN *(Verbena hastata)*

*Parts used:* Entire herb
*Properties:* Alterative, anti-inflammatory, antiperiodic, antispasmodic, diaphoretic, expectorant, nervine, purgative (mild)
*Primary nutrients:* Calcium, manganese, vitamins C and E

Blue vervain has been used for thousands of years. The Chinese used blue vervain to treat malaria, dysentery, and congestion. It was used during the Middle Ages to help cure plagues. Native Americans used blue vervain as a natural tranquilizer for treating nervous conditions as well as female problems. Modern research in Germany supports the use of blue vervain for the nervous system and for pain relief.

Research also shows that blue vervain has pain-relieving and anti-inflammatory properties that relieve respiratory inflammation and are calming for coughs. This herb works to fight mucus, especially for coughs associated with colds. Herbalist Dr. Edward E. Shook recommended using it to treat all diseases of the spleen and liver. It is also used to restore circulation and alleviate menstrual symptoms, epilepsy, indigestion, and dyspepsia.

## PRIMARY APPLICATIONS

| | |
|---|---|
| Asthma | Bronchitis |
| Circulation, poor | Colds |

| | |
|---|---|
| Colon problems | Congestion |
| Convulsions | Coughs |
| Fevers | Flu |
| Gastric disorders | Indigestion |
| Insomnia | Liver disorders |
| Lung congestion | Nervous conditions |
| Pneumonia | Seizures |
| Stomach, upset | Throat, sore |
| Uterine problems | Worms |

## SECONDARY APPLICATIONS

| | |
|---|---|
| Catarrh | Constipation |
| Diarrhea | Dysentery |
| Earaches | Epilepsy |
| Gallstones | Headaches |
| Kidney problems | Malaria/ague |
| Menstrual symptoms | Mucus, excessive |
| Pain | Skin diseases |
| Sores | Spleen ailments |

# BONESET (Eupatorium perfoliatum)

*Parts used:* Entire herb
*Properties:* Alterative, anti-inflammatory, antiperiodic, antiviral, diaphoretic, emetic, febrifuge, purgative (mild), nervine, stimulant
*Primary nutrients:* Calcium, magnesium, PABA, potassium, vitamins C and B-complex

Native Americans used this valuable herb for colds, flu, and fevers. They introduced boneset to the settlers in the New World. Boneset was listed in the U.S. Pharmacopoeia from 1820 through 1916 and in the National Formulary from 1926 through 1950. It has been used to restore strength in the stomach and spleen, and as a tonic for acute and chronic fevers. In fact, Dr. Edward E. Shook felt that boneset was beneficial for every kind of fever humans are subjected to and that it had never failed in overcoming influenza.

Research has shown that boneset contains antiseptic properties and promotes sweating to help in cases of colds and flu. It has also been shown to contain antiviral properties and strengthens the immune system by enhancing the secretion of interferon. Other studies have found boneset effective against minor viral and bacterial infections by stimulating the white blood cells.

In addition, it has been used to treat indigestion and pain and may also contain some mild anti-inflammatory agents to help with conditions such as arthritis.

## PRIMARY APPLICATIONS

| | |
|---|---|
| Chills | Colds |
| Coughs | Fever |
| Flu | Malaria |
| Pain | Rheumatism |
| Typhoid fever | Yellow fever |

## SECONDARY APPLICATIONS

| | |
|---|---|
| Bronchitis | Catarrh |
| Jaundice | Liver disorders |
| Measles | Mumps |
| Rocky Mountain | Scarlet fever |
| spotted fever | Throat, sore |
| Worms | |

# BORAGE (Borago officinalis)

*Parts used:* Leaves
*Properties:* Blood purifier, diaphoretic, febrifuge, galactagogue, purgative (mild)
*Primary nutrients:* Calcium and potassium

Ancient Celtic warriors often drank wine flavored with borage before going into battle because of its reputation of enhancing courage and strength. During the Middle Ages, the leaves and flowers were combined with wine to relieve melancholy, and the Roman scholar Pliny thought this herb was useful for treating depression and lifting the spirits. Along similar lines, John Gerard, the sixteenth-century herbalist, regarded borage as an herb to comfort the heart and increase joy.

Along with its mood-boosting properties, borage is often used to treat bronchitis because of its soothing effect and ability to reduce inflammation and detoxify the body. It is known to help heal the mucous membranes of the mouth and throat and stimulates activity in the kidneys and adrenal glands to rid the body of catarrh.

Borage is also useful for restoring vitality during recovery from an illness. It is helpful for treating problems of the digestive system and has been used to increase quantity and quality of mother's milk.

Virgin borage oil contains essential fatty acids, especially a concentration of gamma-linolenic acid (GLA). This fatty acid can account for as much as 26 percent of the oil's content, and it is the best-known source of concentrated GLA. This plant is known to stimulate the adrenal glands to help the body during stressful times.

### PRIMARY APPLICATIONS

| | |
|---|---|
| Bronchitis | Congestion |
| Eyes, inflammation | Fevers |
| Heart problems | Lactation, absent |
| Mucus, excessive | Rashes |

### SECONDARY APPLICATIONS

| | |
|---|---|
| Blood impurities | Colds |
| Gastric disorders | Insomnia |
| Jaundice | Lung disorders |
| Nervous disorders | Pleurisy |
| Ringworm | Urinary problems |

# BOSWELLIA *(Boswellia serrata)*

*Parts used:* Resin
*Properties:* Analgesic, anti-inflammatory

The trees in the genus boswellia are known for their fragrant, gummy sap that has many medicinal uses, especially as anti-inflammatories. The frankincense of biblical fame was probably an extract from the resin of the tree *Boswellia sacra*. Boswellia, also known as boswellin, has a long history of use in Ayurvedic healing. Its resin, called salai guggal, has been used to treat asthma, arthritis, various inflammatory conditions, and to relieve joint pain and pain resulting from sports injuries. It may also be helpful for treating back pain and some chronic intestinal disorders.

Boswellic acids are the principal compounds thought to be at the root of boswellia's anti-inflammatory properties. These components are believed to inhibit enzymes that induce pain and inflammation.

There have been a few studies conducted on boswellia's effect on sports injuries and arthritis, and some have shown that boswellic acids may contain anti-inflammatory benefits that are as powerful as those found in ibuprofen and aspirin. In one study of rheumatoid arthritis patients, pain and swelling were reduced following three months of boswellia treatment. Boswellia users have occasionally reported mild gastrointestinal distress, such as heartburn and nausea, but there are no reports of serious side effects.

This herb has a long tradition of safe and effective use as a mild anti-inflammatory to alleviate pain and stiffness and enhance mobility without serious side effects, but further research is needed to confirm the long-term safety and effectiveness of this promising extract. Boswellia is best taken as needed to reduce pain and stiffness, rather than regularly as a maintenance herb.

### PRIMARY APPLICATIONS

| | |
|---|---|
| Arthritis | Asthma |
| Inflammatory conditions | Joint pain |
| Sports injuries | |

# BUCHU *(Barosma betulina)*

*Parts used:* Leaves
*Properties:* Alterative, antibacterial, antibiotic, antilithic, antirheumatic, antiseptic, aromatic, astringent, carminative, diaphoretic, diuretic, lithotriptic, nephritic, stimulant, stomachic
*Primary nutrients:* Bioflavonoids

Buchu is a plant indigenous to South Africa and has been used by a tribe of that region, the Hottentots, for thousands of years for just about every ailment. When the Dutch settled in the area, they began using buchu for conditions such as urinary problems, kidney stones, arthritis, and muscle aches. Henry T. Helmbold, known as the Buchu King, patented an extract of buchu and advertised it in 1847 for a myriad of problems such as inflammation of the kidneys, diabetes, bladder problems, and venereal disease.

The leaves of the plant contain an oil that promotes urination. It is excellent for the urinary tract because it absorbs excessive uric acid and reduces bladder irritations. Buchu is also believed to have a healing influence on all chronic complaints of the genitourinary tract. In fact, it has been used to treat enlarged prostate glands and irritation of the urethra membrane. Buchu is also an ingredient in some over-the-counter diuretics because it relieves bloating symptoms associated with PMS.

Buchu may also be helpful in the first stages of diabetes. Buchu acts as a tonic, astringent, and disinfectant of the mucous membranes. Although no clinical studies have substantiated the effects of buchu, herbalists have had success for years. These herbalists attribute the antibacterial activity in the buchu to its diosphenol content. Flavonoids found in buchu may contribute to its diuretic properties.

## PRIMARY APPLICATIONS

| | |
|---|---|
| Catarrh, bladder | Kidney disorders |
| Prostate problems | Urethritis |

## SECONDARY APPLICATIONS

| | |
|---|---|
| Bed-wetting | Cystitis |
| Diabetes, early stages | Edema |
| Gallstones | Rheumatism |
| Urinary incontinence | Yeast infections |

# BUCKTHORN *(Rhamnus frangula)*

*Parts used:* Bark, berries, and root
*Properties:* Alterative, anthelmintic, antineoplastic, antirheumatic, bitter, blood purifier, diuretic, emetic, febrifuge, purgative (mild)
*Primary nutrients:* Vitamin C

Buckthorn, a bitter herb for expelling impurities, has been used in Europe for hundreds of years as a potent laxative for purging the body. The Cherokee Indians used buckthorn as a cathartic and for skin problems. The seventeenth-century herbalist Nicholas Culpeper recommended the bruised buckthorn leaves to stop bleeding when applied to a wound.

Buckthorn is a well-known and powerful laxative, but it is also helpful for cleansing the liver and gallbladder. Buckthorn works by stimulating the flow of bile from the liver to the gallbladder. If taken hot, it

will produce perspiration and lower a fever. An ointment made with the herb will help relieve itching.

There has been some evidence of antitumor effects of buckthorn, but there is no recent research to substantiate the information. Future studies may prove it is beneficial.

Buckthorn should not be abused. Follow directions to avoid gastrointestinal cramping.

## PRIMARY APPLICATIONS

| | |
|---|---|
| Bleeding | Constipation, chronic |
| Fevers | Gallstones |
| Gastric disorders | Liver disorders |
| Poisoning, lead | |

## SECONDARY APPLICATIONS

| | |
|---|---|
| Appendicitis | Edema |
| Gout | Hemorrhoids |
| Itching | Parasites |
| Rheumatism | Skin diseases |
| Warts, external | |

# BUGLEWEED *(Lycopus virginicus)*

*Parts used:* Entire plant
*Properties:* Alterative, antirheumatic, antithyroid, astringent, bitter, diuretic, emmenagogue, hemostatic, narcotic (mild), sedative
*Primary nutrients:* Hydrocinnamic acid derivatives, lithospermic acid, flavonoids

Bugleweed, one of the mildest and most effective narcotics, is a member of the mint family. It is found growing in moist areas of the eastern United States. Bugleweed is used to relieve aches and pains. It contains compounds known to contract the tissues of the mucous membranes, relieving and reducing fluid discharges. Bugleweed is also used to treat enlargement and overactivity of the thyroid gland. It helps relieve symptoms such as tightness of breathing, heart palpitations, and shaking. Research has confirmed the benefits of bugleweed for treating hyperthyroidism.

Bugleweed has been used successfully to treat problems related to the heart. It works as a cardiac tonic to stabilize a rapid or irregular heartbeat due to certain nervous conditions. It is similar to digitalis, lowering the pulse and equalizing circulation. It helps to relieve and soothe the irritations of a cough. It helps improve circulation and tone the heart. It is especially valuable when treating a weak heart due to edema.

## PRIMARY APPLICATIONS

| | |
|---|---|
| Coughs | Fever |
| Hyperthyroidism | Indigestion, nervous |
| Menstruation, excessive | Nervous disorders |

## SECONDARY APPLICATIONS

| | |
|---|---|
| Asthma | Bleeding |
| Bronchitis | Bruises, traumatic |
| Colds | Diabetes |
| Goiter | Heart problems |
| Hemorrhages | Lungs, fluid |
| Nosebleeds | Pneumonia |
| Sores | Tuberculosis |
| Ulcers | Uterine problems |

# BURDOCK (*Arctium lappa*)

*Parts used:* Root
*Properties:* Alterative, antineoplastic, antirheumatic, blood purifier, demulcent, diaphoretic, diuretic, vulnerary
*Primary nutrients:* Carbohydrates, copper, iodine, iron, PABA, protein, silicon, sulfur, vitamins A, B-complex, C, E, and P, zinc

Burdock was once widely known as a cleansing agent for both the blood and bowels. In fact, it is still known as one of the best blood purifiers of all herbs. Many Native American tribes used burdock for skin ailments and a wide variety of other diseases. The Chinese used it to lower blood sugar levels as well as to dispel wind and heat evils, and Europeans used burdock pounded in wine during the fourteenth century to treat leprosy.

Burdock is recommended during pregnancy and for various female complaints because of its ability to aid in hormone balance and to prevent water retention. It is also used to promote kidney function. It contains high amounts of insulin, a form of starch,

which is responsible for some of its healing properties and carbohydrate metabolism.

Modern scientific research has uncovered diuretic properties and tumor inhibitors in burdock in studies done on animals. Burdock may also inhibit mutations in cells that are exposed to mutation-causing chemicals that can lead to cancer. It has been found to contain antibiotic and antifungal properties. Research done in Germany has found fresh burdock root contains polyacetylenes effective in killing bacteria and fungi. In vitro tests have found burdock extracts to have some activity against HIV.

It is beneficial for skin disorders, kidney problems, arthritis, and gout. Burdock root has been used to treat breast cancer, glands, intestines, knees, lips, liver, sinus, stomach, tongue, and uterus in Chile, China, India, Canada, and Russia.

## PRIMARY APPLICATIONS

| | |
|---|---|
| Acne | Allergies/hay fever |
| Arthritis | Blood impurities |
| Cancer | Chicken pox |
| Colds | Constipation |
| Edema | Fevers |
| Hemorrhoids | Hypoglycemia |
| Kidney problems | Liver disorders |
| Lung disorders | Measles |
| Mucus, excessive | Poison ivy/oak |
| Rheumatism | Skin disorders |
| Tonsillitis | Tumors |

## SECONDARY APPLICATIONS

| | |
|---|---|
| Asthma | Back pain, lower |
| Boils | Bronchitis |
| Canker sores | Coughs |
| Cystitis | Dandruff |
| Gallbladder problems | Infection |
| Inflammation | Nervousness |
| Pneumonia | Ulcers |

# BUTCHER'S BROOM
(*Ruscus aculeatus*)

*Parts used:* Rhizome
*Properties:* Anti-inflammatory, diaphoretic, diuretic, lithotriptic, purgative (mild), vasoconstrictor

*Primary nutrients:* Calcium, iron, manganese, niacin, potassium, selenium, sodium, vitamins A, B1, B2, and C, zinc

Butcher's broom is an evergreen shrub found growing abundantly in the Middle East and Mediterranean regions. It also grows in the southern United States. In the past, it was used in Europe, especially Greece, for hemorrhoids, varicose veins, phlebitis, and thrombosis. It was also recommended as a laxative and a diuretic by Dioscorides, an ancient Greek herbalist. Butcher's broom was not widely used in either the United States or Europe until a study conducted in France during the 1950s found vasoconstricting abilities.

In fact, butcher's broom is very useful for circulation problems, which contribute to increasingly large numbers of deaths each year in the United States. It has been used to treat thrombosis or blood clots, arteriosclerosis, hemorrhoids, and peripheral circulation problems and to lower cholesterol because of its ability to strengthen the walls of blood vessels.

Recent studies have verified that this herb contains vasoconstrictive and anti-inflammatory properties. Butcher's broom's effects on varicose veins and hemorrhoids have been tested. It increases circulation to the brain, arms, and legs. Individuals with circulatory problems of the legs and chronic phlebopathy have had improvement with use of butcher's broom extract.

Symptoms such as edema, itching, cramping, and water retention have also been relieved using butcher's broom.

## PRIMARY APPLICATIONS

| | |
|---|---|
| Arteriosclerosis | Blood clots |
| Hemorrhoids | Inflammation |
| Stroke prevention | Thrombosis |
| Veins, varicose | |

## SECONDARY APPLICATIONS

| | |
|---|---|
| Brain circulation, poor | Cramps, leg |
| Edema | Headaches |
| Inflammation, vein | Jaundice |
| Menstrual symptoms | |

# CALENDULA (MARIGOLD)
*(Calendula officinalis)*

*Parts used:* Leaves, flowers, and petals
*Properties:* Alterative, analgesic, anthelmintic, antibacterial, anti-inflammatory, antiseptic, antiviral, astringent, bitter, blood purifier, cholagogue, diaphoretic, diuretic, emmenagogue, hemostatic, stimulant, vulnerary
*Primary nutrients:* Phosphorus and vitamins A and C

Calendula or marigold was thought to have originated in Egypt, but it can now be found throughout the world. The Romans are attributed with naming calendula and grew it mainly because of its beauty and continual blooms, although they did use it as a treatment for scorpion bites. Europeans have used calendula for hundreds of years and planted it in their gardens. The English often added this herb to their stews and soups. Its medicinal value was well known. European settlers brought calendula with them to the New World. It was used during the Civil War to stop bleeding and heal wounds.

Calendula is a well-known first-aid remedy, especially as an ointment for wounds, injuries, scrapes, burns, bruises, sprains, muscle spasms, ulcers, and varicose veins. A tea is used to relieve acute ailments, especially fevers. A poultice can be applied to bleeding hemorrhoids. As a snuff, it can aid in the discharge of mucus from the nose. Some herbalists recommend calendula for the heart and circulation.

This herb has been used extensively, but little research has been done to test its efficacy. Studies done on rats have shown wound-healing potential and definite benefits. Studies in Russia have found that calendula extract can help relieve and heal eye infections in rats. Other in vitro research has found antibacterial and antiviral, as well as immune-stimulating properties. The actual constituents responsible for the wound-healing and anti-inflammatory abilities of calendula have not yet been identified, however.

## PRIMARY APPLICATIONS

| | |
|---|---|
| Bruises, external | Cuts/scrapes |
| Eye infections | Measles |
| Skin diseases/irritations | Wounds |

## SECONDARY APPLICATIONS

| | |
|---|---|
| Anemia | Blood impurities |
| Bronchitis | Cancer |
| Colitis | Cramps, all kinds |
| Diarrhea | Ear infections |
| Fevers | Hemorrhoids |
| Hepatitis | Jaundice |
| Menstruation, absent | Ulcers |
| Veins, varicose | |

# CAPSICUM (CAYENNE)
*(Capsicum frutescens)*

*Parts used:* Fruit
*Properties:* Alterative, antispasmodic, astringent, blood purifier, carminative, diaphoretic, digestive, rubefacient, sialagogue, stimulant, vulnerary
*Primary nutrients:* Calcium, iron, magnesium, phosphorus, potassium, rutin, selenium, sodium, sulfur, vitamins A, B-complex, C, and G, zinc

A physician accompanying Columbus to the West Indies first introduced capsicum to Europe. Though it had been used probably for thousands of years in tropical climates throughout the world, capsicum was first used in Europe after Columbus returned. It was listed in a history book in 1493 as Peter Martyn noted its arrival in Italy. Capsicum was popularized as a natural, powerful stimulant by Dr. Samuel Thomson in the early nineteenth century and then around 1840 by Dr. John Stevens in England, where it was used as a chief ingredient in many of his formulas.

Capsicum was used to sustain the natural heat of the system on which life depends. It was also used to prevent and rid the body of the effects of serious infectious disease. It helps to improve the function of the circulatory system and regulate the heart blood flow. It has also been used to help normalize blood pressure, whether high or low. Capsicum helps cold hands and feet because of its effect on circulation.

Capsicum is often found in combination with other herbs to stimulate their action and improve absorption. Research has verified the benefits of this herb. It restores and stimulates the stomach and intestines, as well as the heart. It is used to help clean and heal the stomach and digestive system. Capsicum is also thought to help lower serum cholesterol levels. It has been used to control pain and bleeding.

Studies indicate that capsicum has the ability to slow fat absorption in the small intestine and increase the metabolic rate and thermogenesis. It may promote the burning of fat in the body.

## PRIMARY APPLICATIONS

| | |
|---|---|
| Arthritis | Bleeding |
| Blood pressure, high/low | Bronchitis |
| Circulation, poor | Colds |
| Congestion | Diabetes |
| Fatigue | Gastric disorders |
| Heart problems | Kidney problems |
| Lung disorders | Phlebitis |
| Rheumatism | Shock |
| Stroke | Throat, sore |
| Tumors | Ulcers |
| Veins, varicose | |

## SECONDARY APPLICATIONS

| | |
|---|---|
| Arteriosclerosis | Asthma |
| Blood impurities | Bruises |
| Burns | Fevers |
| Gas | Infection |
| Jaundice | Lockjaw |
| Malaria/ague | Mucus, excessive |
| Pain | Pancreatic problems |
| Pus discharge | Sinus problems |
| Skin disorders | Spasms |
| Sunburn | Wounds |

# CARALLUMA *(Caralluma fimbriata)*

*Parts used:* Entire plant
*Properties:* Anorectic, energy booster
*Primary nutrients:* Bitters principles, flavone glycosides, megastigmane glycosides, pregnane glycosides, saponins

Caralluma is a succulent plant in the cactus family. It grows wild in Africa, the Canary Islands, India, southern Europe, Sri Lanka, and Afghanistan. It has been used in India for centuries to curb appetite, as a portable food for hunting, and as an endurance-enhancer. It is also used during periods of famine to control appetite.

India's working class uses this plant not only as an appetite suppressant but also to increase energy and endurance. Caralluma can be cooked as a vegetable, pickled, used in chutneys, or eaten raw.

Caralluma seems to block the activity of several fat-promoting enzymes in the body, forcing fat reserves to be burned. A double-blind, placebo-controlled, randomized clinical trial on caralluma extract involving fifty people showed significant reductions in all key indicators of weight loss.

This plant is also thought to affect the appetite-control mechanism of the brain. When we eat, nerves in the stomach send a signal to the brain's hypothalamus, the appetite-controlling center. When the stomach is full, the hypothalamus tells the brain to stop eating. When a person feels hunger, the hypothalamus sends a signal to the brain to eat. By interfering with these signals or perhaps creating a signal of its own, caralluma seems to trick the brain into thinking the stomach is full, even if the person has not eaten.

Patients on caralluma have reported having more energy. They tend to gain lean muscle mass while losing fat. Caralluma not only reduces fat synthesis, it also boosts fat-burning. This makes more energy available to the body.

The plant has no known toxicity or side effects.

## PRIMARY APPLICATIONS

| | |
|---|---|
| Appetite suppressant | Energy, low |
| Obesity | |

# CARAWAY (Carum carvi)

*Parts used:* Root and seed
*Properties:* Anesthetic, antispasmodic, carminative, diuretic, emmenagogue, expectorant, galactagogue, purgative (mild), stimulant, stomachic
*Primary nutrients:* Calcium, cobalt, copper, iodine, iron, lead, magnesium, potassium, silicon, vitamin B-complex, zinc

Caraway seeds have been used both medicinally and as a flavoring in foods, such as rye bread, for

thousands of years by Romans, Germans, and the English. It was generally used to treat flatulence and indigestion and to relieve colic in babies.

Caraway is similar to anise, and both are recommended for the same purposes. It is a powerful antiseptic, especially effective in relieving toothaches. When applied locally to the skin, it also acts as an anesthetic. It can be mixed with other herbs such as mandrake or culver's root to help modify their purgative action. Caraway is also useful for stomach problems and helps prevent fermentation in the stomach. It can help to settle the stomach after taking medication that causes nausea. It also helps to relieve intestinal cramps and colic in babies.

Caraway is known to encourage menstruation and the flow of milk in nursing mothers. It also helps to ease uterine cramps.

## PRIMARY APPLICATIONS

| | |
|---|---|
| Appetite, loss | Colic |
| Cramps, | Gas |
| uterine/intestinal | Gastric disorders |
| Indigestion | Spasms |

## SECONDARY APPLICATIONS

| | |
|---|---|
| Colds | Lactation, absent |
| Menstruation, absent | Stomach, upset |
| Toothaches | |

# CASCARA SAGRADA
*(Rhamnus purshiana)*

*Parts used:* Bark
*Properties:* Alterative, antineoplastic, antispasmodic, hepatic, lithotriptic, purgative (mild)
*Primary nutrients:* Calcium, chlorine, iron, magnesium, manganese, niacin, phosphorus, potassium, selenium, silicon, sodium, vitamins A, B-complex, and C

Native Americans introduced cascara sagrada to the Spanish explorers when they complained of problems with constipation. The Spanish named the herb cascara sagrada, or "sacred bark," and used it as a natural laxative. They brought the herb back to

Spain when they returned. It was admitted to the U.S. Pharmacopoeia in 1877 and is still included as an official medicine.

Cascara sagrada is thought to be one of the best herbs for chronic constipation. It enhances the peristaltic action in the intestines and increases secretions of the stomach, liver, and pancreas. It is also helpful in relieving hemorrhoids because of its nonirritating nature and its softening action on stool.

It is found in many over-the-counter preparations to relieve constipation because it acts on the large intestine to increase the muscular activity in the colon. The anthraquinones in the cascara sagrada are thought to encourage intestinal contraction. It is used to restore natural bowel movement without griping and to restore tone to the bowel.

In addition, an element in the herb known as quinone emodin is being studied for its usefulness in treating lymphocytic leukemia and Walker carcinosarcoma tumor system. More research is necessary before it will be recommended for treatment, but the findings have been promising so far.

Cascara sagrada can be used often and is not considered addictive. Preparations should be made from bark that has been aged at least a year before use. Fresh bark is poisonous and can cause nausea and extreme griping on the intestinal system.

## PRIMARY APPLICATIONS

| | |
|---|---|
| Colon problems | Constipation |
| Gallbladder problems | Gallstones |
| Gas | Gastric disorders |
| Hemorrhoids | Intestinal problems |
| Liver disorders | Worms |

## SECONDARY APPLICATIONS

| | |
|---|---|
| Colitis | Coughs |
| Croup | Dyspepsia |
| Gout | Indigestion |
| Insomnia | Jaundice |
| Mucus, excessive | Pituitary problems |
| Spleen ailments | |

# CATNIP *(Nepeta cataria)*

*Parts used:* Entire herb
*Properties:* Antispasmodic, carminative, diaphoretic, febrifuge, nervine, sedative
*Primary nutrients:* Calcium, magnesium, manganese, organic iron, phosphorus, potassium, selenium, silicon, sodium, vitamins A, B-complex, C, and E

Catnip tea has been used in Europe and China for centuries, perhaps even thousands of years. Catnip was used by Native Americans for soothing colic in infants. It was used to induce sweating without increasing body heat, cure colds and fevers, and as a sedative for pain, restlessness, convulsions, and insomnia. It was official in the U.S. Pharmacopoeia from 1842 to 1882 and in the National Formulary from 1916 to 1950.

Catnip is also used to improve circulation and may help regulate blood pressure. Studies have proven the effectiveness of catnip. It is useful for calming the nerves and helping with anemia and menstrual problems. It also contains some antibiotic properties. It is a mild tonic used for colds, flu, and fevers. It also helps stimulate the appetite. Catnip is a member of the mint family and has similar properties to other mints, such as calming the stomach and aiding in digestion.

## PRIMARY APPLICATIONS

| | |
|---|---|
| Bronchitis | Chicken pox |
| Circulation, poor | Colds |
| Colic | Convulsions |
| Croup | Diarrhea |
| Fevers | Flu |
| Gas | Gastric disorders |

## SECONDARY APPLICATIONS

| | |
|---|---|
| Anemia | Coughs |
| Cramps, | Fatigue |
| menstrual/muscle | Headaches |
| Hemorrhoids | Hiccups |
| Infertility | Insanity |
| Kidney problems | Liver disorders |
| Lung congestion | Menstrual symptoms |
| Miscarriage, preventive | Morning sickness |

Nervousness
Pain
Shock
Sores
Stomach, upset
Vomiting

Nicotine withdrawal
Restlessness
Skin problems
Spasms
Stress

# CAT'S CLAW *(Uncaria tomentosa)*

*Parts used:* Inner bark
*Properties:* Alterative, anti-inflammatory, antineo-plastic, antioxidant
*Primary nutrients:* Alkaloids, glycosides, plant sterols, polyphenols, proanthocyanidins, oxindole, quinovic acid, triterpenes

Cat's claw, or uña de gato, can be found, along with many other medicinal plants, in the rain forests in the highlands of Peru and other South American countries. It takes more than two decades to mature and has been found in trees one hundred feet tall. The vine produces thorns resembling cat's claws that allow the vine to cling to the tree, winding upward toward light in the dense forest regions. Some native Peruvian tribes have used the inner bark and root to cure various ailments such as tumors and arthritis for hundreds of years.

The Peruvians have long recognized the anti-inflammatory capabilities of cat's claw and have used it to treat rheumatism, arthritis, and other inflammatory joint conditions. Clinical research has found that cat's claw does indeed have the ability to reduce inflammation.

Cat's claw can help protect the body from harmful environmental substances such as a high-fat diet, stress, alcohol, cigarette smoke, radiation, chemicals, herbicides, food additives, pesticides, exhaust smoke, air pollution, drug toxicity, and many more. We are often assaulted with potentially dangerous substances without even knowing it. But cat's claw can offer a degree of protection from damage that may occur. It is an amazing herb that can lead to a healthier body.

In fact, cat's claw is indeed promising as an antidote and protection against cancer. A doctor in Peru successfully treated seven hundred patients between 1984 and 1988 with various cancers. Cat's claw has the ability to act as an antioxidant in protecting the body from free-radical damage and destroying or neutralizing carcinogens before they can damage the cells. It may inhibit the growth of cancer cells. It also is recognized in helping support the body during chemotherapy and radiation therapies for cancer.

Cat's claw may be able to remove toxic metabolites and help strengthen the weakened immune system. It has been used successfully to treat individuals suffering from genital herpes, herpes zoster, and AIDS, which are all viral in nature.

Dr. Brent Davis recommends cat's claw for individuals suffering from various stomach and bowel disorders such as diverticulitis, gastritis, hemorrhoids, ulcers, fistulas, parasites, intestinal flora imbalance, and Crohn's disease, to name a few. Bowel problems are thought to be a factor in many different degenerative diseases.

## PRIMARY APPLICATIONS

Cancer
Chemotherapy
Crohn's disease
Intestinal problems
Irritable bowel (IBS)
Parasites
Radiation
Viral infections

Candidiasis
Chronic fatigue
Diverticulitis
Immune system, weak
Lupus
PMS
Ulcers

## SECONDARY APPLICATIONS

Allergies
Bursitis
Constipation
Hormone imbalance

Arthritis
Colitis
Diarrhea

# CELERY *(Apium graveolens)*

*Parts used:* Seed
*Properties:* Alterative, antiseptic, carminative, diuretic, emmenagogue, hypotensive, nervine, purgative (mild), sedative, stimulant (uterine), stomachic
*Primary nutrients:* Calcium, iron, magnesium, phosphorus, potassium, sodium, sulfur, vitamins A, B, and C

Celery grows wild in the marshes near the Mediterranean Sea. The ancient Greeks used celery to make a wine thought to enhance physical performance. It was also used in India and Europe for healing. Celery seeds and stems have long been used in Australia as an acid neutralizer.

Celery has been used to improve digestion and liver function. The organic sodium found in celery can help the stomach and joints.

Celery is often used as a diuretic to alleviate water retention. It has a stimulating effect on the kidneys to promote the flow of urine. It also promotes perspiration, which may help with weight loss when water retention is a problem.

Herbalists have often recommended celery for its calming effect on the nervous system. Studies done on mice have shown the sedative effect of the phthalides in celery. Because of this attribute, celery is often also used for headache and arthritis pain as well as for chemical imbalances.

Research has also found beneficial results of the use of celery juice for hypotensive effects. High blood pressure can lead to serious complications, and some medications to correct the condition have side effects. Studies done on both animals and humans have found blood-pressure-lowering abilities of celery juice.

## PRIMARY APPLICATIONS

| | |
|---|---|
| Arthritis | Back pain, lower |
| Nervousness | Rheumatism |

## SECONDARY APPLICATIONS

| | |
|---|---|
| Bright's disease | Catarrh, postnasal |
| Diabetes | Edema |
| Gout | Headaches |
| Insomnia | Liver disorders |
| Neuralgia | Urine retention |
| Vomiting | |

# CENTAURY (Erythraea centaurium)

*Parts used:* Entire plant
*Properties:* Alterative, aromatic, blood purifier, cholagogue, digestive, emmenagogue, febrifuge, stomachic

Centaury was used anciently to treat intermittent fevers, malaria, and infections from animal bites. Centaury is beneficial for recovery during a long illness because it promotes the appetite and strengthens the digestive system. It also purifies the blood, regulates the gallbladder, and is an excellent tonic. The herb strengthens the bladder of the elderly and helps prevent bed-wetting. Centaury is a preventive for all febrile diseases and helps after a fever. It is also recommended for rheumatism.

## PRIMARY APPLICATIONS

| | |
|---|---|
| Blood impurities | Fevers |
| Gastric disorders | Menstruation, absent |
| Urinary incontinence | |

## SECONDARY APPLICATIONS

| | |
|---|---|
| Bed-wetting | Blood pressure, high |
| Eczema | Gallbladder problems |
| Jaundice | Liver disorders |
| Rheumatism | Ulcers |
| Worms | Wounds |

# CHAMOMILE (Anthemis nobilis)

*Parts used:* Flower
*Properties:* Alterative, anodyne, antibacterial, anti-inflammatory, antineoplastic, antispasmodic, carminative, diaphoretic, febrifuge, nervine, sedative
*Primary nutrients:* Calcium, iron, magnesium, selenium, silicon, tryptophan, vitamins A, C, F, and B-complex, zinc

Chamomile is native to Europe and the Mediterranean regions. The early Egyptians used chamomile for its healing properties for ailments such as ague and malarial chills. The Romans used chamomile for its healing benefits in treating digestive problems and as a sedative. In the well-known story of Peter Rabbit, Peter's mother gave him chamomile tea to calm his nerves. The European countries have used chamomile for centuries for colic in infants and for vomiting because of its antispasmodic properties.

Chamomile is one of the best-known herbs around and is good to have on hand for emergencies. Its sedative qualities are helpful for nervousness and cramps. Chamomile tea is often used to help calm the nerves and reduce stress. A volatile oil compound in chamomile is thought to be responsible for its mild sedative effects. It is also known to be a safe and mild sedative to induce sleep.

One of the most common uses of chamomile is to aid digestion. Recent research has found chamomile to contain properties that aid digestion and relieve indigestion. It works by relaxing and calming the smooth muscle lining of the digestive tract. It actually works as an antispasmodic in relaxing the digestive tract. It is also effective for treating colitis, as well as being used externally for hair, skin, and inflammation. Chamomile contains a natural hormone similar to thyroxine that helps strengthen the hair and skin. Research done in Germany has also found anti-inflammatory properties in chamomile for skin ailments. It helped reduce redness, swelling, and inflammation. This may aid conditions such as burns, wounds, eczema, allergic reactions, and other skin problems. The anti-inflammatory and anti-allergic components are attributed to the flavonoids apigenin and luteolin found in chamomile.

Animal studies also show that chamomile has antihistaminic effects, as well as antiulcer and antibacterial properties. It can help cleanse the liver and promote natural hormones.

## PRIMARY APPLICATIONS

| | |
|---|---|
| Abscesses | Alcoholism |
| Appetite, loss | Bronchitis |
| Circulation, poor | Cramps, menstrual |
| Fevers | Flu |
| Insomnia | Menstruation |
| Muscle pain | Nervousness |

## SECONDARY APPLICATIONS

| | |
|---|---|
| Air pollution, effects of | Anxiety |
| Asthma | Childhood diseases |
| Colds | Colic |
| Colitis | Constipation |
| Coughs | Diarrhea |
| Edema | Drugs, withdrawal |
| Eye, sore | Gallstones |
| Gas | Headaches |
| Indigestion | Jaundice |
| Kidney problems | Measles |
| Mucus, excessive | Pain |
| Spasms | Stomach, upset |
| Teething | Throat, sore |

| | |
|---|---|
| Tumors | Typhoid fever |
| Ulcers, peptic | Urinary problems |

# CHAPARRAL
*(Larrea tridentata, L. divaricata)*

*Parts used:* Leaves and stems
*Properties:* Alterative, anodyne, antibiotic, anti-inflammatory, antineoplastic, antioxidant, antiseptic, bitter, blood purifier, diuretic, expectorant, parasiticide
*Primary nutrients:* Aluminum, barium, chlorine, potassium, protein, silicon, sodium, sulfur

Chaparral is a common shrub found in the desert regions of Mexico and the southwestern areas of the United States. Native Americans used chaparral as a remedy to treat conditions such as bronchitis, arthritis, colds, chicken pox, and stomach pain. In Mexico, chaparral has been used to treat cancer.

Chaparral is a potent healer and cleanser. It has the ability to cleanse deep in the muscle and tissue walls. It works on the urinary tract and lymphatic system as it tones and rebuilds tissue. Studies have found that chaparral works by influencing the body to inhibit unwanted rapid cell growth. It is a strong antioxidant, antitumor agent, painkiller, and antiseptic. It is one of the best herbal antibiotics. Chaparral is also thought to help rid the body of LSD residue to eliminate recurrent flashbacks.

Chaparral is thought to be a powerful antioxidant, able to fight free radicals to prevent damage that may lead to some degenerative diseases and aging. Some studies have found a longer life span in animals and insects given the NGDA (nordihydroguaiaretic acid) in chaparral. No human findings have been confirmed.

At one time, chaparral was thought to be effective in treating cancer. Early studies indicated beneficial results in vitro. Other studies have supported these findings. One study done using rats found that the NDGA found in chaparral was effective in inhibiting aerobic and anaerobic glycolysis and respiration in some types of cancer while not affecting the normal cells. Subsequent studies on cancer patients have not proven successful enough to recommend chaparral for the treatment of cancer. Numerous individuals have claimed success in treating cancer with the use of chaparral. Research is now focusing on the use of NDGA in preventing the formation of cancerous cells. Further research may lead to a more positive outlook on the use of this herb for cancer.

Chaparral was traditionally recommended for treating arthritis. Animal studies have found benefits from the plant's anti-inflammatory, anticarcinogenic, and analgesic properties.

Consult your health-care provider before using chaparral, due to its pontential for liver damage.

## PRIMARY APPLICATIONS

| | |
|---|---|
| Arthritis | Blood impurities |
| Leukemia | Tumors |

## SECONDARY APPLICATIONS

| | |
|---|---|
| Aches | Acne |
| Allergies | Backaches, chronic |
| Boils | Bruises |
| Bursitis | Cataracts |
| Colds | Cuts |
| Eczema | Eyes, weakened |
| Gastric disorders | Hemorrhoids |
| Intestinal problems | Kidney infection |
| Prostate problems | Psoriasis |
| Respiratory problems | Rheumatism |
| Uterus, prolapsed | Venereal diseases |
| Wounds | |

# CHASTE TREE *(Vitex agnus castus)*

*Parts used:* Fruit
*Properties:* Emmenagogue and menorrhagic

Chaste tree, also known as vitex, was used anciently and is mentioned in writings by Hippocrates, Dioscorides, and Theophrastus for a wide variety of ailments related to female health. The use of vitex spread throughout Europe, where it was used for similar conditions. The chaste tree is native to the Mediterranean region and Central Asia. It is a shrub with violet flowers. The dried fruit is the portion used for medicinal purposes.

Chaste tree has traditionally been used for many conditions involving the female reproductive and hormonal systems. It has been used to treat premenstrual syndrome, irregular bleeding, menopausal symptoms, swelling in the breasts, hormonal balance, heavy bleeding, and frequent periods. There is growing evidence as to the use of chaste tree for healing.

The whole fruit extract is used to treat these conditions. Several components are thought to be the active constituents. The activity is thought to center on the pituitary gland in the production of luteinizing hormone, which increases the amount of progesterone in a woman's body.

A common problem for some women approaching menopause is a decrease in the luteal phase. This is thought to be a result of low production of progesterone. There may be an abnormal ratio between estrogen and progesterone. Chaste tree helps balance the hormones estrogen and progesterone, helping to regulate a woman's cycle, including time in between menstruation, bleeding, and length of period.

One German study found beneficial results from the use of chaste tree extract in treating women with gynecological problems. One group of women suffering from PMS was treated with chaste tree liquid extract once a day. The treatment was rated as "good" or "very good" in 92 percent of the participants. Another German study had similar results with a decrease in symptoms such as swelling, tender breasts, irritability, anxiety, cravings, depression, and fatigue. Other studies have also found beneficial results from the use of chaste tree.

## PRIMARY APPLICATIONS

| | |
|---|---|
| Bleeding, excessive | Hormone balance |
| Infertility | Menstrual symptoms |

# CHICKWEED *(Stellaria media)*

*Parts used:* Entire herb
*Properties:* Alterative, anorectic, antineoplastic, blood purifier, demulcent, diuretic, emollient, expectorant, febrifuge, mucilant, nutritive, pectoral, stomachic
*Primary nutrients:* Calcium, copper, iron, manganese, phosphorus, sodium, vitamins C, D, and B-complex, zinc

Chickweed grows abundantly in areas of Europe and North America. The Ojibwe and Iroquois Native American tribes used chickweed as an eyewash and in poultice form to heal wounds. Recently, it has been studied for its abilities to help prevent cancer.

Chickweed is valuable for treating blood toxicity, fevers, and inflammation. Its mucilage elements are known to help with stomach ulcers and inflamed bowels. Chickweed can help dissolve plaque in blood vessels as well as other fatty substances in the body. It acts as an antibiotic in the blood and may be recommended as an anticancer treatment. Some have used chickweed to treat tumors.

It can be used as a poultice for boils, burns, skin diseases, sore eyes, and swollen testes. Chickweed is recommended to aid in weight loss and to break down cellulite. It is a mild herb and has been used as a food as well as medicine.

## PRIMARY APPLICATIONS

| | |
|---|---|
| Appetite, excessive | Bleeding |
| Blood impurities | Convulsions |
| Obesity | Rashes, skin |
| Ulcers | |

## SECONDARY APPLICATIONS

| | |
|---|---|
| Arteriosclerosis | Asthma |
| Bronchitis | Bruises |
| Bursitis | Colitis |
| Constipation | Cramps |
| Eye infections | Gas |
| Hemorrhoids | Lung congestion |
| Mucus, excessive | Pleurisy |
| Poisoning, blood | Testicles, swollen |
| Tissue, inflamed | Water retention |
| Wounds | |

# CHICORY (Cichorium intybus)

**Parts used:** Flowering plant and root
**Properties:** Alterative, anti-inflammatory, blood purifier, diuretic, purgative (mild)
**Primary nutrients:** Vitamins A, C, G, B, K, and P

Chicory originated in Europe, India, and Egypt. The ancient Romans used chicory as a blood purifier and as a food. Chicory was introduced to North America during the late nineteenth century by colonists. It is cultivated in Europe as an additive to coffee or a substitute. The leaves are also added to salads.

Chicory has many of the same constituents as the dandelion. A tea can help eliminate unwanted phlegm from the stomach and can help settle an upset stomach. Regular use of the tea is recommended for gallstones. Chicory is good for conditions caused by excess uric acid such as gout, rheumatics, and joint stiffness. It has also been used as a wash for boils and sores. The sap of the stems can be used to treat poison ivy and sunburns.

One study found that chicory has a mild sedative effect on the central nervous system and may help reduce the stimulating effect of coffee when the two are combined. The lactucin and related compounds in the chicory may be responsible for the sedative effects.

There is also evidence of chicory extract's ability to reduce cardiac rate similar to the drug quinidine. Extracts may be beneficial in treating conditions such as tachycardia, arrhythmias, and fibrillation. The active constituents were not identified, and more research may help to understand its effectiveness. Alcoholic extracts of chicory have been found to have anti-inflammatory activity.

## PRIMARY APPLICATIONS

| | |
|---|---|
| Blood impurities | Jaundice |
| Liver disorders | Phlegm |

## SECONDARY APPLICATIONS

| | |
|---|---|
| Anemia | Arteriosclerosis |
| Arthritis | Congestion |
| Gallstones | Gastric disorders |
| Glandular problems | Gout |
| Infertility | Inflammation |
| Kidney problems | Rheumatism |
| Spleen ailments | |

# CINCHONA *(Cinchona calisaya)*

*Parts used:* Bark
*Properties:* Alterative, antiperiodic, antiseptic, astringent, bitter, febrifuge, oxytocic, stomachic
*Primary nutrients:* Alkaloids (quinine and quinidine)

Colonists from Spain who came to the New World looked for valuable resources and medicinal herbs to send back to the motherland. Jesuit priests often cataloged their findings for the Roman Catholic Church. The cinchona tree was one of their findings. They noticed that the natives would chew the inner bark of the tree and remain free of malaria.

The bark of the cinchona tree is a valuable source of quinine. The drug quinidine was a result of the discovery of quinine. Quinidine is used to alleviate atrial fibrillation and other cardiac arrythmias.

The quinine in the bark contains an alkaloid that suppresses cell enzymes and acts as a disinfectant in cases of malaria and rheumatism. It is also an effective preventive for influenza. It is one of the best tonics for all febrile and typhoid conditions. It strengthens the stomach during convalescence and works on the entire central nervous system. The liquid extract is sometimes used to treat alcoholism.

## PRIMARY APPLICATIONS

| | |
|---|---|
| Fevers, intermittent | Jaundice |
| Malaria | Parasites |

## SECONDARY APPLICATIONS

| | |
|---|---|
| Edema | Flu, preventive |
| Heart palpitations | symptomsMeasles |
| Menstrual | Nervous disorders |
| Rheumatism | Tuberculosis, primary |
| Smallpox | Typhoid fever |

# CINNAMON *(Cinnamomum zeylanicum)*

*Parts used:* Dried bark
*Properties:* Alterative, analgesic, antibacterial, antifungal, antiseptic, astringent, carminative, diaphoretic, emmenagogue, febrifuge, sedative, stimulant, stomachic

*Primary nutrients:* cinnamic aldehyde, eugenol, metholeugenol, starch, sucrose, tannin

Cinnamon has been around for thousands of years and revered as a spice and healing agent. The ancient Egyptians included cinnamon in their embalming oils. It was used in China to treat fever, diarrhea, and menstrual symptoms as far back as 2000 BC. Cinnamon was a major trade commodity during ancient times. Originally, cinnamon grew in the southern regions of Asia.

Cinnamon is used to help relieve upset stomachs, reduce milk flow, stop excessive menstrual flow, and alleviate back pain. Research has found that cinnamon contains components with antifungal and antibacterial capabilities. It is found in some toothpastes, which would help kill some decay-causing bacteria.

Cinnamon is also helpful for promoting healthy blood sugar levels.

## PRIMARY APPLICATIONS

| | |
|---|---|
| Abdominal pain | Candida |
| Diarrhea | Gas |
| Gastric disorders | Indigestion |

## SECONDARY APPLICATIONS

| | |
|---|---|
| Arthritis | Asthma |
| Backaches | Bloating |
| Bronchitis | Cholera |
| Coronary problems | Fevers |
| Menstruation, excessive | Nausea |
| Nephritis | Parasites |
| Psoriasis | Rheumatism |
| Stomach, upset | Vomiting |
| Warts | |

# CLOVES *(Eugenia caryophyllata)*

*Parts used:* Seeds and flower buds
*Properties:* Alterative, analgesic, anodyne, anthelmintic, antibacterial, antiemetic, antifungal, antiseptic, aromatic, astringent, carminative, expectorant, germicide, rubefacient, stimulant, stomachic
*Primary nutrients:* Calcium, magnesium, phosphorus, potassium, sodium, vitamins A, B-complex, and Vitamin C

Cloves have been used for both medicinal and culinary purposes for thousands of years. They grow in warm climates and are cultivated in Tanzania, Sumatra, and South America. Cloves contain one of the most powerful germicidal agents in the herbal kingdom. A few drops of clove oil in water will stop vomiting, and clove tea will relieve nausea. The oil of cloves is also a diffusive stimulant and disinfectant.

Cloves can be used to relieve a toothache when dropped into a cavity and are frequently recommended as a remedy for bad breath. Cloves increase circulation of the blood and promote digestion.

Clove oil has been found to contain antihistaminic and spasmolytic properties. There is also evidence of the volatile oils in cloves containing antibacterial and antifungal properties to inhibit both gram-positive and negative bacteria and fungi. Dentists have used cloves to help relieve toothache and to disinfect root canals. They are found in some toothache remedies.

## PRIMARY APPLICATIONS

| | |
|---|---|
| Breath, odor | Catarrh, bronchial |
| Circulation, poor | Dizziness |
| Earache | Nausea |
| Toothaches | |

## SECONDARY APPLICATIONS

| | |
|---|---|
| Blood pressure, low | Colitis |
| Diarrhea | Dysentery |
| Epilepsy | Gas |
| Indigestion | Pain |
| Palsy | Spasms |
| Vomiting | Sex drive, inhibited |

# COLTSFOOT (Tussilago farfara)

*Parts used:* Flowers and leaves
*Properties:* Alterative, anti-inflammatory, antitussive, astringent, bitter, demulcent, diaphoretic, diuretic, emollient, expectorant, mucilant, pectoral
*Primary nutrients:* Calcium, copper, iron, manganese, potassium, vitamins A, B6, B12, C, and P, zinc

Coltsfoot is another herb that has been around for thousands of years. The ancient Greeks and Romans used coltsfoot for lung conditions. In China, it was used for respiratory disorders such as coughs, asthma, and bronchitis. Europeans also used the herb for lung conditions. The plant is native to Europe but now grows throughout the United States and Canada in sandy soil.

Coltsfoot is a remedy for coughs and other respiratory ailments. It has a calming effect on the throat as well as the brain's cough-activating mechanism. When combined with horehound and marshmallow, it is one of nature's best cough remedies. Coltsfoot contains a high percentage of mucilage and saponins, which have disinfectant and anti-inflammatory effects that ease respiratory problems.

Research on laboratory animals is beginning to confirm the healing benefits of coltsfoot for respiratory ailments. One study found that coltsfoot contains compounds known to help in cases of asthma and other inflammatory conditions. It may help by soothing the respiratory tract as well as increasing the movement of mucus out of the respiratory system.

## PRIMARY APPLICATIONS

| | |
|---|---|
| Asthma | Bronchitis |
| Coughs | Lung problems |
| Mucus, excessive | Whooping cough |

## SECONDARY APPLICATIONS

| | |
|---|---|
| Chills | Colds |
| Diarrhea | Emphysema |
| Hoarseness | Inflammation |
| Pleurisy | Pneumonia |
| Swelling | Tracheitis |
| Tuberculosis | |

# COMFREY (Symphytum officinale)

*Parts used:* Leaves and root
*Properties:* Alterative, anticatarrhal, antitussive, astringent, bitter, demulcent, emollient, expectorant, febrifuge, mucilant, nutritive, vulnerary
*Primary nutrients:* Eighteen amino acids (especially lysine), calcium, copper, iron, magnesium, phosphorus, potassium, protein, vitamins A and C, zinc

Comfrey was used by the Greeks and Romans for wound healing, respiratory ailments, to stop bleeding, and as a poultice to mend broken bones. Nicholas Culpeper, a seventeenth-century English herbalist, recommended comfrey for all wounds external and internal. The Cherokee tribe used the comfrey plant for many ailments.

Comfrey is one of the most valuable herbs known to man. It has been used with success for centuries as a wound healer and bone knitter. It feeds the pituitary with its natural hormone and helps to strengthen the skeletal system. It contributes to the calcium/phosphorus balance by promoting strong bones and healthy skin.

Comfrey helps promote the secretion of pepsin and is a general aid in digestion. It generally has a beneficial effect on all parts of the body. It is one of the finest healers of respiratory ailments and can be used both internally and externally for wounds, sores, and ulcers. It has been used with great success for hemorrhage, whether from the stomach, lungs, bowels, kidneys, or piles.

Comfrey is recommended for just about any part of the body that might be injured to promote rapid healing. It contains allantoin, which helps in stimulating new cell growth and increases cell production. It also helps reduce inflammation, which may aid in healing. In addition, comfrey is a good source of the amino acid lysine, usually lacking in diets that contain no animal protein. Consult a health-care practioner before taking comfrey internally due to the possibility of liver damage.

## PRIMARY APPLICATIONS

| | |
|---|---|
| Anemia | Arthritis |
| Blood impurities | Bones, broken |
| Boils | Bruises |
| Burns | Emphysema |
| Fractures | Lung disorders |
| Sprains | Swelling |

## SECONDARY APPLICATIONS

| | |
|---|---|
| Allergies/hay fever | Asthma |
| Bites, insect | Bleeding |
| Bronchitis | Bursitis |
| Cancer | Colds |
| Colitis | Coughs |
| Cramps, intestinal/leg | Diarrhea |

| | |
|---|---|
| Eczema | Fatigue |
| Gangrene | Gastric disorders |
| Gout | Infection |
| Kidney stones | Pain |
| Pleurisy | Pneumonia |
| Respiratory problems | Sinusitis |

# CORNFLOWER (Centaurea cyanus)

*Parts used:* Entire plant
*Properties:* Alterative, astringent, diuretic

Cornflower was used by the Plains Indians as an antidote for snakebites, insect bites, and stings, because it has properties useful for the nervous system.

The water distilled from cornflower petals has been used as a remedy for weak eyes. The dried powder can be used on bruises. Consumed in the form of wine, the seeds, leaves, or distilled water of the herbs are very good for fighting infectious diseases.

Cornflower is good for ulcers and sores in the mouth. It is also used as remedy for some forms of temporary paralysis. The herb is similar to blessed thistle in its healing benefits. The seeds in cornflower contain glycosides with strong antiseptic properties.

## PRIMARY APPLICATIONS

| | |
|---|---|
| Bites/stings, poisonous | Conjunctivitis |
| Eye disorders | Nervous disorders |
| Ulcers, corneal | |

## SECONDARY APPLICATIONS

| | |
|---|---|
| Dermatitis | Fevers |
| Indigestion | Infection |
| Mumps | Sight, weak |
| Toothaches | |

# CORNSILK (Stigmata maidis)

*Parts used:* Silk
*Properties:* Alterative, antilithic, antiseptic, cholagogue, diuretic, demulcent, lithotriptic, mucilant, stimulant (mild)
*Primary nutrients:* Silicon, PABA, vitamins K and B

Cornsilk was used by the Inca and is thought to have originated in Central America. It was used traditionally to treat urogenital infections. Cornsilk is used for bladder complaints because of its cleansing effect on the urea as it circulates. It is also valuable for the treatment of renal and cystic inflammation. Cornsilk helps with kidney problems, inflamed bladder, and prostate gland problems. It may be helpful for bed-wetting due to a inflamed bladder. It works to rid the body of morbid deposits using its antiseptic properties. Physicians have used cornsilk as a diuretic for conditions of cystitis.

## PRIMARY APPLICATIONS

| | |
|---|---|
| Heart conditions | Kidney problems |
| Urinary incontinence | Urinary problems |

## SECONDARY APPLICATIONS

| | |
|---|---|
| Arteriosclerosis | Bed-wetting |
| Blood pressure, high | Cholesterol, high |
| Cystic irritations | Gonorrhea |
| Obesity | Prostate problems |

# COUCH GRASS (Agropyron repens)

*Parts used:* Root
*Properties:* Alterative, antibiotic, antiphlogistic, blood purifier, demulcent, diaphoretic, diuretic, emollient, nephritic, pectoral
*Primary nutrients:* Calcium, magnesium, potassium, silicon, sodium, vitamins A, C, and B-complex

Native American tribes such as the Cherokee and Iroquois used couch grass to treat ailments such as a sore back, painful urination, and edema. Historically, it has been used for its beneficial effects on the urinary system.

Couch grass is most commonly used to treat conditions of the urinary tract. It has a soothing and diuretic influence that will increase the flow of the discharge of urine. It is especially useful for cystitis and the treatment of catarrhal diseases of the bladder. It has been known to help eliminate stones and gravel from the kidneys and bladder. Couch grass extracts are recommended for their antibiotic effects against a variety of bacteria and molds.

## PRIMARY APPLICATIONS

| | |
|---|---|
| Blood impurities | Catarrhal conditions |
| Cystitis | Jaundice |
| Kidney disorders | Rheumatism |

## SECONDARY APPLICATIONS

| | |
|---|---|
| Back pain, lower | Bright's disease |
| Bronchitis | Constipation |
| Eyes, weakened | Fevers |
| Gout | Kidney stones |
| Lung disorders | Prostate problems |
| Skin diseases | |

# CRAMP BARK (Viburnum opulus)

*Parts used:* Bark and berries
*Properties:* Alterative, antiabortive, antispasmodic, astringent, diuretic, emmenagogue, nervine, sedative
*Primary nutrients:* Calcium, magnesium, potassium, vitamins C and K

Cramp bark is considered a very valuable herb for its use as a female regulator and to relieve cramps during menstruation. Early American practitioners used cramp bark to relieve cramps, which is where it got its name. It has been recommended by herbalists to help with pregnancy, after-pains cramps, and especially for the nervous discomforts of pregnancy.

It is recognized as a uterine sedative and an antispasmodic to relax the uterus and ovaries. It has been used to treat women when threatening miscarriage due to nervous afflictions. It can be used to treat cramps anywhere in the body.

In Russia, the berries, fresh or dried, are used as a pulse regulator to treat high blood pressure, heart problems, coughs, colds, lung problems, kidney problems, and bleeding ulcers. Externally, a decoction of flowers has been used for eczema and other skin conditions.

## PRIMARY APPLICATIONS

| | |
|---|---|
| Asthma | Convulsions |
| Cramps, uterine/leg | Heart palpitations |
| Hypertension | Nervousness |
| Spasms | Urinary problems |

## SECONDARY APPLICATIONS

| | |
|---|---|
| Childbirth after-pains | Colic |
| Constipation | Dysentery |
| Epilepsy | Fainting |
| Gallstones | Gas |
| Jaundice | Lockjaw |
| Ovarian irritations | Rheumatism |

# CRANBERRY (*Vaccinium macrocarpon*)

*Parts used:* Fruit
*Properties:* Antibiotic, anti-inflammatory, diuretic
*Primary nutrients:* Iron, potassium, vitamins B and C

Cranberries are native to areas of Europe, North America, and Asia. In the United States, they are grown mainly in cool, northern areas of the coast in the Northwest and Northeast. Cranberries are grown commercially in Massachusetts, New Jersey, Washington, Wisconsin, and Oregon. American sailors during the nineteenth century stored cranberries on their ships to prevent scurvy, which is caused by a lack of vitamin C.

Researchers in Germany began studying the medicinal properties of cranberries around 1840. They noticed a correlation between a lower incidence of urinary tract infections and the European cranberry. Those individuals who consumed cranberries had hippuric acid in their urine. The speculation was that the increased acidity prevented infections.

The fruit and juice of the cranberry are mainly used to treat bladder and urinary tract infections. The primary bacteria associated with urinary tract infections is *E. coli*, which prefers an alkaline environment in which to grow. Studies have found that certain properties of cranberries make urine more acidic, and this reduces the likelihood of bacteria adhering to the lining of the urinary tract.

The usual course of action when treating urinary infections is antibiotics. This treatment is often not productive, especially for those individuals who suffer from recurrent infections. Antibiotics may solve the problem temporarily, but they can cause other difficulties such as vaginal yeast infections.

One study involved giving patients with active urinary tract infections sixteen ounces of cranberry juice per day. Beneficial effects were seen in 73 percent of the subjects. Another study published in the *Journal of the American Medical Association*, March 9, 1994, found beneficial effects in using cranberry juice to control urinary tract infections. The cranberry-drinking group were found to be 58 percent less likely to have the bacteria known to cause the infections in their urine. The study found beneficial results in older women from the cranberry drink in preventing urinary tract infections.

Studies done at Weber State University in Utah have found substances in cranberries that can inhibit the adherence of *E. coli* bacteria to the bladder wall. This activity is similar to Tamms-Horsfall glycoprotein, which is a compound known to surround the *E. coli* and prevent it from attaching to the bladder wall. Individuals who have high levels of this glycoprotein are less likely to suffer from UTIs.

## PRIMARY APPLICATIONS

| | |
|---|---|
| Cystitis | Kidney problems |
| Urinary problems | |

## SECONDARY APPLICATIONS

| | |
|---|---|
| Bed-wetting | Colds |
| Urinary incontinence | |

# CULVER (*Veronicastrum virginicum*)

*Parts used:* Root
*Properties:* Alterative, bitter, blood purifier, cholagogue, emetic, hepatic, purgative (mild)
*Primary nutrients:* Magnesium, potassium

Culver's root was used by Native Americans and introduced to the colonists as they settled in the New World. A Dr. Culver first introduced the root to the colonists, so it was named Culver's root.

Culver's root has a gentle, relaxing effect on the liver. It is also considered an alterative for the stomach and indigestion. It helps with intestinal indigestion, purifies the blood, and removes catarrhal obstructions and congestion in a mild, natural way. It helps relieve constipation and improve bowel function, especially if due to poor biliary flow. It helps clean old debris from the bowels. Culver's root should be taken with an herb such as fennel to help expel gas. It is recommended that Culver's root be used in its dried state because the fresh root may be too harsh.

## PRIMARY APPLICATIONS

| | |
|---|---|
| Blood impurities | Diarrhea |
| Gastric disorders | Liver disorders |

## SECONDARY APPLICATIONS

| | |
|---|---|
| Fevers | Poisoning, food |
| Syphilis | |

# DAMIANA *(Turnera aphrodisiaca)*

*Parts used:* Leaves
*Properties:* Alterative, aphrodisiac, diuretic, nervine, stimulant, purgative (gentle)
*Primary nutrients:* Calcium, potassium, protein, selenium, sodium, vitamins A, C, and B-complex, zinc

Native Americans of northern Mexico used damiana for nervous and muscular weaknesses. The ancient Mayans used this herb as an aphrodisiac, for lung conditions and dizziness, and as a body cleaner. Damiana was introduced in the United States in 1874 by a druggist in Washington, D.C. It was promoted as a powerful aphrodisiac. It has been used as an alterative for the nervous system and sexual dysfunction.

Traditional uses of damiana include nervousness, fatigue, hormone balance, female disorders, and increasing sexual function. It is used most often for treating female disorders such as problems with menopause and strengthening the reproductive organs. It has been found to help with infertility in both males and females, by strengthening the egg in the female and increasing the sperm count in the male. Damiana helps to revitalize the body when in a state of exhaustion. It can also be found in some cough formulas and is used to treat colds and flu and to stimulate the central nervous system. It is also a great alterative for the brain.

Studies have concluded that damiana has a beneficial effect on sexual debility and nervous tension.

The leaves contain beta-sitosterol and some aromatic oils that may be responsible for the stimulant effect and the building of the sexual and reproductive systems. Damiana strengthens the nerves and brain. It is also used for chronic fatigue and exhaustion, both mental and physical. It is excellent when used in formulas with herbs such as ginseng, suma, sarsaparilla, and saw palmetto.

## PRIMARY APPLICATIONS

| | |
|---|---|
| Aphrodisiac | Bronchitis |
| Emphysema | Frigidity |
| Hormone imbalance | Hot flashes |
| Menopausal symptoms | Parkinson's disease |
| PMS | |

## SECONDARY APPLICATIONS

| | |
|---|---|
| Asthma | Constipation |
| Cough | Depression |
| Exhaustion | Headaches |
| Nervousness | Prostate problems |
| Sex drive, low | |

# DANDELION *(Taraxacum officinale)*

*Parts used:* Leaves and roots
*Properties:* Alterative, antacid, blood purifier, cholagogue, diuretic, hepatic, lithotriptic, purgative (mild), stomachic
*Primary nutrients:* Fructose (roots), glucose (roots), magnesium, manganese, nutritive salts (all), phosphorus, potassium, selenium, vitamins A, B-complex, and C, zinc

This herb has a long history of use, although some consider the dandelion to be a pesky weed. The dandelion is native to Greece and thrives, as many of us know, under just about any conditions. It is considered a great survival food because of its protein, vitamin, and mineral content. Europeans have used dandelion for at least five hundred years to treat fevers, diarrhea, fluid retention, liver congestion, and skin ailments. The Chinese began mentioning dandelion around the seventh century to treat breast problems, liver disease, and digestion. Arabian physicians described it under the name of

Tarakhshagun around the tenth century.

The dandelion is a great herb for building the blood and helping with anemia. It promotes circulation, strengthens the arteries, restores gastric juices after severe vomiting, and reduces cholesterol levels. Dandelion is also used as a diuretic and for diabetes. It has the ability to cleanse obstructions and stimulate the liver to detoxify poisons. The juice from the stem can be applied and allowed to dry to treat warts.

Modern research has proven the efficacy of dandelion. Studies on humans and laboratory animals have shown that the rhizomes and roots increase the flow of bile, which is beneficial for liver disorders, hepatitis, bile duct inflammation, gallstones, jaundice, and the bile duct. Dandelion works to increase bile production in the liver, which in turn increases the flow to the gallbladder, as well as contracting and releasing stored bile in the gallbladder.

In Germany, where herbal medicines are much more mainstream than in the United States, dandelion is often prescribed by physicians to increase bile flow and prevent gallstones. It can help with arthritis, as it stimulates the uric acid elimination from the body. It helps nourish and cleanse the blood, liver, and spleen. It is also useful for treating anemia, because it contains many nutrients. Dandelion is used to heal connective tissue and stop degeneration. Another study using mice and rats found that dandelion greens contain diuretic effects much greater than other herbal diuretics. There was also a marked weight loss, probably due to water loss. Dandelion is thought to have cancer- and infection-fighting potential.

## PRIMARY APPLICATIONS

| | |
|---|---|
| Acne | Anemia |
| Arthritis | Asthma |
| Blisters | Blood impurities |
| Blood pressure, high | Cholesterol, high |
| Fatigue | Gallbladder problems |
| Hepatitis | Jaundice |
| Kidney problems | Liver disorders |
| PMS | Weight conditions |

## SECONDARY APPLICATIONS

| | |
|---|---|
| Age spots | Bronchitis |
| Constipation | Corns |
| Cramps, intestinal | Dermatitis |
| Diabetes | Eczema |
| Fever | Gas |
| Gastric disorders | Gout |
| Hemorrhage | Indigestion |
| Infections | Metabolism, slow |
| Pancreas | Psoriasis |
| Rheumatism | Skin conditions |
| Spleen ailments | Ulcers |
| Warts | |

# DEVIL'S CLAW
*(Harpagophytum procumbens)*

*Parts used:* Leaves and roots
*Properties:* Alterative, anti-inflammatory, antilithic, antirheumatic, blood purifier, diuretic, lithotriptic, stimulant
*Primary nutrients:* Calcium, iron, magnesium, manganese, phosphorus, potassium, protein, selenium, silicon, sodium, vitamins A and C, zinc

For centuries, devil's claw has been used in Africa to treat various ailments without any harmful side effects. It has been used to help with joint pain, liver ailments, kidney disorders, arthritis, rheumatism, hardening of the arteries, and stomach problems.

Devil's claw has traditionally been used for arthritis, rheumatism, diabetes, arteriosclerosis, liver disorders, and kidney and bladder problems. It is considered to be a great cleanser for removing impurities. Regular use may help to improve hardened vascular walls. Even a healthy individual may benefit from using devil's claw once a year to cleanse the body of impurities.

Research has indicated that devil's claw may help relieve gout and joint pain. A German study found that the plant has anti-inflammatory properties comparable to the anti-arthritic phenylbutazine. It is highly regarded in some European countries as a treatment for inflammatory conditions such as arthritis and gout. Another study showed that devil's claw taken as a tea may be beneficial in lowering cholesterol and fat levels.

## PRIMARY APPLICATIONS

| | |
|---|---|
| Arteriosclerosis | Arthritis |

Blood impurities
Diabetes
Headaches
Kidney problems
Pollution, effects of
Urinary problems

Cholesterol, high
Gastric disorders
Inflammation
Liver disorders
Rheumatism

## SECONDARY APPLICATIONS

Gallbladder problems
Gout

Gallstones
Malaria

# DONG QUAI *(Angelica sinensis)*

*Parts used:* Root
*Properties:* Alterative, antibacterial, antineoplastic, antispasmodic, blood purifier, estrogenic, hypotensive, immunostimulant, purgative (mild), sedative
*Primary nutrients:* Essential minerals (all), iron, magnesium, manganese, nicotinic acid, phosphorus, potassium, silicon, sodium, vitamins A, B12, B-complex, C, and E, zinc

Dong quai has been used by the Chinese since the beginning of time and was recorded in the Herbal of ShenNung. It was regarded highly throughout Asia for menstrual cramps, irregular periods, and other gynecological problems. It was used as an alterative for all female problems. Dong quai, also known as angelica, is native to China.

Dong quai has been used extensively for its ability to help with female disorders. It has been called the "queen of female herbs." It contains constituents for nourishing the female glands and strengthening all internal body organs and muscles. It has been used to help with irregular menses, lack of menses, painful menses, and abnormal menses. It is also used to help during pregnancy to nourish the fetus in the womb. It has a tranquilizing effect on the central nervous system and nourishes the blood and brain cells. It helps dissolve blood clots and increases circulation.

Modern scientific research has shown that this herb is able to stimulate as well as inhibit uterine muscles. Dong quai is attributed with being able to increase energy and strengthen the system while creating a sense of well-being. It is used for all

female complaints, including PMS, menopausal symptoms, cramps, backaches due to menstrual cramps, and hot flashes.

It has also been used to improve digestion and assimilation, strengthen the nervous system, aid in stroke recovery, purify the blood, dissolve blood clots, improve circulation, stimulate production of interferon, and boost the immune system. The coumarin compounds found in dong quai have been shown to stimulate white cell function and enhance immune system function. Clinical research has proven dong quai to exhibit antitumor, antifungal, immunostimulant, and antibacterial properties. It contains antibacterial activity against both gram-negative and gram-positive bacteria. Dong quai has been proven to contain estrogenic activity, which is responsible for female characteristics. Dong quai also possesses properties that have a dilating effect on blood vessels. This may help in treating conditions such as hypertension and angina. Many herbalists use dong quai as a brain nourisher.

## PRIMARY APPLICATIONS

Anemia
Blood impurities
Glandular problems
Menopausal symptoms
Nervousness
Uterine problems

Bleeding, internal
Childbirth pain
Hot flashes
Menstrual symptoms
Spasms, muscle

## SECONDARY APPLICATIONS

Angina
Arteriosclerosis
Bruises
Cramps, uterine
Gastric disorders
Hypertension
Insomnia
Lung disorders
Pain
Skin conditions

Arthritis pain
Back pain, lower
Chills
Diabetes
Headaches
Hypoglycemia
Pain, abdominal
Metabolism, slow
Plague
Tumors

# ECHINACEA *(Echinacea purpurea)*

*Parts used:* Root, flowers, and leaves
*Properties:* Adaptogen, alterative, antibiotic, anti-

neoplastic, antiseptic, antiviral, blood purifier, carminative, demulcent, digestive, sialagogue, stimulant, vulnerary

*Primary nutrients:* Calcium, iodine, iron, potassium, sulfur, vitamins A, C, and E

Echinacea was used by Native Americans for toothaches, snakebites, insect stings, and infections. Some individual tribes used echinacea for headaches, swollen glands, and stomach cramps. It was highly regarded and used more than any other herb for illness and injury. The early colonists were very interested in herbs such as echinacea for their use in healing and relied on the natives to learn of the medicinal plants. Dr. John King mentioned the benefits as a blood purifier and alterative in his medical journal in 1887. Echinacea lost favor during the early twentieth century, but this herb was rediscovered around 1980 and is very popular for treating colds and flu.

Echinacea is used for many different ailments. It is used as a blood purifier against strep and staph infections. It is known to fight chemical toxic poisoning in the body. It has been used as a treatment for candida yeast infections and also has the ability to kill fungus. It is beneficial for blood poisoning, ulcers, tuberculosis, pyorrhea, childhood diseases, spinal meningitis, and gangrene. Echinacea is probably the best-known herbal immune booster. It has been found to help with many immune functions. Research is ongoing as to the immune-strengthening effects of echinacea. It has the ability to affect many different immune functions.

Echinacea is known to stabilize the white blood cell count in the body. It contains antiviral properties that are known to increase the activity of the leukocytes (white blood cells), allowing them to do their job of fighting and destroying toxic organisms that invade the body. It also is known to increase the red blood cell counts, which help remove waste from the body. It contains antiseptic properties, helping cleanse and reduce pain with external and internal injuries.

Hundreds of studies have been done to examine the healing abilities and benefits of echinacea. Extracts of echinacea root have been found to help stimulate the production of interferon and other immune activators. They have been found in numerous studies to help enhance the immune response.

One of the greatest benefits of echinacea may be its ability to help prevent and shorten the duration of the common cold and flu. Most everyone is plagued with a bout of the flu or a cold during the winter months, but maybe these bouts can be prevented, or at least lessened in severity. One study found that when participants taking echinacea extract did become infected, they recovered more quickly and their symptoms were less severe than the placebo group.

Another favorable use for echinacea may be in the treatment of some forms of cancer and tumors. Along with its ability to improve immune function, echinacea may help stimulate macrophages to fight tumor cells. Studies have found some anticancer activity in echinacea in animal studies. Research has also found echinacea to be effective in fighting tumor and infectious disease. Cancer patients undergoing radiation treatments generally suffer from a reduced white blood cell count. Echinacea may help to increase the white blood cells for these individuals.

## PRIMARY APPLICATIONS

| | |
|---|---|
| Acne | Blood impurities |
| Boils | Ear infection |
| Glandular problems | Immune system, weak |
| Infection | Lymphatic problems |
| Mouth sores | Mucus, excessive |
| Peritonitis | Poisoning, blood |
| Prostate problems | Skin disorders |
| Wounds | |

## SECONDARY APPLICATIONS

| | |
|---|---|
| Bites | Bronchitis |
| Cancer | Diphtheria |
| Eczema | Fevers |
| Flu | Gangrene |
| Gastric disorders | Gingivitis |
| Hemorrhages | Laryngitis |
| Pyorrhea | Strep throat |
| Syphilis | Throat, sore |
| Typhoid fever | Tonsillitis |

# ELDERBERRY *(Sambucus nigra)*

*Parts used:* Berries
*Properties:* Diaphoretic, diuretic, hydragogue, laxative, purgative
*Primary nutrients:* Calcium, iron, phosphorus, vitamins C, B1, B2, B6

Elderberry grows in Europe, West and Central Asia, and North Africa. The tree can reach thirty feet in height. It has small, yellowish-white flowers that bloom in May and June, and blue-black berries that grow in clusters and ripen in autumn.

For more than twenty-five hundred years, black elderberry has been used to treat influenza, coughs, and colds. Elderberry juice is said to trigger the body's powers of resistance, aiding the restoration and maintenance of good health. Practitioners of folk medicine have long valued elderberry for its benefits as a diaphoretic, diuretic, hydragogue, laxative, purgative, and gargle. It has been used to treat colds, epilepsy, gout, headache, influenza, jaundice, palsy, rheumatism, scrofula, skin eruptions, and syphilis.

A few studies in the 1980s produced persuasive evidence for elderberries' usefulness against influenza viruses. Two active components were isolated from elderberry proteins. Both compounds fight various strains of influenza by destroying the virus's ability to reproduce itself. In one study, a syrup was made from elderberry extract, and a double-blind trial was performed on patients infected with influenza during an outbreak in southern Israel. In the patients who received the elderberry syrup, 20 percent had significant improvement in symptoms within twenty-four hours. In forty-eight hours, 75 percent were much improved, and in seventy-two hours, 90 percent were completely cured. The placebo group took at least six days before any significant improvement was seen. The patients receiving elderberry extract had more antibodies than those given the placebo, indicating their immune function had been enhanced.

## PRIMARY APPLICATIONS

| | |
|---|---|
| Colds | Epilepsy |
| Gout | Headache |
| Influenza | Jaundice |
| Palsy | Rheumatism |
| Scrofula | Skin eruptions |
| Syphilis | |

# ELDER FLOWER *(Sambucus nigra)*

*Parts used:* Flower
*Properties:* Alterative, anti-inflammatory, diaphoretic, expectorant, febrifuge, purgative (mild), stimulant
*Primary nutrients:* Vitamins A and C with bioflavonoids

Elder flower has been used for hundreds of years for medicinal purposes as well as a flavoring. In *Anatomy of the Elder*, written in 1644, the elder flower is listed as a valuable plant for seventy different classes of diseases, including rheumatism. Native Americans used this herb as a drink for rheumatism, neuralgia, sciatica, and back pain. Dr. Edward Shook considered elder flower to be one of the greatest and most versatile herbs in the treatment of disease. Elder flower was found in the U.S. Pharmacopoeia from 1831 to 1905.

Elder flower has been used to reduce a fever by increasing blood circulation and promoting sweating. It is used for detoxifying the body at the cellular level. It also contains constituents known to act as a sedative and relieve pain. This herb works as an expectorant to relieve mucus and to reduce inflammation. It is used in herbal formulas. When combined with goldenseal and yarrow, it is known to speed healing. It is combined with mullein to help heal lung congestion and asthma. It is also used as an eyewash along with eyebright and goldenseal.

Research has found the properties of elder flower to be useful for acute diseases. It is beneficial in the treatment of colds, flu, tonsillitis, laryngitis, rheumatic fever, and hay fever. Research on animals indicates a moderate anti-inflammatory activity in elder flower. The flavonols in the flower may also work as a diuretic to relieve water retention. Some of the compounds found in the elder flower were found to aid in protecting the liver from damage experimentally induced in animals.

## PRIMARY APPLICATIONS

| | |
|---|---|
| Allergies/hay fever | Asthma |
| Bronchitis | Colds |
| Congestion, sinus | Fevers |
| Pneumonia | |

## SECONDARY APPLICATIONS

| | |
|---|---|
| Cancer | Ear infections |
| Eye infections | Flu |
| Gas | Gastric disorders |
| Hemorrhoids | Inflammation |
| Inflammation, brain | Joints, swollen |
| Nervousness | Skin diseases |
| Ulcers | Wounds |

# ELECAMPANE *(Inula helenium)*

*Parts used:* Root
*Properties:* Alterative, antiasthmatic, antibacterial, anticatarrhal, antiseptic, astringent, diaphoretic, diuretic, expectorant, stimulant
*Primary nutrients:* Calcium, magnesium, potassium, sodium

Hippocrates stated that this herb was a stimulant to the uterus, kidneys, stomach, and brain. Elecampane was used by the Romans and Greeks to help with digestion, chest complaints, and many other ailments. Native Americans used the plant for bronchial and lung ailments. The dried root was official in the U.S. Pharmacopoeia and listed as being beneficial for the respiratory organs, skin disease, digestion, and liver problems. Dr. Edward Shook suggested using elecampane for lung diseases such as catarrhal infections, tuberculosis, coughs, asthma, and to dissolve phlegm.

Traditionally, elecampane has been used to treat chest congestion and bronchial coughs. It helps expel mucus and control excessive coughing and chest congestion. It aids in controlling inflammation in the respiratory tract and soothes the tissues. Herbalists now generally recommend elecampane for respiratory ailments. It also contains antiseptic and antibacterial properties. Elecampane has also been used to treat intestinal worms, edema, digestive problems, skin problems, tooth decay, and gum

disorders. It is often found in combination with other herbs.

Scientific research has found in clinical experiments that the extract of elecampane contains a powerful antiseptic and bactericide that is particularly effective against tuberculosis. Dr. Shook's studies had the same results. It has also been proven to be effective in lung problems, digestion, and liver disorders. Noted early herbalist and vegan Jethro Kloss found it useful for coughs, asthma, and bronchitis. It seems to strengthen, cleanse, and tone the mucous membranes of the lungs and stomach. European studies have found that elecampane contains properties to help expel worms and parasites from the body.

## PRIMARY APPLICATIONS

| | |
|---|---|
| Bronchitis, chronic | Convulsions |
| Coughs | Emphysema |
| Lung ailments | |

## SECONDARY APPLICATIONS

| | |
|---|---|
| Appetite, loss | Asthma |
| Catarrh, bladder | Colic |
| Consumption | Cramps |
| Diarrhea | Gastric disorders |
| Menstrual symptoms | Mucus, excessive |
| Phlegm | Poison |
| Tuberculosis | Urinary problems |
| Whooping cough | Worms |

# EPHEDRA *(Ephedra sinensis)*

*Parts used:* Entire herb
*Properties:* Anorectic, antiasthmatic, anticatarrhal, astringent, blood purifier, decongestant, diaphoretic, expectorant, stimulant
*Primary nutrients:* Iron, potassium, selenium, silicon, sodium, vitamins A, C, and B-complex

The Chinese have used ephedra, known as ma huang, for thousands of years in formulas used to treat acute diseases such as colds, flu, bronchitis, and pneumonia. Native Americans used the milder American species for its healthful properties to treat various ailments.

Ephedra contains properties similar to adrenaline, though it's much less potent. It helps increase energy and boost circulation. More oxygen is supplied to muscle tissue to increase performance. It stimulates the nervous system and acts directly on muscle cells. It is a bronchial dilator and decongestant. Ephedra is beneficial for relieving congestion, asthma, and some allergies. Ma huang (ephedra) is used in China as an excellent energy booster to replace caffeine.

Some of the alkaloids found in ephedra are effective in treating mild to moderate asthma and hay fever. Ephedrine, a component of ephedra, is found in many over-the-counter cold and allergy medications. Ephedra is often used as a bronchiodilating agent that helps relieve congestion from colds, flu, bronchitis, and asthma. It is an excellent treatment for chronic and acute asthma.

Recent studies with humans and laboratory animals have shown ephedrine to be beneficial in promoting weight loss. Although ephedrine has an appetite-suppressing effect, its main mechanism for promoting weight loss appears to be found in its thermogenic abilities to increase the metabolic rate of brown adipose tissue and to enhance the body's ability to burn fat. Its weight-reducing effects are greatest in those who have a low basal metabolic rate. One study using ephedrine helped with weight loss with a 14 percent reduction in body weight and a 42 percent loss of body fat. Complementary herbs combined with ephedrine may enhance the weight-loss process. Caffeine is sometimes found in herbal weight-loss combinations along with ephedra. Studies have found that more weight loss occurs with the combination. Ephedra may increase blood pressure and heart rate. For this reason, it is not recommended for individuals with heart disease or hypertension. Also, people taking monoamine oxidase inhibitors (MAOIs) should totally avoid all ephedra products.

## PRIMARY APPLICATIONS

| | |
|---|---|
| Asthma | Blood impurities |
| Bronchitis | Bursitis |
| Colds | Hay fever |
| Headaches | Kidney problems |
| Sinus problems | Venereal diseases |

## SECONDARY APPLICATIONS

| | |
|---|---|
| Arthritis | Bleeding, internal |
| Depression | Diphtheria |
| Drugs, overdose | Fever |
| Menstrual symptoms | Muscle problems |
| Nosebleeds | Pain |
| Pneumonia | Skin disorders |

# EUCALYPTUS *(Eucalyptus globulus)*

*Parts used:* Oil from leaves, roots, and bark
*Properties:* Antibacterial, anti-inflammatory, antiperiodic, antiseptic, antispasmodic, astringent, deodorant, expectorant, germicide, rubefacient, stimulant
*Primary nutrients:* Aldehyde, bitter resin, eucalyptol, tannins

With more than five hundred different species, the eucalyptus plant, which grows abundantly on the Australian continent, has a rich history of use. The roots of the eucalyptus tree hold large amounts of water, so the aborigines and early settlers used this as a water source during the dry season in the outback. In fact, it was the Australian aborigines who first discovered the medicinal value of eucalyptus oil.

Eucalyptus has potent antiseptic properties. Oil extracted from the leaves works to prevent infection and is helpful against poisonous germs. It is recommended by herbalists to treat skin ailments. It is a germicide with antiseptic and astringent properties. Eucalyptus oil has various abilities. It can be sniffed to clear sinus congestion, mixed with water to make an insect repellent, and a small drop on the tongue can help relieve nausea. Eucalyptus is often used to treat respiratory ailments. A few drops can be added to a humidifier to relieve symptoms of bronchitis, asthma, croup, and chest congestion. The oil can also be rubbed on the back or chest to relieve lung congestion. Eucalyptus oil is also used externally as a deodorant. Because of eucalyptus oil's high concentration, it should be mixed with a carrier oil when used either externally or internally.

The leaves of the eucalyptus contain eucalyptol, which has been studied for its healing value. One Russian study involving laboratory animals found eucalyptol effective in killing influenza and some bacteria. The antibacterial properties may help prevent infection from occurring when applied to wounds.

**PRIMARY APPLICATIONS**

| | |
|---|---|
| Bronchitis | Lung disorders |
| Neuralgia | Sores, external |

**SECONDARY APPLICATIONS**

| | |
|---|---|
| Asthma | Boils, external |
| Burns | Cancer |
| Croup | Diphtheria |
| Fever | Indigestion |
| Malaria | Mucus, excessive |
| Nausea | Paralysis |
| Pyorrhea | Throat, sore |
| Typhoid fever | Ulcers, external |
| Uterus, prolapsed | Worms |
| Wounds | |

# EVENING PRIMROSE
*(Oenothera biennis)*

*Parts used:* Bark, leaves, and oil
*Properties:* Astringent and sedative
*Primary nutrients:* GLA (gamma-linolenic acid), magnesium, potassium

Native Americans in North America used evening primrose oil for healing. The Iroquois, Cherokee, and Ojibwe tribes all used this herb for various conditions such as hemorrhoids, weight loss, and bruises. The European settlers learned from the natives and applied a poultice of the fresh herb to wounds and used a tea of the root and leaf for an upset stomach.

Evening primrose stimulates the liver, spleen, and digestive system. It reduces alimentary toxins that result from a faulty diet and adversely affect the central nervous system. Evening primrose slows down the speed at which cholesterol is made in the body and has been found effective in lowering cholesterol levels, inhibiting the formation of clots, and lowering blood pressure in individuals with mild to moderate hypertension. It also works to open blood vessels and relieve pain from angina. Evening primrose oil prevents inflammation and can help control arthritis pain. It has been used in Europe to treat multiple sclerosis.

Research in Britain has concluded that evening primrose oil may help in treating PMS, mastalgia, multiple sclerosis, atopic eczema, some diabetes conditions, and cardiovascular disease. Some women who suffer from PMS have lower levels of GLA, gamma-linolenic acid. Evening primrose oil may help by adding GLA to the body, which may offer relief from mood swings, headaches, sore breasts, and other symptoms of PMS.

Evening primrose oil has been approved for use internally and externally for eczema in England. Beneficial results were seen in a double-blind study involving the use of evening primrose oil to treat eczema. Some research suggests the use of the oil for multiple sclerosis. It may aid in stabilizing the condition, slowing progression, and offering relief. R. H. S. Thompson, a British scientist, found in his research that MS patients had low levels of linoleic acid in their systems. Other research suggests that it may also be beneficial for diabetics and individuals suffering from rheumatoid arthritis.

**PRIMARY APPLICATIONS**

| | |
|---|---|
| Blood pressure, high | Nervous problems |
| Obesity | Prostate problems |
| Rheumatoid arthritis | Skin disorders |

**SECONDARY APPLICATIONS**

| | |
|---|---|
| Alcoholism | Allergies |
| Cancer | Colds |
| Cramps, uterine | Depression |
| Gastric disorders | Glaucoma |
| Headaches | Hyperactivity, children |
| Intestinal problems | Migraines |
| Obesity | Skin irritations |
| Ulcers | |

# EYEBRIGHT *(Euphrasia officinalis)*

*Parts used:* Entire plant
*Properties:* Alterative, anti-inflammatory, antiseptic, astringent, bitter, stimulant (liver)
*Primary nutrients:* Copper, iodine, iron, silicon, vitamins A, B, B-complex, C, D, and E, zinc

The white petals of the eyebright have a red or purple tinge that may resemble bloodshot eyes. This appearance is thought to be the reason for the use of eyebright in treating eye irritations since the Middle Ages. Theophrastus and Dioscorides both prescribed topical applications for eye infections.

Eyebright has been the herb of choice for treating eye irritations for centuries. It is beneficial for conditions involving the mucous membranes. As an eyewash, it can help relieve eye irritations or eyestrain. Antiseptic properties help fight eye infections. Traditional uses include eye problems such as failing vision, eye inflammation, eye ulcers, conjunctivitis, and eyestrain. Eyebright will strengthen all parts of the eye and provide an elasticity to the nerves and optic devices responsible for sight. Eyebright is also stimulating to the liver to help in cleansing the blood.

While numerous herbalists have recommended the use of eyebright for conditions of the eye, no research is available to substantiate the claims.

## PRIMARY APPLICATIONS

| | |
|---|---|
| Blood impurities | Cataracts |
| Colds | Conjunctivitis |
| Eye disorders/infections | Eyestrain |
| Glaucoma | |

## SECONDARY APPLICATIONS

| | |
|---|---|
| Black eyes (compress) | Congestion, sinus |
| Coughs | Hay fever |
| Headaches | Hoarseness |
| Memory loss | Sties |

# FALSE UNICORN
(*Chamailirum luteum*)

*Parts used:* Root
*Properties:* Alterative (stimulating), anthelmintic, aphrodisiac, diuretic, emetic (large doses), estrogenic, stimulant
*Primary nutrients:* Cadmium, cobalt, copper, molybdenum, sulfur, vitamin C, zinc

False unicorn was widely used by Native Americans for all female disorders. Women chewed the root of the plant to prevent miscarriage. The tea was used as an alterative and anthelmintic by some early physicians. Midwives have relied on the use of false unicorn to prevent miscarriage. It was used for infertility problems.

It has been used for both male and female problems associated with infertility. Sterility may be a problem, and one cause may be unhealthy membranes in the uterus unable to support a growing fetus. False unicorn can help restore health and muscle tone to the uterus. It can be used as a general tonic for strengthening the uterus and female reproductive system. It is used for menopausal symptoms because of its effect on the uterus, headaches, and depression. False unicorn may help with male impotency and prostate problems. It is also recommended as an overall tonic. It seems to help strengthen the mucous membranes and aids a sensitive stomach. It is also a strong antiseptic, useful for getting rid of intestinal worms and parasites, and promotes urine discharge.

Scientific research has shown that the steroidal saponins have a normalizing effect on the ovaries. False unicorn has been shown to have estrogenic activity and to help with female complaints.

## PRIMARY APPLICATIONS

| | |
|---|---|
| Colic | Coughs |
| Kidney problems | Menopausal symptoms |
| Miscarriage, tendency | Prostate problems |
| Uterine problems | |

## SECONDARY APPLICATIONS

| | |
|---|---|
| Appetite loss | Bright's disease |
| Depression | Edema |
| Gastric disorders | Headaches |
| Nausea | Parasites |
| Sterility | Urinary incontinence |

# FENNEL (*Foeniculum vulgare*)

*Parts used:* Seeds
*Properties:* Anorectic, antacid, anti-inflammatory, antimicrobial, antispasmodic, carminative, diuretic, estrogenic, expectorant, galactagogue, sedative (children), stimulant
*Primary nutrients:* Calcium, magnesium, niacin, potassium, sodium, sulfur, vitamins A, C, B1, and B2

Fennel is native to southern areas of Europe and Asia Minor. It is now cultivated in the United States and Great Britain. It was used anciently in many civilizations. Fennel was used in ancient Egypt to aid digestion and flatulence. In Italy, it was used to bring surgical patients out of anesthesia. Hippocrates and Dioscorides recommended fennel to increase milk production in nursing mothers. The ancient Greeks used it for weight reduction. The seventeenth-century herbalist Nicholas Culpeper also recommended fennel for losing weight.

Fennel helps with weight reduction by suppressing the appetite. It aids in stabilizing the nervous system and may be used as a sedative for small children. Fennel is used to expel phlegm from the throat, eliminate toxins from the body, and purify the blood. It is known to fortify the immune system and to be good for the eyes. Fennel also aids digestion, improves night vision, relieves gas, expels worms, improves the quality of milk in nursing mothers, and cleans the bladder and liver. Fennel has been used to stimulate menstruation. It helps to soothe the smooth muscles of the digestive tract, aiding in digestion and related problems.

Research has found the seeds to have estrogenic effects on the genital organs of female and male rats. Fennel has been found to promote the production of milk in nursing mothers. It is good for digestion, colic, and other stomach complaints. It contains essential oils similar in composition to catnip and peppermint.

## PRIMARY APPLICATIONS

| | |
|---|---|
| Abdominal cramps | Colic |
| Gas | Gastric disorders |
| Indigestion | Intestinal problems |
| Weight-related conditions | |

## SECONDARY APPLICATIONS

| | |
|---|---|
| Appetite, excessive | Asthma |
| Constipation | Convulsions |
| Coughs | Cramps, uterine |
| Gout | Kidney ailments |
| Lactation, absent | Liver disorders |
| Lung disorders | Nervous disorders |

# FENUGREEK
*(Trigonella foenum-graecum)*

*Parts used:* Seeds
*Properties:* Alterative, anticatarrhal, anti-inflammatory, antiseptic, aphrodisiac, astringent, bitter, demulcent, emollient, expectorant, febrifuge, galactagogue, mucilant, vulnerary
*Primary nutrients:* Choline, iron, lecithin, minerals, protein, vitamins A, B1, B2, B3, and D

Fenugreek is one of the oldest herbal remedies. It was used as both a cooking spice and a medicinal remedy. It was originally native to southwestern Asia and used for inflamed bowels and stomach problems because of its bowel-lubricating abilities. The Greeks used fenugreek for respiratory problems. Fenugreek was used in both the East and West and was thought of as one of the most effective medicinal herbs. Fenugreek plants were fed to sick animals to improve their health.

Fenugreek has a reputation of being able to dissolve hardened masses of accumulated mucus in the body. It helps rid the lungs of mucus and the bronchial tubes of phlegm. Fenugreek combined with lemon juice and honey can help soothe the throat and reduce fever. It also helps expel waste through the lymphatic system. Fenugreek is known to contain antiseptic properties that help kill infections in the lungs. It is also recommended for treating an inflamed gastrointestinal system. Fenugreek contains 30 percent mucilage that may be used as a poultice on wounds, inflammations, boils, and skin ailments. Patent medicine manufacturer Lydia Pinkham designed a formula during the late nineteenth century containing fenugreek and touted as the "miracle medicine" for all gynecological problems. Some studies have found that fenugreek does stimulate the uterus and contains a constituent, diosgenin, similar to estrogen.

Studies on diabetic animals have found fenugreek seeds help reduce urinary glucose levels. The active ingredient seems to be the defatted portion of the seed, which has the alkaloid trogonelline, nicotinic acid, and coumarin. When the defatted seeds were added to the insulin treatment of diabetic dogs, a decrease in insulin dose was noted. Fenugreek contains choline and liptropic, which aid in dissolving cholesterol and lowering cholesterol levels. Animal studies have shown beneficial results in lowering serum cholesterol levels. It helps reduce mucus in cases of asthma and sinus and bronchial congestion. There is evidence of anti-inflammatory activity in fenugreek extracts in animal studies. This may explain why some individuals with arthritis have been helped with fenugreek.

## PRIMARY APPLICATIONS

| | |
|---|---|
| Allergies | Appetite, loss of |
| Catarrh, bronchial | Cholesterol, high |
| Diabetic retinopathy | Gas |
| Gastric disorders | Lung infections |
| Mucus, excessive | Throat, sore |

## SECONDARY APPLICATIONS

| | |
|---|---|
| Abscesses | Anemia |
| Asthma | Body odor |
| Boils | Bronchitis |
| Cancer | Eyes, swollen |
| Fevers | Gallbladder problems |
| Heartburn | Inflammation |
| Sinus problems | Ulcers |
| Uterine problems | Water retention |

# FEVERFEW (*Chrysanthemum parthenium*)

*Parts used:* Leaves and flowers
*Properties:* Alterative, analgesic, anti-inflammatory, antimicrobial, aromatic, bitter, carminative, emmenagogue, febrifuge, nervine, parasiticide, purgative (mild), stimulant, vasodilator
*Primary nutrients:* Iron, niacin, manganese, phosphorus, potassium, selenium, silicon, sodium, vitamins A and C, zinc

Feverfew has been used for the treatment of various ailments for thousands of years. References to feverfew are etched in history. Dioscorides, an ancient Greek herbalist, recommended the use of feverfew almost two thousand years ago. He valued the herb for childbirth, fevers, melancholy, and congestion of the lungs. He also suggested it for "all hot inflammations and swellings," which may refer to arthritis. John Hill, MD, suggested in 1772 that feverfew be used to treat painful headaches. Many believe that feverfew got its name from its use as a remedy for bringing down fevers, but this has been found to be incorrect. Actually, the name feverfew came from the traditional Old English name for feverfew, featherfew. Featherfew came from the feather-shaped leaves of the feverfew plant.

Feverfew has long been used as a natural remedy for pain relief and is considered an excellent remedy for migraines. Feverfew was used to treat any kind of pain. The herb also helped with chills and fever. It aids in relieving colds, dizziness, tinnitus, and inflammation from arthritis. It works gradually and with a gentle action that allows the body to heal itself.

Research done in 1959 by Soucek, Herout, and Sorm isolated a sesquiterpene lactone, parthenolide, from the feverfew plant. This is thought to be the major active constituent in feverfew that helps prevent migraines. Other sesquiterpene lactones found in the plant may also be responsible for its activity. Various studies have found a wide range of the active constituent, parthenolide, from feverfew samples around the world. There must be adequate amounts of parthenolides in order to receive beneficial effects from the feverfew. According to the above study, it appears that the amounts vary considerably. Clinical studies done using feverfew have used preparations ranging from 0.4 percent to 0.8 percent.

Probably the most popular use of feverfew is in the prevention of migraine headaches. Those given the placebo had an increase in frequency and severity of headaches, nausea, and vomiting. Those given the feverfew capsules had no increase in frequency or severity of migraines. A randomized, double-blind, placebo-controlled, crossover study involved seventy-two volunteers with one group receiving capsuled, dried feverfew leaves and the other group a placebo. The group taking feverfew showed less severity of attacks and a reduction in symptoms associated with migraines, such as vomiting. There was a definite improvement in the group using feverfew, with no serious side effects. Some forms of migraines are thought to be associated with abnormal platelet behavior. Feverfew has been found to help restrain the release of serotonin from platelets, preventing a migraine from occurring.

Feverfew may be a useful treatment in cases of rheumatoid arthritis because of its ability to inhibit the formation of inflammation-promoting compounds such as prostaglandins and leukotrienes. It seems to have similar properties to nonsteroidal anti-inflammatory agents (NSAIDs), which include aspirin, but feverfew may actually be more effective with fewer potential complications. Some of the studies involving feverfew and migraines have shown that feverfew may also lower blood pressure.

## PRIMARY APPLICATIONS

| | |
|---|---|
| Chills | Colds |
| Fever | Headaches |
| Headaches, sinus | Inflammation |

## SECONDARY APPLICATIONS

| | |
|---|---|
| Aches | Ague |
| Allergies | Anxiety |
| Arthritis | Bites, insect |
| Circulation, poor | Dizziness |
| Gastric disorders | Headaches, nervous |
| Hot flashes | Indigestion |
| Menopausal symptoms | Menstruation, absent |
| Nervousness | Tinnitus |
| Vertigo | |

# FIGWORT (Scrophularia nodosa)

*Parts used:* Leaves, stems, and roots
*Properties:* Alterative, anodyne, anti-inflammatory, antineoplastic, bitter, demulcent, diuretic, purgative (mild), parasiticide, stimulant

Figwort is generally used as a skin medication for eczema, scabies, tumors, and rashes. But it also provides hormone-like materials that help soothe the digestive organs. It has diuretic properties and can help clean the kidneys. Figwort is sometimes used to treat circulatory disorders and may aid in the treatment of varicose veins. It is recommended to lower high blood pressure. Figwort can be used as a poultice for ulcers, piles, scrofulous glands in the neck, sores, wounds, and toothaches.

## PRIMARY APPLICATIONS

| | |
|---|---|
| Abrasions | Athlete's foot |
| Cradle cap | Fever |
| Impetigo | Indigestion |
| Restlessness | Skin diseases |

## SECONDARY APPLICATIONS

| | |
|---|---|
| Anxiety | Burns |
| Cuts | Eczema |
| Hemorrhoids | Insomnia |
| Kidney problems | Menstruation, light flow |
| Nightmares | Worms |

# FLAXSEED (Linum usitatissimum)

*Parts used:* Seeds
*Properties:* Antineoplastic, demulcent, emollient, expectorant, mucilant, purgative (mild), vulnerary
*Primary nutrients:* Calcium, essential fatty acids, potassium

Flax has been around since the beginning of civilization. The early Swiss used the strong fibers for weaving. The Egyptians decorated their tombs with carvings of the flax plant and wrapped mummies in linen because of the high esteem they felt for this plant. The fibers of the flax plant were a main source of clothing in biblical times. Even Christ was believed to have been buried in linen. Hippocrates recommended the use of flaxseed oil for inflammations of the mucous membranes. Charlemagne, during the eighth century in France, required his subjects to eat the seeds to remain healthy.

Flaxseed has many medicinal properties. The oil has been used as a remedy for colds, coughs, sore throats, mucus, congestion, lung conditions, and as an expectorant. It is soothing on the mucous membranes. It has also been used to treat asthmatic conditions.

Flaxseed is a mild, natural laxative. It provides roughage to aid the body when constipation is a problem. It is also healing on the stomach and intestines. Flaxseed oil is recommended for gastritis, ulcers, and heartburn. The tea can be used to help in detoxifying the liver and purifying the blood.

Flaxseed oil is also thought to aid in reducing the clotting tendency of the blood, which may lower the risk of heart attacks as well as reducing cholesterol levels in the blood. It is also used for reducing inflammation and for urinary tract irritations. A poultice of crushed flaxseed is sometimes used to treat sprains or burns. Studies continue as to the benefits of flaxseed, but there is enough evidence to recommend considering this great herb for increased health.

Studies have been done supplementing flaxseed oil in the diets of individuals with multiple sclerosis. Results in two of three studies found that linoleic acid supplementation slowed the increase of disability and reduced the severity of relapses. Since flaxseed oil contains both linoleic acid and alpha-linolenic acid (an omega-3 oil), it is highly recommended for MS, because they both are readily incorporated into brain lipids and thought to help normalize the activity of the immune system. Patients suffering from MS have been found to have abnormalities of the immune system function.

Unrefined, cold-pressed flax oil is considered to be the richest vegetable source of omega-3 oils, which are essential fatty acids (EFAs). These are useful for balancing the hormones in the body to aid in the weight-loss process. EFAs help improve the function of the glands, which can help in weight loss. Some individuals on low- or no-fat diets experience symptoms of fatigue and periods of no weight loss. This could be due in part to the absence of EFAs in the diet. A small amount of EFAs in the diet can actually help in the weight-loss process.

Two cancer researchers working independently found that adding omega-3 oils such as flaxseed to the cancer treatment regimen helped dissolve tumors faster. The oils aided in immune enhancement on a cellular level. Flaxseed may also help with other conditions to bolster the immune function, such as heart disease, AIDS, and arthritis. Adding flaxseed to the diet may also help with kidney disease, ulcerative colitis, asthma, hives, psoriasis, and migraines.

Flaxseed contains lignans, a type of fiber that has antiestrogenic activity. One study done at the National Cancer Institute followed vegetarian women and indicated a correlation between a high amount of lignans in the blood and a lower risk for breast cancer. It has also been discovered that people living in countries where flaxseed is consumed in high amounts have a lower risk for developing breast and colon cancer. Stabilized flaxseed has a higher content of lignans than any other food.

Flaxseed is also beneficial for preventing heart disease and lowering cholesterol levels. One study found that ground flaxseed added to the diet may reduce the incidence of heart disease. Another study found that flaxseed mucilage extracted and given to diabetics can improve their glucose metabolism 28 percent.

## PRIMARY APPLICATIONS

| | |
|---|---|
| Arthritis | Cardiovascular health |
| Cholesterol, high | Constipation |
| Immune disorders | Multiple sclerosis |
| Skin disorders | |

## SECONDARY APPLICATIONS

| | |
|---|---|
| Bronchitis | Cancer |
| Colds | Gallstones |
| Heart, weak | Jaundice |
| Liver | Lung disorders |
| Rheumatism, muscular | Tumors |

# GARCINIA (Garcinia cambogia)

*Parts used:* Fruit
*Properties:* Anorectic, anticatarrhal, astringent, demulcent, thermogenesis

Garcinia is a little-known fruit that grows extensively in India and Thailand. It has been used for centuries as a condiment. *Garcinia cambogia* is also known as Malabar tamarind or Gorikapuli. It is about the size of an orange and orange in color but looks similar to an acorn squash in appearance. There are approximately two hundred different species of garcinia, but only a few contain the needed component. Scientists have identified the natural compound found in garcinia, hydroxycitric acid. It can help curb appetite, reduce food intake, and slow the body's fat production.

The active component in garcinia, hydroxycitric acid (HCA), is similar to citric acid found in citrus fruits such as oranges, lemons, and grapefruit. The garcinia fruit is approximately 50 percent HCA. Hydroxycitric acid seems to have potent fat-fighting properties. It is known to block the formation of fatty tissue, resulting in less storage of fat. The rind of the garcinia fruit contains high amounts of hydroxycitric acid. It inhibits citrate lyase, which is an enzyme that is required to manufacture body fat. The HCA combines with citrate lyase, leaving less of the enzyme available to form body fat. This action also speeds up the fat-burning process. Some studies have found that fat production may actually be reduced by as much as 70 percent when taking HCA.

Studies have found significant weight-loss benefits on animals and humans when using garcinia. One study involved fifty obese patients. They were given 500 mg of garcinia rind daily, along with 100 mg of chromium. This was also combined with a low-fat diet. The individuals taking the garcinia/chromium lost an average of eleven pounds. The control group reported only a four-pound weight loss.

Garcinia has been found to be beneficial in curbing the appetite, which aids in weight control and obesity. One animal study found appetite reduction in lean and fat rats and mice. The animals ate less, and when HCA was added to their diets, their body fat decreased, but the body protein was unaffected.

Garcinia is also thought to help burn fat through thermogenesis. When there is not enough thermogenic activity, weight gain can result. The thermogenic activity in garcinia helps increase heat production, specifically in the brown fat, which is the body fat surrounded by blood vessels and energy cells. The brown fat is harder to lose because it requires more heat (thermogenesis) to burn.

## PRIMARY APPLICATIONS

Appetite, excessive   Obesity
Weight-related conditions

# GARLIC *(Allium sativum)*

*Parts used:* Bulb
*Properties:* Adaptogen, alterative, antibiotic, anticoagulant, antifungal, antineoplastic, antiseptic, antispasmodic, blood purifier, diaphoretic, digestive, expectorant, febrifuge, rubefacient, stimulant, vulnerary
*Primary nutrients:* Calcium, iron, magnesium, manganese, phosphorus, potassium, selenium, sodium, sulfur, vitamins A, B-complex, and C

Garlic is well known for its health benefits. It is a perennial plant and a member of the lily family. The bulb is used for medicinal purposes. It was used by the ancient Hebrews, Greeks, Romans, Chinese, and Egyptians. The Chinese used garlic at least three thousand years ago for various ailments. While building the pyramids, Egyptians ate garlic to increase their strength and endurance. Hippocrates suggested it for the treatment of uterine cancer. Native Americans used garlic to fight abdominal cancer. The Europeans used garlic during the plague years to provide immunity. Historically, the main uses of garlic were to treat colds, coughs, toothaches, earaches, diarrhea, infection, arteriosclerosis, headaches, dandruff, tumors, worms, and hypertension.

Garlic is nature's antibiotic. It is effective against bacteria that may be resistant to other antibiotics, and it stimulates the lymphatic system to throw off waste material. Unlike other antibiotics, garlic does not destroy the body's natural flora. Instead, it has the ability to stimulate cell growth and activity, thus rejuvenating all body functions. It opens up blood vessels and reduces hypertension. Garlic is a health-building and disease-preventing herb.

Research has discovered even more benefits of garlic. Louis Pasteur found that garlic contains antibiotic properties. Albert Schweitzer used garlic when in Africa for treating amoebic dysentery and as an antiseptic in preventing infections. Garlic is now known to be effective in inhibiting bacterial growth. Garlic has been found to be effective in inhibiting the growth of many different strains of mycobacterium. Garlic also contains broad-spectrum capabilities for fighting bacteria, viruses, worms, and fungi. Garlic extracts have been found to contain antifungal activity, which may help in cases of candidiasis.

Several studies link garlic to lower incidence of cardiovascular disease. Garlic has been found to reduce cholesterol and triglyceride levels in the blood, lower blood pressure, increase immunity, and reduce the blood's clotting ability. Research using the results of many separate studies suggests that eating the equivalent of one-half to one clove of garlic daily can decrease total serum cholesterol levels by approximately 9 percent. German researchers found anticoagulant capabilities with garlic. Garlic was able to benefit individuals suffering from peripheral arterial occlusive disease, blood clots in the legs.

Garlic contains antitumor properties, and studies have shown it has the ability to inhibit the growth of cancer-causing nitrosamine. A questionnaire was given to 41,837 women aged fifty-five to sixty-nine regarding their eating habits, and they were monitored over a period of five years for health problems. The women who consumed the greatest amount of garlic had a decreased risk of colon cancer. The National Cancer Institute has recommended adding more garlic, onions, and other similar vegetables to the diet in order to lower the risk of developing stomach cancer. A study reported on 1,695 individuals, approximately one-third of whom had stomach cancer. Results showed that garlic may be toxic to some cancer cells and may encourage the immune system to spot the invaders and destroy them. This allows for a natural immune process for destroying tumor cells.

Garlic is thought to stimulate the lymphatic system in ridding itself of toxins. Studies by Dr. Eric Block have found that garlic will lower cholesterol, prevent blood clotting, protect the liver from drugs and toxins, kill parasites and worms, and protect the cells from free-radical and radiation damage. The Russians consider garlic to be a natural antibiotic and consume it regularly. Garlic is often used to prevent disease and heal the body. It is nourishing for the body, especially the heart, circulation, stomach, spleen, and lungs. It has been used to stimulate circulation and to help the immune system function more effectively. It may help prevent some forms of cancer, heart disease, strokes, and infections.

## PRIMARY APPLICATIONS

| | |
|---|---|
| Asthma | Blood impurities |
| Blood pressure, high | Bronchitis |
| Cancer | Candidiasis |
| Circulation, poor | Colds |
| Colitis | Coughs |
| Diseases, infectious | Ear infections |
| Fevers | Flu |
| Fungus | Gastric disorders |
| Heart disease | Indigestion |
| Infection | Liver disorders |
| Lung disorders | Parasites |
| Poisoning, blood | Prostate problems |
| Respiratory problems | Staph/strep infections |

## SECONDARY APPLICATIONS

| | |
|---|---|
| Acne | Allergies |
| Arthritis | Childhood diseases |
| Diabetes | Diarrhea |
| Edema | Emphysema |
| Gallbladder problems | Hypoglycemia |
| Insomnia | Kidney ailments |
| Pneumonia | Rheumatism |
| Sinus problems | Ulcers |
| Warts | Worms |

# GENTIAN (Gentiana lutea)

*Parts used:* Root
*Properties:* Alterative, anthelmintic, anti-inflammatory, antiseptic, antispasmodic, blood purifier, emmenagogue, febrifuge, hepatic, sialagogue, stimulant, stomachic, vulnerary
*Primary nutrients:* Inositol, iron, manganese, niacin, silicon, sulfur, vitamins F and B-complex, zinc

In Ancient Rome, gentian was used as a stomach tonic and to aid in digestion. Gentian is native to Europe and western Asia. It was generally consumed as a tea or alcoholic beverage. Gentian was an official drug in the United States Pharmacopoeia from 1820 to 1955 and was used as a gastric stimulant. At one time, it was used and acclaimed by medical science as being very beneficial for mankind.

It is used to reduce fevers by cooling the system. Gentian contains a bitter principle, amarogentin, which stimulates the glands, including the adrenals and the thyroid. It helps in the production of bile, which can have a positive effect on the liver and gallbladder. Gentian is also used to clean the bowels, stimulate the pancreas, stimulate circulation, aid in the digestive process, and help with female problems. Gentian has historically been used to treat wounds and been taken internally for inflammation from arthritis, jaundice, and a sore throat. It is considered a great herb for strengthening the entire body and for use as a tonic when combined with other herbs.

Modern research by German scientists confirms that it is useful as a digestive aid. Herbal bitters, including gentian, are recommended as a treatment for indigestion. The bitter taste receptors in the tongue are known to stimulate the digestive processes by increasing the flow of gastric juices and bile. The alkaloid gentianine, found in gentian, contains anti-inflammatory activity in animal studies.

## PRIMARY APPLICATIONS

| | |
|---|---|
| Appetite loss | Circulation, poor |
| Gastric disorders | Indigestion |
| Jaundice | Liver disorders |

## SECONDARY APPLICATIONS

| | |
|---|---|
| Anemia | Blood impurities |
| Colds | Constipation |
| Cramps, stomach | Diarrhea |
| Dysentery | Fevers |
| Gas | Gout |
| Heartburn | Menstruation, absent |
| Nausea | Spleen ailments |
| Urinary problems | Worms |
| Wounds | Yeast infections |

# GINGER *(Zingiber officinale)*

*Parts used:* Root
*Properties:* Alterative, antacid, anti-inflammatory, carminative, diaphoretic, diuretic, emmenagogue, febrifuge, rubefacient, sialagogue, stimulant
*Primary nutrients:* Calcium, iron, magnesium, phosphorus, potassium, protein, sodium, vitamins A, B-complex, and C

Ginger has been used medicinally for thousands of years. It was first used in the tropical Asian climates. The Greek historian Dioscorides recommended ginger to stimulate the production of digestive juices and to combat chills and colds. The Chinese have used this herb for many ailments, including colds, nausea, and indigestion. The Spaniards are credited with introducing ginger to America during the sixteenth century. Ginger was listed in the U.S. Pharmacopoeia from 1820 to 1873.

Ginger is thought to have blood-thinning properties and the ability to lower blood cholesterol levels. It is a blood stimulant and cleansing herb. It is also used for respiratory problems such as colds, sore throats, bronchitis, congestion, headaches, and pain. Ginger is also known to help with nausea, kidney problems, heart problems, fever, vomiting, cramps, and in herbal combinations to aid in the effectiveness of other herbs. Ginger is well known for its medicinal properties. It is used for numerous ailments, including menstrual symptoms, inflammation, arthritis, high cholesterol, liver problems, gastrointestinal problems, and motion sickness.

Recent studies are convincing concerning the value of ginger. Ginger contains terpenses that are chemically similar to those found in camphor and turpentine. Researchers claim that there are two natural antibiotics found in ginger. It has been found to inhibit the growth of bacteria. It has the ability to relieve dizziness and motion sickness, may help in preventing heart attacks, and contains anti-inflammatory agents. One study involved seven patients with rheumatoid arthritis who had tried numerous conventional drugs providing only temporary or partial relief. All of the patients reported significant improvement, pain relief, reduction in swelling, and improved mobility from the ginger therapy. Other studies have found similar results, with 75 to 100 percent of the patients having relief and improvement from ginger supplementation.

Ginger is probably best known for its positive effect on the gastrointestinal system. In one study, powdered ginger was found to be more effective in treating motion sickness than some common over-the-counter treatments, without causing drowsiness. Out of thirty-six volunteers, the twelve who were given ginger did better than the twelve who received an over-the-counter preparation or the twelve who received a placebo. Ginger root contains zingibain, which is a digestive enzyme beneficial for digestion. Morning sickness often associated with the early months of pregnancy may be eased with ginger root. A study found that women suffering from this condition preferred ginger treatment over a placebo.

## PRIMARY APPLICATIONS

| | |
|---|---|
| Bronchitis | Childhood diseases |
| Circulation, poor | Colds |
| Colic | Colitis |
| Cramps, stomach | Diarrhea |
| Dizziness | Fatigue |
| Fevers | Flu |
| Gas | Gastric disorders |
| Headache | Heart problems |
| Indigestion | Morning sickness |
| Motion sickness | Nausea |
| Throat, sore | Vomiting |

## SECONDARY APPLICATIONS

| | |
|---|---|
| Colon problems | Coughs |
| Cramps, uterine | Hemorrhage |
| Intestinal problems | Kidney problems |
| Paralysis | Sinus problems |
| Toothaches | |

# GINKGO *(Ginkgo biloba)*

*Parts used:* Leaves
*Properties:* Adaptogen, alterative, antioxidant, antiseptic, stimulant
*Primary nutrients:* Bioflavonoids

Ginkgo has received much attention in the past decade. It has been revered throughout China and other areas of Asia for thousands of years. But its popularity has increased in Western countries, with evidence mounting from research done and currently under way. Interest in the benefits of ginkgo on conditions associated with aging such as Alzheimer's, memory loss, dementia, and circulatory disorders has led to an increase in sales.

Ginkgo is often used to increase the blood flow to the brain, improving memory problems such as in Alzheimer's, to prevent strokes, and to increase blood circulation through vasodilation. Because of the improved circulation, it is thought to improve ear conditions, help blood flow to the retina, aid in preventing muscular degeneration, reduce frequency of asthma attacks, and help transplant recipients avoid rejection.

Considerable research and clinical trials have been done on ginkgo, and the results have been positive. Medical professionals in Germany and France often prescribe ginkgo. More than three hundred studies have already been conducted, with more in progress. Ginkgo has been found to aid in arterial blood flow, blood flow to the brain, dementia, brain function, senility, vertigo, heart arrhythmias, tinnitus, depression, memory, and intermittent claudication.

The ability of ginkgo to boost brain function has been documented extensively. The increase in the oxygen supply to brain cells is an important factor, as the brain is the body's most sensitive organ to oxygen deprivation. Ginkgo has been used to improve electrical transmission in nerves and to supply more oxygen and nutrients to brain cells. Studies have demonstrated an increase in the rate of nerve transmissions with the addition of ginkgo extract. Ginkgo's effect on the brain and circulatory system disorders seems very promising for many conditions.

Ginkgo has also been found to be effective in treating migraine headaches. Ginkgo extract was given to individuals suffering from migraines in 1975. Eighty percent of the patients showed improvement or were cured of the condition.

Dementia resulting from poor blood flow to the brain has also been helped with ginkgo extract. Senile dementia is often recognized by depression, memory problems, and unusual fatigue. Recent studies involving ginkgo have shown therapeutic value in treating dementia. Ginkgo can help improve circulation to the brain tissue, improving brain function.

Some forms of depression seem to occur in response to cerebral vascular insufficiency. A study done involving patients aged fifty-one to seventy-eight found beneficial results with the addition of ginkgo extract. They had all been given antidepressants earlier, with little help.

Blood platelet aggregation, or clotting, can cause serious problems such as strokes, heart attacks, and coronary thrombosis. Ginkgo has been found to reduce the tendency for the platelets to stick together and prevent them from forming clots in the arteries and veins.

The nervous system and brain are particularly sensitive to free-radical damage because of the high percentage of unsaturated fatty acids. The antioxidant activity of ginkgo extract has been found to be particularly powerful on these areas, as well as the eye and the retina. This can help with conditions such as retinopathy cataracts and macular degeneration. The central nervous system contains fat lipids in the cell membranes that are often attracted by free radicals. Ginkgo can help protect these cell membranes and prevent conditions which can occur in the brain and nervous system often associated with aging, such as memory loss.

Research has shown ginkgo to be useful in treating irregular heartbeats. One of the active glycosides in ginkgo is ginkgolide B. A study led by M. Koltai tested the use of ginkgolide B along with widely recommended antiarrythmic drugs. The experiment monitored the individuals' heart rates, blood pressure, and aortic and coronary flow. The ginkgo was beneficial in aiding with arrhythmias caused by ischemia (oxygen deprivation of the heart). Ginkgo extract was comparable to the pharmaceutical drugs in activity.

Consult your health-care practitioner before taking gingko with blood thinners such as coumadin.

## PRIMARY APPLICATIONS

| | |
|---|---|
| ADHD | Alzheimer's disease |
| Attention span, lack of | Blood clots |
| Cardiovascular disorders | Circulation, poor |
| Dementia | Dizziness |
| Edema | Impotence |
| Inflammation | Ischemia |
| Memory loss | Mental clarity, lack of |
| Multiple sclerosis | Muscular degeneration |
| PMS | Raynaud's disease |
| Senility | Stress |
| Stroke | Tinnitus |

## SECONDARY APPLICATIONS

| | |
|---|---|
| Allergies | Angina |
| Anxiety | Arthritis |
| Asthma | Cancer |
| Carpal tunnel syndrome | Coughs |
| Depression | Equilibrium, lack of |
| Eye problems | Hearing problems |
| Hemorrhoids | Lung disorders |
| Migraines | Mood swings |
| Toxic shock syndrome | Transplant rejection |
| Veins, varicose | Vascular problems |
| Vertigo | |

# GINSENG

Siberian (*Eleutherococcus senticosus*)
Korean (*Panax schin-seng*)
Wild American (*Panax quinquefolium*)

*Parts used:* Root
*Properties:* Adaptogen, alterative, aphrodisiac, stimulant, stomachic
*Primary nutrients:* Calcium, iron, magnesium, manganese, niacin, phosphorus, potassium, riboflavin, silicon, sodium, sulfur, thiamine, tin, vitamins A, B12, and E

Ginseng is one of the oldest and most beneficial herbs in the world. It is probably the most popular herb used in traditional medicine. In Shen-Nung's Pharmacopoeia (AD 206–220), it was rated the highest and most potent of herbs. People in northern China began using ginseng thousands of years ago. Early herbalists recognized the shape of ginseng as resembling a human figure. They felt this was a sign that the root was valuable for healing the entire body. It is often referred to as the "man root" and is the subject of many legends and folk history. Proponents of the "Doctrine of Signatures," a centuries-old theory about the divine indication of uses for plants, felt that because of the root's shape, it could heal any disorder in the body. The Chinese were so enthralled with the ginseng root that they even fought wars over the land used for growing ginseng.

There are many different varieties of the ginseng plant grown throughout the world that are used for traditional medicine. All of the most common species of plants known as ginseng have similar reactions in the body. The Latin name for ginseng is *Panax ginseng*, from the Greek word meaning "all healing." The North American variety, *Panax quinquefolium*, is thought to have similar properties to the Asian plant. Siberian ginseng (*Eleutherococcus senticosus*), grown in Russia, is not considered to be "true ginseng," though scientists have reported common pharmacological features to *Panax ginseng*.

Ginseng has often been referred to as an adaptogen herb. It helps normalize and adjust the body, restoring and regulating natural immune response. The word *adaptogen* is derived from the Greek word *adapto*, to adjust, and the suffix *gen*, producing. It helps produce adjustments as needed in the body. This function is done without side effects or harm to the body. Ginseng, as an adaptogen, has been used to help normalize blood pressure, whether high or low. It helps increase or slow output to restore equilibrium. Adaptogens help modify the effects of environmental and internal stresses from various sources such as chemical pollutants, radiation, some poisons, weather, temperature changes, poor diet and exercise, and emotional stress. It is used for many ailments and even thought of as a universal cure-all that promotes longevity in general.

Many studies have been done in a variety of countries to determine the effectiveness of ginseng. Incomplete results have occurred in some instances. There have been enough credible studies done to now determine that high-quality ginseng plants do contain active constituents known to be beneficial. Research has shown that the roots are effective against bronchitis and heart disease.

A study done in the late 1950s and early 1960s by Brekhman and Dardymov in Russia involved an experiment with Soviet soldiers. Some were given an extract of ginseng and others a placebo before running a three-kilometer race. Those given the ginseng ran faster with less fatigue than those given the placebo. Another study gave radio operators either a ginseng extract or a placebo. The group given the ginseng performed better with fewer mistakes. A study involving mice followed the results when the mice were put in cold water and forced to swim for a long period of time. The mice given the ginseng were able to swim longer than the control group.

A study in the *American Journal of Chinese Medicine* reported that ginseng seemed to help moderate the effects of a high-cholesterol diet in both rats and humans. This is encouraging because of the positive effect of reducing blood cholesterol levels in the prevention of cardiovascular disease.

Another study found that rats exposed to radiation damage lived twice as long when given ginseng. Their blood showed less damage from the radiation. Ginseng has been found to actually protect cells from radiation damage. When damage does occur from radiation exposure, ginseng is thought to speed the healing process. Radiation exposure is considered by some natural health advocates to be one of the most dangerous stress agents on the immune system.

Hypoglycemic activity has been reported from studies conducted, which may be beneficial for diabetics. It is interesting to note that ginseng increases serum cortisol levels in nondiabetics, yet it reduces serum cortisol levels in diabetics. This is beneficial for diabetics. It is also another example of the adaptogenic properties of ginseng.

There has been a lot of interest in the reported aphrodisiac effects of ginseng. It is often marketed as a sexual stimulant. Yet the results of most studies have been inconclusive. Ginseng seemed to increase the sperm count in rabbits as well as the egg-laying of hens in some studies. A Korean study found the mating behavior of rats to increase with ginseng. Ginseng has been used for thousands of years to strengthen the male reproductive system. It is highly recommended alone or in combinations for male and female health.

There are at least thirteen known triterpenoid saponins, referred to as ginsenosides, in ginseng. These are thought to be the most important active constituents. Many other components, thought to be minor, have also been isolated. The composition of each plant varies greatly according to the age, location, species, and curing method. Some of the plants tend toward stimulating and warming effects, referred to as yang in Chinese traditional medicine, while others are relaxing and cooling, referred to as yin.

## PRIMARY APPLICATIONS

| | |
|---|---|
| Age spots | Appetite loss |
| Asthma | Blood pressure, high |
| Depression | Endurance, lack of |
| Fatigue | Fevers |
| Hemorrhage | Hormone imbalance |
| Sexual stimulant | Stress |

## SECONDARY APPLICATIONS

| | |
|---|---|
| Aging | Anemia |
| Bleeding | Blood diseases |
| Bronchitis | Cancer |
| Concentration, lack of | Gastric disorders |
| Indigestion | Inflammation |
| Impotence | Insomnia |
| Liver disorders | Lung disorders |

| Menopausal symptoms | Menstrual symptoms |
| Radiation, effects of | Ulcers |
| Vitality, lack of | |

# GLUCOMANNAN
*(Amorphophallus konjak)*

*Parts used:* Root
*Properties:* Anorectic, antacid, cholagogue, digestive, nutritive, purgative
*Primary nutrients:* Calcium, iron, magnesium, manganese, niacin, phosphorus, selenium, silicon, sodium, vitamins A, C, B1, and B2, zinc

Glucomannan is derived from the extracted mucilage of the konjac root. It is part of the same family as yams, without calories. It is a 100 percent natural form of fiber. Its principal use is as a bulking agent to promote the feeling of fullness.

Glucomannan helps reduce cholesterol, maintain regularity, and promote intestinal health. It also aids in normalizing blood sugar levels, relieving stress on the pancreas, and discouraging blood sugar abnormalities such as hypoglycemia. Glucomannan absorbs toxic substances produced during digestion and elimination. It binds toxic materials and eliminates them before they can be absorbed into the bloodstream. Studies show that glucomannan and lecithin together reduce cholesterol levels. Lecithin breaks down fat and cholesterol, while glucomannan eliminates them from the body. Glucomannan expands to about fifty times its original volume when taken with a glass of water.

Diabetic patients have reported benefits with glucomannan. One study followed patients who were given glucomannan daily for ninety days. At the end of the period, their mean fasting glucose levels fell by 29 percent. Most participants reduced their insulin requirements. Glucomannan may also help cholesterol levels. Animal studies have found significant reduction in cholesterol levels in rats when given this herb.

## PRIMARY APPLICATIONS

| Blood sugar disorders | Cholesterol, high |
| Constipation | Diverticulitis |
| Hemorrhoids | Obesity |

## SECONDARY APPLICATIONS

| Atherosclerosis | Blood pressure, high |
| Diabetes | Gastric problems |
| Hypoglycemia | Pancreatic problems |

# GOLDENSEAL *(Hydrastis canadensis)*

*Parts used:* Rhizome and root
*Properties:* Adaptogen, alterative, anthelmintic, antibiotic, antiperiodic, antiseptic, cholagogue, emmenagogue, hepatic, nephritic, stomachic, purgative (mild)
*Primary nutrients:* Calcium, copper, iron, manganese, phosphorus, potassium, sodium, vitamins A, B-complex, C, E, and F, zinc

The Native Americans used goldenseal for a tonic, sore throats, eye infections, ulcers, and even arrow wounds. It was used as an insect repellent and as a pesticide for crops. It was also boiled in water and used externally for skin conditions. The dried root was official in the U.S. Pharmacopoeia from 1831 to 1842 and was readmitted in 1863 to 1936.

Goldenseal has been used traditionally for many different conditions, such as boosting the glandular system, hormone imbalance, congestion, inflammation, female problems, infection, bronchitis, menstrual problems, catarrh of the bladder, gastritis, ulcers, bowel stimulation, antiseptic, and as an immune system builder. It is not recommended for those with low blood sugar or pregnant women.

Recent studies have found goldenseal to be beneficial against viruses and infections. It contains the alkaloids hydrastine and hydrastinine, which have strong astringent and antiseptic benefits on the mucous membranes. The berberine found in goldenseal—as well as in barberry, Oregon grape, and goldthread—is effective against infections of the mucous membranes, including the mouth, throat, and sinuses. It has been found to kill toxic bacteria in the intestinal tract such as giardiasis, found in streams in North America. It can help relieve diarrhea in cases of giardiasis, amoebiasis, or other gastrointestinal infections.

The antibiotic properties of goldenseal are due to the alkaloid content, including berberine, which has been found to be effective against organisms such as *Staphylococcus spp.*, *Streptococcus sp.*, *Chlamydia spp.*, *Salmonella typhi*, *Diplococcus pneumonia*, and *Candida albicans*. Goldenseal has a long history of use for fighting colds and flu viruses. The berberine content is an effective natural antibiotic and immune stimulant. It may also help prevent a candida infection that may result from antibiotic use. It is thought to help strengthen the immune system. It may work by increasing the blood supply to the spleen, enabling the spleen to function and release compounds known to strengthen immune function. In England, some herbalists consider goldenseal to be the "wonder remedy" for digestive problems. Goldenseal is recommended for use after the onset of a cold rather than as a preventive agent. It is often found in cold remedy combinations.

## PRIMARY APPLICATIONS

| | |
|---|---|
| Bronchitis | Circulation, poor |
| Colds | Colitis |
| Colon problems | Coughs |
| Diarrhea | Eye infections |
| Gonorrhea | Gum disease |
| Hemorrhages | Hemorrhoids |
| Infection | Inflammation |
| Intestinal problems | Kidney problems |
| Liver disorders | Menstruation, excessive |
| Membrane infections | Mouth sores |
| Nosebleeds | Throat, sore |

## SECONDARY APPLICATIONS

| | |
|---|---|
| Allergies/hay fever | Asthma |
| Bright's disease | Burns |
| Chicken pox | Constipation |
| Earaches | Eczema |
| Fever | Flu |
| Gallbladder problems | Gastric disorders |
| Gastritis | Glandular problems |
| Heart conditions | Herpes |
| Membrane irritation | Nausea |
| Nervous disorders | Ringworm |
| Skin disorders | Spleen ailments |
| Tonsillitis | Urinary problems |

# GOTU KOLA *(Hydrocotyle asiatica)*

*Parts used:* Entire herb
*Properties:* Alterative, antiasthmatic, antispasmodic, blood purifier, diuretic, nervine
*Primary nutrients:* Catechol, epicatechol, magnesium, theobromine, vitamin K

Gotu kola has been used in India and the islands of the Indian Ocean for centuries as a tonic and medicinal remedy. It was believed to increase longevity and improve energy. Anciently, it was used to treat leprosy, calm the nerves, increase mental and physical power, stimulate and rejuvenate the brain, prevent nervous disorders, and avoid mental fatigue and senility.

Gotu kola is considered to be one of the best herbal tonics. A tonic is a substance that works to put the body into balance, so that everything is working properly. An herbal tonic helps promote an optimum state in the body systems. Gotu kola gradually builds the nervous system as a nervous system tonic. It has been used for many different ailments, including nervous disorders, deficient mental function, memory problems, epilepsy, and schizophrenia. It works by cleansing and purifying the blood by neutralizing acids and helps the body defend itself against toxins.

Studies have shown that an ingredient in gotu kola, asiaticoside, speeds the healing of wounds. It is considered a blood cleanser and is also effective for diseases of the lungs and leprosy. It stimulates the capillaries and helps improve brain function, varicose veins, and hypertension.

Gotu kola is often used to increase mental function and performance. Many studies have confirmed the usefulness of gotu kola in improving brain function, and it is commonly prescribed in Europe and India for this purpose. Research done in India found the water extract of fresh leaves to help improve memory and learning. It was also found to help overcome the negative effects associated with stress and fatigue.

Other clinical trials in India have found that gotu kola can help increase the IQ and mental ability of mentally retarded children. The children involved in the study showed improved mental capacity as well as improved behavior. It was given to the children in combination with capsicum and ginseng. This improved behavior and mental capacity can help individuals with mental and learning disabilities achieve a higher quality of life.

Another study found improvement in the memory of rats when given gotu kola extract. The learned behavior retention improved dramatically in the rats. The conclusion of the study was that gotu kola improves learning and memory.

Some natural health professionals recommend gotu kola for ADHD. Gotu kola is considered food for the brain and nervous system and can help improve brain function, which can benefit children suffering from ADHD. Many have reported great improvement from using gotu kola, such as improved memory and mental alertness and longer attention span.

Gotu kola was used anciently to heal wounds and soothe cases of leprosy. Probably the first studies done using gotu kola were with cases of leprosy. The asiaticoside content of gotu kola has been used for years in Europe and the Far East to cure leprosy and tuberculosis. Studies done recently on gotu kola have centered on this healing ability. Gotu kola seems to be able to accelerate the healing of wounds and skin diseases. It has been shown to be beneficial in helping repair tissue after surgery and trauma. It has the ability to strengthen the veins and repair connective tissue. It also nourishes the motor neurons.

Researchers in Madagascar began modern studies on gotu kola in 1949. An extract was injected into leprosy patients directly on nodules and ulcerated areas. The extract was found to aid in dissolving the covering to promote eventual healing in the subjects. This opened the door for the use of gotu kola for healing skin ailments. There have also been excellent results from studies done in treating burn patients with second- and third-degree burns due to boiling water, electrical current, or gas explosions. The gotu kola extract helped limit the swelling and shrinking of skin, which is a result of burning. It reduced infections and scarring and increased healing time.

Gotu kola contains two saponin glycosides known as brahmoside and brahminoside, which are known to promote relaxation. A study done on animals showed that large doses caused a sedative action.

## PRIMARY APPLICATIONS

| | |
|---|---|
| Aging | Arteriosclerosis |
| Blood pressure, high | Circulation, poor |
| Fatigue | Heart problems |
| Hypoglycemia | Leprosy |
| Memory loss | Mental problems |
| Nervousness | Senility |

## SECONDARY APPLICATIONS

| | |
|---|---|
| Blood impurities | Depression |
| Dysentery | Fevers |
| Headaches | Insomnia |
| Liver ailments | Menopausal symptoms |
| Pituitary problems | Psoriasis |
| Rheumatism | Schizophrenia |
| Thyroid problems | Tonsillitis |
| Toxins, effects of | Tuberculosis |
| Veins, varicose | Vitality, lack of |
| Wounds | |

# GUARANA (*Paullinia cupana*)

*Parts used:* Seeds
*Properties:* Anorectic, astringent, febrifuge, narcotic, nervine, nutritive, stimulant

Guarana was used by some Native American tribes as an energy source when traveling for long distances and periods of time. A South American legend tells of the use of guarana by the Incas hundreds of years before the Europeans colonized. Guarana was an important part of the social life of the Amazon Indians. They used it for energy, as an aphrodisiac, and to treat conditions such as malaria and dysentery. Some Japanese soldiers during World War II chewed guarana to increase stamina and alertness.

Guarana is most noted for its caffeine content. It is a stimulant on the nervous system. Guarana is one of the richest sources of caffeine, containing between 3 and 5 percent by dry weight. Because of this, it should be used with caution. Caffeine can be harmful and addictive. It causes stimulation to the heart and increased blood flow.

Guarana is sometimes used to lose weight. The caffeine content is thought to work as an appetite suppressant. It may be found in combination with other herbs in weight-loss formulas. Use with caution.

## PRIMARY APPLICATIONS

| | |
|---|---|
| Alertness, lack of | Energy, lack of |
| Stamina, lack of | Weight conditions |

# GUMWEED *(Grindelia squarrosa)*

*Parts used:* Flowering top and leaves
*Properties:* Antispasmodic, bitter, demulcent, diuretic, expectorant, stimulant (lungs), sedative
*Primary nutrients:* Cadmium, lead, selenium, tin, zinc

Gumweed has a wide variety of uses, but it is most commonly used to treat respiratory problems that accompany colds and wheezing due to asthma. It has been used to reduce spasms, bronchial irritations, and nasal congestion associated with asthma and whooping cough. Gumweed is used to treat poison oak and ivy as well as other skin disorders. It can be used to treat inflammation, skin eruptions, wounds, burns, and rashes with a poultice. Gumweed should not be used by individuals with a history of heart problems.

## PRIMARY APPLICATIONS

| | |
|---|---|
| Asthma | Bronchitis |
| Cystitis | Poison ivy/oak |
| Psoriasis | Skin disorders |
| Whooping cough | |

## SECONDARY APPLICATIONS

| | |
|---|---|
| Blisters | Burns |
| Dermatitis | Eczema |
| Emphysema | Flu |

# GYMNEMA *(Gymnema sylvestre)*

*Parts used:* Leaves and roots
*Properties:* Antiperiodic, diuretic, stomachic

Gymnema has been used medicinally for centuries throughout the world, but it has only recently gained popularity in the Western world. It grows naturally in Africa and India. It is traded all over the world. The leaves are the part generally used, but the root seems to supply some medicinal properties. It is a vinelike, woody plant that grows on bushes and small trees. It is a member of the milkweed family.

Ayurvedic physicians have used gymnema to treat ailments such as stomach problems, diabetes, and urinary disorders for more than two thousand years. Gymnema is also known as gurmar, a Hindu name meaning "sugar destroyer." These early physicians found that chewing some of the leaves helped the individual lose a taste for sweets.

Modern scientific research has confirmed that the active ingredient, gymnemic acid, blocks the taste of sugar as well as blocking sugar's absorption by the body. It is also thought that gymnema suppresses the taste of saccharin and cyclamate, two common artificial sweeteners. A study published in 1986 suggests that the extract of gymnema can significantly increase liver and pancreatic function. This is promising for diabetes, obesity, hypoglycemia, allergies, anemia, and osteoporosis.

Gymnema is used to block the passages from which sugar is normally absorbed so the calories are not absorbed and blood sugar levels are not so drastically affected. It is thought to block the body's desire for sweets. One study found a link between the taste buds and the absorption of sugar in the intestines. The taste-bud tissue structure that detects sugar is similar to the structure of tissue in the intestines. Gymnemic acid found in gymnema has a molecular structure similar to sugar. These molecules fill in the receptor locations on the taste buds temporarily, which prevents the taste buds from being activated by the sugar eaten. The same basic thing happens in the intestines. The gymnemic acid fills in the receptors in the intestines, preventing absorption.

One of the most promising uses of gymnema may be in cases of diabetes. Studies on animals have been done showing a reduction of blood sugar levels after the consumption of gymnema extract. It may help reduce the amount of insulin needed by diabetic individuals on insulin therapy. It is found in combinations associated with controlling blood glucose levels and metabolism. It seems to be successful in some cases of diabetes.

Gymnema has also been found to actually improve liver and pancreatic function.

Gymnema has proven over time to be a nontoxic remedy. It is used for many conditions, including diabetes, digestion, urinary tract problems, obesity, hypoglycemia, allergies, anemia, cholesterol, and hyperactivity. This herb may be a useful remedy in the concern over sugar and sugar-related problems, as well as many other ailments.

## PRIMARY APPLICATIONS

| | |
|---|---|
| Diabetes | Hyperactivity |
| Hypoglycemia | |

## SECONDARY APPLICATIONS

| | |
|---|---|
| Allergies | Anemia |
| Cholesterol, high | Gastric disorders |
| Indigestion | Obesity |
| Weight conditions | |

# HAWTHORN *(Crataegus oxycantha)*

*Parts used:* Berries and flowers
*Properties:* Alterative, antispasmodic, astringent, cardioalterative, diuretic, sedative, vasodilator
*Primary nutrients:* Choline, inositol, vitamins A, B-complex, and C with bioflavonoids

Hawthorn berries were used by the ancient Greeks for heart disease. The Greeks and Romans looked to hawthorn as a source of happiness and hope for the future. The Chinese used the berries for digestion and circulatory problems. Christian legend says that the crown of thorns placed on the head of Christ was made from hawthorn. For centuries in England, the crushed fruit or leaves were used as a poultice for their drawing powers to remove thorns and splinters. Native Americans found hawthorn useful for rheumatism and heart problems.

Hawthorn contains many different constituents that work together to benefit the heart and body. It can feed and strengthen the heart and arteries. It seems to work on the heart muscle to make it work more effectively and may even help a damaged heart. It contains some mild sedative properties, which can help when heart disorders are due to stress and with insomnia. It has been used to treat and prevent arteriosclerosis, rapid heartbeat, feeble heartbeat, enlarged heart, angina, and breathing difficulties due to lack of oxygen in the lungs. Some recommend using hawthorn to protect against disease before symptoms occur.

Hawthorn is noted for its ability to regulate arterial blood pressure. It increases the strength of the heart muscle and works to increase coronary blood flow. It aids in reducing the heart rate and lessens the heart's workload.

Studies indicate the extract dilates the blood vessels, resulting in reduced peripheral resistance. It may also have further cardioprotective effects that become pronounced after prolonged use. Research done involving 132 patients found substantial positive results with hawthorn. The participants were stage two stable heart failure patients. Exercise tolerance was improved. Shortness of breath and fatigue after exercise were reduced by 50 percent. There was also a reduction in systolic blood pressure. The researchers noted that for maximum effect, hawthorn must be used for one to two months. Cardiac improvement accelerates with long-term use and relatively high doses, according to Chinese studies involving animals.

One of the most positive facts about hawthorn is its safety. Hawthorn is thought to be safe for long-term use, without side effects. Some experiments have found that hawthorn dilates the blood vessels, lowers blood pressure, and strengthens the heart. German physicians commonly prescribe hawthorn to treat minor heart problems. Hawthorn also contains a mild sedative effect. This may contribute to a healthy heart. Stress, anxiety, and nervousness are often associated with heart conditions.

## PRIMARY APPLICATIONS

| | |
|---|---|
| Angina | Arrhythmia |
| Arteriosclerosis | Blood pressure, |
| Heart conditions | high/low |
| Heart palpitations | Hypoglycemia |

## SECONDARY APPLICATIONS

| | |
|---|---|
| Arthritis | Blood clots |
| Edema | Hypertension |

Insomnia         Liver disorders
Rheumatism       Sleeplessness
Stress

Diabetes                    Obesity
Weight loss

# HOODIA *(Hoodia gordonii)*

*Parts used:* Stem
*Properties:* Anorectic, aphrodisiac, mood enhancer

Hoodia is a leafless, spiny plant, a succulent (not actually a cactus) in the milkweed family. It grows in South Africa and Namibia. It thrives in very high temperatures and takes years to mature. Bushmen from the Kalahari Desert in southern Africa, the most ancient band of nomadic hunter-gatherers on earth, have used hoodia for centuries to help stave off hunger during long treks in the desert. They eat bite-size chunks to ward off thirst and curb their appetites on long hunting trips in the wilderness.

The first supplements containing a hoodia compound were introduced in the United States early in 2004 as an aid for obesity and weight loss. Hoodia's appetite-suppressing component is a molecule similar to glucose, only stronger. This component has been dubbed P57, and it appears to send a signal to the hypothalamus that tricks the body into thinking it is no longer hungry. The P57 compound seems to increase the amount of adenosine triphosphate (ATP) in nerve cells in the hypothalamus, the brain's control center for regulating thirst, hunger, and temperature. ATP is an energy-producing molecule created from glucose, the brain's preferred fuel. When levels of ATP are increased in hypothalamic nerve cells, those nerve cells fire as if you had just eaten, even if you haven't.

Some people say hoodia works immediately for them, quelling appetite within twenty or thirty minutes of taking the capsules. More often, people require up to two weeks of taking regular doses before they notice results, which include a reduced interest in food, a prolonging of the time after a meal before being hungry again, feeling full more quickly, and a general sense of well-being.

Studies of the effects and safety of hoodia are continuing in the United States and abroad. The prospects for future development of this herb look promising indeed.

# HOPS *(Humulus lupulus)*

*Parts used:* Flower
*Properties:* Alterative, anodyne, antibacterial, antibiotic, antineoplastic, carminative, cholagogue, galactagogue, nervine, sedative, stomachic, vulnerary
*Primary nutrients:* Chlorine, copper, fluorine, iodine, iron, lead, magnesium, manganese, sodium, vitamin B-complex, zinc

The seventeenth-century herbalist Nicholas Culpeper suggested using hops to open obstructions of the liver and spleen, cleanse the blood, loosen the belly, cleanse the veins, and provoke urine. The Romans used hops as a food. Gerard, a famous herbalist, recommended using the buds in salads. Native American tribes found hops to be of value: The Mohicans used it as a sedative and for toothaches, and the Menominee tribe used hops as a cure-all. The lupulin found in hops is described as a sedative and hypnotic drug and was recognized in the U.S. Pharmacopoeia from 1831 to 1916. Hops are probably most often used in the production of beer.

Hops are best known for their sedative action. They are also used for their antibiotic properties, which are beneficial for sore throats, bronchitis, infections, high fevers, delirium, toothaches, earaches, and pain. Hops seem to be strong but safe to use. Their main uses are to alleviate nervous tension and promote a restful sleep. They have been used to relieve insomnia naturally. A poultice of hops is recommended for inflammation, boils, tumors, and swelling. Hops have been used as a stimulant to the glands and muscles of the stomach and also as a relaxant on the gastric nerves. They also have a relaxing influence on the liver and gall duct and a laxative effect on the bowels.

Studies indicate hops as having sedative properties. They are known to be fast-acting, soothing, and calming on the nervous system. Hops are one of the nervine herbs and aid in promoting sleep. Certain constituents of the plant have been found to contain sedative and hypnotic effects. Hops are also used for their antispasmodic effects. Hops contain antibacterial properties, validating some of their historical uses.

## PRIMARY APPLICATIONS

| | |
|---|---|
| Appetite loss | Bronchitis |
| Delirium | Gastric disorders |
| Headaches | Hyperactivity |
| Indigestion | Insomnia |
| Lactation, absent | Nervousness |
| Pain | Sexual desire, excessive |

## SECONDARY APPLICATIONS

| | |
|---|---|
| Alcoholism | Anxiety |
| Blood impurities | Coughs |
| Cramps, intestinal | Dizziness |
| Earaches | Fevers |
| Gas | Indigestion |
| Jaundice | Kidney stones |
| Liver disorders | Menstrual symptoms |
| Menopausal symptoms | Neuralgia |
| Restlessness | Rheumatism |
| Skin disorders | Sleeplessness |
| Toothache | Ulcers |
| Venereal diseases | Water retention |
| Whooping cough | Worms |

# HOREHOUND (*Marrubium vulgare*)

*Parts used:* Entire plant
*Properties:* Alterative, anti-inflammatory, antitussive, aromatic, bitter, diaphoretic, diuretic, expectorant, purgative (mild), stimulant, stomachic
*Primary nutrients:* Iron, potassium, sulfur, vitamins A, B-complex, C, E, and F

Horehound has been around for thousands of years. The Romans used horehound in a combination as an antidote for poison. Galen, an ancient Greek physician, first recommended horehound for use in treating respiratory conditions. Early European physicians also used horehound in treating respiratory ailments. Early settlers to North America brought with them horehound to treat coughs, colds, and tuberculosis. It was also used to treat hepatitis, malaria, and intestinal worms, and to promote menstruation and sweating. It is most commonly used to treat colds and coughs, to soothe the throat and loosen mucus in the chest. It is a well-known lung and throat remedy.

Warm infusions will relieve congestion and hyperemic conditions of the lungs by promoting an outward flow of blood. In large doses, horehound will work as a mild laxative. Applying the dried herb topically has been recommended for use in herpes simplex, eruptions, eczema, and shingles.

The marrubiin (premarrubin) content of horehound is thought to be responsible for its ability to stimulate bronchial mucosa secretions, according to German research done in 1959. Horehound can be used as a safe and effective expectorant.

## PRIMARY APPLICATIONS

| | |
|---|---|
| Asthma | Colds |
| Coughs | Croup |
| Lung ailments | Mucus, excessive |
| Phlegm | Respiratory problems |

## SECONDARY APPLICATIONS

| | |
|---|---|
| Bronchitis | Diseases, infectious |
| Earaches | Eczema, external |
| Fevers | Glandular problems |
| Jaundice | Menstruation, absent |
| Shingles, external | |

# HORSERADISH
(*Cochlearia armoracia*)

*Parts used:* Root
*Properties:* Antibiotic, antineoplastic, antiseptic, bitter, carminative, diaphoretic, digestive, diuretic, expectorant, hepatic, parasiticide, purgative (mild), rubefacient, sialagogue, stimulant, stomachic
*Primary nutrients:* Calcium, iron, phosphorus, sodium, vitamins A, B-complex, and P

Horseradish has been cultivated for at least two thousand years. It was brought to America by early settlers and used to treat conditions such as pain from sciatica, colic, and intestinal worms.

Horseradish has an antibiotic action that is recommended for respiratory and urinary infections.

The volatile oil in horseradish works as a nasal and bronchial dilator. It has been used internally to clear nasal passages, alleviate sinus problems, help with digestion, work as a diuretic, aid with edema and rheumatism, and cleanse various body systems. It has also been used to stimulate digestion, metabolism, and kidney function. It helps promote stomach secretions to aid digestion. It can be used as a compress for neuralgia, stiffness, and pain in the back of the neck. It also is used as a parasiticide.

## PRIMARY APPLICATIONS

| | |
|---|---|
| Appetite, loss of | Circulation |
| Coughs | Edema |
| Mucus, excessive | Sinus problems |
| Tumors, skin/internal | Worms |

## SECONDARY APPLICATIONS

| | |
|---|---|
| Arthritis | Asthma |
| Bronchitis | Congestion |
| Gout | Jaundice |
| Kidney problems | Membranes, irritated |
| Neuralgia | Palsy |
| Rheumatism | Skin conditions |
| Water retention | Wounds |

# HORSETAIL *(Equisetum arvense)*

*Parts used:* Herb
*Properties:* Alterative, antilithic, antineoplastic, astringent, diuretic, emmenagogue, galactogogue, lithotriptic, nephritic, nutritive, vulnerary
*Primary nutrients:* Flavonoids, iodine, iron, manganese, PABA, pantothenic acid, silicon, sodium, vitamin E

Chinese and Asian cultures have used horsetail in healing. During times of famine, the Romans ate the horsetail shoots. Native Americans used horsetail, also known as shavegrass, as a diuretic for kidney problems, cancer, and dropsy to increase blood circulation. The Hopi tribe in New Mexico mixed horsetail and cornmeal as a mush and in their bread. The horsetail plant is one of the oldest plants on the earth, approximately two hundred million years old. It used to be a giant fernlike plant. There are around twenty species of the original plant living today. They are small in comparison to the original plant and are usually considered to be a nuisance. The species *Equisetum arvense* is the most common in North America. It is a small perennial fern plant.

Horsetail is thought to aid the immune system and the nervous system because of its silica content. The nerves contain almost the same amount of silica as does the albumin in the blood. The pancreas is especially rich in silica. It is found combined with fluorine in the enamel of the teeth. Hair needs silica to grow, and it is needed as a protection for the skin and cell walls. Horsetail aids in treating urinary tract problems. It contains silicic acid, which helps with circulation of the blood. Horsetail is also credited with helping coagulate the blood and decreasing blood flow. A decoction applied externally will stop bleeding of wounds and aid in healing. It can be used as a mouthwash for mouth infections. Horsetail is often found in calcium combinations. It is helpful in building the skeletal system and improving bone structure. The silica in horsetail aids in healing bones, keeping the arteries clean, and facilitating the absorption of calcium by the body.

Horsetail is known to have antibiotic properties and contributes to the overall healing process. Horsetail is also thought to help with bleeding, urinary and prostate disorders, bed-wetting, skin problems, and lung disease. There is a weak diuretic effect found in horsetail, probably due to the equisetonin and the flavone glycosides.

## PRIMARY APPLICATIONS

| | |
|---|---|
| Arthritis | Circulation, poor |
| Diabetes | Glandular problems |
| Hair, weak | Kidney stones |
| Nails, weak | Nervousness |
| Osteoporosis | Parasites |
| Rheumatism | Urinary problems |

## SECONDARY APPLICATIONS

| | |
|---|---|
| Edema | Eyestrain |
| Gas | Gout |
| Heart problems | Hemorrhage |
| Incontinence | Liver disorders |
| Membrane irritations | Neuralgia |
| Palsy | Skin disorders |
| Tumors | Water retention |

# HO-SHOU-WU
*(Polygonum multiflorum)*

*Parts used:* Root
*Properties:* Alterative, antineoplastic, antiviral, diuretic, stimulant, vasodilator
*Primary nutrients:* Calcium, iron, magnesium, manganese, phosphorus, potassium, selenium, silicon, sodium, vitamins A, B-complex, and C, zinc

Ho-shou-wu is an herb valued and used by the Chinese for centuries. It is used to promote longevity, for liver and spleen disorders, and to strengthen the heart. It is an herb to benefit the whole body. Ho-shou-wu is a member of the smartweed family, which includes knotweed, bistort, and buckwheat.

Ho-shou-wu is a tonic for the endocrine glands and will help improve health, stamina, and resistance to disease. It is an ingredient in some longevity herbal formulas. Ho-shou-wu is thought to be a cardiovascular strengthener and a tonic for the endocrine glands, liver, and kidneys. It is used to help with premature graying of hair, backaches, pain of knee joints, neurasthenia, and bruises. The properties of ho-shou-wu are similar to those of ginseng. It should be used over a period of time for the best results.

Recent scientific research has found that ho-shou-wu has properties to aid in lowering cholesterol, reducing inflammation, strengthening the heart, and performing antiviral activities. It is considered an antitoxic and nerve-calming herb.

## PRIMARY APPLICATIONS

| | |
|---|---|
| Hair, premature gray | Impotence |
| Infertility | Muscles, weak |
| Nervousness | |

## SECONDARY APPLICATIONS

| | |
|---|---|
| Aging | Anemia |
| Arteriosclerosis | Arthritis |
| Backaches | Blood disorders |
| Bone problems | Bruises |
| Cancer | Circulation, poor |
| Colds | Constipation |
| Diabetes | Diarrhea |
| Dizziness | Gout |

| | |
|---|---|
| Heart problems | Hypoglycemia |
| Inflammation | Knee/joint pain |
| Liver disorders | Menstrual symptoms |
| Spleen ailments | Tumors |

# HYDRANGEA *(Hydrangea arborescens)*

*Parts used:* Leaves and root
*Properties:* Alterative, antilithic, antirheumatic, astringent, diuretic, purgative (mild), nephritic, sialagogue
*Primary nutrients:* Calcium, iron, magnesium, phosphorus, potassium, sodium, sulfur

The Cherokee and the early American settlers used a decoction of hydrangea with great success for calculous diseases. Dr. Edward E. Shook considered this herb remarkable and thought its curative powers were better than any other herb. He considered it a powerful solvent of stone and calculous deposits in the renal organs. It contains alkaloids that act like cortisone without the side effects and has similar cleansing powers to those of chaparral.

Herbalists have found this herb to be gentle and effective as a remedy. It cleans toxins from the body by cleansing the kidneys. Hydrangea works to increase the flow of urine to remove stones and the pain associated with kidney stones. It can help stop infection and dissolve hard deposits in the veins and urinary organs. It is thought to help with rheumatic conditions, work as a diuretic, help with bed-wetting, and treat lymphatic conditions.

Because hydrangea leaves contain cyanide, take only under the supervision of a health-care provider.

## PRIMARY APPLICATIONS

| | |
|---|---|
| Arthritis | Cystitis |
| Gallstones | Gonorrhea |
| Gout | Kidney stones |
| Rheumatism | Uterine problems |

## SECONDARY APPLICATIONS

| | |
|---|---|
| Arteriosclerosis | Backaches |
| Edema | Inflammation |
| Kidney problems | Pain |
| Paralysis | |

# HYSSOP *(Hyssopus officinalis)*

*Parts used:* Entire herb
*Properties:* Carminative, diaphoretic, expectorant, febrifuge, galactagogue, pectoral, stimulant
*Primary nutrients:* Diosmine, flavonoids, marrubin, tannins

In ancient Babylon, hyssop tea was used to reduce fever and for sore throats, colds, lung infections, and eye infections. Hippocrates recommended hyssop for pleurisy. The word *hyssop* is of Greek origin, meaning "holy herb." The Bible contains references to hyssop, although the actual identity of the plant is in question. Jewish priests used hyssop to cleanse the temple more than two thousand years ago. During the seventeenth and eighteenth centuries, hyssop was used to reduce perspiration and to treat dropsy and jaundice. Colonists brought hyssop to the New World and used it to treat colds and chest congestion.

Hyssop is most often used for lung ailments and fevers. Hyssop is useful for lung disorders such as bronchitis, chest congestion, hay fever, tuberculosis, and asthma. It helps relax and expel phlegm from the lungs and relieve coughing. It helps promote sweating to expel toxins through the skin. A mold that produces penicillin grows on the leaves of the plant and may contribute to its healing abilities. Hyssop also contains essential oils that can help build resistance to infectious disease. The leaves can be applied directly to a wound to stop infection and promote healing. Hyssop is usually found in combination with other herbs.

It is a member of the mint family and is thought to aid in digestion and help relieve gas. Hyssop has a history of use as a body purifier. It is strengthening on the immune system and works as a blood pressure regulator. Some of the volatile oils found in hyssop may be responsible for its use in treating sore throats and as an expectorant. It is thought to be effective for mild irritations. Hyssop has also been studied for the treatment of herpes simplex virus. It has been found to inhibit the growth of the virus, which is probably due to the tannin content.

## PRIMARY APPLICATIONS

| | |
|---|---|
| Congestion | Coughs |
| Hay fever | Lactation, absent |
| Lung ailments | Mucus, excessive |
| Phlegm | Wheezing |
| Worms | |

## SECONDARY APPLICATIONS

| | |
|---|---|
| Asthma | Blood pressure, high |
| Bronchitis | Bruises |
| Catarrh, intestinal | Cuts |
| Ear ailments | Edema |
| Epilepsy | Fevers |
| Hoarseness | Jaundice |
| Kidney problems | Lice |
| Sore throat | Spleen ailments |

# ICELAND MOSS *(Cetraria islandica)*

*Parts used:* Entire plant
*Properties:* Alterative, antacid, antiemetic, demulcent, expectorant, galactagogue, mucilant, nutritive, pectoral
*Primary nutrients:* Calcium, iodine, phosphorus, potassium

Iceland moss is actually a lichen and not a moss. It has been used for centuries as a cure for all kinds of chest ailments. It is used to nourish and strengthen sickly children, invalids, and the elderly. Iceland moss is generally used for all types of chest ailments. It has been used beneficially to treat tuberculosis. The high mucilage content of Iceland moss is probably responsible for its soothing effect. It has been used to treat stomach complaints such as gastritis, vomiting, digestive problems, and heartburn. It may help just about anywhere the mucous membranes are irritated. It contains properties similar to those of Irish moss.

## PRIMARY APPLICATIONS

| | |
|---|---|
| Anemia | Bronchitis |
| Congestion | Coughs |
| Gastric disorders | Indigestion |
| Lactation, absent | Lung disorders |
| Mucus, excessive | |

## SECONDARY APPLICATIONS

| | |
|---|---|
| Diarrhea | Dysentery |
| Fevers | Gastritis |
| Hoarseness | Lactation, absent |
| Tuberculosis | |

# IRISH MOSS *(Chondrus crispus)*

*Parts used:* Entire herb
*Properties:* Alterative, antineoplastic, demulcent, emollient, expectorant, nutritive
*Primary nutrients:* Calcium, iodine, phosphorus, potassium, sodium, sulfur, vitamins A, D, E, F, and K

Irish moss, also known as "carrageen moss," is a seaweed first found in Ireland and used since the earliest days and is held in high esteem. The most important component of Irish moss is the pectins known as carageenan. The mucilage content makes it effective for conditions of the skin and mucous membranes. In 1831, it was promoted by Dr. Todhunter in Ireland.

It is high in iodine and considered a valuable food as well as a therapeutic agent. It is beneficial for respiratory ailments such as bronchitis and lung congestion. It is able to absorb excess liquid and remove it from the body and eliminate toxins from the bowel. It is also used to help soften and moisturize the skin tissue. It helps with stomach conditions and for strengthening the glandular system. It is beneficial for all chronic conditions because it is rich in vitamins and minerals to aid the body in healing itself. Because of its nutritional value, Irish moss is beneficial for individuals recovering from illness. It is soothing to inflamed tissues and for lung and kidney ailments. Irish moss is high in iodine, which aids the glandular system.

Studies indicate a correlation between Irish moss and an ability to reduce gastric secretions, high blood pressure, and ulcers. Evidence points to Irish moss as an effective treatment for gastric and duodenal ulcers, along with other marine plants.

It contains fifteen of the eighteen elements that compose the human body.

## PRIMARY APPLICATIONS

| | |
|---|---|
| Bronchitis | Glands |
| Goiters | Lung problems |
| Thyroid problems | |

## SECONDARY APPLICATIONS

| | |
|---|---|
| Cancer | Coughs |
| Diarrhea | Intestinal problems |
| Mucus, excessive | Parathyroid problems |
| Pneumonia | Radiation, effects of |
| Tuberculosis | Tumors |
| Ulcers | Urinary problems |
| Veins, varicose | Weight conditions |

# JOJOBA *(Simmondisia chinensis)*

*Parts used:* Oil
*Properties:* Emollient
*Primary nutrients:* Chromium, copper, iodine, silicon, vitamins E and B-complex, zinc

Jojoba was used by Native Americans in Arizona, California, and northern Mexico for the hair and as a tonic for the body. It is a valuable crop for some Native American tribes in those areas. Jojoba is found in shampoos, conditioners, moisturizers, and sunscreens.

Jojoba oil, made from the seeds of the plant, has traditionally been used by Native Americans to promote hair growth and relieve skin problems. Jojoba helps remove the deposits of sebum that cause dandruff and scalp disorders. It tends to make the scalp less acidic.

The wax found in the jojoba oil has been found in one study to aid in treating acne and psoriasis. It has traditionally been used successfully for this purpose, along with healing minor skin irritations. One study found that rabbits fed jojoba oil had a reduction of 40 percent in their blood cholesterol levels. The reason or component responsible for this activity is not known.

## PRIMARY APPLICATIONS

| | |
|---|---|
| Dandruff | Hair loss |
| Psoriasis | Scalp, dry |

## SECONDARY APPLICATIONS

| | |
|---|---|
| Abrasions | Acne, vulgaris |
| Athlete's foot | Cuts |
| Eczema | Pimples |
| Seborrhea | Sores, mouth |
| Warts | Wrinkles |

# JUNIPER *(Juniperus species)*

*Parts used:* Berries
*Properties:* Anodyne, antispasmodic, aromatic, astringent, carminative, diuretic, emmenagogue, nephritic, stimulant
*Primary nutrients:* Copper, sulfur, vitamin C

In ancient Greece, juniper berries were used as a diuretic. In Europe, the scent of juniper berries was used to help ward off the plague. The seventeenth-century herbalist Nicholas Culpeper suggested using juniper as an appetite stimulant. Native Americans used juniper berries as a survival food during the cold winter months. They would dry and grind the berries, then make them into cakes. Some tribes roasted the berries, ground them, and used them as a coffee substitute. Jethro Kloss recommended using the tea for kidney, prostate, and bladder disorders, and for dropsy and digestive diseases. The berries and oil were listed in the U.S. Pharmacopoeia from 1820 to 1873 and in the National Formulary until 1960.

Juniper berries contain a volatile oil that has traditionally been used to treat conditions of the urinary tract. Juniper berries are often used to increase the flow of urine. They are beneficial for ridding the body of uric acid, which may crystallize in the kidneys. They are also used to dissolve kidney stones and sediment in the prostate. Juniper berries are recommended for treating digestive problems, indigestion, gas, and to cleanse the blood. The berries may help stimulate the appetite. Juniper contains a natural insulin that helps restore the pancreas when no permanent damage has occurred. Juniper may be applied directly to wounds as a poultice for healing and infection prevention.

One study done using animals has found juniper berries to be an effective diuretic. The berries are thought to stimulate the flow of urine and the filtration process. The volatile oils found in the juniper berries increase the glomerular filtration rate of the kidneys. Juniper berries are often used for their diuretic properties. Juniper is not recommended for use by pregnant women as it may also increase uterine contractions.

## PRIMARY APPLICATIONS

| | |
|---|---|
| Adrenal gland problems | Bed-wetting |
| Bleeding | Colds |
| Diabetes | Edema |
| Hypoglycemia | Infection |
| Kidney infections | Kidney stones |
| Pancreatic problems | Uric acid irritations |
| Urinary problems | Uterine problems |
| Water retention | |

## SECONDARY APPLICATIONS

| | |
|---|---|
| Acne | Ague |
| Allergies/hay fever | Arthritis |
| Arteriosclerosis | Bites, insects/snakes |
| Blood impurities | Bursitis |
| Catarrhal inflammation | Colic |
| Coughs | Convulsions |
| Cramps, stomach/uterine | Cystic fibrosis |
| Fungus | Gas |
| Gonorrhea | Gout |
| Gums, bleeding | Menstruation, irregular |
| Mucus, excessive | Prostate problems |
| Rheumatism | Scurvy |
| Sores | Tuberculosis |
| Typhoid fever | Urinary incontinence |
| Worms | |

# KAVA KAVA *(Piper methysticum)*

*Parts used:* Root
*Properties:* Alterative, analgesic, anesthetic, antifungal, antiseptic, antispasmodic, aphrodisiac, diuretic, sedative
*Primary nutrients:* Calcium and magnesium

Many island communities in the Pacific such as Polynesia, Micronesia, and Melanesia used kava kava in their ceremonial drinks as a mild sedative and relaxant. They used it to relax the body and mind and to promote a restful sleep. It is considered to be an important herb for pain relief. It is beneficial for insomnia and nervous conditions.

This herb is recommended as a strong muscle relaxant. It is considered to be one of the most powerful of the herbal muscle relaxants. Kava kava is used as an analgesic sedative, for rheumatism, for insomnia, and to relax the body.

Research has found kava kava to contain anticonvulsant and muscle-relaxing properties in animal studies. This may be beneficial for people with stress-related muscle tension or seizures. Individuals who drink kava kava relate feeling a sense of tranquillity and sociability. It helps achieve a feeling of well-being and relaxation. Kava kava seems to have an advantage over drugs often prescribed for anxiety and insomnia in that it does not seem to lose effectiveness over time. Several studies have shown significant benefit for individuals suffering from anxiety. This is extremely promising for individuals requiring long-term therapy for anxiety disorders. Kava is not addictive and is free of associated complications, unlike many of the medications routinely prescribed.

Another benefit of kava may be as an analgesic for pain relief. The chewed leaves cause numbness in the mouth. This anesthetic activity is similar to cocaine and lasts longer than benzocaine.

## PRIMARY APPLICATIONS

| | |
|---|---|
| Insomnia | Nervousness |

## SECONDARY APPLICATIONS

| | |
|---|---|
| Anxiety | Asthma |
| Bronchitis | Fatigue |
| Pain | Rheumatism |
| Uterine infections | Vaginitis |
| Venereal diseases | |

# KELP *(Fucus vesiculosus)*

*Parts used:* Entire plant
*Properties:* Alterative, antacid, antibiotic, demulcent, diuretic, hypotensive, mucilant, nutritive, hypotensive

*Primary nutrients:* Aluminum, barium, bismuth, boron, calcium, chlorine, chromium, cobalt, copper, gallium, iodine, iron, lithium, magnesium, manganese, nickel, phosphorus, potassium, silicon, silver, sodium, strontium, sulfur, tin, titanium, vanadium, vitamins A, B-complex, C, E, G, S, and K, zinc, zirconium

Kelp is a principal source of natural iodine and is used extensively by the Japanese. The Polynesians also use kelp as a regular part of their diet. Dr. Bernard Russell, an English physician in 1750, used burned, dried kelp to treat his patients suffering from goiter. In 1862, it was used with success by Dr. C. Dupare to treat obesity.

Traditionally, kelp has been used for its rich abundance of iodine to treat thyroid disorders, whether underactive or overactive. It is a great promoter of glandular health and regulates metabolism. It has a reputation for increasing the rate at which calories are burned. Kelp is used to rid the body of toxins and radioactive material by preventing their absorption. It promotes the growth of healthy tissue, skin, hair, and nails. It is also able to improve the cardiovascular system, nervous system, and mental alertness and alleviate kidney, bladder, prostate, and uterine difficulties.

The ocean water contains one of the richest sources of the vital life-sustaining mineral elements known to science. Kelp extracts and assimilates the mineral elements from the ocean water and converts them into a usable form for humans. This plant is thought to provide nourishment, enhance the immune system, aid in hormone balance, and restore strength. Kelp has been proven to contain antibiotic properties. It is thought that the brominated phenalic compounds in kelp are responsible for killing both gram-negative and gram-positive bacteria. Kelp has natural iodine to nourish the thyroid. The Japanese eat kelp regularly and have an extremely low rate of thyroid disease. Kelp helps increase energy through regulation of metabolism and may help reduce fat in the body. Kelp is full of nutrients to nourish the entire body. Kelp can also help prevent the absorption of some radioactive elements known to cause tumors, cancer, and leukemia in adults and children.

Kelp contains nearly thirty minerals.

## PRIMARY APPLICATIONS

| | |
|---|---|
| Adrenal gland problems | Arteries, weak |
| Colitis | Complexion, unhealthy |
| Eczema | Energy, lack of |
| Fatigue | Goiter |
| Infection | Metabolism, slow |
| Nails, weak | Obesity |
| Pituitary problems | Pregnancy problems |
| Radiation, effects of | Skin, unhealthy |
| Thyroid problems | |

## SECONDARY APPLICATIONS

| | |
|---|---|
| Acne | Anemia |
| Arthritis | Asthma |
| Blood pressure, high | Cancer |
| Diabetes | Gallbladder problems |
| Gas | Gastric disorders |
| Glandular problems | Headaches |
| Heart problems | Hypothyroidism |
| Indigestion | Kidney problems |
| Morning sickness | Nervous disorders |
| Pancreatic problems | Prostate problems |
| Tumors | Vitality, lack of |

# KUDZU *(Pueraria omeiensis)*

*Parts used:* Root, flowers
*Properties:* Anti-inflammatory, antileukemic, antimicrobial
*Primary nutrients:* Daidzein, daidzin, genistein, puerarin

Kudzu is native to southern Japan and southeast China. It is a climbing perennial vine that can grow to heights of nearly one hundred feet in trees, but also invades lower vegetation. Kudzu plants grow as much as twelve inches per day, or sixty feet in one season. The vine can reach one hundred feet in length. It was brought to the United States from Asia more than a century ago and is sometimes called "the plant that ate the South," due to its alarmingly prolific growth in the southeastern United States.

Kudzu has been used for more than thirteen hundred years, perhaps longer. The leaves can be used raw in salad or cooked, the flowers can be dipped in batter and fried, and the starchy roots can be cooked similarly to any root vegetable.

The roots are traditionally ground into a powder and used for herbal medicines. Asian healers have used kudzu for alleviating allergies, colds, flu, chest pain, high blood pressure, tinnitus, vertigo, and other complaints. Kudzu contains a variety of isoflavones, including daidzein (anti-inflammatory and antimicrobial), daidzin (a cancer fighter), and genistein (antileukemic). Kudzu is a unique source of the isoflavone puerarin, which may boost blood flow to the heart and brain.

More recently, Chinese practitioners have successfully used kudzu to minimize alcohol cravings and hangovers. Research undertaken in the 1990s showed that daidzin and daidzein reduced alcohol consumption in rodents that had been bred to crave alcohol. These two elements restrain the enzymes vital to metabolizing alcohol. However, findings of a small study in humans published in the February 2000 issue of the *Journal of Alternative and Complementary Medicine* showed that doses smaller than those used in the China studies did not help human alcoholics avoid drinking. More studies are needed to determine kudzu's value as a treatment for alcoholism.

Kudzu root can also influence neurotransmitters in the brain and has been beneficial for migraine and cluster headaches. There are no known drug or nutrient interactions associated with kudzu. This plant has been used for centuries in Asia without harmful effects.

## PRIMARY APPLICATIONS

Alcoholism
Allergies
Chest pain
Colds
Headache
High blood pressure
Influenza
Tinnitus
Vertigo

# LADY'S SLIPPER
*(Cypripedium pubescens)*

*Parts used:* Root
*Properties:* Antispasmodic, nervine, sedative
*Primary nutrients:* Calcium, magnesium, vitamin B-complex

Native American tribes used lady's slipper as a sedative and nerve medicine. The early settlers also found this herb valuable for insomnia and female problems. It was in the U.S. Pharmacopoeia from 1863 to 1916 as an antispasmodic and nerve medicine.

Lady's slipper is used for all diseases of the nervous system. It is one of the best and safest nervine herbs in the plant kingdom. Its action is slow yet effective. Lady's slipper acts primarily on the medulla of the brain, helping regulate breathing, sweating, saliva, and heart function. It is also used as a pain reliever. It may help with brain damage, epilepsy, stroke, cystic fibrosis, and muscular dystrophy. It is an excellent pain remedy for discomfort associated with muscular problems. It is often used as a nervine herb to calm the nerves and relieve stress, tension, insomnia, and anxiety. Lady's slipper is also used for fevers, headaches, depression, stomach ailments, and hyperactivity in children.

## PRIMARY APPLICATIONS

| | |
|---|---|
| Chorea | Insomnia |
| Nervousness | Pain |
| Restlessness | |

## SECONDARY APPLICATIONS

| | |
|---|---|
| Abdominal pain | Afterbirth pain |
| Anxiety | Colic |
| Cramps, uterine/stomach | Cystic fibrosis |
| Epilepsy | Headaches, nervous |
| Menstrual symptoms | Muscle spasms |
| Neuralgia | Tremors |
| Typhoid fever | |

# LEMON GRASS *(Cymbopogon citratus)*

*Parts used:* Leaves
*Properties:* Astringent, blood purifier, carminative, expectorant, febrifuge
*Primary nutrients:* Vitamins A and C

Lemon grass is included in South American folk medicine for pain, stomach disorders, and fevers. Lemon grass is used in China for a variety of ailments, including headaches, colds, stomach disorders, abdominal cramps, and rheumatic complaints. In India, the leaves are used for rheumatism and as an antiseptic.

Lemon grass has an astringent or tightening effect on tissues of the body. This helps stop or slow discharge from mucous membranes, which makes the herb useful for infants and children. It is a mild herb. Lemon grass is also recommended with a periodic cleanse as a blood purifier. It may help relieve stress, menstrual cramps, headaches, and dizziness. Lemon grass tea is generally used for colds, flu, and fever.

## PRIMARY APPLICATIONS

| | |
|---|---|
| Colds | Fevers |
| Gastric disorders | Indigestion |

## SECONDARY APPLICATIONS

| | |
|---|---|
| Blood impurities | Blood pressure, high |
| Boils | Colic |
| Gas | Headaches |
| Kidney problems | Liver disorders |
| Menstruation, absent | Nausea |
| Nervousness | Spleen ailments |
| Urinary problems | Vomiting |

# LICORICE *(Glycyrrhiza glabra)*

*Parts used:* Root
*Properties:* Alterative, antibacterial, anticatarrhal, anti-inflammatory, antiviral, cholagogue, demulcent, estrogenic, expectorant, purgative (gentle), sialagogue
*Primary nutrients:* Biotin, chromium, iodine, lecithin, manganese, niacin, pantothenic acid, phosphorus, vitamins E and B-complex, zinc

Licorice has a long history of use. It has been used medicinally for thousands of years by the Egyptians, Romans, Greeks, and Chinese. It is thought to have originated in the Middle East. It was highly esteemed by the Egyptians. They used it to quench thirst and as a sweetener in drinks. It has a history of use in Europe since around the sixteenth century. The Chinese thought of licorice as a great detoxifier. They continue to use it for strength and endurance. Hippocrates, Theophrastus, and Pliny all wrote about the benefits of licorice. It was used for sore throats, menstrual cramps, fever, arthritis, respiratory problems, and hypoglycemia. It was thought to have been introduced to Native Americans by the English settlers. They used it to treat earaches, colds, lung congestion, and to disguise the taste of bitter herbs.

Licorice is thought to work as a stimulant on the adrenal glands and as a natural source of a hormone similar to cortisone. Licorice is thought to help with the production of cortin hormone, which helps when coping with stress. Licorice contains glycyrrhizin and glycyrrhetinic acid, which help stimulate interferon in the body. Interferon is essential for protecting the immune system. Licorice is thought to help the body in preventing and healing disease. It is also used by some to help increase energy. Licorice is used for lung, throat, and chest complaints. It is a common ingredient in many cough syrups and cough drops. It contains glycosides that have the ability of purging excess fluid from the lungs, throat, and body. The saponin content is thought to be responsible for the expectorant action. It has the ability to loosen phlegm in the respiratory tract and help the body expel mucus. It has a reputation for being effective in relieving coughs. Licorice is a good source of isoflavones and phytoestrogens. It is often used to treat female problems. It may stimulate menstruation in females not experiencing normal ovulation.

Studies done using animals have found that licorice does contain anti-inflammatory and antiarthritic properties. It also has been found to exhibit antibacterial and some mild antiviral activity in vitro. Licorice is used for female problems with the reproductive system, such as menopause and menstrual cramps. In one study, women not ovulating were successfully treated with licorice root. Licorice may also be useful for protecting against and healing ulcers, as well as treating hepatitis. It is being studied as a therapy for Addison's disease, which involves inadequate adrenal function. The glycyrrhizin in licorice stimulates the adrenal cortex to produce aldosterone. Addison's disease involves abnormally low function of the adrenal cortex.

Licorice may also help in healing gastric and duodenal ulcers. Licorice helps stimulate the defenses that prevent ulcers from forming. It seems to stimulate the increase of cells that protect the lining of the gastrointestinal system. It is also used to help heal inflammations of the intestinal tract. There are some precautions when taking licorice: It may increase blood pressure in some and cause water retention.

## PRIMARY APPLICATIONS

| | |
|---|---|
| Addison's disease | Adrenal problems |
| Blood impurities | Colds |
| Coughs | Diabetes |
| Drugs, withdrawal | Ear infections |
| Energy, lack of | Fatigue |
| Hoarseness | Hyperglycemia |
| Hypoglycemia | Lung disorders |
| Sex drive, inhibited | Throat, sore |
| Vitality, lack of | |

## SECONDARY APPLICATIONS

| | |
|---|---|
| Abscesses | Age spots |
| Allergies | Arteriosclerosis |
| Arthritis | Asthma |
| Bronchitis | Circulation, poor |
| Constipation | Cushing's disease |
| Dizziness | Edema |
| Emphysema | Endurance, lack of |
| Fevers | Flu |
| Heart problems | Impotence |
| Liver disorders | Menopausal symptoms |
| Phlegm | Ulcers |

# LILY-OF-THE-VALLEY
*(Convallaria majalis)*

*Parts used:* Flowers, leaves, and rhizome
*Properties:* Alterative, diuretic, cardiac, mucilant, purgative (mild)
*Primary nutrients:* Calcium, iron, potassium, rutin

Dr. Edward Shook recommended lily-of-the-valley as a valuable cardiac tonic. He said that it acts similarly to digitalis without the cumulative effects of that drug. He also suggested it for slowing the action of the heart, increasing heart contractions, as a diuretic, and as a remedy for dropsy involving a faulty heart. Nicholas Culpeper, another well-known herbalist, treated brain weakness and memory problems with this herb.

Lily-of-the-valley contains glycosides used to treat heart disorders—much the same as digitalis, but without the side effects. It can also help with water retention that often accompanies heart problems. It can help strengthen the heart and arteries.

Scientific research has found that lily-of-the-valley contains twenty cardiac glycosides. This may account for its use to treat heart conditions such as valvular heart disease, dropsy, and cardiac debility. In Europe, it is used extensively for apoplexy, convulsions, dropsy, epilepsy, heart ailments, palsy, and vertigo.

## PRIMARY APPLICATIONS

| | |
|---|---|
| Arrhythmia | Edema |
| Epilepsy | Heart problems |
| Water retention | |

# LOBELIA *(Lobelia inflata)*

*Parts used:* Entire plant
*Properties:* Analgesic, anodyne, antiasthmatic, anticatarrhal, antispasmodic, astringent, decongestant, diaphoretic, diuretic, emetic (small doses), emmenagogue, expectorant, nervine, purgative (mild), sedative
*Primary nutrients:* Cobalt, copper, iron, lead, selenium, sodium, sulfur

Some herbalists consider lobelia to be one of the most valuable herbs available to humankind. Early-nineteenth-century physician Samuel Thomson recommended lobelia as a muscle relaxant during childbirth and as a poultice for wounds. He called it the most powerful, certain, and harmless relaxant that has ever been discovered. He considered relaxation to be a big part of the healing process in the majority of diseases. Many early herbalists agreed with this theory and used this herb in their treatments.

Lobelia is one of the most powerful relaxant herbs in the plant kingdom. Its healing powers include the ability to remove congestion from within the body, especially in the blood vessels. It is also good for bronchial spasms as a relaxant. Lobelia can be used externally as a poultice with slippery elm to heal abscesses or boils. Water needs to be taken along with lobelia to aid in the elimination of toxins from the body. Lobelia is also thought to reduce the desire for tobacco, as its action resembles a mild form of nicotine. This is a powerful herb to relax the nervous system. It increases the flow of urine and perspiration, and this aids in the reduction of fever. Lobelia is a powerful antispasmodic for the respiratory system, allowing for the flow of oxygen. Lobelia is beneficial for spasms, convulsions, epilepsy, and nervous conditions. It is relaxing for the croup and coughs. It is also helpful in expelling phlegm from the lungs.

The activity of lobelia is thought to be due to its alkaloid content, mainly lobeline. It works to stimulate the respiratory centers. It is most effective when applied topically. It may possibly help as a smoking deterrent. Lobelia first stimulates the central nervous system, then relaxes it. Normal dosage causes dilation of the bronchioles and an increase in respiration. Overdose is not advised as it may cause respiratory depression, as well as other undesirable symptoms. Lobelia is considered useful for heart and lung conditions as an expectorant and cardiac decongestant on one hand and an antispasmodic relaxant on the other. Many similarities exist between the Chinese herb tian nan xing, tuber arisaemae, and lobelia.

## PRIMARY APPLICATIONS

| | |
|---|---|
| Abscesses | Arthritis |
| Asthma | Bronchitis |
| Colds | Congestion |
| Convulsions | Cough |
| Croup | Earaches |
| Ear infections | Epilepsy |
| Fevers | Lockjaw |
| Lung disorders | Miscarriage tendency |
| Mucus, excessive | Nervousness |
| Pain | Pneumonia |

Poisoning, food          Whooping cough
Worms

## SECONDARY APPLICATIONS

Allergies                Childhood diseases
Circulation, poor        Colic
Constipation             Eczema
Headaches                Heart problems
Hepatitis                Hydrophobia
Palsy                    Pleurisy
Poisoning, blood         Poison ivy/oak
Rabies                   Rheumatism
Ringworm                 Scarlet fever
Shock                    Spasms
Syphilis                 Teeth, pain
Tetanus                  Tonsillitis
Toothaches               Vomiting
Wounds

# MACA (*Lepidium meyenii*)

*Parts used:* Root
*Properties:* Aphrodisiac
*Primary nutrients:* Calcium, iron, linolenic acid, magnesium, oleic acid, palmitic acid, polysaccharides, selenium

Maca, sometimes called Peruvian ginseng, is a plant that has been cultivated in the high, barren plateaus of the central Andes in Peru for approximately two thousand years. Related to the turnip and radish, it is traditionally eaten as a root vegetable. Few other plants can thrive at such high elevations. This hardy plant grows well only in cold climates with relatively poor-quality soil. Although it has been grown outside the Andes, these varieties may not have the same potency. Dried maca root is highly nutritious, comparable to rice and wheat. It contains 10 percent protein and is rich in essential minerals.

Maca has long been connected to sacred fertility rites. Its use was first recorded by Spanish settlers who arrived in Peru in the 1500s. Legend has it that when the Spanish explorers arrived, their livestock were weak and not reproducing. The Incas advised the Spaniards to feed maca to their animals. The

Spaniards did, and their livestock regained health and fertility. Spanish writers mention Inca warriors fortifying themselves with boiled maca root before battle and using it as fuel for endurance sports. During Spanish colonization, this plant was even used as currency.

Maca is often used to restore energy, vitality, and fertility. It may help increase libido, regulate hormones, boost energy, improve memory, and curb depression.

There is much anecdotal evidence of benefits for sexual function, and some research has been done in this area. In a study published in the April 2000 issue of *Urology*, male rats that were given maca mated more often than those given a placebo. Sterols found in maca may act on the glands that produce hormones (the hypothalamus, pituitary, and adrenals), which could mean improved energy and libido. Small-scale studies on men have demonstrated that maca extracts can increase sex drive and enhance semen quality. Larger studies are needed to confirm these findings, particularly of men with sexual dysfunction and infertility. No studies have yet shown an effect on sex hormone levels. No toxic effects have been noted.

## PRIMARY APPLICATIONS

Depression               Hormonal regulation
Libido                   Low energy
Memory loss

# MAGNOLIA (*Magnolia officinalis*)

*Parts used:* Bark
*Properties:* Anti-allergic, anti-angiogenic, antianxiety, antiasthmatic, antioxidant, antistress
*Primary nutrients:* Eudesmol, honokiol, magnolol

The magnolia tree is native to the mountains and valleys of China, where its bark has been used since AD 100 in traditional Chinese medicine. Known as houpu or hou po, the aromatic bark contains magnolol and honokiol, two polyphenolic compounds that have been shown to possess antianxiety and antiangiogenic benefits. Magnolia bark also has demonstrated antiallergic and antiasthmatic activity. It has traditionally been used to treat low energy, emotionally based digestive disturbances, stress, and anxiety.

More recent claims connect magnolia's antistress properties with regulation of the stress hormone cortisol. Elevated cortisol levels have been linked to diabetes, obesity, osteoporosis, low immunity, and memory problems. The magnolol and honokiol found in magnolia are thought to be key to its cortisol-lowering benefits. Magnolol generally is present from 2 to 10 percent; honokiol occurs at 1 to 5 percent. Magnolia also contains just under 1 percent of the essential oil eudesmol, a triterpene that may provide antioxidant value.

Japanese researchers have found that magnolol and honokiol are a thousand times more powerful than alpha-tocopherol (vitamin E) as antioxidants. Other scientists have found that magnolol and honokiol can have a beneficial effect on the brain by controlling the activity of various neurotransmitters and enzymes.

Many studies in animals have shown that honokiol depresses the central nervous system at high doses but is a non-sedating antistressor at lower doses. Thus a low dose of magnolia bark extract may relax you without making you sleepy, while a higher dose may put you to sleep. Compared to medicines such as Valium, honokiol seems to be as effective at relieving anxiety without the potent sedative activity of these drugs, suggesting that magnolia bark extract is a better alternative. No toxic effects have been found with traditional use of magnolia, but high doses can cause drowsiness.

## PRIMARY APPLICATIONS

| | |
|---|---|
| Allergies | Anxiety |
| Asthma | Depression |
| Digestion, poor | Energy, lack of |
| Stress | |

# MANDRAKE *(Podophylluim peltatum)*

*Parts used:* Root
*Properties:* Alterative, anthelmintic, antirheumatic, cholagogue, diaphoretic, emetic, hepatic, parasiticide, purgative (mild)

The American variety of mandrake is a very strong glandular stimulant. It is used for chronic liver diseases, skin problems, bile flow, digestion, and the elimination of obstructions. Mandrake is often combined with supporting herbs to regulate liver and bowels, for uterine disorders, and for intermittent fevers. It is being studied as a natural plant cure for cancer. It is a powerful herb and should be used with caution and avoided during pregnancy.

## PRIMARY APPLICATIONS

| | |
|---|---|
| Bowels, lower | Cancer |
| Constipation | Fevers |
| Indigestion | Intestinal problems |
| Liver disorders | Worms |

## SECONDARY APPLICATIONS

| | |
|---|---|
| Asthma | Diarrhea |
| Gallstones | Hay fever |
| Headaches | Jaundice |
| Nervousness | Pain, chronic |
| Poisoning, lead | Rheumatism |
| Tuberculosis, primary | Skin problems |
| Syphilis | Typhoid fever |
| Vomiting | Warts |

# MANGOSTEEN
*(Garcinia mangostana)*

*Parts used:* Fruit
*Properties:* Antioxidant
*Primary nutrients:* Benzophenones, flavonoids, lactones, phenolic acids

The mangosteen is a tropical evergreen tree that grows to be about ten to twenty-five meters tall. These trees are native to Malaysia and other parts of Southeast Asia. Mangosteen fruit is valued for its delicate flavor. Sometimes called the "queen of fruits," it has been described as the tastiest fruit in the world. The fruit has a smooth, thick, firm rind that turns from pale green to dark purple or reddish-purple as it ripens. It is rich in antioxidants known as xanthones, compounds that may provide immune and cardiovascular benefits. Antioxidants help protect cells from damage by free radicals.

For hundreds of years, Southeast Asians have used the mangosteen, especially the rind, to treat infections, alleviate pain, reduce fever, and help with a variety of ailments. Researchers publishing in peer-reviewed journals have discovered more than forty xanthones in mangosteen. There is much anecdotal evidence of health benefits, but these have yet to be proven in human studies.

In one study, six xanthones found in mangosteen were tested in vitro on a variety of carcinomas. One xanthone called garcinone E had powerful cancer-fighting effects on cancer cells of the liver, stomach, and lung. In another study, a substance derived from mangosteen called gamma-mangostin was found to inhibit the first step in the process of creating free radicals in rat cells.

Mangosteen is thought to be helpful with protecting against free radicals, boosting immunity, aiding joint flexibility and decreasing joint inflammation, reducing allergies, and preventing cancer.

## PRIMARY APPLICATIONS

| | |
|---|---|
| Allergies | Cancer |
| Immune function | Joint flexibility |
| Joint inflammation | Mental support |

## MANGOSTEEN JUICE BLENDS

To further enhance the healing and healthful properties of mangosteen, some products are available that include other botanicals, such as grapeseed, blueberries, sea buckthorn, green tea, grapes, and lycium. These additional ingredients have abundant quantities of xanthones, flavonoids, amino acids, polyphenols, anthocyanins, and carotenoids, which add a powerful antioxidant complement to mangosteen, "the queen of fruits."

# MARJORAM *(Origanum vulgare)*

*Parts used:* Entire plant
*Properties:* Alterative, antiseptic, antispasmodic, carminative, diaphoretic, emmenagogue, expectorant, rubefacient, stimulant
*Primary nutrients:* Calcium, iron, magnesium, niacin, phosphorus, potassium, riboflavin, silicon, sodium, thiamine, vitamins A, B12, and C, zinc

Marjoram was used by the ancient Greeks, who made garlands of it for weddings and funerals. It was thought to be precious to Aphrodite, the goddess of love. Greek couples wore wreaths of marjoram around their necks. The legend was that if marjoram was applied to the skin before sleep, you would dream of your future spouse. It was used as an antidote for snakebites and to treat rheumatism, muscle and joint pain, and sprains. Roman herbalists found that marjoram was beneficial for treating an upset stomach. Nicholas Culpeper, a seventeenth-century English physician, prescribed the herb for the brain, stomach, phlegm, and chest complaints. Marjoram was introduced into America by early colonists.

Traditionally, marjoram was used as a stimulant and carminative. It is useful for conditions such as asthma, coughs, and various spasmodic afflictions. Marjoram helps to strengthen the stomach and intestines. It is used as an antidote for narcotic poisons and for convulsions and dropsy. It is recommended as a digestive aid, tranquilizer, and cough suppressant.

Marjoram does work as an antispasmodic, aiding in settling the stomach and soothing the digestive tract. It works on the smooth muscle lining of the digestive tract as well as on the uterine muscles for menstrual cramps. It is not recommended for pregnant women.

## PRIMARY APPLICATIONS

| | |
|---|---|
| Colic | Coughs |
| Cramps, abdominal | Headaches, nervous |
| Indigestion | Respiratory problems |

## SECONDARY APPLICATIONS

| | |
|---|---|
| Asthma | Bed-wetting |
| Convulsions | Diarrhea |
| Edema | Fevers |
| Gas | Gastritis |
| Measles | Nightmares |
| Nausea | Neuralgia |
| Poisoning, narcotic | Seasickness |
| Toothaches | Urinary incontinence |

# MARSHMALLOW
*(Althaea officinalis)*

*Parts used:* Root
*Properties:* Alterative, anticatarrhal, anti-inflammatory, antilithic, demulcent, diuretic, emollient, expectorant, galactagogue, lithotriptic, mucilant, nutritive, vulnerary
*Primary nutrients:* Calcium, iodine, iron, pantothenic acid, sodium, vitamins A and B-complex

The name *althaea* is derived from the Greek *altho*, which means to cure. Marshmallow has been used as food and medicine since ancient Egyptian times. One of the herbs found in the grave of a Neanderthal man in a cave in Iraq was marshmallow. It was used anciently for irritated throats and intestinal tracts. Europeans used marshmallow for bronchitis, colds, and coughs because of its soothing and healing properties. Native Americans used it to treat snakebites and wounds.

Marshmallow helps expel phlegm and relaxes the bronchial tubes while soothing and healing. It aids in healing lung ailments such as asthma and inflammation. The soothing and healing properties of the mucilage in marshmallow make it a valuable herb for many lung ailments. It is also useful on sore throats, infections, diarrhea, dysentery, skin irritations, and for coughs. Marshmallow is a powerful anti-inflammatory and anti-irritant, which makes it good for the joints and the gastrointestinal tract. Used as a poultice with cayenne, it can help with gangrene, blood poisoning, burns, bruises, and wounds.

Research has found that the mucilaginous properties of marshmallow yield a soothing effect on the mucous membranes. A study done on animals showed some indication of a reduction in blood sugar levels and hypoglycemic activity. This may be beneficial for diabetics.

## PRIMARY APPLICATIONS

| | |
|---|---|
| Asthma | Bed-wetting |
| Bleeding | Boils |
| Bronchitis | Emphysema |
| Kidney problems | Lung congestion |
| Nervous disorders | Pneumonia |
| Urinary incontinence | Urinary problems |
| Uterine problems | Whooping cough |
| Wounds | |

## SECONDARY APPLICATIONS

| | |
|---|---|
| Allergies | Breast problems |
| Burns | Constipation |
| Coughs | Diabetes |
| Diarrhea | Dysentery |
| Eyes, sore | Gangrene |
| Gastric disorders | Glandular problems |
| Inflammation | Intestinal problems |
| Kidney stones | Lactation, absent |
| Liver disorders | Membranes, irritated |
| Mucus, excessive | Skin disorders |

# MILK THISTLE *(Silybum marianum)*

*Parts used:* Seeds
*Properties:* Alterative, antioxidant, galactagogue, hepatic, stimulant
*Primary nutrients:* Bioflavanoids

Milk thistle was used in Europe as a well-known remedy for liver problems and as a digestive aid. The early Roman writer Pliny the Elder (AD 23–79) explains how the juice of milk thistle mixed with honey was used for carrying off bile. In 1597, Gerard, an herbalist, said that milk thistle was one of the best remedies for liver-related diseases. It was also given to nursing mothers to improve milk production, but there has been no research substantiating this treatment.

The liver is an extremely important organ in the body. It filters toxic material from the body, preventing accumulation that can lead to disease and even death. The vital functions of the liver are often overlooked but nevertheless are extremely important. It is essential to keep the liver working properly. Milk thistle has been proven to be very beneficial for liver function. Observations have shown that milk thistle extract can help reverse both acute and chronic liver problems, such as cirrhosis and viral hepatitis. The bioflavonoid content may account for antioxidant properties in milk thistle. It has also been found to help heal the liver from damage occurring from alcohol toxicity. It has been used to treat many different liver ailments, such as fatty liver disorders, chronic hepatitis, inflammation of the bile ducts, hardening of the liver, and cirrhosis. It is also thought to actually help liver regeneration when part of the liver is removed.

Milk thistle has a complex of compounds known as silymarin that includes silybin, silydianin, and silychristin. These substances are known to protect the liver against some toxins and help increase the function of this important organ. Silybin is used as an antidote to the deadly deathcap mushroom, which is known to destroy liver cells. The deathcap species is one of the most toxic of liver poisons and has up to a 50 percent death rate. In one study, sixty patients suffering from deathcap poisoning were treated with silybin, with incredible results. None of the participants died. Silymarin is an effective remedy if administered within forty-eight hours of ingestion. It seems to occupy the receptor sites to protect the cell membranes. It not only works to treat serious liver conditions, but it also prevents damage from occurring. It contains amines, thyramine and histamine, that are known to help stimulate the production and flow of bile. Researchers have found that silymarin works almost exclusively on the kidneys and liver. It probably moves in a cycle from blood plasma to the liver bile and concentrates in the liver cells. It counteracts the destructive activity of poisons or toxins that enter the body. The properties of milk thistle have been confirmed in animal studies to be a protection in liver disorders. Rats and dogs injected with liver-destructive toxins were protected with silymarin. Other studies indicate that milk thistle is beneficial for severe liver disorders such as hepatitis and cirrhosis, as well as general liver restoration, protection, and strengthening.

Milk thistle stimulates protein synthesis.

## PRIMARY APPLICATIONS

| | |
|---|---|
| Cirrhosis | Hepatitis |
| Jaundice | Kidney problems |
| Liver disorders | |

## SECONDARY APPLICATIONS

| | |
|---|---|
| Alcoholism | Appetite loss |
| Blood pressure, high | Boils |
| Chemotherapy | Depression |
| Epilepsy | Fatty deposits |
| Gas | Heartburn |
| Heart problems | Hemorrhages |
| Hypoglycemia | Indigestion |
| Lactation, absent | Menstrual symptoms |
| Radiation, effects of | Skin diseases |
| Veins, varicose | Toxins, effects of |

# MISTLETOE

*(Phorandendron flavescens* and *Viscum flavescens)*

*Parts used:* Entire plant
*Properties:* Alterative, antineoplastic, antispasmodic, diuretic, emetic, emmenagogue, hypotensive, nervine, sedative, stimulant
*Primary nutrients:* Cadmium, calcium, cobalt, copper, iodine, iron, magnesium, potassium, sodium, vitamin B12

Mistletoe is a plant full of holiday tradition. Many individuals, while celebrating Christmas, hang mistletoe over a doorway. Those caught under the mistletoe are entitled to a kiss. The history of mistletoe is full of mystery and intrigue. Pagan traditions were difficult to suppress with the spread of Christianity. Mistletoe was banned in some Christian nations, but many brought old rites, such as the use of mistletoe, into their homes as a part of the Christmas celebration. The Druids, or ancient priests of the Celts, cut mistletoe from the sacred oak and gave it away as charms. Early Europeans used mistletoe in their ceremonies, which probably started the traditional use of mistletoe today.

Mistletoe is a plant that grows as a parasite on the trunks and branches of trees. It is often difficult to get rid of. It is an evergreen with leathery leaves and small yellow flowers that bloom in February and March. The seeds are scattered by birds as they fly away with seeds attached to their beaks, which they then clean on other trees.

The medicinal properties of mistletoe are well known. There are two varieties, European and American mistletoe. They are of the same family but vary somewhat in their effects. Some studies comparing the two types have found similar pharmacological effects. The stems and leaves contain related compounds.

European mistletoe *(Viscum album)* is an ancient herb with many medicinal properties. It has been used to control high blood pressure and arteriosclerosis due to the choline and acetylcholine-tyramine substances in the plant. This causes a lowering of the blood pressure. Studies have found that this variety of mistletoe has antineoplastic and antitumor activity in vitro. Lung and liver tumors were reduced in animal studies using mistletoe extract. Limited human studies have found beneficial results. Mistletoe has been used to stop hemorrhaging, especially for postpartum and intestinal bleeding. It is also considered to be a nervine antispasmodic when taken in small doses. It should be noted that mistletoe is considered to be poisonous by some individuals and should be used with caution. The leaves of the young twigs are the Parts used medicinally. The berries are poisonous in both varieties and should be kept away from children.

American mistletoe *(Phoradendron flavescens)* is generally thought to raise blood pressure. It is a powerful stimulant to smooth muscles and increases the contractions of the intestines and uterus. It has been used as a circulatory and uterine stimulant. The American variety is not as widely used as European mistletoe.

## PRIMARY APPLICATIONS

| | |
|---|---|
| Blood pressure, high | Chorea |
| Circulation, poor | Convulsions |
| Epilepsy | Hemorrhages, internal |
| Menstruation, excessive | Nervousness |
| Spleen ailments | |

## SECONDARY APPLICATIONS

| | |
|---|---|
| Arteriosclerosis | Arthritis |
| Asthma | Blood impurities |
| Cholera | Delirium |
| Gallbladder problems | Heart problems |
| Hypertension | Hypoglycemia |
| Infection | Migraines |
| Neuralgia | Poisoning, blood |
| Rheumatism | Skin inflammation |
| Tumors | Wounds |

# MUGWORT *(Artemisia vulgaris)*

*Parts used:* Root, leaves
*Properties:* Abortifacient, anthelminthic
*Primary nutrients:* Lipophilic flavonoids, sesquiterpene lactones

Mugwort, native to Europe, Asia, and northern Africa, is also sometimes called felon herb, St. John's plant, chrysanthemum weed, and wild wormwood. The plant's root has a history of medicinal use. Mugwort was used in the ancient world as a treatment for fatigue and to guard travelers from evil spirits and wild animals. Roman soldiers are said to have placed mugwort in their sandals to keep their feet energized. Chewing mugwort leaves was supposed to curb fatigue. Mugwort is sometimes confused with wormwood *(Artemisia absinthium)*.

Popular in witchcraft, mugwort is said to promote lucid dreaming and astral travel. Smoking or eating mugwort before going to sleep is supposed to make dreams more intense and help the dreamer remember them upon waking.

Mugwort contains wormwood oil, thujone, flavonoids, triterpenes, and coumarin derivatives. Thujone is toxic. Expectant mothers particularly should avoid consuming large amounts of mugwort. The plant is recommended less often now due to toxicity concerns.

Mugwort still has a role in traditional Chinese medicine in an aged, pulverized, and recompounded form in which it is used to correct breech birth presentation. However, a randomized, controlled study in 2005 was inconclusive. Mugwort can cause uterine contractions, so it has been used to induce abortion.

Mugwort leaves have been recommended for colic, diarrhea, constipation, stomach cramps, weak digestion, worm infestation, and persistent vomiting. Mugwort has been used to stimulate secretion of bile and gastric juices; as a laxative, liver tonic, and sedative; to promote circulation; and for hysteria, epilepsy, convulsions in children, and menstrual problems. Mugwort root has been used as a tonic to boost strength and energy. Combined with other ingredients, it has been used for neuroses, neurasthenia, depression, hypochondria, irritability, restlessness, insomnia, and anxiety.

## PRIMARY APPLICATIONS

Anxiety
Colic
Constipation
Depression
Diarrhea
Digestion
Epilepsy
Hysteria
Insomnia
Menstrual problems
Vomiting
Worms

# MULLEIN (*Verbascum thapsus*)

*Parts used:* Leaves
*Properties:* Analgesic, anticatarrhal, antispasmodic, antitussive, astringent, demulcent, diuretic, expectorant, mucilant, vulnerary
*Primary nutrients:* Calcium, iron, potassium, sulfur, vitamins A, B-complex, and D

Dioscorides suggested using mullein to treat eye problems, tonsillitis, coughs, stings, and toothaches. Mullein was introduced to America by the early European settlers. Native Americans used it to treat lung problems, and some tribes smoked the leaves to treat asthma. It was used during the Civil War for respiratory ailments and was made into a syrup for coughs. Dr. Edward Shook called mullein a great herb in treating tuberculosis and other lung problems.

Traditionally, mullein is well known for its use in treating respiratory disorders such as asthma, bronchitis, coughs, tuberculosis, and congestion. It can help loosen mucus from the respiratory and lymphatic systems. It nourishes and strengthens the lungs. Other uses of mullein include to relieve pain, soothe hemorrhoids, treat burns and bruises, and to induce sleep. It has a calming effect on inflamed tissues and irritated nerves. Mullein helps control coughs, cramps, and spasms. The tea has been used for dropsy, sinusitis, swollen joints, and can be applied to mumps, tumors, a sore throat, and tonsillitis. Though mullein has been used traditionally for

centuries, little is known of the healing components of the herb.

Modern research has found that the saponins, mucilage, and tannins contribute to the soothing topical effect of the plant. These properties are ideal for treating lung ailments, coughs, colds, asthma, whooping cough, and emphysema. Mullein is also suggested for pain, as a sleep aid, a laxative, and to get rid of warts. One study found that mullein inhibits the growth of bacteria known to cause tuberculosis in vitro.

## PRIMARY APPLICATIONS

| | |
|---|---|
| Allergies/hay fever | Asthma |
| Bleeding, bowels/lungs | Bronchitis |
| Colds | Congestion, sinus |
| Coughs | Croup |
| Diarrhea | Dysentery |
| Earaches | Emphysema |
| Glandular problems | Hemorrhages |
| Insomnia | Joints, swollen |
| Lung disorders | Lymphatic congestion |
| Membranes, irritated | Nervousness |
| Pain | Pleurisy |
| Pulmonary disease | Tuberculosis |

## SECONDARY APPLICATIONS

| | |
|---|---|
| Bruises | Constipation |
| Diaper rash | Edema |
| Eye problems | Intestinal problems |
| Menstrual symptoms | Mumps |
| Skin disorders | Throat, sore |
| Toothaches | Tumors |
| Venereal diseases | Ulcers |
| Warts | Wounds |

# MUSHROOMS
(*Maitake, Shiitake, Reishi, Kombucha*)

Mushrooms have emerged as a medicinal food with merit. Used for thousands of years in Asia, these exotic fungi offer great value to the body in preventing illness, healing, and maintaining health.

The numerous varieties of mushrooms have many different characteristics. Some are tasty, others are bitter; some are highly toxic, some work as hallucinogenics, while others possess valuable medicinal properties. In fact, one of the fastest-growing areas in herbal medicine is the use of mushrooms and other fungi. There is growing interest in the importance of the mushroom as a healing food.

The polysaccharides in mushrooms are thought to be the constituent responsible for their medicinal properties. These polysaccharides are able to stimulate the immune response against viral and bacterial diseases. They may even help with life-threatening diseases such as cancer, cardiovascular disease, HIV, free-radical damage, liver problems, and immune-related conditions. Many have benefited from the healing abilities of mushrooms.

# MAITAKE *(Grifola frondosa)*

*Parts used:* Cap and stem
*Properties:* Adaptogen, antineoplastic, antiviral, cardioalterative, immunostimulant

The maitake mushroom, also called "dancing mushroom," "hen in the woods," and "cloud mushroom," is found growing in temperate climates with deciduous forests. These mushrooms grow on trunks or stumps of trees. They are found growing wild in eastern Canada and the northeastern and mid-Atlantic area of the United States. Maitake thrives in northeastern Japan and parts of Europe. The mature plant can weigh as much as twenty pounds.

The maitake mushroom is growing in popularity. It is interesting to note that only twenty years ago, this variety of mushroom was not cultivated or well known. Some Japanese research has shed light on the use of maitake for healing a variety of ailments. Now it is becoming more important in the field of natural health as evidence points to its beneficial effects.

As with other medicinal mushrooms, the maitake is rich in polysaccharides. Polysaccharides are complex natural sugars that appear to have great benefits in healing. The powerful polysaccharide found in maitake is the beta-1.6 glucan, which works to stimulate the immune response. It is a powerful adaptogen, able to help the body heal. These important constituents are able to strengthen the immune system to fight disease.

Studies have found that the maitake mushroom can reduce blood pressure in laboratory experiments on animals. Human studies have also shown impressive results. One study conducted in 1994 at the Ayurvedic Medical Center in New York involving individuals with mild to moderate hypertension found a reduction in blood pressure of 5 to 20 percent in a one-month trial. Another study found that three out of four patients with hypertension showed reduction in their blood pressure while taking 3 grams to 5 grams per day of maitake. Maitake may help lower blood cholesterol levels, which is a major factor in fighting and preventing heart disease.

Maitake contains properties to protect the liver from damage and may even reverse damage that has already occurred. It has demonstrated a hepatoprotective effect to protect the liver from toxins and potential damage. It also has been found to help protect the liver from the detrimental effects of hepatitis.

Cancer continues to be a leading cause of death in the Western world. Human studies have found that the D-fraction polysaccharides in maitake may help treat various types of cancer, such as stomach, lung, liver, and leukemia. The D-fraction component has been found to inhibit carcinogenesis and metastasis. Studies have found in animals that the maitake aided in reducing tumor growth by 90 percent when injected into the abdominal cavity. The immune-stimulating properties increase the protection of interleukin-1, which may be responsible for the anti-tumor abilities.

Maitake was the first mushroom found that inhibited the activity of HIV in laboratory studies. Research done at the National Cancer Institute in Bethesda, Maryland, and in Japan has discovered the ability of the maitake extract to kill the HIV virus. It is the first mushroom to have this ability confirmed in the laboratory. It appears that the maitake can stimulate the action of T cells and prevent them from being destroyed by HIV.

## PRIMARY APPLICATIONS

| | |
|---|---|
| AIDS/HIV | Blood pressure, high |
| Cancer | Heart disease |
| Immune system | Liver disorders |
| Tumors | |

# SHIITAKE *(Lentinus edodes)*

*Parts used:* Stems and caps
*Properties:* Adaptogen, antineoplastic, immuno-stimulant

Shiitake is probably the most popular of all the exotic herbs. This mushroom has been a major contributor to medicine in Asian culture for thousands of years. The large shiitake mushroom grows on dead or dying broad-leaf trees in the temperate mountain regions of Asia. It is prized for its great flavor and nutritional value.

Shiitake is high in B-complex vitamins, including B1, B2, B12, niacin, and pantothenic acid. It also contains protein, enzymes, and eight essential amino acids. The shiitake mushroom is full of nutritional value. These B vitamins are necessary for cell energy and hormone production.

Research has found shiitake to be useful for conditions such as cancer, heart disease, AIDS, flu, tumors, viruses, high blood pressure, obesity, and aging. Shiitake's healing properties are gaining popularity.

Much of the research on shiitake has centered on the polysaccharide lentinan. It is found in the root and cell wall of the plant. Lentinan has a triple helix structure. This shape is thought to be important to the healing properties of shiitake. The lentinan has been found to stimulate the production of T-lymphocytes and interleukin. Interleukin is known to be essential in stopping cancer cell growth and viruses.

Lentinan is a polysaccharide found in shiitake that has been through extensive clinical trials. It is now an approved drug in Japan for treating cancer patients, along with chemotherapy. Dr. Goro Chihara, who isolated the lentinan in shiitake, feels that cancer research should focus on improving the defense mechanism in the individual and on working to restore homeostasis to encourage resistance to disease. Results of studies have shown that shiitake can help prolong the life of cancer patients in advanced stages with minimal side effects.

When taken by animals and humans either orally or by injection, shiitake has been found to possess strong antitumor activity. This action is not directly related to "killing" the cancer, which is the action of chemotherapy. Rather, it helps stabilize and enhance the body's immune system to fight the abnormal cells. It helps the body produce more interferon to defend itself from viruses and potentially harmful matter. Lentinan helps stimulate the T cells and macrophages, which ingest the foreign invaders.

A substance in shiitake has been found to lower cholesterol levels in the blood. High blood cholesterol levels have been linked to many serious conditions, such as arteriosclerosis, heart disease, and stroke. Eritadenine is the constituent in shiitake that is thought to help lower these levels. Rats fed a high-cholesterol diet were found to lower their cholesterol levels by 25 to 45 percent in only a few days. Using the whole herb is thought to produce similar results.

One Japanese study fed human volunteers 90 grams per day of fresh shiitake. Butter was added to their diets, and their cholesterol levels were still lowered by an average of 12 percent.

Shiitake mushroom is also being studied for use with HIV-infected patients. Research has found that shiitake extract aids in promoting macrophages and the growth of bone marrow cells to help stimulate the immune system, which may help slow the development of AIDS symptoms for individuals infected with HIV.

## PRIMARY APPLICATIONS

| | |
|---|---|
| Aging | AIDS/HIV |
| Allergies | Blood pressure, high |
| Cancer | Cholesterol, high |
| Diabetes | Fatigue |
| Heart disease | Immune deficiencies |
| Nervous disorders | |

# REISHI *(Ganoderma lucidum)*

*Parts used:* Body and stem
*Properties:* Adaptogen, alterative, antineoplastic, antiviral, immunostimulant, nervine

Reishi is another remarkable mushroom with healing properties. It affects many different ailments. It has particular benefits as a blood cleanser, supporter of the immune system, strengthener of the circulatory system, helper with tumors and allergies, and in aiding the body when under stress.

The reishi is a bitter mushroom with a dark, glossy exterior. It is found growing in wooded mountain regions of high humidity and little light. It is rarely found growing in the wild, as it is generally found on only two to three out of ten thousand trees. The spores are very hard, which makes germination difficult. Commercial cultivation has allowed the benefits of reishi to reach the general population.

Reishi has not gained popularity because of its taste, but it has long been used as a healing agent. It has been used in China and other Asian countries for thousands of years. The Chinese have looked to reishi as a spiritual healer, and it also has a following among students of meditation, yoga, and tai chi.

There are many different varieties of reishi. Some include the akashiba or red reishi, kuroshiba or black reishi, aoshiba or blue reishi, shiroshiba or white reishi, kishiba or yellow reishi, and the murasakishiba or purple reishi. It is thought that all of the varieties contain the same health benefits. Akashiba is the variety that is cultivated, and because of its abundance, it is used for most research that has been conducted.

Beta D-glucan is one component in reishi found to stimulate the activity of the immune system. It contains antitumor activity and may help fight different types of cancer, such as sarcoma. This polysaccharide found in reishi has shown immunostimulating, antitumor, and antistress activity in animals.

Reishi can be very beneficial for the heart and circulatory system. One study found that reishi extract can lower blood cholesterol levels as well as blood pressure. Reishi was also used to help improve the condition of heart patients by improving coronary heart disease, palpitations, pain, and edema. Other research has found reishi to improve both hypertension and hypotension, improve blood circulation, and reduce incidence of stroke and cardiac problems.

Some other active components of reishi have been found to help in treating allergies. They are similar in structure to steroid hormones and help in treating allergy symptoms. Reishi inhibits the release of histamines, and this can help with allergies, asthma, and other respiratory problems.

Along with other medicinal mushrooms, reishi has been found to help slow the progression of HIV into AIDS. It helps protect T cells to fight the disease. The polysaccharides have been shown to increase the production of white blood cells to fight the infection.

Reishi, as well as other mushrooms, has been found beneficial in treating cancer patients. Studies done at the Cancer Research Center in Moscow have found reishi extract to be a host defense potentiator. This involves increasing the activity of the immune system in order to fight the disease. The beta-D glucan in reishi helps fight different types of cancer.

## PRIMARY APPLICATIONS

| | |
|---|---|
| Aging | AIDS/HIV |
| Allergies | Cancer |
| Fatigue | Immune system |
| Heart disease | Respiratory problems |

# KOMBUCHA

*Parts used:* Entire plant
*Properties:* Antibacterial, antibiotic, antifungal, immunostimulant

Kombucha, also known as Manchurian tea or mushroom, is not officially a member of the fungi family. It is actually a symbiotic culture of genus Saccharomyces yeast and xylinum bacteria. It dates back as far as two thousand years in east Asia. It was originally used for healing in Japan, China, and Korea. Kombucha use spread with the beginning of trade. Merchants took the kombucha to Russia and then to Eastern Europe. Though not technically a fungus, it contains many similar healing properties and is often recommended along with members of the mushroom family.

Kombucha is usually placed in a nutrient solution of distilled water, black tea, and sugar. It then undergoes chemical changes beneficial for human consumption. Chemical reactions occur that are very complex. The kombucha feeds on sugar, producing glucuronic acid, lactic acid, vitamins, amino acids, and some antibiotic solutions. The healing properties are thought to be due to the production of glucuronic acid, B-complex vitamins, C vitamins, and lactic acid.

Russian research has uncovered the presence of substances in the kombucha tea that contain antibiotic properties. The tea was found to prevent the growth and colonization of other yeasts and bacteria.

Kombucha is thought to help with a wide variety of conditions. It seems to have a detoxifying effect on the entire body, which makes it beneficial for invigorating the whole body.

German research led by Dr. Valentin Koehler found that kombucha has the ability to increase the function of the immune system by boosting levels of interferon.

## PRIMARY APPLICATIONS

Immune deficiencies        Toxins, effects of

# MUSTARD *(Sinapis alba)*

*Parts used:* Seeds
*Properties:* Alterative, analgesic, blood purifier, carminative, digestive, diuretic, emetic, expectorant, irritant, rubefacient, stimulant
*Primary nutrients:* Calcium, cobalt, iodine, iron, manganese, phosphorus, potassium, sulfur, vitamins A, B1, B2, B12, and C

Mustard was used by the ancient Greeks for its medicinal value as well as a flavoring. The Romans also used the herb. They added crushed seeds to wine for a spicy flavor. English herbalists John Parkinson and Nicholas Culpeper both recommended mustard for ailments such as epileptic seizures and toothaches. It was used by Native Americans and early colonists for rheumatism and muscle pain.

Mustard is a strong stimulating herb. It promotes the appetite and stimulates the gastric mucous membranes to aid in digestion. An infusion of the mustard seed stimulates urine and helps promote menstruation. It is also a valuable emetic for narcotic poisoning because it empties the stomach without depression of the system. Mustard is often used externally as a plaster or poultice for sore, stiff muscles. A mustard plaster may be used to treat congestion, warm the skin, and clear the lungs.

## PRIMARY APPLICATIONS

Indigestion          Liver disorders
Lung disorders

## SECONDARY APPLICATIONS

Appetite loss            Arthritis
Blood impurities         Breath, odor
Bronchitis               Emphysema
Feet, sore               Fevers
Gas                      Hiccups
Kidney problems          Pleurisy
Pneumonia                Snakebites
Sprains                  Throat, sore

# MYRRH
*(Balsamodendron myrrha or Commiphora myrrha)*

*Parts used:* Resin
*Properties:* Alterative, antibiotic, antimicrobial, antiseptic, astringent, carminative, emmenagogue, expectorant, stimulant
*Primary nutrients:* Chlorine, potassium, silicon, sodium, zinc

Myrrh was valued anciently as a fragrance and healing agent. Ancient Egyptian women used the burned myrrh to rid their homes of fleas. The Chinese used myrrh to heal wounds and for menstrual problems, bleeding, hemorrhoids, and ulcerated sores. It is mentioned frequently throughout the Bible: In the Old Testament, it is referred to in the preparation of the holy ointment (Exodus 30:23). In Esther 2:15, myrrh is used as a purification herb for women, and in Psalm 45:8, it is a perfume.

Myrrh is a powerful antiseptic. Like echinacea, it is a valuable cleansing and healing agent. Myrrh works on the stomach and colon to soothe and heal inflammation. Myrrh provides vitality and strength to the digestive system. It stimulates the flow of blood to the capillaries. It helps speed the healing of the mucous membranes, including the gums, throat, stomach, and intestines. It can be applied to sores and works as an antiseptic. It can help promote menstruation, aid digestion, heal sinus problems, soothe inflammation, and speed the healing process.

Research has verified the use of myrrh as an antiseptic. It is sometimes added to mouthwash and toothpaste. Myrrh has also been found to have mild astringent and antimicrobial properties. Myrrh contains silymarin, which protect the liver from chemical toxins and help increase liver function.

## PRIMARY APPLICATIONS

| | |
|---|---|
| Asthma | Bronchitis |
| Colds | Colitis |
| Colon problems | Cuts |
| Emphysema | Gangrene |
| Gastric disorders | Gums, sore |
| Hemorrhoids | Herpes |
| Hypoglycemia | Indigestion |
| Infection | Lung diseases |
| Mucus, excessive | Pyorrhea |
| Sinus problems | Sores, mouth/skin |
| Tonsillitis | Toothaches |

## SECONDARY APPLICATIONS

| | |
|---|---|
| Abrasions | Arthritis |
| Boils | Breath, odor |
| Canker sores | Coughs |
| Diarrhea | Diphtheria |
| Eczema | Gas |
| Menstrual symptoms | Nervous conditions |
| Phlegm | Rheumatism |
| Scarlet fever | Thyroid problems |
| Tuberculosis | Ulcers |
| Wounds | Yeast infections |

# NETTLE *(Urtica dioica)*

*Parts used:* Leaves and root
*Properties:* Alterative, antiseptic, astringent, blood purifier, diuretic, expectorant, galactagogue, hemostatic, nutritive
*Primary nutrients:* Calcium, chlorophyll, chromium, copper, iron, manganese, potassium, protein, silicon, sodium, sulfur, vitamins A, C, D, E, F, and P, zinc

Nettle is native to Europe and is also found throughout the United States and into Canada. It was cultivated in Scotland for use in making a durable cloth. Nettle is so rich in chlorophyll that the English used it to make a green dye for camouflage paint during World War II.

Nettle is recognized as one of the most useful of all plants. It contains alkaloids that neutralize uric acid. Decreasing uric acid helps reduce symptoms of conditions such as gout and rheumatism. The astringent activity of nettle helps decrease bleeding. Nettle is rich in iron, which is vital to good circulation. It helps reduce high blood pressure. Tannin found in the nettle root has been used as part of an astringent enema to shrink hemorrhoids and reduce excess menstrual flow. Nettle became popular for its use in irritating the skin of an inflamed area and increasing the flow of blood to reduce inflammation. The stinging action of the nettle is caused by a histamine reaction created by the formic acid in the hairs. Nettle has a reputation for use in cases of asthma and other respiratory conditions.

German physicians recommend the use of nettle root extract for treating urinary retention due to benign prostatic hypertrophy, based on evidence from clinical studies. Other studies have found that nettle root can increase the excretion of chlorides and urea from the urine. The diuretic activity has been confirmed in animal studies. The diuretic properties may be due to the high potassium content, but this has not been verified. A study conducted at the National College of Naturopathic Medicine in Portland, Oregon, found evidence of nettle for treating hay fever. Freeze-dried capsules, 300 mg, were used. There was significant relief from hay fever symptoms in the participants. These capsules are not available to the public.

## PRIMARY APPLICATIONS

| | |
|---|---|
| Bleeding, external/internal | Blood impurities |
| | Blood pressure, high |
| Bronchitis | Diarrhea |
| Rheumatism | |

## SECONDARY APPLICATIONS

| | |
|---|---|
| Anemia | Asthma |
| Circulation, poor | Eczema |
| Hay fever | Hemorrhoids |
| Hives | Kidneys, inflamed |
| Menstruation, excess | Mouth sores |
| Nosebleeds | Skin disorders |
| Vaginitis | |

# NOPAL
*(Opuntia streptacantha, Opuntia ficus-indica)*

*Parts used:* Leaves
*Properties:* Antiasthmatic, astringent, laxative, pectoral, vermifuge
*Primary nutrients:* Mucilage, pectin, phytochemicals

Nopal is another name for the prickly pear cactus. The broad, thick, succulent leaves of the cactus are used for medicinal purposes. Nopal is most commonly found in the southwestern United States.

In Mexico and among Native Americans, dethorned nopal stems are used as food. Early settlers peeled the stems and used them in wound dressings. The gel from the cactus pads would soften the skin, lessening tension against the wound and alleviating pain. Nopal juice is valued as an anti-inflammatory diuretic. Practitioners of folk medicine recommend its use for painful urination. West Coast Indians traditionally ate the mashed pulp of the cactus to ease childbirth. The pulp was also used as a lung remedy and a cardiac aid.

Nopal contains numerous phytochemicals. Among its components are pectin, mucilage, and gums that aid the digestive system. Nopal also contains nutrients that inhibit bowel absorption of dietary fat and excess sugars. Nopal fortifies the liver and pancreas, enhancing insulin's ability to move glucose from the blood into cells, where it produces energy. Researchers have also found nopal to have hypoglycemic benefits in rabbits. This could be helpful for people with diabetes. Other studies have found that nopal lowers serum levels of LDL cholesterol and triglycerides. It may also inhibit cancer growth and prevent cancer development. Laboratory animals treated with cactus juice show increased immune response regarding tumor growth, Epstein-Barr virus, and suppressed immune function.

## PRIMARY APPLICATIONS
Cancer
Diabetes
Digestive aid
High cholesterol
Immune function

# OATSTRAW *(Avena sativa)*

*Parts used:* Stem
*Properties:* Alterative, demulcent, nervine, nutritive, vulnerary
*Primary nutrients:* Calcium, phosphorus, silicon, vitamins A, B1, B2, and E

Oats are thought to have been cultivated for approximately two thousand years. They were brought to the New World by the English colonists and are used extensively in the United States today. Oatmeal is a popular breakfast cereal in many American homes. Oats do well in places with harsh climates, such as Ireland and Scotland, where the grain has been a staple for many years.

Oatstraw is rich in silica, which is found in the nervous system. The brain and nerves need silica. Oatstraw tea is often used to calm the nerves and seems to work rapidly. It may aid relaxation and relieve insomnia and depression. Oatstraw can help strengthen a weak nervous system. It is very relaxing to the body and can help with aches and pains. It can help strengthen the lungs and loosen lung mucus, which can help with colds, allergies, and asthma. The silica in oatstraw is thought to aid in expelling phlegm and mucus buildup in the lungs and bronchial tubes. Oatstraw contains avenin, an alkaloid that stimulates the neuromuscular system. It helps strengthen nerves and muscles. Oatstraw taken regularly can help build the immune system. The silica content may help strengthen the body against disease. It is helpful for building the body and promoting a feeling of well-being. It can nourish the body and aid in the healing process. In homeopathy, a tincture is made from the fresh flowering plant and is used for arthritis, rheumatism, paralysis, liver infections, and skin diseases.

Oatstraw is found in many herbal calcium formulas. It is beneficial for depression, liver, kidneys, exhaustion, insomnia, in lowering blood sugar levels, for skin conditions, and for many other ailments. Oatstraw is a powerful stimulant and rich in nutrients to strengthen the body. It contains antiseptic properties and is an excellent tonic for the whole body. Oatstraw can help with physical fatigue, nervous conditions, depression, and colds.

Oat bran has been studied and found to help reduce cholesterol levels. It may also help reduce high blood pressure.

## PRIMARY APPLICATIONS

| | |
|---|---|
| Appetite loss | Arthritis |
| Bed-wetting | Hair, weak |
| Heart problems | Indigestion |
| Insomnia | Nervousness |
| Urinary problems | |

## SECONDARY APPLICATIONS

| | |
|---|---|
| Boils | Bones, weak |
| Bursitis | Constipation |
| Eyes, itchy | Fingernails, weak |
| Gallbladder | Gout |
| Kidney problems | Liver disorders |
| Lung disorders | Pancreatic problems |
| Paralysis | Rheumatism |
| Skin conditions | Urinary incontinence |

# OREGON GRAPE

*(Berberis aquifolium)*

*Parts used:* Rhizome and root
*Properties:* Alterative, antiseptic, blood purifier, cholagogue, hepatic, nephritic, nutritive, purgative (mild)
*Primary nutrients:* Copper, manganese, silicon, sodium, vitamin C, zinc

Oregon grape tonics were first introduced as medicinal remedies in the late nineteenth century. They were marketed as blood purifiers.

Oregon grape is well known for the treatment of skin diseases caused by toxins in the blood. This is because it stimulates the action of the liver and is one of the best blood cleansers. It also mildly stimulates thyroid function. Oregon grape aids in the assimilation of nutrients, promotes digestion, and is a tonic for all glands.

## PRIMARY APPLICATIONS

| | |
|---|---|
| Acne | Blood conditions |
| Blood impurities | Eczema |
| Jaundice | Liver disorders |
| Psoriasis | Staph infections |

## SECONDARY APPLICATIONS

| | |
|---|---|
| Arthritis, rheumatoid | Bronchitis |
| Constipation, chronic | Hepatitis |
| Herpes | Intestinal problems |
| Kidney problems | Leucorrhea |
| Lymphatic problems | Rheumatism |
| Strength, lack of | Syphilis |
| Uterine problems | Vaginitis |

# PAPAYA *(Carica papaya)*

*Parts used:* Fruit, juice, and seeds
*Properties:* Anti-inflammatory, digestive, expectorant, nutritive, parasiticide, stomachic
*Primary nutrients:* Calcium, iron, magnesium, phosphorus, potassium, sodium, vitamins A, B, C, D, E, G, and K

Papaya was used by natives of the Caribbean after a heavy meal to aid digestion. Meat was wrapped in papaya leaves to cook, making the meat tender. Europeans introduced papaya to the tropical regions of Asia, where it is now cultivated. Native Americans from Central America used the juice of the plant to remove warts, tumors, and corns.

Papaya contains papain, an enzyme that breaks down protein into a more digestible form. It also aids the digestion of fats and carbohydrates. Eating the fruit after a meal can help with digestion. Papaya is also valued as a blood-clotting agent. The leaves have been wrapped around ulcerated skin and open wounds to encourage healing. Papaya seeds are combined with honey to expel worms and reduce enlargement of the liver and spleen. A paste made from the seeds can be applied to the skin to heal ringworm. Papaya juice has been used to dissolve corns, warts, and pimples.

Along with improving digestion, papaya extracts have been found to offer prevention from stomach ulcers in animal studies. The subjects were given high doses of ulcer-causing drugs, and some were given papaya. The ones given papaya developed significantly fewer ulcers. This may prove beneficial for individuals who rely on medications that can cause ulcers.

## PRIMARY APPLICATIONS

| | |
|---|---|
| Bites, insect | Colon problems |
| Gas | Indigestion |
| Intestinal problems | |

## SECONDARY APPLICATIONS

| | |
|---|---|
| Allergies/hay fever | Blood clots |
| Burns | Constipation |
| Gastric disorders | Hemorrhage |
| Sores | Wounds |

# PARSLEY *(Petroselinum staivum)*

*Parts used:* Leaves
*Properties:* Antibacterial, antifungal, antilithic, antirheumatic, antiseptic, antispasmodic, carminative, diuretic, emmenagogue, expectorant, galactagogue, hepatic, lithotriptic, nervine, parasiticide, purgative (gentle), stimulant
*Primary nutrients:* Calcium, chlorophyll, cobalt, copper, iron, potassium, riboflavin, silicon, sodium, sulfur, thiamine, vitamins A, B, and C

Parsley leaves were used by both the ancient Greeks and Romans to flavor and garnish foods. Galen, an ancient Greek physician, recommended parsley for epilepsy and water retention. It was also used as a breath freshener. By the Middle Ages, parsley was well known as a healing remedy for a variety of conditions. The seventeenth-century herbalist Nicholas Culpeper prescribed parsley for water retention, menstruation problems, kidney stones, bladder conditions, and coughs.

Parsley is often recommended as a preventive herb. It is so nutritious that it increases resistance to infections and disease. The roots and leaves are very good for all liver and spleen problems caused by jaundice and venereal diseases. Parsley is effective in treating the kidneys by providing essential nutrients that help cleanse the blood filtering system. It helps protect and strengthen the urinary tract. It is a mild and gentle diuretic. As a diuretic, parsley can help reduce high blood pressure. Parsley is said to contain a substance in which cancerous cells cannot multiply. It should not be used during pregnancy, as it may bring on labor pains and can dry up mother's milk after birth.

Studies done using parsley have found diuretic properties. The apiol and myristicin in the seeds and oil are thought to be the active components responsible for the diuretic activity. In Germany, parsley tea is often prescribed to help reduce high blood pressure. Diuretics are sometimes used to treat this condition. Parsley may also be used to treat congestive heart failure when water retention is a problem. But any use of parsley should be monitored and supervised by a physician. In Russia, a product containing 85 percent parsley juice is used to induce contractions during labor. Apiol and myristicin are thought to stimulate uterine contractions. In vitro studies have found some mild antibacterial and antifungal activity in parsley extracts.

## PRIMARY APPLICATIONS

| | |
|---|---|
| Blood impurities | Cystitis |
| Gallstones | Jaundice |
| Kidney inflammation | Lactation, absent |
| Urine retention | |

## SECONDARY APPLICATIONS

| | |
|---|---|
| Allergies/hay fever | Arthritis |
| Asthma | Back pain, lower |
| Blood pressure, low | Breath, odor |
| Cancer | Coughs |
| Conjunctivitis | Gonorrhea |
| Gout | Indigestion |
| Liver disorders | Menstruation, absent |
| Nerve problems, sciatic | Pituitary problems |
| Prostate problems | Rheumatism |
| Thyroid problems | Tumors |
| Veins, varicose | Venereal diseases |

# PARTHENIUM
*(Parthenium integrifolium)*

*Parts used:* Leaves, roots
*Properties:* Antiperiodic, emmenagogue, lithotriptic
*Primary nutrients:* Sesquiterpene esters

Parthenium, also called American feverfew, prairie dock, or wild quinine, is a perennial herb found in the eastern United States. The fresh leaves were traditionally used by the Catawba Indians in a poultice to treat burns. Europeans who settled in the Midwest discovered that Native Americans used parthenium for sore throats and coughs.

Parthenium is a valuable medicinal herb. It is used as an antiperiodic, emmenagogue, and lithotriptic. It has been used in folk medicine to treat debility, fatigue, respiratory infection, gastrointestinal infection, and venereal disease. Parthenium is currently used by herbalists for lymphatic congestion, colds, ear infections, sore throats, fevers, and Epstein-Barr virus. The tops of the plant are bitter and are used as a substitute for quinine to treat intermittent fevers.

Parthenium has been studied in many European laboratories and clinics. This research indicates that the herb stimulates the immune system. Parthenium contains the sesquiterpene esters echinadiol, epoxyecinadiol, echinaxanthol, and dihydroxynardol. These components enhance the ability of the blood cells to digest foreign particles and help heal wounds. The plant seems to be a liver-stimulating bitter that helps detoxify the blood.

Studies have shown that parthenium can activate natural killer cells and other immune cells. The herb has often been sold as (or combined with) echinacea for more than fifty years. Both plants are in the sunflower family, and their roots are strikingly similar. Many people have been finding these parthenium products beneficial.

## PRIMARY APPLICATIONS

Burns
Colds
Ear infections
Epstein-Barr virus
Fatigue
Fever
Gastrointestinal infections
Lymphatic congestion
Respiratory infections
Sore throats
Venereal disease

# PASSION FLOWER
(*Passiflora incarnata*)

*Parts used:* Herb
*Properties:* Anodyne, anti-inflammatory, antispasmodic, diaphoretic, nervine, sedative
*Primary nutrients:* Calcium and magnesium

Passion flower is very soothing on the nervous system and for conditions such as insomnia, hysteria, anxiety, and hyperactivity. It is also useful for eye conditions such as inflammations, dimness of vision, and eye irritations. Native Americans used passion flower as a tonic and a poultice for bruises and injuries. The Aztecs used it as a sedative and for pain. The juice was used for sore eyes and the crushed plant tops and leaves for treating hemorrhoids and skin eruptions. It was listed in the National Formulary from 1916 to 1936. R. Swinburne Clymer, MD, referred to passion flower as the opium (nonpoisonous and not dangerous) of the natural physician.

Passion flower depresses the central nervous system to help with insomnia, anxiety, and nervousness and may be useful in lowering high blood pressure. Combinations containing valerian and passion flower are considered very useful as a natural tranquilizer. Passion flower is thought to be safe for children as well as the elderly.

Passion flower contains complex substances that work on the nervous system as a sedative. The components responsible for the overall effect are not specifically known, although maltol, ethyl-maltol, and flavonoids are thought to contribute. Most research has focused on the sedative action, with good results. The extract of passion flower has been found to reduce locomotor activity and prolong sleep. One of the active ingredients of the plant is thought to be passiflorine, which has some similar activity to morphine. It contains anti-inflammatory properties that may be useful for those suffering from arthritis. Another possible benefit of passion flower is its ability to kill a wide variety of organisms, such as yeasts, molds, and bacteria. As an antispasmodic, passion flower works on the digestive system smooth muscles as well as the uterine muscles, making it effective as a digestive aid and for menstrual cramps.

Passion flower contains calcium and magnesium, both essential for the nervous system.

## PRIMARY APPLICATIONS

| | |
|---|---|
| Alcoholism | Anxiety |
| Asthma, spasmodic | Blood pressure, high |
| Eye infections | Eye tension |
| Fevers | Headaches |
| Insomnia | Menopausal symptoms |
| Nervousness | Neuralgia |

## SECONDARY APPLICATIONS

| | |
|---|---|
| Bronchitis | Convulsions |
| Depression | Diarrhea |
| Dysentery | Epilepsy |
| Eyestrain | Menstruation, painful |
| Muscle spasms | Pain |
| Parkinson's disease | Restlessness |
| Seizures | Vision, poor |

# PAU D'ARCO (*Tabebuia avellanedae*)

*Parts used:* Inner bark

*Properties:* Adaptogen, alterative, analgesic, antifungal, antimicrobial, antineoplastic, antiviral, astringent, blood purifier

*Primary nutrients:* Calcium, iron, magnesium, manganese, phosphorus, potassium, selenium, sodium, vitamins A, B-complex, and C, zinc

In South America, this herb was known for its healing powers by the Callaway tribe. They called the herb taheebo and have been using it for more than one thousand years. Pau d'arco was used anciently by the Inca civilization's medicine men. Traditions passed down through the generations included the use of pau d'arco. In the Santo André Hospital in Rio de Janeiro, Brazil, pau d'arco has been used to treat cancer and other illnesses since the 1970s. Pau d'arco has become a well-known herb for healing and protecting the body from disease.

This tall tree grows high in the Andes and can weather the worst storms because of its hard wood and deep roots. Pau d'arco is found in the inner bark of the red lapacho tree. Most of the trees surrounding the red lapacho eventually become covered with spores that lead to fungus, and this will eventually kill the trees. But the red lapacho seems to be able to resist the spores. This may be a factor in pau d'arco's ability to heal the body and resist disease.

There seems to be some evidence of antitumor properties in pau d'arco. Many individuals have taken this herb when undergoing radiation and chemotherapy in order to strengthen the body and help prevent the side effects associated with these treatments. Pau d'arco seems to be a powerful alterative and blood builder. It has the ability to increase the hemoglobin and red corpuscles in the blood. It gives the body greater vitality by increasing the resistance to disease. It seems to aid the body by giving it the energy and strength to defend itself and resist disease. It is also known to help inhibit the growth of tumors while increasing the growth of normal tissue. It is used to aid in the assimilation of nutrients and the elimination of waste matter. Pau d'arco is often referred to as the "everything" herb because of its uses for many disorders. Pau d'arco has been used by many along with other medications. There seem to be no problems associated with the combination. It is used to help counteract the side effects of some medications and is thought to reduce liver damage caused by some drugs. Herbalists have used pau d'arco to treat many conditions. It is effective as an immune system enhancer and can aid in treating conditions such as cancer, leukemia, tumors, and blood disorders. It is also used to treat the pain of arthritis and for diabetes, candidiasis, herpes, liver ailments, hypoglycemia, and assimilation of nutrients.

Studies have found that the quinone lapachol, a component of pau d'arco, has antimicrobial and antiviral properties. It also seems to have an antitumor effect without any toxic side effects. Other components, including beta-lapachone, hydroxynapthoquinone, alpha-lapachone, and xyloidone, are effective against numerous viruses, bacteria, and fungi, including herpes, influenza, poliovirus, and many others. Dr. Theodoro Meyer, a researcher at the National University of Tucumán in Argentina, discovered the substance xyloidin, which is able to kill viruses. Xyloidin is also beneficial in inhibiting the causative agents of dysentery, tuberculosis, and anthrax.

## PRIMARY APPLICATIONS

| | |
|---|---|
| AIDS/HIV | Blood impurities |
| Cancer | Candidiasis |
| Diabetes | Eczema |
| Herpes | Hodgkin's disease |
| Immune system | Leukemia |
| Liver disorders | Pain |
| Prostate problems | Rheumatism |
| Toxemia | Tumors |

## SECONDARY APPLICATIONS

| | |
|---|---|
| Allergies | Anemia |
| Arthritis | Asthma |
| Bronchitis | Circulation, poor |
| Colitis | Constipation |
| Diarrhea | Fevers |
| Gastritis | Hemorrhages |
| Infection | Intestinal problems |
| Lung disorders | Lupus |
| Nephritis | Psoriasis |
| Skin disorders | Ulcers |
| Urinary problems | Venereal diseases |

# PAWPAW *(Asimina triloba)*

*Parts used:* Bark, roots, twigs, seeds
*Properties:* Antimicrobial, antitumor, cytotoxic, pesticidal
*Primary nutrients:* Acetogenins, alkaloids

Pawpaw, also known as custard apple, prairie banana, Ozark banana, or poor man's banana, is a small tree native to the eastern United States. The name probably comes from the Spanish word *papaya*, perhaps due to pawpaw fruit's similarity to that fruit. The fruit of this tree is nutritious, with a flavor similar to banana or mango, and it contains more protein than most fruits.

The earliest written record of pawpaws is in the de Soto expedition's report of 1541. They found Native Americans growing it east of the Mississippi River. Lewis and Clark relied heavily on pawpaws during their journey. Chilled pawpaw fruit was one of George Washington's favorite desserts, and Thomas Jefferson planted it at Monticello.

The bark, which contains alkaloids, was traditionally used as a medicine. In homeopathy, pawpaw is used as a treatment for scarlet fever and skin rashes. Researchers are studying components of the bark and leaves for potential anticancer benefits. The roots, bark, twigs, and seeds of the pawpaw tree are rich in acetogenins, which are known for their antibacterial, antitumor, cytotoxic, pesticidal, immunosuppressive antimalarial, and antifeedant benefits. No animal or clinical studies have been done yet, but scientists have performed some in vitro research. These studies have demonstrated that specific acetogenins found in pawpaw extract show powerful cytotoxic potential against lung, breast, and colon cancer.

Although pawpaw has been used in homeopathy, higher doses can be toxic because of the extract's cytotoxic and pesticidal properties.

## PRIMARY APPLICATIONS

Cancer
Scarlet fever
Skin rashes

# PEACH *(Prunus persica)*

*Parts used:* Bark, seed, and leaves
*Properties:* Alterative, antibiotic, antiseptic, antispasmodic, astringent, carminative, demulcent, diuretic, emmenagogue, expectorant, nervine, parasiticide, purgative (mild), sedative, stomachic

The peach has a long history of use in China. It was used anciently for its therapeutic value. The seed of the peach contains some cyanide, which is thought to be low enough in content by some herbalists to produce therapeutic value without being toxic.

The peach contains curative powers. The powdered, dried leaves have been used to heal sores and wounds. Peach contains strengthening powers for the nervous system and has mild sedative properties. It is useful for chronic bronchitis and chest complaints because of its expectorant properties. It also stimulates urine flow and has anticancer properties.

## PRIMARY APPLICATIONS

| | |
|---|---|
| Bronchitis, chronic | Cancer |
| Congestion, lung | Kidney problems |
| Nausea | Urinary problems |
| Water retention | |

## SECONDARY APPLICATIONS

| | |
|---|---|
| Blood impurities | Constipation |
| Gastric disorders | Insomnia |
| Jaundice | Morning sickness |
| Mucus, excessive | Nervousness |
| Parasites | Sores |
| Uterine problems | Whooping cough |

# PENNYROYAL *(Hedeoma pulegioides)*

*Parts used:* Entire plant
*Properties:* Alterative, antispasmodic, antivenomous, aromatic, carminative, decongestant, diaphoretic, diuretic, emmenagogue, nervine, oxytocic, parasiticide, sedative, stimulant, stomachic

European settlers brought pennyroyal to the New World. They found that Native Americans were using the American variety of pennyroyal for repelling insects, for skin irritations, and many of the same ailments as their own variety. The herb was also used to soothe the stomach and relieve cold symptoms. Pennyroyal found in America and Europe have similar properties. The European variety is thought to be much more potent.

Pennyroyal contains a volatile oil that works to remove gas from the stomach. It can be consumed as a tea or used as a footbath. If taken a few days before menstruation is due, it can help increase a suppressed flow. A tea is also beneficial in relieving cold symptoms and promoting perspiration. The herb has a strong, minty odor and is used externally to repel insects such as fleas, flies, and mosquitoes.

Pennyroyal oil is very concentrated and has been linked to toxic results. The oil has been associated with abortions and convulsions, with deaths resulting. The oil is thought to irritate the uterus, causing uterine contractions. The action is not predictable and is potentially dangerous. The oil should be used only externally as a natural insect repellent. The herb is suggested for use as a decongestant for coughs and colds. Tea made from the herb is not associated with toxicity. It is a member of the mint family and helps relax the digestive tract and soothe the stomach.

## PRIMARY APPLICATIONS

| | |
|---|---|
| Bronchitis | Childbirth pain |
| Colds | Colic |
| Cramps, uterine | Fevers |
| Gas | Lung infections |
| Menstruation, absent | |

## SECONDARY APPLICATIONS

| | |
|---|---|
| Convulsions | Coughs |
| Cramps, abdominal | Delirium |
| Earache | Flu |
| Gout | Headaches |
| Leprosy | Measles |
| Migraines | Mucus |
| Nausea | Phlegm |
| Pleurisy | Pneumonia |
| Smallpox | Sunstroke |
| Toothaches | Tuberculosis |
| Ulcers | Uterine problems |
| Vertigo | |

# PEPPERMINT *(Mentha piperita)*

*Parts used:* Leaves and oil
*Properties:* Antibacterial, anti-inflammatory, antispasmodic, aromatic, carminative, diaphoretic, rubefacient, stimulant
*Primary nutrients:* Copper, iodine, inositol, iron, magnesium, niacin, potassium, silicon, sulfur, vitamins A and C

The Romans and Greeks used mint in some of their sacred rites. It was highly regarded for medicinal purposes. The Romans used mint as a stomach aid and to promote digestion. The Greeks also used this herb for many different ailments. Mint abounds in stories from Greek mythology. Native Americans used peppermint leaf tea as a carminative, to prevent vomiting, nausea, and fevers. Peppermint is native to Europe. There are many different variations of the peppermint, and it is thought to be a hybrid between spearmint and water mint.

Peppermint leaf is one of the great herbal remedies and useful to have around the house. It is easy to grow, either in the garden or the home. It contains a warming oil that is effective as a nerve stimulant. The oil aids in increasing oxygen in the blood and works to clean and strengthen the entire body. Peppermint works as a sedative on the stomach. It has been found to contain properties that stimulate the flow of bile and help settle the stomach after vomiting. It is beneficial for nausea, chills, colic, fevers, gas, and diarrhea. It has a cleansing, soothing, and relaxing effect on the body. Herbalists have long recommended peppermint for digestive problems. It is also used for convulsions in infants, to increase respiration, for colds, and to strengthen the entire body.

The menthol in peppermint is thought to be the major component responsible for its medicinal value. Plants contain between 50 and 78 percent menthol. Research has found numerous volatile oils in peppermint that possess antibacterial activity in vitro. Just how effective peppermint will be in clinical studies has yet to be determined. The oil of peppermint is also thought to soothe gastrointestinal contractions and help relieve gas. The volatile oils produce relaxation on the smooth muscles. This may help with conditions such as irritable bowel, abdominal pain, and other gastrointestinal complaints. Research conducted in 1979 found that peppermint oil capsules were effective in treating irritable bowel syndrome. One study done using laboratory mice found peppermint leaf extract to produce a mild sedative effect. In animal studies, the azulene in peppermint oil has been found to contain anti-inflammatory properties.

## PRIMARY APPLICATIONS

| | |
|---|---|
| Appetite loss | Colds |
| Colic | Digestion |
| Fever | Gas |
| Headaches | Heartburn |
| Nausea | Nerves |
| Shock | Spasms, bowel |
| Vomiting | |

## SECONDARY APPLICATIONS

| | |
|---|---|
| Chills | Cholera |
| Constipation | Convulsions |
| Cramps, stomach/uterine | Depression |
| Dizziness | Flu |
| Heart problems | Insomnia |
| Menstrual symptoms | Morning sickness |
| Motion sickness | Neuralgia |
| Shingles | Sores, mouth |
| Spasms, stomach | Throat, sore |

# PERIWINKLE

*(Vinca major; Vinca minor)*

*Parts used:* Entire plant
*Properties:* Antineoplastic, astringent, hemostatic, nervine, sedative

Periwinkle has been used for centuries in different areas of the world to treat a variety of conditions. Periwinkle grows in temperate climates and is often grown as an ornamental plant. In India, periwinkle juice from the leaves is applied to bee stings and bug bites. The plant grows well in Hawaii, and the extract has been applied to wounds to stop bleeding. Periwinkle grows in South America and has been used for various medicinal purposes. Native healers in Madagascar used periwinkle for cancer. Two anticancer drugs, vincristine sulfate and vinblastine sulfate, were developed from the periwinkle plant after the herbal healers in Madagascar were studied.

Periwinkle is considered a good binder and can be chewed to stop bleeding in the nose or mouth. Historically, it has been used for female complaints such as excessive menstrual bleeding and uterine discharge, as well as aiding blood coagulation in wounds. It is also effective in treating colitis, diarrhea, hemorrhoids, high blood pressure, headaches, migraines, nervous conditions, and diabetes.

Research supports the claims that periwinkle has anticancer attributes. Anticancer agents in periwinkle have been used to treat Hodgkin's disease, leukemia, and cancer of the lungs, liver, and kidneys, as well as other types of cancer.

## PRIMARY APPLICATIONS

| | |
|---|---|
| Cancer | Diabetes |
| Hemorrhoids | Nervousness |
| Ulcers | |

## SECONDARY APPLICATIONS

| | |
|---|---|
| Bleeding | Congestion |
| Constipation, chronic | Cramps |
| Dandruff | Diarrhea, chronic |
| Hemorrhages, internal | Leukemia |
| Menstrual bleeding | Mucus, excessive |
| Nightmares | Skin disorders |
| Sores | Toothache |

# PHELLODENDRON
*(Phellodendron amurense)*

*Parts used:* Bark
*Properties:* Antibacterial, antifungal, anti-inflammatory, antiparasitic, immunosuppressive
*Primary nutrients:* Berberine, jactorrhizine, palmatine, phellodendrine

Phellodendron is a tree native to east and northeast Asia. It is not related to the houseplant philodendron. Phellodendron has been used in traditional Chinese medicine and is a popular element in Chinese herbal combinations. The plant's inner bark is used medicinally.

The Chinese have used phellodendron in formulas for gastrointestinal problems, inflammatory ailments, as an antibacterial, for swollen joints in the legs, and for jaundice. Phellodendron bark is often used along with other herbs.

Phellodendron's alkaloid phytochemicals include berberine, which has antibacterial and antifungal activity; jactorrhizine, which may be anti-mutagenic; phellodendrine, which may act as an immune suppressant; and palmatine, which may be a vasodilator. Berberine is likely the most active component, as it is well known for its antifungal, antiparasitic, and anti-inflammatory benefits.

Phellodendron has been used to treat diabetes, meningitis, pneumonia, tuberculosis, eye infections, and cirrhosis of the liver. Phellodendron has exhibited antibacterial and anti-inflammatory activity when used topically. The herb shows pronounced effectiveness against many kinds of candida. It may also be useful as an immunosuppressive; laboratory animals that had transplants and were given phellodendron had fewer organ rejections.

Several studies have supported phellodendron's efficacy as an anti-inflammatory. Berberine is thought to prevent the production of enzymes that initiate inflammatory responses in the body. The herb has also shown usefulness as an ulcer remedy. Research on phellodendron in diabetes treatment showed the herb was able to limit the damage done to the eyes and kidneys as the disease progressed.

High doses of phellodendron may cause nausea and vomiting. Its high berberine content means it should not be taken by pregnant women or those with heart and circulation problems.

## PRIMARY APPLICATIONS

| | |
|---|---|
| Cirrhosis, liver | Diabetes |
| Eye infections | Gastrointestinal issues |
| Jaundice | Meningitis |
| Pneumonia | Swollen joints, legs |
| Tuberculosis | |

# PINE *(Pinus maritima)*

*Parts used:* Bark and oil
*Properties:* Anti-inflammatory, antineoplastic, antioxidant, rubefacient, stimulant
*Primary nutrients:* Vitamin C and bioflavonoids

Various tribes of Native Americans relied on the bark of pine trees to treat a number of disorders. Because of its marvelous healing benefits, the Annedda pine was called the "tree of life." Diaries written by the noted explorer Jacques Cartier in 1535 reveal early medicinal uses for pine tree bark. Cartier and his crew, caught in the bitter snows of Quebec while navigating the St. Lawrence River, came down with scurvy while living on hard biscuits and cured meat. Several men died before they were approached by Quebec Indians, who prepared a tea from the bark of a pine tree. The men drank the tea, applied poultices to their wounds, and were soon healed. The recovery that they considered miraculous is actually a result of the vitamin C and bioflavonoids in the bark. A French professor, Jacques Masquelier, discovered Cartier's account and became intrigued with studying pine tree extract. From the extract, he isolated a certain kind of proanthocyanidin flavonoid later found to have antioxidant attributes.

Pine bark extract has become an important herbal remedy because of its antioxidant power. It binds with collagen fibers and helps restore skin elasticity as well as protecting it from free-radical damage, thereby preventing excess and premature wrinkles. Studies done on proanthocyanidin flavonoids found an anti-enzyme effect that prevents the breakdown of collagen and elastin. This effect is what keeps the skin firm and youthful.

Pine tree bark also protects capillaries from free-radical damage that can cause phlebitis, varicose veins, and bruising. Those suffering from skin conditions such as psoriasis can also benefit from pine bark extract.

In addition to its antioxidant power, pine bark extract is a natural anti-inflammatory that can help heal joint pain associated with such things as arthritis and sports injuries. It also helps control and prevent edema and bursitis.

Eyesight is another important area where pine bark extract can help. It reduces the risk of and treats diabetic retinopathy. Studies have determined its benefits in improving night vision as well. In one study, there was a marked improvement in visual performance in the proanthocyanidin (pycnogenol) group over a placebo group.

Pine bark extract may also aid in inhibiting cellular mutations such as tumors. Some reports have found that pycnogenol can help prevent cellular deterioration in breast tumors and cardiovascular disease. There is also evidence of antiulcer properties that may help prevent the formation of undesirable chemicals in the stomach.

Other conditions that benefit from pine bark proanthocyanidin therapy include autoimmune disorders such as lupus, neural problems such as Parkinson's disease and multiple sclerosis, and vascular problems, including heart disease, atherosclerosis, and strokes. Common complaints such as insomnia, flu, and even the common cold have been treated with pine bark extract. It is beneficial for memory, longevity, and the prostate, and its stimulant properties decrease the production of histamines in allergic reactions such as hay fever.

## PRIMARY APPLICATIONS

| | |
|---|---|
| Allergies/hay fever | Arthritis |
| Atherosclerosis | Brain dysfunction |
| Cancer | Circulation, poor |
| Diabetic retinopathy | Heart disease |
| Sports injuries | Ulcers |
| Vision, poor | |

## SECONDARY APPLICATIONS

| | |
|---|---|
| Arthritis, rheumatoid | Colds |
| Edema | Flu |
| Insomnia | Memory loss |
| Multiple sclerosis | Osteoarthritis |
| Phlebitis | Prostate problems |
| Skin conditions | Stroke |
| Veins, varicose | Viruses |

# PLANTAIN *(Plantago major)*

*Parts used:* Leaves and seeds
*Properties:* Alterative, anti-inflammatory, antiseptic, antispasmodic, antivenomous, astringent, blood purifier, demulcent, diuretic, emollient, expectorant, febrifuge, mucilant, parasiticide, purgative (gentle), vulnerary
*Primary nutrients:* Calcium, potassium, sulfur, trace minerals, vitamins C, K, and T

Plantain is one of the most commonly used plants in the world. From England to the New World, plantain was known for its medicinal properties, and its popularity continues to grow. Plantain seeds are related to psyllium seeds and are often used for the same purposes.

The outer layer of the seeds of plantain contains mucilage, a product that swells up when moist. These seeds help lower cholesterol levels. However, plantain is most known for its gastric benefits. It neutralizes stomach acids and normalizes stomach secretions. Fresh plantain juice has been used to treat mild stomach ulcers. It helps absorb toxins from the bowels and promotes normal bowel function. It is a bulk laxative and, when mixed with water, increases in mass. Studies have confirmed the value of plantain as a mild laxative. In subjects tested, plantain decreased intestinal transit time.

In addition to its intestinal uses, plantain can help with bladder infections and kidney problems, as well as bed-wetting in children.

As an expectorant, plantain ingested in tea clears the head and ears of congestion. The tea is also a beneficial treatment for chronic lung problems in children.

The herb is known for its ability to neutralize poisons in the body. Patients with poison ivy were treated topically with crushed plantain leaves. Itching was eliminated and the condition did not spread in those treated. In addition, the leaves, when applied to a bleeding surface, can stop hemorrhaging. The astringent properties in plantain help stop bleeding and promote healing in wounds.

As an anti-inflammatory, plantain can help with problems such as edema and hemorrhoids. Other conditions plantain has been used for include nerve problems, fevers, burns, eye pain, and jaundice.

## PRIMARY APPLICATIONS

| | |
|---|---|
| Bed-wetting | Bites, snake |
| Cystitis | Diarrhea |
| Intestinal problems | Kidney problems |
| Lung disorders, chronic | Neuralgia |
| Poisoning, blood | Poison ivy |
| Sores | Ulcers |
| Urinary incontinence | Wounds |

## SECONDARY APPLICATIONS

| | |
|---|---|
| Bites, insects | Bronchitis |
| Burns | Cholesterol, high |
| Colitis | Coughs |
| Cuts | Dysentery |
| Edema | Epilepsy |
| Eyes, sore | Fevers |
| Gas | Hemorrhages, external |
| Hemorrhoids | Infections |
| Jaundice | Leucorrhea |
| Menstruation, excessive | Respiratory problems |
| Tuberculosis, primary | Skin conditions |
| Stings | |

# PLEURISY (Asclepias tuberosa)

*Parts used:* Root
*Properties:* Alterative, anodyne, antispasmodic, carminative, diaphoretic, diuretic, emetic, expectorant, febrifuge, nervine, purgative (mild), stimulant

Pleurisy root was named because of its use for treating lung conditions. "Pleurisy" is derived from the Greek root *pleura*, or "lung membranes." As the name implies, this herb is valuable for treating pleurisy, because it relieves chest pain and eases breathing difficulties. It was used by Native Americans, and they introduced it to the European settlers, who were suffering from numerous respiratory problems.

Pleurisy root works primarily as an expectorant. It helps expel phlegm from bronchial and nasal passages. It opens lung capillaries, thereby aiding the release of mucus that thins discharge. This process reduces lung congestion and improves breathing.

Aside from its pulmonary uses, pleurisy root is also used as a gentle tonic for the stomach pain caused by gas, indigestion, and dysentery.

In addition, pleurisy root acts as a powerful diaphoretic to increase body temperature and open pores to induce perspiration. It has also been used against poisoning and acute rheumatism. However, it is not recommended for children.

## PRIMARY APPLICATIONS

| | |
|---|---|
| Asthma, spasmodic | Bronchitis |
| Dysentery, acute | Emphysema |
| Fevers | Indigestion |
| Lung disorders | Pleurisy |
| Pneumonia | |

## SECONDARY APPLICATIONS

| | |
|---|---|
| Croup | Diseases, contagious |
| Flu | Gas |
| Kidney problems | Measles |
| Mucus, excessive | Perspiration, absent |
| Poisoning | Rheumatism, acute |
| Scarlet fever | Tuberculosis |
| Typhus | |

# PRICKLY ASH
*(Xanthoxylum americanum)*

*Parts used:* Bark and berries
*Properties:* Alterative, anthelmintic, antiasthmatic, antispasmodic, astringent, blood purifier, sialagogue, stimulant

Prickly ash was used by some Native American tribes for toothaches and infection and subsequently appeared in the U.S. Pharmacopoeia from 1829 to 1926 and in the National Formulary from 1916 to 1947 as a treatment for rheumatism. Prickly ash was used in the South during cholera and typhus epidemics with positive results. Prickly ash is often used in combination with other herbs.

The nineteenth-century herbalist Samuel Thomson considered it a valuable natural stimulant against problems like rheumatism, cold hands and feet, ague, and fever. It stimulates circulation, which is essential for a healthy body. Prickly ash can help impaired circulation, such as cold extremities and joints. It can also help with arthritis and lethargy, not only because of its stimulant action, but also because it shows promise as a means for enhancing the immune system and relieving exhaustion.

Used as a poultice, prickly ash helps speed the healing of wounds and prevents infection. It helps increase the production of saliva, eliminating mouth dryness. Its bitter and sweet qualities help heal deficiencies of the heart, lungs, spleen, and intestines and strengthens them. For example, it has been used to treat ulcers, asthma, and colic.

Prickly ash also is used to aid digestion, to relieve feminine problems such as premenstrual cramps, and to treat sexually transmitted and skin diseases.

## PRIMARY APPLICATIONS

| | |
|---|---|
| Circulation, poor | Fevers |
| Paralysis | Sores, mouth |
| Ulcers | Wounds |

## SECONDARY APPLICATIONS

| | |
|---|---|
| Ague | Arthritis |
| Asthma | Blood impurities |
| Cholera | Colic |
| Cramps, uterine | Diarrhea |
| Edema | Gas |
| Gastric disorders | Indigestion |
| Lethargy | Liver disorders |
| Rheumatism | Tuberculosis, primary |
| Skin diseases | Syphilis |
| Thyroid problems | Typhus |

# PSYLLIUM *(Plantago ovata)*

*Parts used:* Seeds
*Properties:* Demulcent, mucilant, purgative (mild)
*Primary nutrients:* Fiber, bulking agents

Psyllium was used by Native Americans as an eyewash and to treat sprains and abrasions. It was also (and continues to be) used as a laxative to help relieve constipation. Psyllium contains aucubine, enzymes, fats, glycosides, mucilage, and protein.

Psyllium, taken internally, is an excellent remedy for many problems of the digestive system. It can help prevent autointoxication from the reabsorption of toxins into the bloodstream by removing the toxins if used over a period of time. Because psyllium prevents toxin reabsorption, it gives added protection to the colon, which helps the body fight disease and illness. Psyllium also works as a lubricant on the intestinal tract and helps with diarrhea.

Studies have also suggested psyllium as a useful treatment for irritable bowel syndrome. IBS refers to an overly sensitive colon that responds to stress. Psyllium may help by soothing, healing, and aiding in the elimination of toxins from the colon. It has also been suggested for diabetics. It produces copious mucilage to soothe and heal the large intestines and clean the colon. It does not irritate the delicate mucous membranes, but works to strengthen and restore the tissues. Jethro Kloss suggested using psyllium in cases of colitis and anal ulcers.

Psyllium is a safe alternative to drug therapy for chronic constipation when used properly. The husks from the psyllium seeds are an excellent source of insoluble and soluble fiber and serve as an intestinal cleanser and stool softener. Psyllium is also a hydrophilic bulking agent, which means that it increases several times in size when combined with water. This happens because one of the main components of psyllium is mucilage—a thickening and stabilizing agent that swells in water. The swelling of psyllium in the intestines helps increase the peristaltic activity of the bowel, which bulks up stool and promotes bowel movement. For this reason, it is important to drink plenty of water when taking psyllium. Mucilage also helps soothe and heal inflamed tissue in the intestinal tract.

Research has found psyllium to be beneficial for lowering cholesterol and for strengthening the heart. An article in the *Journal of the American Medical Association* in 1988 suggested using dietary modifications, such as the addition of psyllium, to lower cholesterol levels before turning to drug therapy. Adding mucilage, such as that found in psyllium, to the diet can successfully reduce serum cholesterol levels, because recent studies on psyllium and other forms of fiber have found that mucilage in fiber inhibits cholesterol production. Not only does psyllium (taken before meals) reduce bad cholesterol and triglyceride levels, it also increases levels of good cholesterol.

Using psyllium externally can help with skin inflammation and irritation. Simply make a poultice of crushed psyllium seeds (crush the whole seed). Psyllium is also a great drawing agent and is recommended for drawing the pus out of boils and sores.

## PRIMARY APPLICATIONS

| | |
|---|---|
| Cholesterol, high | Colon problems |
| Constipation | Diverticulitis |

## SECONDARY APPLICATIONS

| | |
|---|---|
| Cystitis | Diarrhea |
| Dysentery | Gonorrhea |
| Hemorrhage | Inflammation |
| Intestinal tract irritation | Irritable bowel (IBS) |
| Skin irritations | Toxins, effects of |
| Ulcers | Urinary problems |

# PUMPKIN *(Cucurbita pepo)*

*Parts used:* Seeds and oil
*Properties:* Anthelmintic, demulcent, diuretic, nutritive, parasiticide, purgative (mild)

*Primary nutrients:* Amino acids, beta-carotene, magnesium, zinc, essential fatty acids, vitamin E, and carotenoids.

In the United States, the pumpkin is associated with autumn holidays such as Halloween and Thanksgiving. The seeds are generally thrown away as waste; however, pumpkin seeds and their oil can be used for their beneficial properties—especially for ridding the body of intestinal parasites.

Studies have shown that various squash, including pumpkin, have special parasite-fighting capacities. Although researchers are not exactly sure what compound in pumpkin seeds expels the worms, the seeds are well known for their ability to do so quickly and safely, even in children. The seeds work best when a laxative is taken an hour after use.

The seeds are also used to strengthen the prostate gland and promote male hormone function. They have been used to treat an enlarged prostate. Myosin is also found in pumpkin seeds and is known to be essential for muscular contractions.

Applying the oil of the pumpkin seed to wounds, burns, and chapped skin is soothing and helps heal injured skin.

## PRIMARY APPLICATIONS

| | |
|---|---|
| Intestinal problems | Parasites |
| Tapeworm | |

## SECONDARY APPLICATIONS

| | |
|---|---|
| Burns | Gastric disorders |
| Nausea | Prostate problems |
| Roundworms | Skin, chapped |
| Uterine problems | Wounds |

# PYGEUM *(Prunus africana)*

*Parts used:* Bark
*Properties:* Anti-inflammatory, diuretic, hormonal
*Primary nutrients:* Fatty acids

Pygeum is commonly partnered with saw palmetto and found in herbal combinations for the prostate gland. It was used by natives of tropical South Africa to treat uterine disorders and prostate problems in combination with milk or palm oil, and it comes from the bark of an African evergreen tree.

Pygeum contains compounds known for their ability to reduce inflammation of the prostate because of their lipophilic effects. Many European physicians prescribe pygeum for benign prostatic hyperplasia (BPH), which can cause urination problems. It is used not only to treat existing prostate problems, but also as a preventive measure for promoting prostate health.

There is also evidence that pygeum can help counteract problems of male infertility and impotence. Because it promotes health in the underlying condition of the prostate, pygeum can promote sexual health and function as a by-product, as well as boosting energy and fighting fatigue. It is also known to improve the composition of semen. Pygeum has been known to cause stomach irritation.

## PRIMARY APPLICATIONS

| | |
|---|---|
| Prostatitis | Prostate enlargement |
| Prostate problems | Urination problems |

## SECONDARY APPLICATIONS

| | |
|---|---|
| Circulation, poor | Energy, lack of |
| Fatigue | Impotence |

# QUASSIA *(Picrasma amara)*

*Parts used:* Bark
*Properties:* Alterative, anthelmintic, bitter, emetic, febrifuge, stomachic
*Primary nutrients:* Calcium, potassium, sodium

Quassia is a great healer of the sick. It is a powerful herb, and if taken in excess, it can be an emetic, irritant, depressant, and produce nausea. However, if taken in small doses, it can actually speed recovery in the body.

Quassia is best known for its gastrointestinal attributes. It is considered one of the best remedies for moving noxious substances, which can remain in the alimentary canal as a result of improper digestion, out of the body. It kills roundworms and pinworms and is also a good tonic to help with stomach problems.

Not only does quassia aid digestion, it helps with constipation and can stimulate appetite. It is recommended for anorexics, convalescents, and the elderly. Additionally, it is said to be a good remedy for alcoholics who need help losing the taste for alcohol. It is also beneficial to the eyes, because it promotes liver health.

Other uses for quassia include dandruff (external use), fevers, constipation, dyspepsia, and rheumatism.

## PRIMARY APPLICATIONS

| | |
|---|---|
| Appetite, lack of | Fevers |
| Gastric disorders | Indigestion |
| Worms | |

## SECONDARY APPLICATIONS

| | |
|---|---|
| Alcoholism | Constipation |
| Dandruff | Dyspepsia |
| Rheumatism | |

# QUEEN OF THE MEADOW
*(Eupatorium purpureum)*

*Parts used:* Leaves and rootstock
*Properties:* Alterative, anti-inflammatory, antirheumatic, astringent, diuretic, hepatic, immunostimulant, lithotriptic, nephritic, nervine, stimulant
*Primary nutrients:* Vitamins A, C, and D

Queen of the meadow is also known as "gravel root," for its ability to loosen and dissolve kidney stones (from the older term *gravel*), and "joe-pye weed," after a medicine man who used it to treat typhus. The Iroquois and Cherokees used queen of the meadow primarily as a diuretic, but also as a burn poultice and for ailments of the genitourinary tract.

It is often recommended for various urinary tract ailments. Queen of the meadow contains anti-inflammatory properties that work with the urinary tract to aid urine flow. It is used not only for kidney and bladder infections, but also for those suffering from Bright's disease or cystitis.

Queen of the meadow also helps with water retention and joint pain caused by uric acid deposits.

These attributes should appeal to women who suffer from PMS and individuals with rheumatism, arthritis, edema, gout, backaches, sprains, strains, and pulled ligaments and tendons. Studies support the use of queen of the meadow for arthritis, rheumatism, and gout. It also has been used by women during childbirth.

Queen of the meadow has properties that enable it to clear the body of waste products and clean it out. The juice of the rootstock can be applied externally as an astringent. A European species related to this herb has been studied and found to contain immunostimulant properties that help against viral infections.

## PRIMARY APPLICATIONS

| | |
|---|---|
| Arthritis | Bright's disease |
| Bursitis | Cystitis |
| Gallstones | Gout |
| Kidney infections | Neuralgia |
| Rheumatism | Ringworm |
| Uterine problems | Water retention |

## SECONDARY APPLICATIONS

| | |
|---|---|
| Backaches | Childbirth |
| Diabetes | Edema |
| Headaches | Menstrual bloating |
| Nervous disorders | Prostate problems |
| Sprains | Strains |
| Typhus | Viruses |

# RED CLOVER *(Trifolium pratense)*

*Parts used:* Flowers

*Properties:* Alterative, antibiotic, antispasmodic, blood purifier, nutritive, sedative, stimulant, vulnerary

*Primary nutrients:* Calcium, cobalt, copper, iron, magnesium, manganese, nickel, selenium, sodium, tin, vitamins A, C, B-complex, F, and P

Red clover (also called wild clover, purple clover, meadow clover, honeysuckle clover, or cow grass) is a member of the pea family commonly found in pastures, lawns, along roadsides, and in meadows. Many consider it a nuisance and try to eliminate it from their lawns, although this may not be easily accomplished because of its hearty nature.

The use of red clover probably originated in Europe, where it was used as an expectorant and a diuretic. It was also burned as incense to invoke the spirits of the deceased—some even wore the leaves of red clover as charms against evil. Early Christians revered the red clover because they associated its three leaves with the Trinity. The ancient Chinese dried the flowers and put them in pillows to help relax the body and mind. Native Americans used red clover as an infusion gargle for sore throats, whooping cough, and asthma. They used it on children because it was a milder, safer way to fight debilitating childhood diseases.

Red clover has been used for treating cancer, bronchitis, nervous conditions, spasms, and toxins in the body. Herbalists consider it to be a blood cleanser and recommend this mild herb in formulas when using a cleansing program. As an expectorant, it is often mixed with honey and water to make a cough syrup. It is also a mild sedative and useful for spasmodic conditions, bronchitis, wheezing, and fatigue. Since red clover is mild, it can be used by children.

Studies indicate red clover contains some antibiotic properties beneficial against several bacteria, including the one that causes tuberculosis. In addition, red clover has a long history of use in treating cancer. Researchers at the National Cancer Institute have found anticancer activity in red clover—including daidzein and genistein activity. Although the findings are preliminary and the use of red clover as a cancer treatment has not been validated, research continues and is promising.

Red clover has also been used externally to treat skin problems such as acne, psoriasis, eczema, and even vaginal irritation, in addition to topical application on burns, boils, sores, and ulcers. Documented uses of red clover for treating AIDS, syphilis, and leprosy also exist. It can be applied externally to help soothe lymphatic swelling or as an eyewash.

## PRIMARY APPLICATIONS

| | |
|---|---|
| Acne | AIDS/HIV |
| Athlete's foot | Blood impurities |
| Bronchitis | Cancer |

Eczema
Liver disorders
Psoriasis
Spasms

Leukemia
Nervous disorders
Skin disorders
Toxins, effects of

## SECONDARY APPLICATIONS

Arthritis
Boils
Childhood diseases
Constipation
Cramps, muscle
Flu
Gastric disorders
Leprosy
Rheumatism
Syphilis
Tuberculosis
Urinary infections
Whooping cough

Asthma
Burns
Colds
Coughs
Fatigue
Gallbladder
Indigestion
Lymphatic irritations
Sores
Throat, sore
Ulcers
Vaginal irritations
Wounds

# RED RASPBERRY *(Rubus idaeus)*

*Parts used:* Leaves
*Properties:* Alterative, analgesic, antiemetic, antiseptic, antispasmodic, antiviral, astringent, galactagogue, homeostatic, oxytocic, stimulant
*Primary nutrients:* Calcium, iron, manganese, phosphorus, vitamins A, B, C, D, E, F, and G

Henry Box, a famous English herbalist, praised red raspberry as the best gift God ever gave to women. He said, "If the pains of childbirth are premature, it will make all quiet. If the mother is weak, it will abundantly strengthen her, cleanse her, and enrich her milk." Red raspberry is rich in iron and calcium and contains phosphorus and manganese—all helpful supplements in a woman's diet. Not only is red raspberry excellent for a safe and easy childbirth, it is also recommended for a weak stomach. It even helps relieve the discomfort of morning sickness because it contains tannins that are effective for nausea, vomiting, and diarrhea.

Red raspberry has traditionally been used for women, especially during pregnancy, to strengthen the uterus, prevent nausea and hemorrhage, reduce pain during childbirth, and enrich colostrum found in breast milk. Its use for pregnant women is supported by physicians throughout Europe, since it helps strengthen the entire reproductive system (although excess dosages should be avoided while pregnant). For women who are not pregnant, red raspberry can help with menstrual problems as well as miscarriage or a prolapsed uterus.

Scientific research has proven the value of red raspberry for women. One of the properties discovered, fragarine, was found to have a relaxing effect on the pelvic and uterine muscles. An early study using animals found uterine relaxant activity in red raspberry. It is also proven to have a balancing effect on hormone levels and has been shown to promote tissue healing, especially in the cervix. Because of the healing aspects of the leaves, they are also used for after-birth pains.

Red raspberry helps soothe the stomach and gastrointestinal system, and it is a wonderful herb for treating children for colds, diarrhea, colic, fever, and other childhood diseases. Studies indicate that red raspberry contains antiviral properties to help fight viral diseases such as herpes and the flu.

The soothing properties of red raspberry are also helpful—especially when it is applied externally to sores and skin irritations, and it has been used to promote healthy skin, teeth, and bones, as well as heart health. It can also be used as an eyewash. As a refrigerant, using red raspberry in water with honey can help with fevers.

## PRIMARY APPLICATIONS

Bowel problems
Diarrhea
Flu
Membranes, irritated
Miscarriage, tendency
Mouth sores
Pregnancy, discomfort

Childbirth pains
Fevers
Heart problems
Menstrual symptoms
Morning sickness
Nausea
Vomiting

## SECONDARY APPLICATIONS

Breast-feeding
Canker sores
Colds
Constipation
Diabetes
Gastric disorders
Hemorrhoids

Bronchitis
Cholera
Colic
Coughs
Dysentery
Hemorrhages
Herpes

| Indigestion | Lactation, absent |
|---|---|
| Leucorrhea | Measles |
| Nervous conditions | Prostate problems |
| Rheumatism | Stomach ailments |
| Teething | Throat, sore |
| Ulcers | Uterine problems |
| Uterus, prolapsed | Wounds |

# REDMOND *(Montmorillonite)*

*Parts used:* Clay
*Properties:* Anthelmintic, antiseptic, emollient

Redmond clay is used externally for skin problems such as acne. It is good to have around for stings, bug bites, and for expelling worms from the intestinal tract. It also helps heal muscle sprains and wounds. It can be used for fevers and will quickly absorb poisons in the stomach if taken with a glass of water.

## PRIMARY APPLICATIONS

| Skin conditions | Stings, bee |
|---|---|

## SECONDARY APPLICATIONS

| Acne | Bites, insect |
|---|---|
| Poisoning | Worms |

# RHODIOLA *(Rhodiola rosea)*

*Parts used:* Root
*Properties:* Adaptogen, anticarcinogenic, antioxidant

Sometimes called golden root, arctic root, or rose root, rhodiola grows at high elevations in the arctic areas of Europe and Asia. It has been used in folk medicine in Russia and Scandinavia for centuries. Swedish researchers think the Vikings used rhodiola regularly, and a bouquet of the plant may still be presented today to a bride and groom in Siberia to ensure a bountiful marriage.

Rhodiola root is an adaptogen, and studies of its medicinal benefits have been performed in France, Sweden, Norway, Germany, the Soviet Union, and Iceland. Currently in Russia it is used as a tonic and treatment for fatigue, lack of concentration, and poor memory, and to increase worker productivity. In Sweden and other Scandinavian nations, it is used to enhance the capacity for mental work and as a general strengthener.

A recent review in *Herbalgram, the Journal of the American Botanical Council,* stated that numerous studies of rhodiola in vitro and in animals and humans have shown that it helps combat fatigue, stress, and the harmful effects of oxygen deprivation; it can also protect against cancer and increase immunity.

Other research on rhodiola has shown that the herb can help boost learning capacity, enhance memory, regulate menstrual periods, help with infertility, reduce chemotherapy side effects, enhance libido, aid erectile dysfunction, improve thyroid function, expand endurance, and protect against environmental toxins.

Rhodiola seems to work differently in the body than other adaptogens, such as Siberian ginseng. Rhodiola appears to act on key neurotransmitters in the brain, including dopamine and serotonin. An imbalance of these chemicals is thought to be behind such illnesses as chronic fatigue syndrome, fibromyalgia, and seasonal affective disorder (SAD). Some herbalists think rhodiola may help regulate levels of these neurotransmitters, alleviating these ailments. In contrast, most other adaptogens appear to fortify the body's reserves by increasing the production of stress-fighting hormones from the adrenal glands.

Irritability and insomnia may be a risk with high doses of rhodiola. Also, a recent study showed that rhodiola has an estrogenic effect in rats that had their ovaries removed. This estrogenic activity might increase the risk of estrogen-related cancers in humans, such as those of the breast and uterus.

## PRIMARY APPLICATIONS

| Cancer | Endurance |
|---|---|
| Fatigue | Immune function |
| Infertility | Libido |
| Memory, poor | Menstrual irregularity |
| Stress | Thyroid function |

# RHODODENDRON
*(Rhododendron caucasicum)*

*Parts used:* Leaves
*Properties:* Antibacterial, antioxidant
*Primary nutrients:* Caffeic acid, chlorogenic acid, flavonoids, phenylpropanoids, polyphenolics, proanthocyanidins

The Republic of Georgia, formerly part of the Soviet Union, is reputed to have an abundance of healthy, long-lived elders. A traditional Russian toast goes something like, "May you have the good health and long life of a Georgian." One of the reasons for this supposed longevity may be the daily consumption of a beverage known as alpine tea, which is made from the leaves of *Rhododendron caucasicum*.

Grown at high altitudes in the Caucasus Mountains, rhododendron (also called "alpine snow rose") contains polyphenolics, including flavonoids and proanthocyanidins.

Years of Russian and Georgian research suggest rhododendron can increase cardiovascular function and boost blood supply to the muscles and brain. It also is an antibacterial. It has detoxicant properties, guarding against capillary fragility, and is a top-notch free-radical scavenger. Studies have shown that rhododendron inhibits or neutralizes the activity of the enzyme hyaluronidase, a known initiator of colon cancer.

One Soviet study showed that rhododendron lowered blood pressure, improved coronary circulation, reduced serum cholesterol, and eliminated chest pain. Another Soviet study showed increased discharge of uric acid and pain relief in sufferers of severe gout. Research in Georgia found a marked reduction of symptoms in depressed patients.

Rhododendron's inhibition of hyaluronidase activity also has possible benefits for osteoarthritis, perhaps by blocking that enzyme's abnormal release from the cartilage cells, a release that leads to cartilage breakdown.

Rhododendron has demonstrated antioxidant properties, dietary fat-blocking activity, and anti-inflammatory and antiallergy actions. Modern studies have shown that rhododendron can guard against and treat cardiac dysfunction, blood vessel damage, and lung damage; help regulate blood pressure, pulse, and cholesterol levels; help prevent brain and eye degeneration; slow down arthritis progression; prevent and treat gout; inhibit fat absorption; help dissolve stored fat; fortify blood vessels; protect and detoxify the liver; increase the availability of vitamin E in the blood; and reduce the activity of viruses and bacteria.

## PRIMARY APPLICATIONS

| | |
|---|---|
| Allergies | Arthritis |
| Cancer | Cardiovascular issues |
| Depression | Gout |
| Infections | Obesity |

# RHUBARB *(Rheum palmatum)*

*Parts used:* Root
*Properties:* Alterative, antibacterial, antibiotic, anti-inflammatory, antimicrobial, antineoplastic, astringent, diuretic, hepatic, hypotensive, parasiticide, purgative (mild), sialagogue, stomachic, vulnerary
*Primary nutrients:* Calcium, cobalt, iron, nickel, phosphorus, potassium, sodium, sulfur, tin, vitamins A, B-complex, and C

Rhubarb was brought to the New World from Europe and used as a laxative, because in large doses, it cleans intestinal irritants and checks diarrhea with its astringent action.

Rhubarb is useful when the stomach is weak and the bowels are relaxed because it acts as a gentle cathartic. When taken in small doses, rhubarb acts as a blood cleanser and builder. It is very useful in toxic blood conditions caused by excessive intake of meat. It is helpful for individuals suffering from anemia and jaundice. It is also a mildly stimulating alterative for the liver, gall bladder, and mucous membranes of the intestines. It can be used as a digestive aid.

## PRIMARY APPLICATIONS

| | |
|---|---|
| Blood, toxic | Colon problems |
| Diarrhea | Liver disorders |

## SECONDARY APPLICATIONS

| | |
|---|---|
| Anemia | Colitis |
| Constipation | Dysentery |

| | |
|---|---|
| Indigestion | Jaundice |
| Gallbladder problems | Gastric disorders |
| Headaches | |

# ROSE HIPS *(Rosa species)*

*Parts used:* Fruit
*Properties:* Antiseptic, antispasmodic, astringent, blood purifier, nutritive, stomachic
*Primary nutrients:* Calcium, iron, potassium, silica, sodium, sulfur, vitamins A, B-complex, C, D, and E

Native Americans used rose hips as food, because it was available all year round. Scurvy was uncommon among them because of the vitamin C and bioflavonoids in this herb. The bioflavonoids aid the body's absorption of vitamin C. Modern research has recognized the value of rose hips for its vitamin C content. Rose hips also is rich in vitamins E, A, and B-complex. It has some vitamin D and contains iron, calcium, sodium, potassium, sulfur, and silica. Because of this benefit, rose hips is often used as a survival food.

Rose hips is useful for acute diseases, such as childhood diseases, as well as colds, flus, and fevers. Studies have found that the vitamin C content in rose hips helps relieve symptoms and shortens the duration of the common cold. It is useful for preventing and healing infections.

Rose hips has been found to have a mild laxative and diuretic effect. This is thought to be due to the presence of malic and citric acids or the purgative glycosides. The Swiss herbalist Father Kunzle recommended the use of rose hips to expel kidney stones. Rose hips fruit has also been used for stress-related problems, female complications such as PMS, skin irritations, and heart and circulation health, as well as a cancer treatment.

## PRIMARY APPLICATIONS

| | |
|---|---|
| Adrenal gland problems | Blood impurities |
| Cancer | Childhood diseases |
| Circulation, poor | Colds |
| Constipation | Exhaustion |
| Fevers | Flu |
| Headaches | Infection |

| | |
|---|---|
| Nervousness | PMS |
| Sores | Stress |
| Throat, sore | Vitamin C deficiency |

## SECONDARY APPLICATIONS

| | |
|---|---|
| Arteriosclerosis | Bites |
| Bladder problems | Bruises |
| Colic | Coughs |
| Cramps | Diarrhea |
| Dizziness | Earaches |
| Emphysema | Heart problems |
| Hemorrhoids | Kidney problems |
| Mouth sores | Psoriasis |
| Stings | |

# ROSEMARY *(Rosmarinus officinalis)*

*Parts used:* Leaves
*Properties:* Alterative, analgesic, anodyne, anti-inflammatory, antioxidant, antiseptic, aromatic, astringent, carminative, diaphoretic, nervine, stimulant, stomachic
*Primary nutrients:* Calcium, iron, magnesium, phosphorus, potassium, sodium, vitamins A and C, zinc

In Greek history, rosemary was thought to help strengthen the brain and improve memory. Rosemary became a symbol of remembrance. Europeans used rosemary leaf for headaches, pain, and stomachaches. Rosemary is currently used as a seasoning spice all over the world.

Rosemary is a strong stimulant that works mainly on the circulatory system and the pelvic region. It is an excellent tonic for the heart and as a treatment for high blood pressure. It is also excellent for various female ailments, such as irregular menses and uterine pain, and is a good tonic for the reproductive organs. In Germany, rosemary is already approved for use in cases of indigestion and rheumatic disorders, as well as externally for circulatory problems.

In addition, rosemary is a powerful herbal remedy to strengthen the nervous system. It can help relieve depression and is also recommended for headaches associated with the nervous system, stress headaches, and migraines. It can be used as a cooling tea when there is restlessness, nervousness, and insomnia.

Rosemary can be taken in the early stages of colds and flu as a warm infusion. Rosemary, sage, and vervain in equal parts make an antiseptic drink for fevers. Rosemary can also be applied externally to wounds of all kinds, including bites and stings. In addition, it has been used to prevent premature baldness by stimulating increased activity of the hair follicles. Rosemary extract has also been found to work as an insect repellent and an eyewash.

Anticancer activity has been found in rosemary. Extracts contain carnosic and labiatic acid, thought to be responsible for the antioxidant properties. Animal studies reported a lower incidence of experimentally induced mammary tumors from rosemary extract, though human studies have not been done and its therapeutic value is not entirely known.

## PRIMARY APPLICATIONS

| | |
|---|---|
| Cancer | Halitosis |
| Headaches | Heart problems |
| Indigestion | Migraines |
| Pelvic and uterine pain | Stomach disorders |

## SECONDARY APPLICATIONS

| | |
|---|---|
| Blood pressure, high | Circulation problems |
| Colds | Convulsions |
| Depression | Eczema |
| Edema | Fevers |
| Flu | Gallbladder ailments |
| Gas | Gastric disorders |
| Hair loss | Insomnia |
| Liver disorders | Memory, loss of |
| Menstrual symptoms | Nervousness |
| Prostate problems | Restlessness |
| Rheumatism | Spasms |
| Sores, open | Stings |
| Wounds | |

# RUE (Ruta graveolens)

*Parts used:* Entire plant
*Properties:* Anthelmintic, antispasmodic, emetic, sedative
*Primary nutrients:* Vitamin P

Rue is native to Europe but has been cultivated and naturalized in the United States. It has been used since ancient times to help prevent the plague and as an insect repellent.

Rue can be used for a variety of ailments. It has the ability to expel poisons from the body and has been used to treat snake, scorpion, spider, and jellyfish bites. Rue has also been found very effective in preserving sight by strengthening the ocular muscles. The volatile oils found in rue are thought to be responsible for its antispasmodic effects on smooth muscles. This quality also helps those women who suffer from premenstrual cramps and those who suffer from hypertension and strained muscles. Rue's calming effects on the nervous system are also a plus for those who have muscle pain, as well as those suffering from neuralgia or sciatica.

Rue helps remove deposits that are liable to form with age in the tendons and joints, especially in the wrist, and helps harden bones and teeth. Additionally, rue contains large amounts of rutin, vitamin P, which is known for its ability to strengthen the capillaries and veins. These elements can aid people with arteriosclerosis or poor circulation and even help those who bruise easily, are prone to varicose veins, or get chronic nosebleeds. However, because of its emetic properties, rue should not be used before meals or taken by pregnant women.

## PRIMARY APPLICATIONS

| | |
|---|---|
| Aches, joints | Blood pressure, high |
| Cramps, uterine | Hypertension |
| Muscles, strained | Nervous disorders |
| Neuralgia | Sciatica |
| Tendons, strained | Trauma |

## SECONDARY APPLICATIONS

| | |
|---|---|
| Arteriosclerosis | Bruising easily |
| Circulation, poor | Colic |
| Convulsions | Coughs |
| Croup, spasmodic | Earaches |
| Epilepsy | Eye problems |
| Insanity | Malaria |
| Metabolism, slow | Nerve problems |
| Nosebleeds, chronic | Poisons |
| Typhoid | Veins, varicose |
| Whooping cough | Worms |

# SAFFLOWER (*Carthamus tinctorius*)

*Parts used:* Flowers
*Properties:* Alterative, analgesic, anti-inflammatory, carminative, diaphoretic, digestive, diuretic, emmenagogue, purgative (mild)
*Primary nutrients:* Essential fatty acids, vitamin K

Safflower is native to the Middle East but is now cultivated throughout Europe and the United States. Safflower has been used since the Middle Ages, and perhaps before, primarily for dying fabrics red and yellow. It contains a significant amount of vitamin K.

Safflower has gained popularity in the past few years because of the unsaturated oil found in its seeds. In fact, it contains one of the highest percentages of unsaturated fatty acids of any oil. Research has confirmed that the addition of safflower oil does aid in reducing cholesterol levels in the blood. Safflower contains essential fatty acids that help maintain the central nervous system function.

Safflower is also a good remedy for jaundice and other liver and gallbladder problems. It can be used for fevers and various childhood diseases and has the ability to remove hard phlegm from the body, clear the lungs, and help in pulmonary tuberculosis. Safflower can also help improve digestion and colon function. It can help reduce lactic acid accumulations for athletes, and its diaphoretic qualities help with fevers and other conditions that can be eased by perspiration.

## PRIMARY APPLICATIONS

| | |
|---|---|
| Colon dysfunction | Delirium |
| Fevers | Gastric disorders |
| Gout | Indigestion |
| Jaundice | Lactic acid buildup |
| Liver disorders | Nervous system issues |
| Phlegm | Sweating |
| Uterine problems | |

## SECONDARY APPLICATIONS

| | |
|---|---|
| Boils | Chicken pox |
| Gallbladder problems | Heart, weak |
| Measles | Menstrual symptoms |
| Mumps | Poison ivy |
| Tuberculosis, pulmonary | |

# SAFFRON (*Crocus sativus*)

*Parts used:* Flowers
*Properties:* Alterative, anodyne, antineoplastic, antispasmodic, aphrodisiac, blood purifier, carminative, diaphoretic, emmenagogue, expectorant, sedative, stimulant
*Primary nutrients:* Calcium, lactic acid, phosphorus, potassium, sodium, vitamins A and B12

The Greeks and Chinese used saffron as a royal dye because of its yellow color, and wealthy Romans used saffron to perfume their homes. It was used medicinally in Europe between the fourth and eighteenth centuries, besides being used in the kitchen.

Nicholas Culpeper in his 1649 book *The Complete Herbal* recommended using saffron for the heart, brain, and lungs. He also suggested it for acute diseases such as smallpox and measles and for hysteric depression. In the *Materia Medica and Pharmacology* by Dr. David Culbreth in 1917, saffron was characterized as a pain reliever and was said to promote perspiration and gas expulsion and ease painful menstruation, as well as relieving eye infections and encouraging sore eruptions.

Saffron is soothing to the stomach and colon and aids in the digestive process by acting as a blood purifier. It helps stimulate circulation and regulates the spleen, heart, and liver. It also helps reduce inflammation; treats arthritis, gout, bursitis, kidney stones, hypoglycemia, and chest congestion; and improves circulation and promotes energy. Take small doses internally for coughs, gas, and colic and to stimulate appetite, or apply externally in a salve for gout.

Saffron may even help reduce cholesterol levels, because it neutralizes uric acid buildup in the system. In a recent study, rabbits fed crocin, a component of saffron, had a significant reduction in cholesterol and triglyceride levels, and in Valencia, Spain, saffron is eaten daily, and little heart disease occurs among the inhabitants. Evidence points to the fact that saffron increases oxygen diffusion from the red blood cells. And not only does it discourage uric acid buildup, it also inhibits the accumulation of lactic acid. It may, therefore, help prevent heart disease.

Research done on saffron suggests the ingredient crocin may have the potential to act as an anticancer agent in studies done in vitro and in animals. One study done in vitro using saffron extract found that tumor colony cell growth was limited by inhibiting the cellular nucleic acid synthesis. Other research on cancer has found that saffron given orally assisted in increasing the life span of mice with a variety of laboratory-induced cancers. Use strong caution when using saffron, as it is a poison and can be fatal.

## PRIMARY APPLICATIONS

| | |
|---|---|
| Fevers | Gout |
| Indigestion | Liver disorders |
| Measles | Perspiration, excessive |
| Phlegm | Psoriasis |
| Rheumatism | Scarlet fever |
| Stomach acid | |

## SECONDARY APPLICATIONS

| | |
|---|---|
| Appetite loss | Arthritis |
| Blood impurities | Bronchitis |
| Cancer | Colds |
| Conjunctivitis | Coughs |
| Fatigue | Gas |
| Headaches | Heartburn |
| Hemorrhages, uterine | Hyperglycemia |
| Hypoglycemia | Insomnia |
| Jaundice | Kidney stones |
| Menstrual symptoms | Skin diseases |
| Tuberculosis | Ulcers |
| Water retention | Whooping cough |

# SAGE (Salvia officinalis)

*Parts used:* Leaves
*Properties:* Alterative, antigalactagogue, antihydrotic, antioxidant, antiseptic, antispasmodic, aromatic, astringent, carminative, diaphoretic, digestive, febrifuge, parasiticide, stimulant, vulnerary
*Primary nutrients:* Calcium, phosphorus, potassium, silicon, sodium, sulfur, vitamins A, B-complex, and C

The Latin name for sage is *salvia*, which means healthy, and this plant was highly revered for its healing benefits in the Mediterranean, where it originated. Although it now grows in many areas throughout the globe, it should not be confused with the brush sage that grows in desert areas.

Dried sage leaves are often used as culinary spices. Sage is, and has been, a staple in many households and is traditionally used to prolong life. It is used in a lotion to heal sores and other skin ailments. The fresh leaves are chewed as a remedy for infections of the mouth and throat, and gargling with sage can help a sore throat. Sage helps with excessive mucus discharge, nasal drip, sores, and excessive saliva secretions, and its antipyretic qualities have been known to help with fevers, night sweats, and related problems.

Sage is also beneficial for mental exhaustion and for increasing the ability to concentrate. It improves memory and has been used on some forms of mental illness. It has also been used to treat digestive disorders such as ulcers, nausea, and diarrhea, and it is used topically as an antiseptic for sores, sore gums, and even as a teeth cleaner or hair tonic.

Sage has been found in clinical studies to contain antioxidant properties. The labiatic acid is thought to be the active constituent. There is evidence of some antimicrobial activity as well. Research using laboratory animals has found antispasmodic activity in sage extracts, which may account for its use as a digestive aid.

People with seizure disorders should use sage only under the supervision of a health-care provider.

## PRIMARY APPLICATIONS

| | |
|---|---|
| Coughs | Diabetes |
| Fevers | Gastric disorders |
| Gums, sore | Indigestion |
| Infection | Lactation, absent |
| Memory impairments | Mental illnesses |
| Mouth sores | Nausea |
| Nervous conditions | Night sweats |
| Sores | Throat, sore |
| Worms | |

## SECONDARY APPLICATIONS

| | |
|---|---|
| Bites, snake | Blood infections |
| Colds | Cystitis |
| Diarrhea | Dysentery |
| Flu | Hair loss |
| Headaches | Kidney stones |
| Laryngitis | Lung congestion |
| Mucus discharge | Nasal drip |
| Palsy | Parasites |

| | |
|---|---|
| Phlegm | Sinus congestion |
| Skin disorders | Tonsillitis |
| Ulcers | Yeast infections |

# ST. JOHN'S WORT
*(Hypericum perforatum)*

*Parts used:* Entire herb
*Properties:* Alterative, antifungal, antineoplastic, antispasmodic, astringent, blood purifier, diuretic, nervine, sedative, vulnerary
*Primary nutrients:* Bioflavonoids

St. John's wort is a perennial shrub with multiple bright-yellow flowers. It is generally found in open fields throughout Europe and the United States that are sunny and dry, and it is often found growing in the wild in northern California and southern Oregon. It has been used for thousands of years to heal and strengthen the body.

Many in ancient Greece and the Middle Ages felt that St. John's wort contained magical properties. Dioscorides, Pliny, and Hippocrates all used this herb medicinally for many ailments. The flowers "bleed" a bright red juice when pressed between the fingers, which led to the belief that it symbolizes the blood of Christ or the blood of St. John.

Nicholas Culpeper mentioned St. John's wort in his book *The Complete Herbal*, published in 1649. He suggested using it for conditions such as malaria, worms, injuries, bruises, open obstructions, swelling, sciatica, and as an antidote to poison, venom, or infection. It was used in Europe during Crusade battles to treat war injuries.

St. John's wort has been used to rid the chest and lungs of mucus in cases of bronchitis and other related problems. It is used to treat nervous system conditions such as neuralgia, as well as anxiety and nervous tension. It can help relieve pain; reduce swelling; treat abscesses, burns, bruises, and insect bites; and ease the pain of rheumatism and arthritis. A German patent for an ointment containing an extract shortens the healing time for burns by acting as a strong antiseptic: "According to the report, first-degree burns healed in forty-eight hours when treated with the ointment, while second- and third-degree burns healed three times faster than burns treated by conventional methods, and did so without forming scars."

St. John's wort is also used as an excellent blood purifier. In addition, it is recommended for bed-wetting, colds, and gastric ulcers.

St. John's wort is used extensively in Europe and Russia and is currently official in the pharmacopoeias in many Eastern European countries. Studies have found that it contains diuretic properties, strengthens the capillaries, dilates coronary arteries, prevents tumors, helps with diarrhea and viruses, and kills germs. It has antifungal properties and is effective for nervous disorders. St. John's wort contains bioflavonoids, including rutin, quercetin, and hyperoside, which may explain its effect on the arteries and capillaries. It is also a very promising herb for the immune system and for protecting the circulatory system.

In fact, St. John's wort is currently being studied as a treatment against HIV infection. It has been shown in studies to contain anti-HIV activity. One study showed significant improvement in T cell count of HIV patients who took hypericin daily. Their T cell count increased 13 percent after one month. Another study followed eighteen HIV patients, of which sixteen stayed with the program. Of those sixteen, only two acquired an infection during the forty months of observation. This is significant, since infections often occur in HIV patients because of a compromised immune system. The patients' T cell counts were stable or even increased during the observation period. St. John's wort is known to combat all sorts of infections: bacterial, fungal, and viral, in vitro.

However, European physicians most commonly recommend St. John's wort for cases of mild to moderate depression. In fact, its greatest role has been as an antidepressive agent. There have been at least twenty-eight controlled studies in Europe. One German study conducted by Muldner and Zoller involved fifteen depressed women who were given a standard extract of St. John's wort. The group was found to have less anxiety, show more interest in their surroundings, and have fewer symptoms associated with clinical depression. St. John's wort also relieved symptoms of anxiety, insomnia, and feelings of worthlessness.

St. John's wort is contraindicated with birth-control pills and prescription antidepressants. It also increases skin photosensitivity.

## PRIMARY APPLICATIONS

| | |
|---|---|
| AIDS/HIV | Arthritis |
| Bed-wetting | Bronchitis |
| Cancer | Childbirth, after-pains |
| Circulatory problems | Depression |
| Lung congestion | Menstrual symptoms |
| Nerve pain | Poisoning |
| Rheumatism | Swelling |
| Tumors | Urinary incontinence |
| Uterine problems | Viruses |

## SECONDARY APPLICATIONS

| | |
|---|---|
| Abscesses | Anemia |
| Anxiety | Bites, insect |
| Bleeding | Blood impurities |
| Boils | Bruises |
| Burns | Colds |
| Coughs | Diarrhea |
| Dysentery | Fevers |
| Gallbladder ailments | Gout |
| Headaches | Heart problems |
| Hemorrhaging | Insomnia |
| Jaundice | Melancholy |
| Menopausal symptoms | Nervous conditions |
| Palsy | Skin problems |
| Spasms | Ulcers |
| Worms | Wounds |

# SARSAPARILLA *(Smilax ornata)*

*Parts used:* Root
*Properties:* Alterative, anti-inflammatory, antiseptic, aromatic, blood purifier, carminative, diaphoretic, diuretic, febrifuge, stimulant
*Primary nutrients:* Copper, iodine, iron, manganese, silicon, sodium, vitamins A, B-complex, and C, zinc

Sarsaparilla is native to the Pacific regions of Mexico, along the coast to Peru. The root is commonly used to make root beer.

Sarsaparilla is often used in glandular balance formulas; components in sarsaparilla aid in the production of testosterone and progesterone. Sarsaparilla also stimulates metabolism, aids digestion, and improves the appetite. It has been used to help with gas and edema, among other related conditions. In addition, research shows that sarsaparilla contains diuretic activity and increases the elimination of chlorides and uric acid.

Sarsaparilla is beneficial for skin ailments such as psoriasis, eczema, and leprosy, according to various studies. It also works as an anti-inflammatory by increasing circulation to rheumatic joints and helps relieve arthritis and other inflammatory conditions.

Sarsaparilla also stimulates breathing when congestion occurs and helps purify the blood.

## PRIMARY APPLICATIONS

| | |
|---|---|
| Aches/pains, joint | Arthritis |
| Blood impurities | Eczema |
| Gas | Glandular problems |
| Hormone imbalance | Inflammation |
| Psoriasis | Skin diseases |
| Syphilis | |

## SECONDARY APPLICATIONS

| | |
|---|---|
| Age spots | Appetite loss |
| Colds | Congestion |
| Edema | Eyes, sore |
| Fevers | Gout |
| Impotence | Leprosy |
| Menopausal symptoms | Metabolism disorders |
| Parasites, skin | Rheumatism, chronic |
| Ringworms | Tuberculosis, primary |
| Sores | |

# SAW PALMETTO *(Serenoa repens)*

*Parts used:* Fruit
*Properties:* Alterative, antiseptic, aphrodisiac, diuretic, sedative
*Primary nutrients:* Vitamin A

Native American tribes in the South used saw palmetto for sore eyes. The dried root was used to lower high blood pressure, and the crushed root was applied to sore breasts in women. John Lloyd, an early American botanist, noticed that animals eating the berries were fat and healthy. Saw palmetto was listed in the U.S. Pharmacopoeia from 1910 to 1916 and the National Formulary from 1926 to 1950 as being a diuretic, sedative, expectorant, and an analgesic recommended for neuralgia. It has also been known in folk history as an aphrodisiac and sexual stimulant. It was used to treat urination problems, inflammation of the bladder, and prostate enlargement.

Saw palmetto has been used to treat conditions of the genitourinary system. It is also used as an antiseptic, for excessive mucus in the head and sinuses, and for both male and female reproductive organs. Saw palmetto is known for its ability to help with male health. But it also helps with thyroid function, regulating development of the reproductive system, stimulating glandular function, removing excess mucus accumulation in the sinuses, and for colds, sore throat, whooping cough, bronchitis, and asthma. The berries have been useful for improving digestion, increasing weight, and building strength. Saw palmetto has even been reported to increase the size of breasts in women of childbearing age. Saw palmetto is often found in herbal combinations for diabetes, thyroid function, digestion, nutrition, female reproductive problems, and prostate difficulties.

Research has shown that saw palmetto has diuretic properties and is effective in treating an enlarged prostate and other prostate disorders. Many men suffer from prostate problems that affect sexual function, as well as bladder obstructions. One study published in the *Annals of Urology* followed a group of men with enlarged prostate glands. The group taking saw palmetto increased their urine flow rate by 50 percent and reduced the number of times they got up at night to urinate by 45 percent. The group taking the placebo had an increase of 9 percent in their response. Studies on laboratory animals have found the hexane extract of saw palmetto contains antiallergic and anti-inflammatory activity. Proscar is a drug prescribed to treat benign prostatic hyperplasia (BHP). One study comparing it to saw palmetto found better results over a three-month period with saw palmetto in treating the condition.

## PRIMARY APPLICATIONS

| | |
|---|---|
| Gastric disorders | Glandular problems |
| Hormone imbalance | Impotence |
| Indigestion | Prostate problems |
| Reproductive organs | |

## SECONDARY APPLICATIONS

| | |
|---|---|
| Alcoholism | Asthma |
| Bright's disease | Bronchitis |
| Colds | Diabetes |
| Frigidity | Infertility |
| Kidney disorders | Lung congestion |
| Mucus, excessive | Nerve pain |
| Neuralgia | Obesity |
| Throat, sore | Urinary problems |

# SCHIZANDRA (Schizandra chinensis)

*Parts used:* Berries
*Properties:* Alterative, antibacterial, astringent, sedative
*Primary nutrients:* Calcium, iron, magnesium, phosphorus, potassium, selenium, silicon, sodium, vitamin C

Schizandra grows wild in northern China. It has been used as a natural medicine for thousands of years and prescribed by physicians in that region. In the sixteenth century, it was listed in a book on pharmacy written by Li Schizheng. It was used to increase energy, replenish and nourish the viscera (internal abdominal organs), improve vision, boost muscular activity, and soothe both coughs and digestive upsets. Schizandra is an adaptogenic Asian herb gaining popularity throughout the world.

Schizandra helps the body heal itself. It can help increase energy in the cells of the brain, muscles, liver, kidney, glands, nerves, and the entire body. It stimulates the immune system and protects against free-radical damage, radiation, and the effects of sugar, as well as boosting stamina, normalizing blood sugar and blood pressure, and protecting against infections. It has a tonic action on the immune system, as well as other body systems, and can be taken regularly. It can help protect the body from both viral and bacterial infections.

Scientific studies have found that schizandra is antibacterial, stimulant, and protects the liver against toxins. Problems with the liver can lead to immune disorders because of the buildup of toxins. Schizandra also has been found to help allergies, depression, and fatigue in mice. It has been found to protect against the effects of alcohol in laboratory mice. Other studies have found this herb to have a mild regenerative effect on the liver. It has been used effectively in China to treat infectious hepatitis. Schizandra seems to have a liver-protective effect similar to that of milk thistle extracts.

## PRIMARY APPLICATIONS

| | |
|---|---|
| Diabetes | Energy, lack of |
| Fatigue | Impotence |
| Mental alertness, lack of | Nervous disorders |
| Stress | |

## SECONDARY APPLICATIONS

| | |
|---|---|
| Aging | Anxiety |
| Arteriosclerosis | Asthma |
| Blood pressure, high | Coughs |
| Diarrhea | Edema |
| Gastritis | Heart palpitations |
| Hepatitis | Indigestion |
| Infections | Insomnia |
| Kidney disorders | Lung disorders |
| Motion sickness | Radiation, effects of |
| Uterine problems | Vision, poor |

# SEA BUCKTHORN
*(Hippophae rhamnoides)*

*Parts used:* Berries
*Properties:* Anti-inflammatory
*Primary nutrients:* Amino acids, carotenoids, fatty acids, flavonoids, fructose, glucose, vitamins C, E

Sea buckthorn, also known as seaberry or Siberian pineapple, is a small shrub native to a wide swath across Europe and Asia. Southeast Asians have used this plant to treat various diseases for hundreds of years. The ancient Greeks are said to have used sea buckthorn berries to promote weight gain and shiny fur in horses.

Analysis of sea buckthorn's orange berries shows an abundance of vitamins C and E, carotenoids, flavonoids, glucose, fructose, several amino acids, and fatty acids. The berries are used for juices, jams, liquors, and lotions. Oil from the berries has been used to treat inflammation-related ailments such as canker sores, esophagitis, cervicitis, peptic ulcers, and ulcerative colitis. During the Cold War years, horticulturists from the Soviet Union and East Germany came up with new varieties of sea buckthorn with bigger berries and better nutrition.

In traditional Chinese medicine, sea buckthorn is used to boost energy, and Olympic athletes in that country have recently used sea buckthorn-based sports drinks as part of their training. In Russia, sea buckthorn has been used in ointments to help shield cosmonauts from radiation damage while in orbit. The oil contains high amounts of palmitoleic acid, a rare fatty acid found in skin fat that aids cell tissue and wound healing. Some U.S. cosmetics firms put sea buckthorn in their skin creams as a skin protectant and antiaging ingredient.

Herbalists recommend sea buckthorn to boost energy levels, promote wound healing, and shield skin from damage from ultraviolet rays. There is some research on the wound-healing and tissue-protecting properties of sea buckthorn extract. In animal studies, the extract was seen to strengthen cardiac pump function and myocardial contractility in dogs with heart failure. It also seems to improve oxygen use in the hearts of dogs and animal heart cells in test tubes.

Sea buckthorn oils are generally used externally for burns and other skin damage and internally for stomach and duodenal ulcers. There are anecdotal reports of sea buckthorn extract being used to combat tumor growth, high blood pressure, and high cholesterol.

## PRIMARY APPLICATIONS

| | |
|---|---|
| Burns | Canker sores |
| Cervicitis | Colitis |
| Energy, lack of | Esophagitis |
| Skin protection | Ulcers |
| Wounds | |

# SENEGA *(Polygala senega)*

*Parts used:* Root
*Properties:* Diaphoretic, diuretic, emetic, emmenagogue, expectorant, stimulant (large doses), purgative (mild)
*Primary nutrients:* Aluminum, iron, lead, magnesium, tin

Senega root has been recommended by herbalists for treating asthma and bronchitis to expel phlegm. It is used as an expectorant for respiratory problems. It is useful in the second stages of acute bronchial catarrh and pneumonia. Senega root helps thin mucus fluids so they are more easily removed from the body. It is effective for colds, flu, asthma, bronchitis, and most respiratory ailments. It helps in cases of blood poisoning to eliminate toxins from the system. Some recommend the use of senega as an antidote for many poisons.

## PRIMARY APPLICATIONS

| | |
|---|---|
| Asthma | Bites, snake |
| Bronchitis, chronic | Croup |
| Lung congestion | Mucus, excessive |
| Pneumonia | |

## SECONDARY APPLICATIONS

| | |
|---|---|
| Drugs, side effects | Pleurisy |
| Poisoning, blood | Rheumatism |

# SENNA *(Cassia acutifolia)*

*Parts used:* Leaves and pods
*Properties:* Anthelmintic and purgative (mild)
*Primary nutrients:* Calcium, iron, magnesium, manganese, potassium, selenium, silicon, sodium, vitamins A, B-complex, and C, zinc

The American senna has been widely used for its mild purgative effect. Native Americans used it as a drink to reduce fevers, for sore throat, and as a laxative. It was official in the U.S. Pharmacopoeia from 1820 to 1882. The Chinese used senna in their medicine. Senna and other laxatives have been used since prehistoric times for colonic and menstrual obstructions. Senna is found along the Nile River and was used in Arab medicine as an effective and safe laxative. The seventeenth-century herbalist Nicholas Culpeper claimed that senna cleaned the stomach and purged melancholy and phlegm from the head, brain, lungs, heart, liver, and spleen.

Senna is considered a useful laxative. It increases the intestinal peristaltic movements. It has a strong effect on the entire intestinal tract, especially the colon. Many believe that a clean colon can prevent autointoxication and may be an underlying cause of many diseases. Senna is usually combined with other herbs, such as ginger or fennel, to prevent intestinal cramping and get better results. It should not be used if there is inflammation of the stomach, as it may aggravate the problem. It helps tone and restore the digestive system through cleansing. It has been used throughout history and is still used throughout the world.

Senna is a powerful laxative. The anthroquinone glycosides in senna are thought to be responsible for the stimulation of the colon. Laxatives should not be used for extended periods of time.

## PRIMARY APPLICATIONS

| | |
|---|---|
| Constipation | Jaundice |
| Worms | |

## SECONDARY APPLICATIONS

| | |
|---|---|
| Acne | Bile, excessive |
| Breath, odor | Colic |
| Gallstones | Gout |
| Menstrual symptoms | Obesity |
| Rheumatism | Skin diseases |

# SHEPHERD'S PURSE
*(Capsella bursa-patoris)*

*Parts used:* Entire plant
*Properties:* Astringent, diuretic, febrifuge, hemostatic, purgative (mild), stimulant
*Primary nutrients:* Calcium, iron, magnesium, potassium, sodium, sulfur, tin, vitamins C, E, and K, zinc

Shepherd's purse was used anciently by the Greeks and Romans as a laxative. An Italian physician promoted the use of shepherd's purse to stop bleeding. This herb was brought to North America by settlers and is now a common weed. During World War I and World War II, when traditional medications were in short supply, shepherd's purse tea was used out of necessity to control bleeding due to casualties of war.

Shepherd's purse has historically been used for hemorrhaging after childbirth, excessive menstruation, and internal bleeding in the lungs and colon. Properties in shepherd's purse act as a blood coagulant. The herb can be applied externally to sores, wounds, nosebleeds, and bruises. It helps constrict the blood vessels and is used to regulate blood pressure and heart action. It acts as a stimulant and tonic for catarrh of the urinary tract, which is indicated by mucus in the urine.

Some evidence points to shepherd's purse in promoting the coagulation of blood in wounds. It should be remembered that serious bleeding should always have pressure applied, and prompt medical assistance should be sought. Shepherd's purse has also been found to contain components that lower blood pressure and stimulate uterine contractions. For this reason, it should not be used by pregnant women.

## PRIMARY APPLICATIONS

| | |
|---|---|
| Bleeding | Blood pressure, high |
| Ear ailments | Menstrual symptoms |
| Urine, bloody | |

## SECONDARY APPLICATIONS

| | |
|---|---|
| Arteriosclerosis | Back pain, lower |
| Bowels | Constipation |
| Diarrhea | Heart problems |
| Hemorrhages | Kidney problems |
| Uterine problems | Water retention |

# SKULLCAP *(Scutellaria lateriflora)*

*Parts used:* Herb
*Properties:* Alterative, analgesic, antibacterial, antifungal, antispasmodic, febrifuge, nervine, sedative
*Primary nutrients:* Calcium, iron, magnesium, potassium, vitamins C, E, zinc

Skullcap was used by the Cherokee tribe as an emmenagogue and was used historically as an anticonvulsant. Chinese physicians have used an Asian skullcap as a tranquilizer, sedative, and to treat convulsion. In the eighteenth century, it was used as a treatment for rabies by some physicians. It was later recommended by eclectic physicians for insomnia, nervousness, malaria, and convulsions. It was officially listed in the U.S. Pharmacopoeia from 1863 to 1916 and in the National Formulary from 1916 to 1947.

Skullcap may treat a variety of conditions, including pain, anxiety, high blood pressure, and epilepsy. It is well known for its ability to calm the nerves and help with all nervous system conditions. It has also been used to treat infertility, fatigue, inflamed tissues, digestion, coughs, and headaches. Some herbalists consider skullcap to be one of the best nervine herbs available. It has been used as a nerve tonic and can promote a feeling of well-being and promote a relaxed sleep. Some recommend skullcap for problems associated with drug and alcohol withdrawal. It may help lessen the severity of symptoms. Traditional uses have included infertility, regulation of sexual desire, and as a remedy for cramps and pain.

Research done in Europe and Russia has proven the benefits of skullcap as a tranquilizer and mild sedative. It is recommended for use in nervous conditions to induce sleep and relaxation. There is some evidence that the Asian skullcap contains components that inhibit the enzyme sialidase, which is known to increase in certain disease states such as cancer, infections, and inflammations. Another study done in vitro found antibacterial and antifungal activity in skullcap. There is also some early evidence of skullcap in treating high blood pressure. It is used and prescribed widely in Europe. Studies in Japan using animals showed that skullcap could increase levels of good cholesterol and prevent serum cholesterol levels from rising in rabbits fed a high-cholesterol diet. This may suggest skullcap as a heart disease and stroke preventive.

## PRIMARY APPLICATIONS

| | |
|---|---|
| Anxiety | Blood pressure, high |
| Convulsions | Epilepsy |
| Infertility | Insomnia |
| Nerve problems | Restlessness |

## SECONDARY APPLICATIONS

| | |
|---|---|
| Alcoholism | Bites, poisonous |
| Childhood diseases | Chorea |
| Circulation, poor | Coughing |
| Delirium | Drug withdrawal |
| Fevers | Hangover |
| Headaches | Hydrophobia |
| Hypertension | Hypoglycemia |
| Insanity | Neuralgia |
| Pain | Palsy |
| Parkinson's disease | Rabies |
| Rheumatism | Rickets |
| Spasms | Spinal meningitis |
| Thyroid problems | Tremors |
| Urinary problems | |

# SLIPPERY ELM (Ulmus fulva)

*Parts used:* Inner bark
*Properties:* Antacid, antineoplastic, astringent, demulcent, emollient, expectorant, mucilant, nutritive
*Primary nutrients:* Calcium, copper, iodine, iron, phosphorus, potassium, selenium, sodium, vitamins A, F, K, and P, zinc

Slippery elm was used anciently by the Greek physician Dioscorides to help speed the healing of broken bones. Nicholas Culpeper, a seventeenth-century physician, also recommended slippery elm for healing broken bones, balding, and burns. Slippery elm was known by Native Americans and early colonists as a valuable survival food. They used the inner bark as a salve externally for burns and wounds. It was used for colds, coughs, sore throats, wounds, as a poultice to bring boils to a head, and for bowel complaints. Dr. Edward Shook called it one of the most valuable remedies in herbal practice.

Slippery elm contains as much nutrition as oatmeal and provides a wholesome and sustaining food for young children and invalids. Slippery elm has been used mainly to treat gastrointestinal problems, such as stomach and intestinal ulcers, soothing the stomach and colon, indigestion, acidity, and to lubricate the bowels. The mucilage content is thought to help heal ulcers and ulcerated conditions. It was used for asthma, bronchitis, colitis, colon problems, and all lung problems. It is a mild purgative, aiding in elimination.

Studies done on slippery elm have found it to be an excellent demulcent and beneficial for diarrhea, coughs, stomach problems, colitis, and lung problems. The bark of slippery elm contains mucilage that swells in water and can be applied to wounds or taken internally to soothe and heal. Some lozenges for throat irritations contain the powdered bark to soothe the throat and promote healing.

## PRIMARY APPLICATIONS

| | |
|---|---|
| Abscesses | Asthma |
| Bronchitis | Burns |
| Colitis | Colon problems |
| Constipation | Coughs |
| Diaper rash | Diarrhea |
| Gastric disorders | Lung problems |

## SECONDARY APPLICATIONS

| | |
|---|---|
| Appendicitis | Bladder problems |
| Boils | Cancer |
| Croup | Diphtheria |
| Dysentery | Eczema |
| Eye ailments | Fevers |
| Flu | Hemorrhoids |
| Herpes | Inflammation |
| Kidney problems | Pain |
| Phlegm | Pneumonia |
| Sores | Syphilis |
| Throat, sore | Tuberculosis |
| Tumors | Ulcers |
| Uterine problems | Vaginal irritations |
| Warts | Worms |
| Wounds | Whooping cough |

# SPEARMINT (Mentha spicata)

*Parts used:* Leaves
*Properties:* Alterative, antiemetic, antispasmodic, aromatic, carminative, diaphoretic, diuretic, nervine, stimulant, stomachic
*Primary nutrients:* Calcium, iodine, iron, magnesium, potassium, sulfur, vitamins A, B-complex, and C

Spearmint is similar in action to peppermint but milder in its activity. Spearmint was the original mint used for healing. Peppermint is a hybrid of spearmint. This mint was used anciently by the Egyptians, Greeks, and Romans for its medicinal value.

Spearmint is a valuable herb that can be well tolerated by most individuals. It is an excellent herb for the gastrointestinal tract. Spearmint helps settle an upset stomach by soothing the stomach and intestines. It increases circulation in the stomach. It helps control vomiting due to morning sickness during pregnancy. The oil in spearmint leaves works on the salivary glands to aid digestion. It stimulates gastric secretions. It is a gentle and effective remedy for babies with colic. Spearmint also helps relieve smooth muscle spasms, increase blood circulation, promote sweating, and relieve pain.

## PRIMARY APPLICATIONS

| | |
|---|---|
| Colds | Colic |
| Flu | Gas |
| Nausea | Vomiting |

## SECONDARY APPLICATIONS

| | |
|---|---|
| Bladder inflammation | Chills |
| Cramps | Dizziness |
| Edema | Fever |
| Indigestion | Kidney inflammation |
| Kidney stones | Spasms |
| Urine, inhibited | |

# SPIKENARD (Aralia racemosa)

Parts used: Root
Properties: Alterative, blood purifier, expectorant, stimulant

Spikenard tea has traditionally been used by women before labor to make childbirth easier and to help shorten the duration. It is also useful for reducing uric acid buildup and has been combined with other herbs to purify and build the blood. Spikenard has a slight expectorant effect and is useful in cough syrups along with other herbs. The properties of spikenard are similar to ginseng. Russians use the roots of spikenard as a general alterative and stimulant, especially for physical and mental exhaustion.

## PRIMARY APPLICATIONS

| | |
|---|---|
| Asthma | Childbirth |
| Cough | Rheumatism |

## SECONDARY APPLICATIONS

| | |
|---|---|
| Backaches | Chest pains |
| Diarrhea | Hay fever |
| Hemorrhoids | Inflammation |
| Lung congestion | Skin problems |
| Venereal diseases | |

# SQUAW VINE (Mitchela repens)

Parts used: Entire plant
Properties: Alterative (uterine), antiseptic, astringent, diuretic, emmenagogue, galactagogue

Squaw vine was used by Native Americans for just about anything associated with childbearing. The women used squaw vine as a tea during the final weeks of pregnancy. They also drank the tea to help ease childbirth.

Squaw vine strengthens the uterus for a safe and easy childbirth. It is called a uterine tonic, as it helps strengthen and relieve congestion in the uterus and ovaries. It is also valuable for restoring normal menstrual function. Squaw vine contains antiseptic properties that make it ideal for any kind of vaginal infection. It is also a beneficial natural sedative. It is best used in combination with other herbs, such as red raspberry. Squaw vine is recommended for most female ailments. It is also used for dropsy, suppression of urine, diarrhea, sore eyes, water retention, and skin ailments.

## PRIMARY APPLICATIONS

| | |
|---|---|
| Childbirth | Lactation, absent |
| Menstrual symptoms | Uterine problems |

## SECONDARY APPLICATIONS

| | |
|---|---|
| Bites, snake | Diarrhea |
| Eyes, sore | Gonorrhea |
| Hemorrhoids | Insomnia |

Nerve problems
Syphilis
Water retention

Skin problems
Veins, varicose

# STEVIA *(Stevia rebaudiana)*

*Parts used:* Leaves
*Properties:* Sugar substitute
*Primary nutrients:* Calcium, carbohydrates, fibers, iron, magnesium, phosphorus, potassium, protein, rutin, selenium, sodium, vitamins A and C, zinc

Stevia is a small, shrublike plant found growing in Central and South America as well as in southwestern sections of the United States. It grows wild from Argentina to Mexico. It has been used for hundreds of years as a sweetener in South America. It is now being used widely in Japan, where it is used in soy sauce, chewing gum, and soft drinks, as well as other items. It is easily cultivated and grows like a weed, making it attractive to many companies.

Stevia can be beneficial for those who crave sweets. It can be used on cereal, for baking, in herbal teas, in soda, in toothpaste, and in ice cream, to name a few items. Another benefit is that it contains no calories, so it can easily be used to replace artificial sweeteners, which have side effects and cause problems with some individuals. Stevia is becoming increasingly popular in the United States. It can be found in health food stores in liquid or powder form. Most prefer the taste of the powder. It is not affected by heat and can be used in teas or hot water. Stevia is a beneficial herb, not only used as a sweetener, but as a healing agent.

Scientists began experimenting with stevia during World War II, when sugar was in high demand. It was too expensive to manufacture at that time, but modern techniques have made it available. Stevia is an herbal food and contains properties that are useful to the body other than just as a natural sweetener. A study done at Hiroshima University School of Dentistry suggests that stevia may suppress the growth of dental caries. It does not feed bacteria, as sugar does. It has not only been shown to have no harmful effects on diabetics and individuals suffering from hypoglycemia, it may actually help blood sugar levels remain stable. Studies completed seem to show a correlation between stevia and the regulation of blood sugar levels. One study of twenty-four individuals suffering from hypoglycemia showed no signs of intolerance from stevia use. In the studies done, no harmful effects have been reported.

Stevia is high in magnesium, phosphorus, potassium, and selenium. It also contains manganese, silicon, sodium, and small amounts of calcium, iron, and zinc.

## PRIMARY APPLICATIONS

Diabetes
Hypoglycemia
Sugar substitute

Food cravings
Obesity
Tobacco cravings

## SECONDARY APPLICATIONS

Addictions
Hypertension

Cavities
Hypoglycemia

# STILLINGIA *(Stillingia ligustina)*

*Parts used:* Root
*Properties:* Alterative, blood purifier, emetic, expectorant

Stillingia is one of the most powerful herbs known. It is a North American plant that is relatively new in its use as a medicinal agent.

It is an effective glandular-system stimulant and an activator for the liver. It is said to be valuable for ridding the system of toxic drugs caused by chemotherapy. It should be used with caution and is best when combined with other herbs. It has been used to treat tuberculosis, cancer, and cystic fibrosis. Stillingia helps the body digest protein. It can be used for skin disorders such as eczema, acne, and psoriasis.

## PRIMARY APPLICATIONS

Acne
Eczema
Respiratory problems
Syphilis

Blood impurities
Liver disorders
Skin problems

**SECONDARY APPLICATIONS**

| | |
|---|---|
| Bronchitis | Constipation |
| Throat, sore | Uterine problems |

# STRAWBERRY (*Fragaria vesca*)

*Parts used:* Leaves
*Properties:* Blood purifier, galactagogue, purgative
*Primary nutrients:* Calcium, iron, phosphorus, potassium, vitamins A, B-complex, and C

Strawberry aids in the overall health of the body. It acts as a cleanser for the stomach and is useful for bowel troubles. The roots are especially useful for obstinate dysentery. It has been used for eczema, both externally and internally. Discolored teeth or teeth encrusted with tartar can be cleansed with strawberry juice.

This herb is safe and useful for children.

**PRIMARY APPLICATIONS**

| | |
|---|---|
| Blood impurities | Diarrhea |
| Eczema | Intestinal problems |
| Miscarriage, tendency | |

**SECONDARY APPLICATIONS**

| | |
|---|---|
| Acne | Blood pressure, high |
| Bowel problems | Dysentery |
| Fevers | Jaundice |
| Lactation, absent | Nerves |
| Vomiting | |

# SUMA (*Pfaffia paniculata*)

*Parts used:* Bark and root
*Properties:* Adaptogen, alterative, nutritive, stimulant
*Primary nutrients:* Amino acids, germanium, iron, magnesium, minerals, vitamin B-complex

Suma is found in the rain forests of Brazil. It has an ancient reputation among herbalists, shamans, and physicians in Brazil and is used as a tonic, food, wound healer, antidiabetic, and aphrodisiac. Suma has been used as a source of energy, a rejuvenator, a treatment for serious diseases, and for almost all illnesses. It is reported to be more powerful than Siberian ginseng in its activity.

Suma has been used traditionally to strengthen the immune system and to treat immune-related diseases such as cancer, leukemia, Hodgkin's disease, and diabetes. It enhances energy in the body and promotes longevity. It may also help relieve stress on the body, protect against viral infections, restore sexual function, and promote the healing of wounds.

Suma is thought to be valuable in treating diabetes, joint diseases, osteomyelitis, elevated blood cholesterol, uric acid buildup, and a range of cancers. Suma has been found to stimulate the production of estrogen without stimulating an excess. Professor Nobushige Nishimoto researched suma in Japan and found that the root contains pfaffic acid capable of inhibiting certain types of cancerous cells. He also reported that suma has properties that combat anemia, bronchitis, cholesterol, diabetes, fatigue, stress, and other infirmities.

**PRIMARY APPLICATIONS**

| | |
|---|---|
| Cancer | Cholesterol |
| Circulation | Degenerative diseases |
| Diabetes | Fatigue |
| Hormone imbalance | Immune system issues |
| Stress | Vitality, lack of |

**SECONDARY APPLICATIONS**

| | |
|---|---|
| Anemia | Arthritis |
| Bronchitis | Colds |
| Emotional swings | Energy ailments |
| Heart | Hot flashes |
| Hypoglycemia | Joint diseases |
| Menopausal symptoms | Osteomyelitis |
| Osteoporosis | Skin problems |
| Strokes | Tumors |
| Wounds | |

# TEA TREE (*Melaleuca alternifolia*)

*Parts used:* Oil of the leaves
*Properties:* Anesthetic (mild), antibacterial, antimicrobial, antiseptic, disinfectant, fungicide, germicide

*Primary nutrients:* Cinerol, cymones, pinenes, sesquiterpenes, sesquiterpene alcohols, terpinenes, terpineols

Tea tree oil was discovered by Captain James Cook in 1770 while on an expedition to Australia with a botanist, Sir John Banks, who collected samples of the leaves and took them to England for further studies. The aborigines were known to chew on the leaves. Tea tree oil was used as a medicinal agent for cuts, burns, bites, and many skin ailments. Tea tree oil is extracted from the leaves of *Melaleuca alternifolia*, which is a shrublike tree found in the northeast tropical coastal region of New South Wales and Queensland, Australia. There are more than three hundred different varieties of tea tree, but only a few are known to produce the medicinal oil.

Tea tree oil is an important component of the first-aid kit. It can help with many common, minor conditions. Some include athlete's foot, acne, boils, burns, warts, vaginal infections, tonsillitis, sinus infections, ringworm, skin rashes, impetigo, herpes, corns, head lice, cold sores, canker sores, insect bites, repelling insects, and fungal infections. It is truly a remarkable oil with valuable properties for healing and preventing infection. Tea tree oil acts as a mild anesthetic when applied to painful areas and can soothe cuts, burns, and mouth sores. It can help heal as well as reduce scarring. Burn victims in Australia are often treated with tea tree oil to help prevent infection, relieve pain, and speed healing. Tea tree oil can help heal and prevent infections from occurring, and it can be used to prevent bites and stings. Bugs don't like the scent and may stay away.

Tea tree oil contains at least forty-eight different organic compounds. The compounds work together to produce the healing abilities found in the oil. Research done in the 1950s and early 1960s found that tea tree oil is a germicide and fungicide with additional characteristics of dissolving pus and debris. Recent studies have found it effective for thrush, vaginal infections of *Candida albicans*, staph infections, athlete's foot, hair and scalp problems, mouth sores, muscle and joint pain, and boils. Tea tree oil is a valuable antiseptic for skin infections. It is able to penetrate the epidermis to heal from within. Clinical studies have found that tea tree oil can heal quickly and with less scarring than other treatments. The oil is even effective against *Staphylococcus aureus*, which is often difficult to treat and is becoming resistant to antibiotic therapy. Tea tree oil has been found to be effective against many organisms, including *E. coli*, *Candida albicans*, the herpes virus, and many others. Eduardo F. Pena, MD, has studied *Melaleuca alternifolia* oil for its value in treating vaginitis and *Candida albicans*.

Tea tree oil is an effective bactericide. It is safe for healthy tissue. It is a strong organic solvent and will help heal and disperse pus in pimples and wounds. It has been used to neutralize the venom of minor insect bites. It is able to kill bacteria by penetrating the skin layers and reaching deep into abscesses in the gums and even beneath the fingernails. It has been found to have some of the strongest antimicrobial properties ever discovered in a plant.

Research has found that tea tree oil is a very complex substance. Its many different compounds work together in synergy to produce maximum healing power.

## PRIMARY APPLICATIONS

| | |
|---|---|
| Boils | Candidiasis |
| Infections | Joint pain |
| Skin disorders | Staph infections |
| Strep infections | |

## SECONDARY APPLICATIONS

| | |
|---|---|
| Athlete's foot | Bruises |
| Burns | Fungus |
| Insect bites | Mouth sores |
| Muscle pain | Thrush |

# THYME *(Thymus vulgaris)*

*Parts used:* Entire plant
*Properties:* Alterative, antibacterial, antifungal, antiseptic, antispasmodic, aromatic, carminative, diaphoretic, emmenagogue, expectorant, nervine, parasiticide, rubefacient, sedative, stimulant, vulnerary
*Primary nutrients:* Iodine, silicon, sodium, sulfur, vitamins B-complex, C, and D

Thyme was used by the ancient Greeks as a flavoring agent and for its medicinal value. The herb was considered a symbol of bravery during the Middle Ages, when it was used to encourage strength, for nervous conditions, and as an antispasmodic. It was used for respiratory problems such as asthma and whooping cough. The use of thyme spread throughout Europe, and it was brought to the New World with early colonists. The seventeenth-century herbalist Nicholas Culpeper recommended thyme for killing worms in the belly and as an ointment and disinfectant for hot swelling and warts.

Thyme is a powerful antiseptic and general tonic with healing powers. It is used in cases of anemia, lung ailments, and gastrointestinal ailments. It is also used as an antiseptic against tooth decay. Thyme destroys fungal infections such as athlete's foot and skin parasites such as head lice. It has a long history of use as a folk remedy for bronchitis, catarrh, colic, diabetes, fever, leprosy, rheumatism, sore throat, warts, and whooping cough.

Thyme has traditionally been used as an antiseptic. It does contain antibacterial and antifungal properties, according to some studies. There is also evidence of antispasmodic activity, with components thymol and carvacol relaxing the smooth muscles of the digestive tract and uterus.

## PRIMARY APPLICATIONS

| | |
|---|---|
| Bronchitis, acute | Colic |
| Digestion | Gas |
| Gout, external | Headaches |
| Laryngitis | Lung congestion |
| Sciatica | Throat problems |

## SECONDARY APPLICATIONS

| | |
|---|---|
| Appetite stimulant | Asthma |
| Bowel problems | Bruises |
| Diarrhea | Epilepsy |
| Fainting | Fevers |
| Gastritis | Heartburn |
| Hysteria | Infections, internal |
| Mastitis | Menstruation, inhibited |
| Paralysis | Parasites |
| Perspiration, lack of | Rheumatism |
| Sinus problems | Sprains |
| Stomach problems | Uterine problems |

# TURMERIC *(Curcuma longa)*

*Parts used:* Root
*Properties:* Antibacterial, anticoagulant, antifungal, anti-inflammatory, antineoplastic, antioxidant, antiviral
*Primary nutrients:* Antioxidants

Turmeric has been used throughout Southeast Asia and India for thousands of years. It was used for flavoring foods, dyeing fabrics, and medicinally. It was and continues to be an important part of the Indian culture. Ayurvedic medicine in India uses turmeric as a digestive aid and for cleansing, fevers, infections, dysentery, arthritis, and liver problems. Chinese physicians recommended turmeric for hemorrhage, liver conditions, menstrual problems, and congestion. The ancient Greeks also used turmeric for its medicinal benefits. The use of turmeric has never really caught on in North America, but research indicates healing benefits.

Turmeric is a component of curry powder. It was also used to make an orange-yellow dye. There have been many medicinal claims, including a treatment for ringworm, flatulence, hemorrhage, arthritis, fevers, digestion, liver conditions, gallbladder complaints, and lung congestion.

Research has been conducted, primarily in India, documenting some benefits. Curcumin, the yellow pigment in turmeric, helps stimulate the bile flow to aid digestion. There is also evidence of liver-protective properties in curcumin. Animals given liver-damaging drugs received protection from curcumin. One of the benefits of turmeric is its antioxidant properties. Antioxidants protect against free-radical damage, which can lead to cell damage, aging, and numerous diseases. Turmeric helps stop free-radical progression and prevents free radicals from occurring.

Studies have found that turmeric is a stronger antioxidant than vitamins C and E. It may help by improving the body's own antioxidant and anti-inflammatory capabilities. There is also evidence of anticancer activity in turmeric. The curcumin is thought to be the active component to inhibit tumor cell growth. A number of studies have found these results. Curcumin may help restrict the growth of existing tumors and prevent other cancers, including stomach, colon, esophageal, breast, and skin. Anti-inflammatory effects of turmeric have also been studied. There seem to be analgesic and anti-inflammatory benefits for conditions such as arthritis. When compared with nonsteroidal anti-inflammatory medications, the curcumin was as or more effective in treating inflammatory conditions. Other studies have found even more value in turmeric. It contains antibacterial, antifungal, and antiviral properties. There may also be cholesterol-lowering ability to help in preventing heart disease. And there is anticoagulant activity that can help prevent internal blood clots that can lead to stroke or trigger a heart attack.

## PRIMARY APPLICATIONS

| | |
|---|---|
| Arthritis | Cancer |
| Infections | Inflammation |
| Heart disease | Joint pain |
| Liver disease | Stroke |
| Tumors | |

# UVA URSI *(Arctostaphylos uva-ursi)*

*Parts used:* Leaves
*Properties:* Alterative, antibacterial, antilithic, antimicrobial, antiseptic, astringent, diuretic, lithotriptic
*Primary nutrients:* Iron, manganese, trace minerals, vitamin A

Galen, an ancient Greek physician, used uva ursi's leaves to treat wounds and stop bleeding. It has been used by the Chinese for more than one thousand years as a diuretic and antiseptic for the urinary tract. Native Americans knew the value of uva ursi, which is also known as bearberry. They drank the tea of the steeped leaves to strengthen and heal bladder and kidney problems and women's disorders. Uva ursi was admitted to the London Pharmacopoeia in 1763 and the U.S. Pharmacopoeia in 1820, where it was listed until 1963. Dr. Edward E. Shook used it for its diuretic action for diseases of the bladder and kidneys.

Herbalists have recommended uva ursi for strengthening the urinary system and preventing and treating bladder and kidney infections. It can help increase the flow of urine. Uva ursi works to treat many bladder and kidney problems, including pyelitis, nephritis, urolithiasis, cystitis, urethritis, and urinary catarrh. It contains astringent activity to help clean and protect the urinary system. It helps reduce inflammation and aids with diabetes, arthritis, and hemorrhaging.

Uva ursi has been studied and found to contain allantoin, a substance found to be healing and soothing to irritated tissues. Experiments by Romanian scientists in 1980 found it to contain anti-trichomonal, antiviral, and antibacterial properties. The arbutin found in uva ursi may be the active component, with antiseptic and antimicrobial activity. In vitro studies have found beneficial results.

## PRIMARY APPLICATIONS

| | |
|---|---|
| Cystitis | Diabetes |
| Gonorrhea | Kidney infections |
| Nephritis | Spleen ailments |
| Urethritis | |

## SECONDARY APPLICATIONS

| | |
|---|---|
| Arthritis | Bed-wetting |
| Bright's disease | Bronchitis |
| Diarrhea | Digestion |
| Dysentery | Female problems |
| Fevers | Gallstones |
| Gravel | Hemorrhoids |
| Infection | Liver problems |
| Lung congestion | Menstruation |
| Pancreatic ailments | Prostate problems |
| Rheumatism | Uric acid |
| Urinary incontinence | Uterine disorders |
| Vaginal discharge | Venereal disease |
| Water retention | |

# VALERIAN *(Valeriana officinalis)*

*Parts used:* Root
*Properties:* Alterative, antiseptic, carminative, decongestant, diuretic, galactagogue, nervine, sedative
*Primary nutrients:* Calcium, iron, magnesium, manganese, niacin, potassium, selenium, silicon, sodium, vitamins A and C, zinc

Galen, an ancient Greek physician, prescribed valerian as a decongestant. The Greeks also used it for digestion, nausea, and urinary tract disorders. John Gerard, an herbalist, recommended this herb in 1597 for chest congestion, convulsions, bruises, and falls. Native Americans used valerian for healing wounds. Samuel Thomson recommended using valerian as a tranquilizer. It was accepted in the U.S. Pharmacopoeia as a tranquilizer in 1820 until 1942 and in the National Formulary until 1950.

Valerian is beneficial for the heart, lungs, liver, and stomach, as well as the nerves and the brain. It may also help with epilepsy, hysteria, migraines, and eliminating worms. It is a strong nervine herb that produces a calming effect to aid individuals suffering from insomnia, anxiety, muscle spasms, and nervous tension. Valerian is a tonic herb in its effects on the nervous system. It seems to be able to relax and calm when necessary, as well as improving mental acuity and coordination. It is usually recommended for short-term use.

Studies have identified some of the properties of valerian. It has been found to act as a relaxant and is effective for insomnia. The active ingredients found in the root are responsible for relaxing the smooth muscle tissue (those responsible for involuntary muscles) and depressing the central nervous system. Studies have found that valerian can produce a deep, satisfying sleep similar to some sleep aids often prescribed. But valerian has an advantage over medication in that it does not cause the morning grogginess often associated with prescription sleep medications. The valepotriates in the valerian plant are thought to be responsible for its sedative activity. It appears that no single component of valerian is responsible for all of its sedative activity, but that several of the constituents work together.

Research has found valerian to be effective in treating insomnia and reducing sleep latency. It not only reduced sleep latency but also helped reduce the number of night awakenings. Valerian is thought to be safe, and there appear to be no contraindications to its use, even during pregnancy and lactation. Many different studies have confirmed the benefits of valerian for insomnia, anxiety, and stress. It is useful for sleep disorders, especially when they are related to anxiety, nervousness, headache pain, or physical and mental exhaustion. It can help relieve problems without side effects often associated with medication, such as dependency, drowsiness, and morning hangover. One study even found that hyperactive individuals were able to concentrate for longer periods of time when taking valerian.

## PRIMARY APPLICATIONS

| | |
|---|---|
| After-birth pains | Blood pressure |
| Convulsions | Heart palpitations |
| High blood pressure | Hypochondria |
| Hysteria | Muscle spasms |
| Nervous conditions | Pain |

## SECONDARY APPLICATIONS

| | |
|---|---|
| Alcoholism | Arthritis pain |
| Bladder ailments | Bronchial spasms |
| Colds | Constipation |
| Coughs | Cramps |
| Digestion | Drug addiction |
| Epilepsy | Fatigue |
| Fever | Gas |
| Headache | Insomnia |
| Lactation, absent | Measles |
| Menstruation | Palsy |
| Restlessness | Stomach problems |
| Stress | Ulcers |
| Worms | |

# VERVAIN *(Verbena officinalis)*

*Parts used:* Tops
*Properties:* Alterative, antispasmodic, astringent, cholagogue, diaphoretic, emmenagogue, galactagogue, nervine, parasiticide, sedative, stimulant

Vervain is a common plant found growing throughout the world. It has a long history of use. It was used by the ancient Romans medicinally and to purify their temples and homes. Egyptian mythology speaks of vervain. It was used by the Greeks for fevers and plague. Use of vervain spread throughout Europe. As with many herbs, vervain was brought to the New World by colonists. Native Americans were using the American vervain to treat fevers and stomach complaints.

Vervain has been used traditionally to treat many conditions. Some include colds, fevers, intestinal worms, menstrual irregularities, acute diseases, gout, and skin disorders. It is recommended as a nervous system strengthener, for nervous disorders, and for mental stress. It is used for liver conditions and congestion. Modern uses of vervain include fever, depression, gum disease, headache, menstruation problems, and as a relaxant.

Vervain has been found to work on mild pain and inflammation. In small doses, the glycoside verbenin in vervain stimulates the flow of milk.

## PRIMARY APPLICATIONS

| | |
|---|---|
| Colds | Congestion |
| Convulsions | Coughs |
| Fevers | Gum disorders |
| Liver congestion | |

## SECONDARY APPLICATIONS

| | |
|---|---|
| Ague | Asthma |
| Bladder | Bowels |
| Catarrh | Circulation |
| Digestion | Eczema |
| Flu | Gallstones |
| Headache | Hemorrhage |
| Hepatitis | Insect bites |
| Insomnia | Jaundice |
| Lactation, absent | Menstruation |
| Mental stress | Nervousness |
| Skin problems | Stomach disorders |
| Throat ailments | Tuberculosis |
| Uterine problems | Worms |

# VIOLET (Viola odorata)

*Parts used:* Flowers and leaves
*Properties:* Alterative, antiseptic, antispasmodic, demulcent, expectorant, febrifuge, vulnerary
*Primary nutrients:* Vitamins A and C

Violet is another herb with a long history. Both the Romans and Greeks regarded the violet as a valuable plant for its beauty and medicinal uses. Pliny recommended violet for gout, headaches, and dizziness.

Violet is very effective in healing internal ulcers. It is also used internally and externally for tumors, boils, abscesses, pimples, swollen glands, and malignant growths. It is found in some alternative treatments for cancer. The properties of violet leaves and flowers seem to have the ability to reach parts of the body only accessible by the blood and lymphatic fluids. It is useful to aid the respiratory system and for coughs, sore throats, and asthma. Violet is also used to treat headaches. It may help soften hard tumors and cancerous growths.

## PRIMARY APPLICATIONS

| | |
|---|---|
| Asthma | Bronchitis |
| Cancer | Colds, head congestion |
| Coughs | Sinus catarrh |
| Tumors | Ulcers |

## SECONDARY APPLICATIONS

| | |
|---|---|
| Breathing difficulty | Gout |
| Headaches | Sores |
| Syphilis | Throat, sore |

# WATERCRESS (Nasturtium officinale)

*Parts used:* Entire plant
*Properties:* Alterative, antineoplastic, bitter, blood purifier, diuretic, emmenagogue, expectorant, galactagogue, purgative (mild), nutritive, stimulant, stomachic
*Primary nutrients:* Calcium, copper, iodine, iron, manganese, sulfur, vitamins A, B, C, D, E, and G

Watercress was brought by colonists from Europe to prevent scurvy. This plant grows in clear, cold water along the edges of small streams. Native Americans used watercress for liver and kidney problems.

Watercress is used principally as a tonic for regulating metabolism and the flow of bile. It helps increase stamina and physical endurance. Eaten fresh daily, watercress helps purify the blood and supplies essential vitamins and minerals. The juice of the leaves can be applied to the face for freckles and pimples. Watercress soaked in honey has been found beneficial as a cough medicine. This herb is an excellent food for enriching the blood.

Studies have found that the dried leaves contain high amounts of vitamin C.

## PRIMARY APPLICATIONS

| | |
|---|---|
| Anemia | Blood impurities |
| Cramps | Kidney problems |
| Liver complaints | Nervous ailments |
| Rheumatism | |

## SECONDARY APPLICATIONS

| | |
|---|---|
| Acne | Appetite problems |
| Cysts | Eczema |
| Heart ailments | Joints, stiff |
| Kidney stones | Lactation, absent |
| Mental disorders | Tuberculosis |
| Tumors, internal | Uterine cysts |

# WHITE OAK BARK
*(Quercus alba)*

*Parts used:* Bark
*Properties:* Antiseptic, astringent, diuretic, lithotriptic
*Primary nutrients:* Calcium, cobalt, iodine, iron, lead, phosphorus, potassium, sodium, strontium, sulfur, tin, vitamin B12

Native Americans used white oak bark as a poultice for gangrene. The Iroquois used it as an astringent; the Penobscotts used it for bleeding piles; the Houmas crushed the roots and mixed them with whiskey for a liniment to rub on rheumatic parts; the Ojibwe scraped the root bark and inner bark and boiled them for a decoction for diarrhea; the Meskwakis drank the tea to expel phlegm from the lungs; and the Menominees used the bark as an infusion for treating hemorrhoids. The inner bark was listed in the U.S. Pharmacopoeia from 1820 to 1916.

The clotting and shrinking action of white oak bark is useful for tightening gums with loose teeth and for pyorrhea, as well as any gum infection. White oak bark contains strong astringent properties that can be used for both external and internal bleeding. It is an excellent cleanser for the skin and mucous membranes to heal damaged tissues in the stomach and intestines. It has been used for excess stomach mucus, which causes common complaints of sinus congestion and postnasal drip. The stomach is strengthened for better absorption and secretion, thus improving metabolism. It has been used to treat diarrhea, external and internal bleeding, varicose veins, hemorrhoids, and excess mucus. It is used to treat inflamed areas of the skin, mucous membranes, stomach, and intestines. It aids the stomach by increasing the internal absorption and secretion and improving metabolism. White oak is used to aid in normalizing the kidneys, liver, and spleen. It is known to help increase the flow of urine and to aid in cases of kidney stones and gallstones. It is used to help with all kidney problems, including bladder infections and blood in the urine.

This herb has been used as an antidote for drug allergies and in easing the side effects of chemotherapy. It is used as a blood cleanser to help eliminate drugs and toxins in the body.

Research has found that white oak bark has astringent and antiseptic properties. The tannins in white oak bark can bind with substances in the intestinal tract and also help stop bleeding, helping heal tissue that has been damaged due to injury or illness.

## PRIMARY APPLICATIONS

| | |
|---|---|
| Bleeding | Hemorrhoids |
| Menstrual symptoms | Mouth sores |
| Skin irritations | Strep throat |
| Teeth problems | Thrush |
| Ulcers | Varicose veins |
| Worms | |

## SECONDARY APPLICATIONS

| | |
|---|---|
| Bites, insect and snake | Bladder ailments |
| Bruises | Cancer |
| Canker sores | Dental problems |
| Diarrhea | Enema |
| Fevers | Gallstones |
| Gangrene | Gingivitis |
| Glandular swelling | Goiter |
| Gums | Indigestion |
| Jaundice | Kidney ailments |
| Liver ailments | Nausea |
| Prostate problems | Pyorrhea |
| Spleen ailments | Tonsillitis |
| Tumors | Uterine problems |
| Vaginal problems | Venereal disease |
| Vomiting | Wounds |

# WHITE PINE BARK (*Pinus strobus*)

*Parts used:* Bark
*Properties:* Aromatic, astringent, expectorant
*Primary nutrients:* Calcium, copper, iodine, manganese, nickel, sodium, vitamins A and C, zinc

White pines are found growing in forests in the northeastern areas of the United States. Native Americans used the white pine bark for treating colds, coughs, scurvy, kidney ailments, and chest congestion. They soaked the bark in water until it became soft and then applied it to wounds. They also boiled the inner bark saplings and drank the liquid for dysentery. A poultice was applied to wounds to speed healing. The Iroquois and Micmac tribes often used white pine bark in remedies to treat various ailments.

White pine bark has medicinal properties as well as food value. The bark is an excellent expectorant. It helps reduce mucus secretions that occur with the common cold.

## PRIMARY APPLICATIONS

| | |
|---|---|
| Bronchitis | Dysentery |
| Laryngitis | Mucus |

## SECONDARY APPLICATIONS

| | |
|---|---|
| Colds | Croup |
| Flu | Kidney problems |
| Lung congestion | Rheumatism |
| Scurvy | Strep throat |
| Tonsillitis | Whooping cough |

# WILD CHERRY (*Prunus virginiana*)

*Parts used:* Bark
*Properties:* Alterative, antiasthmatic, anticatarrhal, antitussive, aromatic, astringent, bitter, carminative, expectorant, nervine, parasiticide, pectoral, sedative, stomachic, stimulant

Wild cherry bark was used by Native Americans to aid in cases of diarrhea and lung conditions. Colonists followed the example of the natives and used the bark for coughs and congestion.

Wild cherry bark is a very useful expectorant and is a valuable remedy for all catarrhal conditions. It is beneficial for bronchial disorders caused by the accumulation of mucus. Its action is mild and soothing on the mucous membranes and respiratory organs. Wild cherry bark soothes the nerves in the respiratory system to help stop coughs and relieve asthmatic conditions. Wild cherry bark contains a volatile oil that acts as a local stimulant in the alimentary canal and aids digestion. It is a useful tonic for those convalescing because it tones the entire system.

## PRIMARY APPLICATIONS

| | |
|---|---|
| Asthma | Bronchitis |
| Catarrh | Coughs |
| Fever | High blood pressure |
| Mucus, hardened | Phlegm |

## SECONDARY APPLICATIONS

| | |
|---|---|
| Diarrhea | Eyesight |
| Flu | Gallbladder |
| Heart palpitations | Stomach, irritated |

# WILD LETTUCE (*Lactuca virosa*)

*Parts used:* Entire plant
*Properties:* Anodyne, bitter, diuretic, galactagogue, hypnotic, narcotic, nervine

Native Americans used wild lettuce as a tea for lactation. During the nineteenth century, it was used as a substitute for opium and was referred to as the poor man's opium.

Wild lettuce has been used to increase the flow of urine and to soothe sore and chapped skin. The leaves contain sedative properties that act somewhat like morphine, only milder. It is the dried leaves that are used to induce sleep and treat severe nervous disorders. The juice of the plant can be applied to relieve the itching of poison ivy and poison oak. The mild sedative activity helps relieve pain, insomnia, cramps, whooping cough, and bronchitis. It may help relieve pain associated with arthritis.

Early studies attribute the sedative properties to lactucorpicrin and lactucin. This sedative effect may help with sleep problems, restlessness, and nervousness.

## PRIMARY APPLICATIONS

| | |
|---|---|
| Bronchitis | Cramps |
| Nervous disorders | Pain, chronic |
| Whooping cough | |

## SECONDARY APPLICATIONS

| | |
|---|---|
| Asthma | Colic |
| Coughs | Diarrhea |
| Edema | Insomnia |
| Lactation, absent | Spasms |

# WILD YAM (*Dioscorea villosa*)

*Parts used:* Root
*Properties:* Anti-inflammatory, antispasmodic, blood purifier, cholagogue, diaphoretic
*Primary nutrients:* Calcium, iron, magnesium, manganese, phosphorus, potassium, selenium, silicon, sodium, vitamins A, B-complex, and C, zinc

Wild yam was used by Native Americans as a root decoction to relieve the pains of childbirth and to treat muscular rheumatism. The Aztecs used wild yam to treat skin disorders such as scabies and as a poultice for boils. In his book *Back to Eden*, herbalist Jethro Kloss says that wild yam combined with ginger can help in preventing miscarriage.

Wild yam relaxes the muscular fiber, soothes the nerves, and relieves pain, especially in the uterus. It is often used to balance hormones to treat nausea in pregnant women and to aid in preventing miscarriage, cramps, and general pains during pregnancy. It is a blood cleanser and helps strengthen the liver, reduce cholesterol levels, and lower blood pressure. It helps relieve pain associated with gallstones.

Wild yam contains a component known as diosgenin, which is a precursor of progesterone. It has the ability to convert to progesterone, but wild yam does not contain progesterone. One physician found that an herbal formula containing wild yam was 71 percent effective in reducing the total number of symptoms of progesterone deficiency and 100 percent effective in reducing the severity of symptoms.

Studies on animals suggest wild yam contains steroid-like properties that inhibit inflammation. Another study found that natural progesterone supplementation was more effective in preventing osteoporosis than estrogen. A study on progesterone was conducted at Johns Hopkins University. Women who had a progesterone deficiency were over five times more at risk of developing breast cancer than women with normal progesterone levels. The progesterone derived from wild yam closely resembles natural progesterone synthesized in the body. Wild yam, when absorbed by the body, is easily converted into the same molecule as progesterone.

## PRIMARY APPLICATIONS

| | |
|---|---|
| Arthritis | Asthma, spasmodic |
| Bowel spasms | Colic |
| Cramps, uterine | Gas |
| Liver ailments | Morning sickness |
| Muscle pain | Spasms |

## SECONDARY APPLICATIONS

| | |
|---|---|
| Abdominal pain | Blood impurities |
| Boils | Bronchitis |
| Catarrh | Cholera |
| Hiccup | Inflammation |
| Intestinal problems | Jaundice |
| Nausea | Nervousness |
| Pain | Rheumatism |
| Stomach ailments | Ulcers |
| Whooping cough | |

# WILLOW (*Salix*)

*Parts used:* Bark
*Properties:* Alterative, analgesic, anodyne, anthelmintic, anti-inflammatory, antiperiodic, antiseptic, antispasmodic, astringent, diaphoretic, diuretic, febrifuge
*Primary nutrients:* Isorhamnetin, phenolic glycosides, quercetin, salicin, salicylic acid, salinigrin

Willow was recognized for its medicinal value by Dioscorides, the Greek physician, during the first century AD. He recommended the use of willow bark for pain and inflammation. Early Chinese physicians also used willow bark for pain and inflammation. Egyptians considered the willow to be a sign of joy and celebration. Native Americans also recognized the value of willow and used it to treat pain, fevers, and inflammation. They passed on their knowledge to the colonists who moved to the New World.

Willow is valued as a nerve sedative because it has no depressing aftereffects. It works in a manner similar to aspirin, but is gentle on the stomach. Traditionally, a bitter drink was made by steeping willow bark and twigs in water. This drink was used for fevers and chills and as a substitute for chinchona bark. Willow bark extract is helpful in cleansing and healing eyes that are inflamed or infected. It has been called one of the essential first-aid plants. It has strong but benign antiseptic properties and is good for infected wounds, ulcerations, and eczema. The bark contains the glycoside salicin, which is an effective painkiller. Aspirin is a synthetic derivative of this component. Willow is most often used for minor aches and pains in the body.

Salicylic acid was the natural source of synthetic aspirin. Aspirin and willow share many similar analgesic properties. The activity of salicylates reduces pain by acting on sensory nerves and inhibiting the synthesis of prostaglandins that are involved with inflammation.

## PRIMARY APPLICATIONS

| | |
|---|---|
| Eczema | Fever |
| Headache | Nervousness |
| Pain | Rheumatism |
| Sex depressant | Ulceration |

## SECONDARY APPLICATIONS

| | |
|---|---|
| Bleeding | Chills |
| Corns | Dandruff |
| Diarrhea | Dysentery |
| Earache | Flu |
| Gout | Hay fever |
| Heartburn | Impotence |
| Infection | Inflammation |
| Muscle, sore | Night sweats |
| Ovarian pain | Tonsillitis |

# WINTERGREEN
*(Gaultheria procumbens)*

*Parts used:* Leaves and oil
*Properties:* Analgesic, anodyne, antirheumatic, antiseptic, antispasmodic, aromatic, astringent, diuretic, expectorant, rubefacient
*Primary nutrients:* Gaultherin (similar to aspirin), gaultherase, glycoside, tannins

Wintergreen oil contains properties such as methyl salicylate that are similar to aspirin. Native Americans recognized the value of wintergreen. They ground the leaves into a poultice and applied it to painful areas of muscles and joints.

Wintergreen is a fragrant analgesic. It is very valuable when used in small doses. It stimulates the stomach, heart, and respiration. It has a penetrating effect on every cell and acts on the cause of pain. As a tea or hot compress, it is beneficial for headaches, rheumatic pain, sciatica, and pains in the joints and muscles. An infusion may also be used as a gargle for sore throats or as a douche for leucorrhea. Externally, the oil of wintergreen has been used for rheumatism, inflammation, wounds, warts, corns, calluses, cysts, and even tattoo marks.

Taken orally in small doses, wintergreen oil helps stimulate digestion and gastric secretion. Due to the similarities in chemical structure of wintergreen and aspirin, there is potential for some analgesic effect.

## PRIMARY APPLICATIONS

| | |
|---|---|
| Aches and pains | Arthritis |
| Back pain, lower | Gout |
| Headaches, migraines | |

## SECONDARY APPLICATIONS

| | |
|---|---|
| Cystitis | Diabetes |
| Diphtheria | Gas |
| Inflammation | Leucorrhea |
| Rheumatic fever | Sciatica |
| Throat gargle | Urinary system |
| Yeast infections | |

# WITCH HAZEL *(Hamamelis virginiana)*

*Parts used:* Bark
*Properties:* Alterative, anti-inflammatory, antiseptic, astringent, hemostatic, sedative
*Primary nutrients:* Copper, iodine, manganese, selenium, vitamins C, E, K, and P, zinc

Native Americans used witch hazel for cuts, bruises, muscle aches, wounds, and as a general tonic. They also drank a tea for sore throats and to prevent miscarriage, fevers, and colds. They used it in steam baths for coughs and congestion. It was one of the most valued remedies native to America. Colonists adopted the use of witch hazel from the natives. Witch hazel was listed in the U.S. Pharmacopoeia from 1862 through 1916 and the National Formulary from 1916 to 1955 as an astringent and anti-inflammatory.

Witch hazel is used externally as an alcohol extract for insect bites, varicose veins, burns, hemorrhoids, and to stop bleeding wounds. It is used internally to help stop bleeding from the lungs, uterus, and other internal organs. It can be used as a mouthwash for bleeding gums and inflammation in the mouth and throat. Compresses can be applied to the skin to treat headaches, sores, skin irritations, insect bites, sunburn, other burns, and infections. It is a safe treatment with a mild and gentle action.

The leaves and bark of witch hazel contain tannins that are known to have astringent properties. Animal studies have found vasoconstrictive activity in an alcoholic fluid extract.

## PRIMARY APPLICATIONS

| | |
|---|---|
| Bleeding, internal | Gum problems |
| Hemorrhoids | Mucous membranes |
| Varicose veins | |

## SECONDARY APPLICATIONS

| | |
|---|---|
| Bruises | Burns |
| Cuts | Diarrhea |
| Dysentery | Eyes, bags |
| Hemorrhage | Insect bites |
| Menstruation, excess | Muscles, sore |
| Scalds | Sinus ailments |
| Swelling | Tuberculosis |
| Tumors | Venereal disease |

# WOOD BETONY *(Betonica officinalis)*

*Parts used:* Herb
*Properties:* Alterative, analgesic, aromatic, blood purifier, hepatic, hypotensive, nervine, parasiticide, sedative
*Primary nutrients:* Magnesium, manganese, phosphorus

Antonius Musa, an herbalist who was the Roman physician to Caesar Augustus, wrote a book devoted to the value of betony. He suggested it for preserving the liver and bodies of men from epidemic diseases, digestion of meat, weak stomachs, and belching. In 1611, a German pharmacist named Schroeder said that wood betony could help with almost any ailment.

Traditional uses of wood betony include the treatment of nervous disorders; as a sedative; to relieve head and facial pain; as a blood purifier, a liver strengthener, and a gentle laxative; and to treat indigestion. It is used as an effective sedative for children and a good tranquilizer for adults. It works to clean impurities from the blood and opens congested areas of the liver and spleen. Wood betony contains glycosides that contain hypotensive properties. This may help relax the nerves and open constricted blood vessels. This activity may also be responsible for wood betony's abilities in headache pain relief.

Little research has been done on wood betony, but one study found hypotensive activity attributed to the glycoside components. More research needs to be done, but this herb may be useful for pain relief, as a relaxant, for catarrh and fatigue, as a brain enhancer, and as a general alterative.

## PRIMARY APPLICATIONS

| | |
|---|---|
| Delirium | Fevers |
| Headaches | Hysteria |
| Jaundice | Liver problems |
| Migraines | Nervousness |
| Parkinson's disease | Worms |

## SECONDARY APPLICATIONS

| | |
|---|---|
| Anemia | Arthritis |
| Asthma | Bladder problems |
| Bleeding, internal | Blood impurities |

| | |
|---|---|
| Bronchitis | Colds |
| Colic | Consumption |
| Convulsions | Cramps, stomach |
| Diarrhea | Digestion |
| Dropsy | Epilepsy |
| Fainting | Gout |
| Heartburn | Heart problems |
| Indigestion | Insanity |
| Insomnia | Kidney ailments |
| Lung congestion | Menstruation |
| Muscle spasms | Neuralgia |
| Pain | Parasites |
| Rheumatism | Ulcers |
| Varicose veins | Wounds |

# WORMWOOD (*Artemisia absinthium*)

*Parts used:* Herb and leaves
*Properties:* Alterative, anthelmintic, febrifuge, stomachic
*Primary nutrients:* Calcium, cobalt, manganese, potassium, sodium, tin, vitamins C and B-complex

European wormwood has been used in medicine since ancient times. The name was derived from its use as an intestinal anthelmintic to rid the body of parasites. It was used to combat intestinal worms by Dioscorides and Pliny. It was mentioned by Tragus in Brunfels's *Herbal* in 1531, imported to Italy, and mentioned as having its most positive effect upon roundworms. In Germany, wormwood was used as a flavoring for wine. Dr. Edward E. Shook mentioned it as being of great value in melancholia, yellow jaundice, and dropsy. Herbalists value wormwood as a stimulant to promote sweating and improve digestion. It can expel worms and improve liver function.

Wormwood has been used for poor circulation, rheumatism, fevers, colds, and jaundice. Herbalists have also recommended wormwood for indigestion, stomach acidity, and constipation. Wormwood may help stimulate sweating in cases of dry fevers. It has also been used to expel worms, promote menstruation, stimulate uterine circulation, relieve menstrual cramps, and as an insect repellent. Wormwood can be used externally to reduce hair loss. It is usually recommended to be used for only short periods of time and is not for children.

The anthelmintic activity of wormwood is thought to be due to lactones. There may also be some antimalarial properties in wormwood. There is evidence of the thujone content being able to stun roundworms, allowing them to be expelled through normal excretory functions.

People with seizure disorders and pregnant women should not use wormwood.

## PRIMARY APPLICATIONS

| | |
|---|---|
| Constipation | Cramps, menstrual |
| Debility | Digestion |
| Fever | Inflammation, GI tract |
| Jaundice | Liver problems |
| Menstruation, lack of | Stomach problems |
| Worms | |

## SECONDARY APPLICATIONS

| | |
|---|---|
| Appetite problems | Blood circulation |
| Diarrhea | Earaches |
| Edema | Female disorders |
| Gallbladder | Gout |
| Indigestion | Insect repellent |
| Kidney ailments | Morning sickness |
| Nausea | Neuralgia |
| Obesity | Poisons |
| Rheumatism | Swelling |

# YARROW (*Achillea millefolium*)

*Parts used:* Flower
*Properties:* Alterative, antiseptic, astringent, blood purifier, diaphoretic, diuretic, homeostatic, stimulant
*Primary nutrients:* Copper, iodine, iron, manganese, potassium, vitamins A, C, E, F, and K

Yarrow was used anciently by the Greeks and was named after the legendary warrior Achilles. Legend reports that during the conquest of Troy, Achilles applied yarrow to the wounds of his soldiers. It was used anciently for menstrual problems, indigestion, hemorrhoids, and wounds. Yarrow was also used in China for inflammation, bleeding, wounds, and snakebites. Yarrow is native to Europe and Asia.

Nicholas Culpeper, a seventeenth-century English herbalist, suggested yarrow for wounds, inflammation, and bleeding. Colonists probably introduced the use of yarrow to the New World. The Paiutes used it as a tea for a weak stomach. It was used by some Native American tribes for swelling, earaches, bruises, and abrasions. Yarrow was listed in the U.S. Pharmacopoeia from 1863 to 1882 and was recommended for promoting menstruation and for its stimulant properties. Yarrow has been used for just about every ailment in its history and has proven healing properties.

Yarrow is well known for its ability to help stimulate clotting in cuts and abrasions. It may speed healing, relieve inflammation, and reduce the pain of injuries. Yarrow acts as a blood cleanser and is good for colds, fevers, flu, lung disorders, nosebleeds, and perspiration. It also helps regulate and improve the function of the liver. It tones the mucous membranes of the stomach and bowels and aids the glandular system.

The use of yarrow for healing wounds has evidence to back it up. Research has found yarrow extract to contain slight antibiotic properties that may protect an injury from infection. Yarrow has also demonstrated some antispasmodic properties that work to relax smooth muscles in the digestive tract and uterus. This may help with digestion, as well as menstrual cramps, which was a traditional use. A volatile oil in yarrow known as azulene and related compounds have been shown in studies to have anti-inflammatory properties that also help with wound healing, which generally involves some inflammation. The thujone content in yarrow has a slight sedative effect that has been compared to marijuana. In large doses, thujone can be toxic, but recommended amounts of yarrow appear to be safe. Yarrow reportedly has properties to protect the liver from toxic chemical damage and to treat hepatitis. The properties of each species may be affected by the age and environment in which they are grown, causing differences in chemical components.

## PRIMARY APPLICATIONS

| | |
|---|---|
| Blood impurities | Bowels, hemorrhage |
| Catarrh | Colds |
| Fevers | Flu |
| Lung, hemorrhage | Measles |
| Nosebleeds | Perspiration, blocked |

## SECONDARY APPLICATIONS

| | |
|---|---|
| Abrasions | Ague |
| Appetite problems | Bladder ailments |
| Blood pressure | Bright's disease |
| Bronchitis | Bruises |
| Burns | Cancer |
| Chicken pox | Cramps |
| Cuts | Diarrhea, infants |
| Epilepsy | Female disorders |
| Gas | Hair loss |
| Headaches | Hemorrhoids |
| Hysteria | Jaundice |
| Malaria | Menstrual bleeding |
| Mucous membranes | Pleurisy |
| Pneumonia | Rheumatism |
| Skin problems | Smallpox |
| Stomach problems | Typhoid fever |
| Ulcers | Uterine problems |

# YELLOW DOCK (*Rumex crispus*)

*Parts used:* Root
*Properties:* Alterative, antibiotic, astringent, blood purifier, cholagogue, nutritive, purgative (mild)
*Primary nutrients:* Iron (easily digestible form), manganese, nickel, vitamins A and C

Yellow dock was a favorite herb among Native Americans for a variety of ailments, including primary tuberculosis, eruptive diseases, and infections of the eyes, ears, and skin. Many herbalists have used yellow dock for blood and glandular problems, including cancer, leprosy, and lung and bowel bleeding. Yellow dock was listed in the U.S. Pharmacopoeia from 1863 until 1905.

Yellow dock is well known as a blood cleanser, tonic, and builder, helping the liver purify the blood and lymph systems. Modern herbalists recommend yellow dock for anemia, as a blood purifier, for liver congestion, and for skin problems. It is also considered beneficial for toxemia, infections, lymph congestion, ulcers, and wounds. It stimulates elimination, working as a mild laxative, and improves bile flow. Yellow dock nourishes the spleen and liver and has been used to treat jaundice. It is considered one of the best blood builders in the herbal kingdom.

The anthroquinone content of yellow dock may be responsible for its mild laxative effect. Yellow dock has been found to be a good alterative, especially for chronic skin problems. It is useful for leprosy, psoriasis, and cancer.

## PRIMARY APPLICATIONS

| | |
|---|---|
| Anemia | Blood impurities |
| Cancer | Coughs |
| Eyelids, ulcerated | Hives |
| Liver congestion | Rheumatism |
| Skin ailments | |

## SECONDARY APPLICATIONS

| | |
|---|---|
| Acne | Arthritis |
| Bladder problems | Blood disorders |
| Bowels, bleeding | Bronchitis |
| Constipation | Dysentery |
| Dyspepsia | Ear infections |
| Eczema | Energy |
| Fatigue | Fevers |
| Gallbladder ailments | Hay fever |
| Hemorrhoids, external | Hepatitis |
| Jaundice | Leprosy |
| Leukemia | Lymphatic system |
| Scurvy | Spleen ailments |
| Stomach problems | Thyroid gland |
| Tumors | Ulcers |
| Varicose veins | Venereal disease |

# YERBA SANTA
*(Eriodictyon californicum)*

*Parts used:* Leaves
*Properties:* Alterative, antiasthmatic, aromatic, astringent, bitter, blood purifier, carminative, decongestant, expectorant, sialagogue, stimulant, stomachic
*Primary nutrients:* Eriodictyol (expectorant)

Native Americans used yerba santa for various ailments such as colds, coughs, sore throats, congestion, diarrhea, and stomach ailments. The Spaniards who colonized South America learned of the value of yerba santa from the natives and found beneficial results from its action. Yerba santa means "sacred herb" in Spanish.

Yerba santa is a mild but useful decongestant. It is recommended for all forms of bronchial congestion and is an excellent remedy for chest conditions, both acute and chronic. It works as a blood purifier and stimulates all digestive secretions. The fresh or dried leaves of this herb were traditionally used as a poultice for broken bones and bruises. It is also beneficial for pain resulting from rheumatism, tired limbs, swelling, and sores. Yerba santa is a stimulating and rejuvenating herb that helps relieve fatigue. It may also help improve the effectiveness of other herbs.

Little research has been reported, but the thujone found in yerba santa appears to have some expectorant activity.

## PRIMARY APPLICATIONS

| | |
|---|---|
| Asthma | Bronchial congestion |
| Colds | Hay fever |

## SECONDARY APPLICATIONS

| | |
|---|---|
| Bladder catarrh | Blood impurities |
| Coughs | Diarrhea |
| Dysentery | Fever |
| Flu | Hemorrhoids |
| Kidney problems | Laryngitis, chronic |
| Nasal discharge | Rheumatism |
| Stomachaches | Throat, sore |
| Vomiting | |

# YOHIMBE *(Pausinystalia johimbe)*

*Parts used:* Bark
*Properties:* Aphrodisiac

The yohimbe tree is found growing wild throughout tropical coastal west Africa from Nigeria to Gabon. It is a tall evergreen with large, leathery leaves. The inner bark has been used traditionally to treat angina and hypertension. It was also smoked and snuffed by natives for its hallucinogenic effect. In some areas of western Africa, a decoction is used to treat fevers and leprosy. It is also chewed to help relieve a cough. The yohimbe bark was first brought to the attention of the Europeans by early traders. While on their adventures in western Africa, they heard about the yohimbe tree. They became interested in finding and trying the legendary yohimbe bark. They were able to acquire some of the bark and return with it to Europe. Future trips brought more interest in the yohimbe bark, and it soon was in demand.

Yohimbe has gained popularity because of its use as an aphrodisiac. Compounds founds in yohimbe are known to be precursors of testosterone. It is found in some athletic formulas for muscle development and bodybuilding. It may also help with both male and female sexual dysfunction. A form of yohimbine (the active ingredient found in the yohimbe bark) called yohimbien hydrochloride has been used in some prescription formulas to treat erectile dysfunction. Yohimbe dilates blood vessels near the skin, mucous membranes, and sex organs. This may cause fatigue in individuals with low blood pressure; therefore, yohimbe should be avoided by individuals with blood pressure or heart irregularities.

Both the crude bark and the purified compound are used as aphrodisiacs. The yohimbine content is thought to be approximately 6 percent. Other minor alkaloids found in yohimbe bark include ajmaline, alloyohimbine, corynanthine, quebrachine, and tetrahydromethylcorynanthein.

Studies have found that yohimbine works as a treatment for impotent men. Yohimbe is listed in the *Physicians Desk Reference* as a sensual stimulant. It helps increase sexual desire, but the main function is to increase the blood flow to the erectile tissue. It has been found to be effective in treating both organic (physiological) and psychogenic (mental) forms of impotence. The aphrodisiac effects associated with yohimbe are related to this dilation. It increases the blood flow and enlarges the vessels in the sexual organs, as well as increasing reflex excitability in the lower spinal cord. Yohimbe has been found to make erections harder and firmer through increased circulation to the area. It is also

thought to aid in maintaining an erection by causing a compression and preventing blood from flowing out of the organ. Vascular disease is known to be a major factor in many cases of impotence. Atherosclerosis in the body also affects the penile artery, reducing circulation to that area. A study done using rats in 1984 gave small doses of yohimbine to sexually active male rats. Though they showed normal sexual activity before, their sexual arousal increased with the addition of the yohimbine. This has led to an increase in studies involving yohimbe and yohimbine, which seem to have a similar effect in human studies. Yohimbine may also help increase the production of norepinephrine in the body, which is known to decrease with age and affects the formation of erections. The adrenaline supply may also increase, which can heighten the male sensual stimulation.

An Italian clinical study was conducted in 1994 using yohimbine for cases of impotence. The individuals involved in the study were suffering from psychogenic forms of impotence due to stress, tension, and fatigue. The group taking the yohimbe had a 71 percent success rate, while the placebo group had only a 22 percent improvement. The placebo group then had the opportunity of trying the yohimbe tablets, and the positive results reached 74 percent among the placebo group. The study also found that yohimbe had the ability of stimulating the male libido.

A recent study published in the *Journal of Urology* tested yohimbine on a group of men who suffered from chronic sexual dysfunction. The improvement rate for men who had suffered impotence for less than two years was 81 percent. They all took a moderate dose of yohimbine for one month. These results are very encouraging, as the improvement was seen quickly. There was also significant improvement for men who had trouble sustaining an erection. They reported fuller and more lasting erections. The results for all the studies have been positive.

Some medical professionals feel that yohimbe should be avoided because of the possible side effects associated with its use. The use of yohimbe should be closely watched and monitored for side effects. Yohimbine is thought to be toxic if ingested in high doses.

## PRIMARY APPLICATIONS

Aphrodisiac              Impotence
Sexual dysfunction

# YUCCA  *(Yucca glauca)*

*Parts used:* Root
*Properties:* Alterative, antibacterial, antirheumatic, astringent, blood purifier, purgative (gentle)
*Primary nutrients:* Calcium, copper, iron, manganese, phosphorus, potassium, vitamins A, B-complex, and C

Yucca is found growing in the southwestern areas of the United States. Native Americans used yucca for arthritis, rheumatism, and as a poultice on breaks and sprains. It was also used for skin disorders and to stop bleeding. The yucca plant was very valuable to the native cultures and was used for making clothing as well as for healing.

Yucca contains saponins that improve the body's ability to produce a natural cortisone to help with inflammation, healing, and pain. Herbalists often recommend yucca for arthritis and rheumatism. It is also used for intestinal problems and to aid digestion. Yucca has an effect on the intestinal flora that may help prevent certain types of harmful bacterial from flourishing. Extracts of yucca are often found in shampoo and soaps. It can be used as a soap and will form a lather when the roots are chopped up with water and rubbed on the skin.

Studies have shown that yucca contains nontoxic steroid saponins that are similar to cortisone. These properties are useful in cases of arthritis, rheumatism, high blood pressure, and high cholesterol levels in the blood. Various arthritic conditions have been successfully treated with yucca saponin extract. Not only were benefits found in reducing pain and inflammation, there was significant reduction in blood pressure, serum cholesterol levels, and the incidence of migraines.

## PRIMARY APPLICATIONS

| | |
|---|---|
| Arthritis | Blood impurities |
| Cholesterol | Rheumatism |

## SECONDARY APPLICATIONS

| | |
|---|---|
| Addison's disease | Bursitis |
| Cancer | Colitis |
| Dandruff | Gallbladder ailments |
| Gonorrhea | Gout |
| Inflammation | Liver problems |
| Skin disorders | Venereal disease |

# NUTRITIONAL SUPPLEMENTS

## ACIDOPHILUS

Each body has its own ecosystem. Trillions of microorganisms live inside everyone. These microorganisms coexist within the body and are necessary for health and vitality by extracting nutrients and protecting the body from detrimental factors. Intestinal microflora, in particular, perform many essential functions and have the ability to change according to environmental and dietary changes.

The intestinal flora can be affected by various elements. The overuse of antibiotics, oral contraceptives, excessive sugar consumption, aspirin, antihistamines, cortisone, prednisone, coffee, and stress can all contribute to an imbalance in the bacterial flora of the gastrointestinal tract.

The term *bacteria* carries a negative connotation, because most individuals associate bacteria with infections and illness. However, intestinal bacteria are necessary for body health and prevention of disease. Even though we traditionally take antibiotics to fight illness, in recent years, different strains of drug-resistant bacteria have emerged due to an overuse and misuse of antibiotics. Antibiotics are sometimes prescribed by physicians even when they are not appropriate.

Antibiotics interfere with the growth of bacteria, both good and bad. Bacteria grow at a very rapid rate, allowing for a whole generation of drug-resistant strains to develop in just a relatively short period of time. Alexander Fleming, who discovered penicillin, warned of the problem that could occur with resistant strains if antibiotics were overused. The weaker bacteria may be killed, while the stronger endure. This causes the strong, resistant bacteria to invade and take hold in the body.

Mitchell L. Cohen, a researcher with the National Center for Infectious Diseases at the Centers for Disease Control, warned about this problem, saying that "unless currently effective antimicrobial agents can be successfully preserved and the transmission of drug-resistant organisms curtailed, the post-antimicrobial era may be rapidly approaching in which infectious disease wards housing untreatable conditions will again be seen. Patients, doctors, scientists, and public health officials must all play their part in finding ways to reduce reliance upon antibiotics."

Despite this recent phenomenon, there are certain types of bacteria which can actually keep negative bacteria under control naturally. *Lactobacillus acidophilus* is one type of bacteria that does this, and it is, in fact, essential to maintaining a healthy intestinal flora.

Acidophilus is the primary friendly bacteria found in the intestinal tract and vagina. It adheres to the intestinal wall and prevents disease-causing bacteria from taking hold. Because these bacteria cover the lining of the intestines, no space is left for detrimental organisms to reside. When the friendly bacteria are compromised, space is made for the invading organisms to take hold.

In addition, the good bacteria eat all the food reserves and starve out the bad bacteria—allowing them to pass through without taking up residence. Acidophilus is also responsible for producing acetic acids that lower the natural pH in the intestines and discourage the growth of the other bacteria, which flourish in a more acidic environment.

*Lactobacillus acidophilus*, along with other beneficial bacteria, produces an antibiotic-like substance that works against other bacteria, viruses, protozoa, and fungi. According to Dr. Khem Shahani, a professor of food science at the University of Nebraska, milk fermented by *Lactobacillus acidophilus* contains an antibiotic he calls "acidophilin." It is a powerful antibiotic with abilities similar to penicillin, streptomycin, and Terramycin. He actually believes that it is more powerful than the antibiotics mentioned.

Friendly bacteria can be replaced and nurtured by changing your diet. For instance, plain yogurt is basically a combination of milk and *Lactobacillus acidophilus*, the friendly bacteria. This is the bacteria that produces lactase, which aids in the process of curdling the milk and giving yogurt its tart flavor. Yogurt containing live cultures of *Lactobacillus acidophilus* has been found effective in treating vaginal yeast infections, infant diarrhea, food poisoning, and in preventing flu infections. Eileen Hilton, MD, a specialist at the Long Island Jewish Medical Center in New York, followed eleven women with chronic yeast infections. They ate one cup daily of yogurt rich in live *Lactobacillus acidophilus*. During the last six months of the study, the women averaged only one yeast infection.

High cholesterol levels have been linked to many serious conditions such as heart disease and cancer. Acidophilus seems promising in helping to lower cholesterol levels. It may work by converting cholesterol to coprostanol, which is not absorbed in the body, thus working to lower overall body cholesterol levels.

A study reported in the *Journal of the American Medical Association* involved 194 hospitalized individuals with constipation problems. The average age of the volunteers was seventy-two, and none of them were being hospitalized for serious illnesses. They were given a daily dose of *Lactobacillus acidophilus* in a yogurt-prune whip dessert. More than 95 percent of the patients soon were off laxatives, as long as they continued eating the nightly dessert.

A study done by Heikki Vapatalo, MD, involved sixteen healthy men taking erythromycin, which is an antibiotic known to cause diarrhea. One group was given two cups daily of yogurt with live cultures and the other pasteurized yogurt. The group with the live cultures recovered in two days from diarrhea, while the other group took eight days to show improvement.

*Lactobacillus bulgaricus* is another type of beneficial bacteria sometimes found in the intestinal tract. Though not always found in the body, it helps to produce lactic acid and has some antibiotic activity. Studies have found that *Lactobacillus bulgaricus* can help to increase immune function, aiding in healing and the prevention of infections.

*Lactobacillus casei ssp. rhamnosus* is a beneficial bacteria similar to acidophilus. Some believe that because of their close similarities, they may have been confused in the past to some degree. This type of bacteria grows rapidly and aids immune response.

*Lactobacillus bifidus* is also often found in the large intestine and vagina. It is often found in the normal intestinal flora of infants and children. For this reason, some children's supplements have been formulated containing this bacteria, along with others. Breast milk has been found to contain *Lactobacillus bifidus*. It has also been found to help protect infants against intestinal infections, to fight overgrowths of candida following antibiotic therapy, and to aid in breaking down lactose for those with lactose intolerance.

*Streptococcus faecium* is another beneficial component of the intestinal tract. It helps to produce large amounts of lactic acid. It reproduces rapidly, is resistant to acidic conditions, contains antibiotic activity, aids in returning the normal flora to the intestinal tract after antibiotic therapy, and is heat-resistant up to 90 degrees Fahrenheit.

## ALPHA LIPOIC ACID

Alpha lipoic acid is one of the latest fatty acid supplements to make the news. It has been used in Europe and is now being tested for its therapeutic value in working as a free radical scavenger. It may be able to improve some degenerative diseases and restore health.

Alpha lipoic acid (ALA) is an antioxidant that is synthesized in the body in very small amounts. It contributes to the energy reaction in mitochondrial electron transport. It is related to the metabolism of glucose into energy. ALA is both fat- and water-soluble, allowing for it to help protect both lipid and aqueous cell structures. As with other nutrients, ALA levels decline with age. A supplement may be necessary to ensure levels for antioxidant protection.

Dr. Lester Packer, a professor at the University of California at Berkeley, believes ALA is the most effective antioxidant available. In the dihydrolipoic form, it is able to neutralize peroxyl and peoxynitrite free radicals. This ability makes ALA a universal antioxidant with incredible benefits in protecting the body.

European physicians have also used ALA for a number of years to treat diabetes-related complications. ALA supplementation has helped to boost glucose uptake in some diabetic individuals while resulting in less insulin dependency. Other research has found evidence of ALA's ability to help prevent protein modifications that occur with elevated blood sugar levels.

Studies have also found that ALA can protect brain tissue on a cellular level. The study involved mice supplemented with ALA. The aging mice given the supplement showed improvement in long-term memory. This may help to prevent a number of age-related disorders of the brain. There also seems to be protection from harmful chemicals that can damage brain cells.

Supplementation of ALA has shown promising results in studies relating to heart disease. Blood cholesterol levels were reduced by 40 percent in individuals taking ALA. This allowed for an increased amount of oxygen supplied to both the heart and liver tissue. ALA also has potential for increasing the survival rate and damage done from strokes. In one study done on rats, some were administered ALA before restricted blood flow. Those given the ALA had an 80 percent survival rate, while the ones who did not get the ALA had a 20 percent survival rate.

There is increasing evidence in a number of areas involving the use of ALA. One study found that animals given ALA had greater protection from chemi-cally induced cataracts. Other benefits may involve HIV patients. It may help to inhibit the action of a certain gene in the AIDS virus that allows for replication. There is also information on the detoxification abilities of ALA. It may help to protect the liver and other organs from damage due to pollutants and radiation.

ALA is easily absorbed in the body, making it particularly valuable as an antioxidant. It seems to contain some of the most potent antioxidant properties available. Research continues so that we can more fully understand the implications of this amazing supplement.

## AMINO ACIDS

Amino acids are the building blocks of every living cell. They are the basis of life itself. Amino acids are the single most important nutrient in the body. They are the building blocks of protein needed to create cells, enzymes, and hormones. If an amino acid is missing, a weakness can develop. Proteins play an essential role in bodily functions. A proper balance of amino acids can benefit the blood, the skin, and the immune and digestive systems.

In nutritional research, amino acids have been neglected, but today amino acids are being recognized as a great power in restoring and maintaining good health. Amino acids aid in the assimilation and utilization of other nutrients, including vitamins and minerals. Amino acid therapy has benefited many ailments, such as arthritis, anxiety, cancer, chronic fatigue, candidiasis, behavioral disorders, attention deficit disorder, autoimmune diseases, chemical sensitivity, learning disorders, eating disorders, hypoglycemia, diabetes, cardiovascular diseases, seizures, headaches, and chronic pain.

Amino acids are divided into essential and nonessential subtitles, but those labels can be misleading, because they are both necessary. Most of the twenty-one identifiable amino acids can be manufactured by the body in the liver. Eight cannot and must be supplied in the diet—isoleucine, leucine, lysine, methionine, phenylalanine, threonine, tryptophan, and valine. Cystine and tyrosine should also be classified as essential, as they are derived from the essential amino acids methionine and phenylalanine. Also, the nonessential amino acids histidine and arginine should be considered essential during growth periods, since they cannot be made by the body fast enough to meet the requirements of the rapid growth of young children.

## Isoleucine

Isoleucine is essential for growth and to fight chronic diseases. It is necessary for hemoglobin formation and is often lacking in the mentally and physically ill. A deficiency of this amino acid affects glycine production, which is a factor in mental retardation. It is also used to synthesize nonessential amino acids and maintain correct nitrogen levels. Isoleucine regulates the function of the thymus, spleen, and pituitary glands.

## Leucine

Leucine is necessary for growth and development. It stimulates brain functions, is essential for blood development, regulates digestion and metabolism, assists the functions of the glandular system, and increases muscular energy levels. It works to lower blood sugar levels. Leucine also complements the function of isoleucine.

## Valine

Valine sparks mental vigor, muscular coordination, and nervous system function and is necessary for glandular function and normal growth of cells. A deficiency could lead to nervous disorders, insomnia, and poor mental health. Valine, isoleucine, and leucine are very similar in structure and are usually referred to as a branched chain.

## Lysine

Lysine strengthens the circulatory system and maintains normal growth of cells. It controls acid/alkaline balance and is one of the building blocks of blood antibodies. Lysine may lessen the incidence of certain types of cancer. Lysine may help control and prevent conditions such as herpes simplex I and II, cold sores, fever blisters, osteoporosis, rickets, dental caries, and digestive disorders. It also helps to regulate the pineal and mammary glands and function of the gallbladder. It is necessary for all amino acid assimilation and also assists in the storage of fats.

Lysine has been found to have therapeutic effects on viral-related diseases. It also has the essential function of ensuring adequate absorption of calcium and the formation of collagen necessary for bone, cartilage, and connective tissue growth. Before lysine can be utilized in the formation of collagen, it needs the assistance of vitamin C. Without vitamin C or adequate protein to supply lysine, wounds would not heal properly and would be more susceptible to infection.

## Methionine

Methionine is important in preventing excessive accumulation of fat in the liver. It also helps to control fat levels in the blood and aids in preventing the buildup of cholesterol on the artery walls. Methionine increases the production of lecithin. It is also necessary for hemoglobin blood development. Methionine contains sulfur to keep hair, skin, nails, and joints healthy. It works with the antioxidant selenium to protect against cancer, free-radical damage, and to slow down the aging process. It combines with choline to add protection against tumor growth. It helps keep the kidneys healthy and functioning properly.

Methionine has been used to treat rheumatic fever, toxemia during pregnancy, digestive disorders, diaper ammonia rash, and blisters. Bottle-fed babies have high ammonia content in their urine that is not often found in breast-fed babies. Methionine may be the antidote. It is an antifatigue agent, works to combat stress, calms the nerves, detoxifies heavy metals, and prevents atherosclerosis.

## Phenylalanine

Phenylalanine is vital for the production of adrenaline. It also enhances vitamin C absorption and uses vitamins C and B6 for its metabolism. It is necessary for the growth and formation of skin and hair pigment. It aids in waste elimination of the kidneys and bladder. Phenylalanine is being investigated as a treatment for mental disorders. It is often used for disorders such as arthritis, migraine headaches, low back pain, whiplash, AIDS, PMS, and Parkinson's disease, and for boosting the immune system, suppressing appetite, strengthening weak blood vessels, and treating eye problems.

## Threonine

Threonine improves the assimilation and absorption of nutrients. It is essential in the prevention and treatment of many forms of mental illness. Threonine is required for new cell development. It works in combination with other amino acids to improve nutrient absorption, prevent fat buildup in the liver when choline is deficient in the diet, and is an important constituent of collagen and the enamel in teeth. It may help with the treatment of mental illness and personality disorders.

## Tryptophan

Tryptophan is an important element for growth of the body and cell tissues. It is necessary for healthy hair and skin. It is a factor in the regulation of sleep and mood patterns. It also assists in the production of gastric juices, improving digestion. Tryptophan helps with blood clotting and is involved with the chemical messages (serotonin) sent from the brain to the pituitary gland. It enhances the function of the immune system. Vitamin B6 is needed to catalyze tryptophan. Niacin and vitamin E enhance and keep tryptophan in the bloodstream.

## Alanine

Alanine's main nutritional function is in the metabolism of tryptophan and pyridoxine. It helps to strengthen cellular structure. In cases of hypoglycemia, it may be useful as a source for glucose production. It has been found to have a cholesterol-reducing effect when used in combination with arginine and glycine.

## Arginine

Arginine is considered an essential amino acid in periods of growth, since it cannot be made by the body fast enough to meet the requirements of young children. It is also important to male sexual health, as 80 percent of the male seminal fluid is made up of arginine. It detoxifies poisonous waste from blood and supports the function of the immune system. Arginine is a chelating agent for manganese. Combined with ornithine, it is involved in weight control. It works with the pituitary gland, which is the master gland involved in burning fat and building muscle tissue. Arginine is also connected with increasing the size and activity of the thymus gland in cases of stress and injury. It may also help to reduce the risk of atherosclerosis. It controls body cell degeneration, is necessary for cell reproduction

and muscle contraction, and assists the body in nitrogen elimination.

## Cystine

Cystine is a sulfur-containing amino acid. It is essential as an antioxidant and free-radical deactivator. It is considered a detoxifying agent, because it bonds to toxic metals such as copper, cadmium, lead, and mercury. Cystine stimulates the body's immune system. It is a powerful aid in fighting radiation and pollution and in extending the life span. Cystine helps to protect and repair.

It protects against acetaldehyde found in air and cigarette smoke. Cystine works with vitamins C, E, A, B1, B5, B6, selenium, and zinc to protect against cellular damage and improve the health of hair and skin. It is also necessary for the utilization of vitamin B6. Cystine is responsible for supplying more than 10 percent of the body's insulin, and it aids in pancreatic health. It stabilizes blood sugar and carbohydrate metabolism. Along with pantothenic acid, cystine is used in the treatment of arthritis and rheumatoid arthritis.

## Glutamine/Glutamic Acid

Glutamine/glutamic acid, along with glucose, is one of the principal fuels for the brain cells. It stimulates mental alertness, improves intelligence, normalizes physical equilibrium, detoxifies ammonia from the brain, improves and soothes erratic behavior in elderly patients, improves the ability to learn, aids memory, helps with behavioral problems and autism in children, stops sugar and alcohol cravings, may improve IQ in mentally deficient children, enhances peptic ulcer healing, and may be used to treat schizophrenia and senility.

## Glycine/Serine

Glycine/serine are essential in the synthesis of nonessential amino acids. Together with arginine, glycine heals trauma injuries and damaged tissue. It is utilized in liver detoxification, promotes energy and oxygen use in the cells, is necessary for biosynthesis of nucleic acids as well as bile acids, enhances gastric acid secretion, and readily converts into serine, which protects fatty sheaths surrounding nerve fibers.

## Histidine

Histidine is considered an essential amino acid, especially during the growth periods of young children. It is fundamental for the maintenance of myelin sheaths. It is necessary for the function of nerve cells in hearing mechanisms. Histidine affects the auditory nerve, and a deficiency can cause deafness and hearing loss. It is important for the formation of glycogen. Histidine is also a vital component of blood and is involved in controlling the mucus level of the digestive and respiratory systems. Histamine is released during trauma and stressful conditions, causing allergies, but as the level of histidine increases, the concentration of histamine decreases. Along with niacin and vitamin B6, histidine is considered a sexual stimulant. It may be used in the treatment of rheumatoid arthritis, cardiocirculatory conditions, anemia, allergies, and stress. It has a vasodilating action, is a good chelating agent, is effective against radiation or heavy metals, and aids in healing allergic conditions. Histidine has been given to cosmonauts to protect against the effects of radiation.

## Asparagine/Aspartic acid

Asparagine/aspartic acid enhances liver function; increases stamina and endurance in athletes; cleanses ammonia from the system, causing resistance to fatigue; and aids in transformation of carbohydrates into cellular energy.

## Proline/Hydroxyproline

Proline is essential for collagen formation and maintenance. It readily transforms into hydroxyproline. Vitamin C aids in the effectiveness of proline. It is useful in wound healing and protects the body tissues from the effects of aging.

## Tyrosine

Tyrosine, in combination with tryptophan, may be a better sleep aid than tryptophan alone. It is involved in the pigment of skin and hair and therapeutically alters brain function, which may make it a useful agent in treating mental illness. Some patients who had previously responded to amphetamines responded well to tyrosine therapy. Tyrosine works synergistically with glutamine, tryptophan, niacin, and vitamin B6 in controlling depression, anxiety, and appetite. Tyrosine combined with phenylalanine may help with weight control. It plays a role in the function of the adrenal, thyroid, and pituitary glands. It may help to create positive feelings, elevate moods, and increase alertness and ambition. It has been combined with tryptophan, niacin, vitamin B6, hops, skullcap, passion flower, and valerian root to aid with alcoholism. It can be used in cases of high blood pressure, the aging of cells, Parkinson's disease, muscle development, allergies, cancer, and irritability.

## Carnitine

Carnitine is considered an accessory nutrient. Its primary purpose is to encourage fat metabolism in the muscles, and it is necessary for the heart, body tissue, and other organs. It is synthesized in the liver by lysine and methionine, together with adequate amounts of vitamins C, B6, B3, and iron. Vitamin C is essential for the conversion process. The need for carnitine increases with strenuous exercise. It improves fat metabolism in the heart and other organs. It may also help in preventing high blood fat and triglyceride levels. Men have a greater need for carnitine than women. There is a possible relation to infertility via inadequate sperm mobility. It is an essential nutrient in newborn infants.

## Glutathione

Glutathione is a tripeptide consisting of three amino acids: cystine, glutamic acid, and glycine. It helps to remove poisons from the body, protect cells from destruction, clean harmful bacteria from the lungs, protect against dust, build immunity, destroy free radicals, and works as a prevention and treatment for a wide range of degenerative diseases. Along with vitamins A, C, E, selenium, and zinc, it may be used to treat chronic asthma, allergies, respiratory problems, pneumonia, poisoning from metals, a toxic liver, and aid in the regression of tumor development. It is a form of cancer prevention, protects the liver from damage due to alcohol, and helps to reduce alcohol cravings.

## Ornithine

Ornithine works with the pituitary gland and helps to secrete large amounts of growth hormones. It aids in the burning of fat and in the building of muscle tissue. It is involved with arginine in weight control. Taking two parts arginine to one part ornithine on an empty stomach at bedtime is thought to work during the night to release growth hormone by the pituitary gland.

## Taurine

Taurine stimulates the production of growth hormone. It is synthesized from methionine and cystine. It is necessary for brain development and function. It is also an essential element for infants not breast-fed, since it is contained in high concentrations in breast milk. Along with zinc, it is associated with eye function. A deficiency in taurine has been linked to epileptic seizures, and it is thought to play a role in controlling seizures. It has a potent and long-lasting anticonvulsive effect and is used with B6 for seizure problems. It is concentrated in the heart, skeletal muscles, and central nervous system. It helps to regulate osmotic control of calcium as well as potassium in the heart muscle. It influences blood sugar levels similar to insulin. In combination with vitamins A and E, it is thought to be of importance in cases of muscular dystrophy. IQ levels in Down's syndrome patients have improved with taurine supplementation, along with vitamins B, C, and E.

## ANTIOXIDANTS

Every day, the body is bombarded with toxic substances that wreak havoc on the normal functions of the immune system. Think of it as an invasion of enemy forces that are kept under control by our own superior protection. These substances enter the body or are by-products of normal bodily functions that create free radicals. The antioxidants, free-radical scavengers, neutralize the free radicals and protect the body.

Recent studies have focused on antioxidant supplements for their ability to protect against conditions such as cancer, heart disease, arthritis, allergies, and aging. Some of these important nutrients include vitamin A (beta-carotene), vitamin C, vitamin E, and selenium. The process that can lead to disease and cellular damage is known as free-radical damage. Antioxidants help to block the free-radical damage and stimulate the immune response. They neutralize free radicals before they can cause damage.

A free radical is a molecule that is incomplete, lacking an electron, and this puts it out of balance. Free radicals do not stay in this state very long but react with other compounds quickly. They are highly reactive, often causing more free-radical reactions that are capable of doing cellular damage, which can lead to disease. Each individual free radical can cause damage to a molecule or an entire cell. Free radicals can damage the cells by damaging the cell membrane. They are now thought to be responsible for many degenerative diseases.

Free radicals can come from the environment (cigarette smoke, pollution, sunlight, radiation, X-rays, chemicals) or be ingested with the food we eat and drink. Most free radicals are produced within the body through normal metabolic processes. The oxygen molecule is the greatest source of free-radical damage. Oxygen, which sustains life, is also responsible for destruction of cells. To some degree, this process is similar to the formation of rust (oxidized iron). Oxygen can actually oxidize molecules in the body, leading to free-radical damage.

Because we don't live in a perfect world, we will ingest some pollutants in the normal cycle of a day. Chemical toxins, pollutants, and pesticides are in the food we eat. Even the water used in irrigation and the air we breathe contain pollutants. It is essential to eat a diet rich in valuable antioxidants, as well as taking supplements to ensure the protection that the body needs to defend itself.

Eat a diet rich in fruits, vegetables, and whole grains, including carrots, sweet potatoes, dark green leafy vegetables, spinach, broccoli, apricots, peaches, tomatoes, oranges, strawberries, green peppers, grapefruit, nectarines, and melons. They contain nutrients full of antioxidants to help the body fight free-radical damage and prevent disease. Supplementing the diet with essential antioxidants may be necessary.

## Vitamin A/Beta-Carotene

Beta-carotene is converted to vitamin A in the body. They both aid the immune system and may destroy carcinogens and prevent free-radical damage. One study found that carotenes protect and inhibit the growth of malignancies in normal cells. Beta-carotene has also been found to enhance the immune system function to protect the body. A survey conducted in 1992 found that individuals with high levels of beta-carotene in the blood had a low incidence of cancer. Beta-carotene may also help to prevent cataracts. Good sources of vitamin A and beta-carotene include carrots, sweet potatoes, nectarines, dark green leafy vegetables, spinach, squash, broccoli, apricots, peaches, and tomatoes.

## Vitamin C

Vitamin C increases the production of interferon. It is a powerful antioxidant, aiding in the neutralization of free radicals. Vitamin C may not prevent the common cold, but it seems to have the ability to reduce the duration and severity of colds and cold symptoms. It is a water-soluble vitamin, which makes it easily assimilated in the blood plasma and other fluids in the body. Vitamin C was found to prevent scurvy, a common condition on sailing vessels, and is essential in the formation of collagen, which binds cells together and is important for body structure.

Vitamin C is also useful in the prevention of heart disease. Potential benefits include increasing levels of "good" cholesterol while preventing the formation of LDL, or "bad" cholesterol. It may also help by making the blood less sticky and reducing the risk of stroke or heart attack. Vitamin C helps to increase immunity and enhances the effects of vitamin E. Vitamin C can be found in oranges, strawberries, melons, green peppers, grapefruit, broccoli, and Brussels sprouts.

## Vitamin E

Vitamin E has been found to be a potent antioxidant. Evidence from research has found that the red blood cells of individuals taking vitamin E aged more slowly than those who did not take the supplement. This may be beneficial for preventing aging and related conditions such as Alzheimer's disease and senility. Vitamin E also shows promise for protection against heart disease. There seems to be an association between vitamin E supplementation and a lower incidence of developing heart disease.

Vitamin E helps to protect the coating around the cells. It helps to enhance and improve the immune response. Food sources of vitamin E include wheat germ, barley, grains, cold-pressed oils, egg yolks, nuts, and legumes. It is found in lesser amounts in green leafy vegetables.

## N-Acetyl-Cysteine (NAC)

N-Acetyl-Cysteine (NAC) is derived from cysteine, a sulfur-containing amino acid. NAC is both produced by the body and absorbed from food. The body's most important cellular antioxidant is glutathione, to which NAC is a precursor. By increasing glutathione levels—and resultant antioxidant levels—NAC can help prevent cancer, enhance immune functioning, reduce fatigue, treat bronchitis, help combat HIV infections, and treat heavy metal poisoning, as well as acetaminophen poisoning.

## Selenium

Selenium is an antioxidant that helps to increase the antibody response to infection. It is an essential trace mineral that is found in all tissues of the body. There is evidence linking selenium to a lower incidence of cancer. Selenium works closely with vitamin E, and they enhance each other's performance. Lower-than-normal levels of selenium have been found in patients suffering from AIDS, multiple sclerosis, arthritis, and cancer, to name a few. Selenium is found in fish, kidney, liver, mushrooms, garlic, and asparagus.

## Superoxide Dismutase (SOD)

Superoxide dismutase (SOD) is an enzyme that has particular value as an antioxidant because it helps to protect against cell destruction. It has the distinct ability to neutralize superoxide, one of the most damaging free-radical substances in nature. Like so many other protective compounds that naturally occur in the body, it decreases with age, making cells much more vulnerable to the oxidants that cause aging and disease. It occurs naturally in broccoli, Brussels sprouts, wheatgrass, and in the majority of green plants.

SOD can help slow the cellular damage caused by aging, and offer some protection against cancer. Two varieties of SOD are available: copper/zinc SOD and manganese SOD. Both work in different ways to provide two types of cellular protection. SOD is sold in pill form and should be enterically coated so that it does not digest in the stomach, but rather in the intestines for better absorption.

## Coenzyme Q10

CoQ10 works as an antioxidant and improves the oxygen uptake on a cellular level. CoQ10 is similar to vitamins E and K in its chemical structure. It is also thought to resemble vitamin E in its ability to function as an antioxidant. It has the ability to neutralize free radicals, which cause damage to the cells. It can be synthesized within the body if a proper nutritional base is available. Supplements may help to reduce heart disease and enhance the immune system.

## Melatonin

Melatonin has been promoted as a sleep aid to encourage and establish a restful sleep. It has also been found to contain powerful antioxidant capabilities. A study done at the University of Texas in San Antonio showed the effects of adding melatonin to white blood cells and then exposing them to radiation. Another group of white blood cells did not have the melatonin added. The ones exposed without melatonin showed chromosome damage; the ones with melatonin did not. The more melatonin added, the more the protection from damage. There seems to be protection from melatonin in its ability to neutralize free radicals. It may also help by activating enzymes to heal the damaged cells faster. There are many immune-related conditions that may benefit from melatonin's antioxidant properties, including heart disease, arteriosclerosis, cancer, tumors, Alzheimer's, emphysema, cataracts, aging, and some neurological problems.

## Pycnogenol

Pycnogenol is a beneficial antioxidant, helping to reduce the risk of cancer, protecting the body against toxins, strengthening the immune system, and preventing premature aging. Pycnogenol contains proanthocyanidin, which is a very bioavailable flavonoid. It is extracted from grapeseed or pine bark. Some experts believe that pycnogenol may be the most potent antioxidant available from nature. Pycnogenol has been found to inhibit cellular mutations such as tumors. One study found that patients suffering from circulatory insufficiencies found benefit from pycnogenols in pain control and vessel elasticity. Supplementing with pycnogenol may help with cardiovascular disease, edema, bruising, aging of skin, diabetes, stress, and many other conditions.

## BEE PRODUCTS
### Bee Pollen

Bee pollen consists of the fine powder in the male seed of a flower blossom. The bees transport it and mix it with nectar for their own nourishment. The pollen grains are collected and eaten by the bees but also pollinate flowers. Bee pollen and honey have been recognized since the beginning of time for their healing benefits. Egyptian records dating back thousands of years have references to honey and its healing potential. Ancient Greek marathon runners recognized the value of bee pollen and used it to increase their strength and endurance. European nations, as well as Asian countries, also revered bee pollen for its medicinal value.

Bee pollen is considered a complete food because it contains every chemical substance needed to maintain life. It is a great supplement for building the immune system and providing energy to the body. It is thought to have the ability to correct the body chemistry and eliminate unhealthy conditions. It is recommended for premature aging, chronic fatigue, prostatitis, low or high blood pressure, indigestion, menopause, allergies, asthma, infertility, and as an immune system enhancer. It can also help to improve concentration and mental function, reduce cholesterol and triglyceride levels, and normalize weight by balancing the body chemistry. Athletes often use this supplement to help increase their strength, endurance, and speed. It is also used to treat hay fever, allergies, and asthma.

Research has found bee pollen to contain properties beneficial to healing, revitalizing, and protecting against radiation therapy. It is a rich source of protein and carbohydrates and can be used as a food supplement. It can help athletes increase their stamina, endurance, and ability. It may also help prevent plaque buildup in the arteries. Bee pollen is well known for increasing mental as well as physical performance. One study found a group of students' mental performance improved significantly with the addition of bee pollen.

Researchers at the Institute of Bee Culture in Bures-sur-Yvette near Paris, along with other scientists throughout Europe, studied the effects of honeybee pollen consumption on human beings. They found exceptional antibiotic properties in the bee pollen. They also found the bee pollen helpful in treating conditions such as fatigue, allergies, bronchitis, sinusitis, colds, balancing the endocrine system, menstrual problems, prostate problems, constipation, colitis, anemia, depression, and hair loss, to name a few.

Bee pollen contains essential fatty acids that are necessary for vital body functions. It contains twenty-one amino acids essential for life and health. It contains enzymes that are responsible for chemical reactions in the body. It contains all vitamins, minerals, and trace minerals. It is considered to be a complete food.

### Royal Jelly

Royal jelly is considered the "crown jewel" of the beehive. It promotes longevity by helping to maintain health, beauty, and youth. It is a potent, highly nutritional, and natural food. It is an incredibly rich, creamy, opalescent white liquid and is synthesized by the worker bees exclusively for the nourishment and cultivation of the queen bee. This remarkable material transforms a common honeybee into a queen bee, extending longevity from six weeks to five years.

Royal jelly is rich in natural hormones and B vitamins. In addition, it contains an impressive array of seventeen amino acids, including eight essential amino acids, and is particularly rich in cystine, lysine, and arginine. Royal jelly is comprised of 16.1 percent aspartic acid, which is absolutely essential for proper tissue growth and regeneration.

Gelatin, another component of royal jelly, is one of the primary precursors of collagen, a potent anti-aging compound that helps to keep the skin youthful while supporting the organs, glands, and muscular systems. It contains vital fatty acids, sugars, sterols, phosphorus compounds, and acetylcholine. Acetylcholine is essential for the proper transmission of nerve impulses and the proper functioning of the endocrine system. A lack of acetylcholine can lead to a susceptibility to a number of nerve disorders, including Alzheimer's disease, Parkinson's disease, and multiple sclerosis.

Royal jelly contains the following properties: antibacterial, antiviral, antibiotic, tonic, nutritive, and antiaging. It is beneficial for the following body systems: immune, cardiovascular, endocrine, integumentary, nervous, reproductive, cellular, skeletal, hepatic, and respiratory.

Aging is inevitable, but the process can be significantly slowed with supplements. Researchers in Argentina have been working scientifically to document the ability of royal jelly to not only slow down tissue deterioration, but to reverse it as well. Consider the story of Noel Johnson, who experienced a rebirth of health at age eighty. Keep in mind that in 1964, at age sixty-five, he was refused life insurance due to a weak and damaged heart and was cautioned to dramatically restrict his physical activity or death could occur. He said, "I stripped down and looked in the mirror. All the classic signs of aging were there. I was forty pounds overweight, with a bulging gut, dull eyes, slack, unused muscle. I looked defeated. I knew I was doing everything wrong, so I decided to teach myself to live right."

In 1989, at age ninety, Johnson wrote a book called *The Living Proof . . . I Have Found the Fountain of Youth*, in which he claimed that his use of bee products, in addition to a solid nutritional program, changed his life. "I have made the products of the beehive the solid foundation of my nutritional program. Although I eat a large variety of whole foods, bee products are an unvarying part of my diet." Since running his first marathon in 1977, his credits include many marathon medals in the senior division and the title of the World's Senior Boxing Champion.

Despite the additional exercise and diet changes, Johnson attributes most of his vitality to bee products: "I discovered the bee's gift at age seventy. These perfect foods have restored my manhood, brought me to full vigor and sexual potency, and continue to nourish every cell in my body. I am improving in every way. I don't spend five cents on medicine."

Royal jelly may help many conditions. Some include menopause, impotence, infertility, chronic fatigue, skin blemishes, wrinkles, immune system problems, viral and bacterial infections, endocrine disorders, hormonal balance, cardiovascular disease, weight control, inflammation, liver ailments, cancer, arthritis, memory, depression, Parkinson's disease, diabetes, asthma, and mental exhaustion.

### Bee Propolis

Bee propolis is considered Mother Nature's fighter and healer. It is another nutrient made by the honeybee. It has the ability to provide protection against infectious invaders, promote healing, regenerate tissue, and provide a superior source of energy and endurance.

Bee propolis is a resinous substance that is gathered by honeybees from deciduous trees' bark and leaves. It is a sticky material that bees very efficiently use to seal hive holes and cracks. This natural glue is cleverly utilized by the industrious honeybees to provide exterior protection to the hive against the invasion of any outside contaminants. Bees purposely place this tacky substance in the areas that lead into the hive to prevent intruders and sterilize bees brushing against it from infection.

Cultures all over the world have recognized the ability of propolis to fight infection, promote healing, and support immune function. It was used in the Soviet Union during World War II for treating battle wounds. The widespread use of propolis in the Soviet Union for infection earned it the appropriate title of "Russian penicillin." Propolis is regarded as the strongest and most powerful natural antibiotic.

Nineteen substances have been found in propolis. These compounds include a number of substances thought belong to the flavonoid family, including betulene and isovanillin. Except for vitamin K, propolis has all the known vitamins. Of the fourteen minerals required by the body, propolis contains them all, with the exception of sulfur. Like royal jelly and bee pollen, propolis also contains a number of unidentified compounds that work together synergistically to create a perfectly balanced nutritive substance. It contains sixteen amino acids. It has the following properties: antibacterial, antiviral, antibiotic, antifungal, antiinflammatory, and antioxidant.

Propolis has the ability to energize the body and restore vigor and stamina. It helps to stimulate the thymus gland. An underactive thymus gland is thought to be responsible for weakness and fatigue in many individuals. Propolis is an excellent supplement to use as a preventive agent for this problem.

Propolis can also help with the following conditions: allergies, bruises, burns, cancer, herpes zoster, fatigue, sore throat, nasal congestion, respiratory ailments, acne, skin disorders, sunburn, shingles, flu, colds, coughs, ulcers, and wounds.

## BLUE-GREEN ALGAE/SPIRULINA

Blue-green algae is well known for its great nutritional value. There are many different species of blue-green algae, including one of the most studied, spirulina. Blue-green algae has the characteristics of both plants and bacteria. It is rich in nutrients that help balance the body chemistry and build resistance to viral diseases. It is known to increase the oxygen utilized by the body. It is beneficial in cases of acute diseases such as colds, flu, and fevers. It is rich in essential amino acids: isoleucine, leucine, lysine, methionine, cystine, phenylalanine, tyrosine, and tryptophan. Amino acids are the building blocks of DNA. They provide material for bones, tissue, organs, hormones, neurotransmitters, and enzymes, and they work to support the immune system. Blue-green algae is high in beta-carotene, which is stored in the liver and used by the body as needed. Beta-carotene protects the lungs against air pollution. It is high in vitamin C, acts as an antioxidant, and is needed by the body on a daily basis. Algae also contains thiamine, riboflavin, niacin, choline, biotin, pantothenic acid, vitamin K, iodine, calcium, phosphorus, magnesium, potassium, copper, iron, manganese, zinc, and sodium.

Blue-green algae is a rich source of chlorophyll, which causes the green color in plants. It is the richest source of chlorophyll. Chlorophyll is a valuable nutrient with medicinal benefits. It helps to inhibit the growth of bacterial, viral, and fungal infections. It also helps to deodorize and sanitize the body. Chlorophyll can help to protect against tooth decay and gum disease. It is a natural anti-inflammatory. It helps to build a weakened body and to strengthen the immune system. It is also important in purifying and building the blood. Chlorophyll promotes the growth of intestinal-friendly bacteria.

Blue-green algae has been found to increase the immune function by stimulating more T-cell activity. It also accelerates the reproduction of macrophages, which are referred to as the killer cells in the immune system. These cells surround and ingest foreign matter, removing it from the body. Algae may help to increase resistance to infections: viral, bacterial, and fungal. One study showed that chlorella can help to increase the interferon production in mice. This helped to protect them from an artificially induced influenza.

Spirulina, a type of blue-green algae, proved to be valuable in reducing cholesterol levels in a Japanese study. Components of the spirulina may help to strengthen the heart and cardiovascular system to protect against cardiovascular disease.

Blue-green algae is also recommended for its ability to detoxify all organs, especially the liver. Its high amounts of chlorophyll can remove toxic buildup and drug deposits from the body. Studies have found that blue-green algae can help to lessen the effects of toxic poisoning from X-rays, ultraviolet light, radiation, and chemical toxins. It can also help to remove heavy metals such as lead and mercury from the body. Research in Japan has shown that spirulina can help stimulate the excretion of some contaminants, including cadmium, lead, and mercury. Another Japanese study followed patients suffering from PCP (polychlorobiphenyl) exposure. They were given daily doses of chlorella for one year. The patients improved dramatically and experienced less fatigue and improved digestion.

Animal studies have found that chlorella contains some antitumor activity. There seems to be protection from mammary tumors, leukemia, ascitic sarcoma, and liver cancer. Protection is probably from the increased interferon production and immune stimulation.

## CETYL MYRISTOLEATE (CMO)

Cetyl myristoleate (CMO) has been studied for its use in protecting against arthritis-related conditions. It is regarded as a natural and safe compound, effective in treating joint damage and inflammation. It is considered to be a nontoxic substance with valuable potential.

CMO is a fatty acid ester consisting of both single- and double-bonded chemical types that is an essential constituent in the majority of plant and animal cells. It can technically be considered a waxy lipid.

Information on CMO came to the forefront with research done at the National Institutes of Health. A species of laboratory mice were protected against developing a laboratory-induced form of arthritis. One study found that rats injected with CMO were protected from joint swelling or inflammation when given an injection of *Mycobacterium butyricum*. The control group all experienced arthritic symptoms.

Scientists theorized that this specific substance acted to protect the joints against induced arthritis.

Swiss albino mice were found to possess a protective agent against arthritis. When they were injected with arthritis-producing substances, they remained free of swelling or pain. Tests isolated the CMO, and extracts were originally made from mice tissue. Technology has allowed for synthetic compounds to be successfully produced in the laboratory.

When CMO is taken in oral form, it is absorbed through the intestinal tract and migrates to the bloodstream to joint receptor sites. While the exact physiological mechanisms involved in CMO therapy are not fully understood, it seems this compound actually alters the immune system response that triggers joint inflammation and causes pain and swelling. The presence of CMO within affected joints seems to block the inflammatory response.

Arthritis triggers inflammation, an immune reaction that initiates the release of certain compounds and biological processes that cause redness, pain, and fluid accumulation. CMO apparently is able to inhibit the inflammatory response in joints. It provides a sort of shield against this immune response. CMO has the ability to inhibit the symptoms of arthritic disease and is also considered an immunizing agent against the development of rheumatoid arthritis.

Patent documentation of CMO includes some uses for this product. It has been used successfully to treat pain from all joints, including knee and hip pain and swelling, as well as finger mobility, limited neck motion, liver inflammation, foot pain, hand eczema, and back pain. The benefits appear to be rapid and effective.

## CHITOSAN

Chitosan is one of the latest additions to help people manage their weight. Chitosan is an amino polysaccharide that basically binds to fats before they can be absorbed by the body and removes them from the body, inhibiting their absorption. It can actually absorb four to five times its own weight in fat. Chitosan is nondigestible and has no caloric value. Plant fibers add bulk to the digestive tract, but chitosan is unique in that it actually binds with the fat in the digestive tract.

Chitin is a precursor to chitosan. It is found most abundantly in the shells of shellfish. Chitosan is made by cooking chitin in alkali. After cooking, the links of the chain of chitosan include glucosamine units, with each containing a free amino group. This allows for the amazing abilities of chitosan.

Chitosan has an unusual history. It has been used for the past thirty years in a water purification process. It has the ability to bind and remove oils, grease, and some fine particulates from water systems. It has also been used on oil spills, making the cleanup process easier.

Then the focus for chitosan shifted toward weight loss, though it has many benefits beyond aiding in weight management. One study done in Helsinki found that individuals taking chitosan over a four-week period lost an average of 8 percent of their body weight. The benefits of chitosan can be improved with the addition of certain nutrients. Ascorbic acid was shown to increase fat loss in chitosan usage. Citric acid also seemed to enhance the ability of chitosan.

Chitosan is also useful in lowering bad cholesterol, LDL, while increasing HDL cholesterol levels. It has been reported to be extremely valuable for lowering LDL without any side effects associated with drug therapy. Further research has found that even with the addition of a diet high in fat and cholesterol, lower cholesterol levels were achieved in studies on animals.

Chitosan seems to be a safe approach to weight management. It is prudent to take supplements such as essential fatty acids and fat-soluble vitamins at a different time from chitosan to ensure their proper absorption.

## CHROMIUM

Chromium is being marketed in formulas as a weight-loss aid. It indeed plays a vital role in a healthy body. It is a trace mineral needed daily by the body. In its active form, it is referred to as glucose tolerance factor, or GTF. It aids in the metabolism and regulation of blood glucose levels. It is also involved in muscle development and energy production. Chromium helps synthesize cholesterol, fats, and protein. It helps stabilize blood sugar levels through insulin utilization. And because of the poor diet of the average American, it is thought to be deficient in most diets. It is estimated that 80 percent of chromium is lost in processed food.

But how does chromium aid weight loss? Chromium, or GTF, helps maintain insulin activity and aids in the utilization of glucose, which leads to appetite suppression. It seems to help with the hunger center in the brain. It may actually reduce false feelings of hunger or cravings for junk food.

Another positive effect of chromium for dieters is the prevention of fluctuation in blood sugar levels. Eating less sometimes causes mood swings because of low blood sugar levels. The stored glycogen can be retrieved for use with the help of chromium. It aids in the production and storage of glycogen.

Chromium is probably more widely known for recent studies linking it to a reduced risk of heart disease. It may help prevent plaque buildup in the arteries. Low levels of chromium are thought to be a risk factor for developing heart disease. It also may help increase the beneficial HDL cholesterol and aid in lowering LDL cholesterol. Chromium is also being studied with regard to diabetes. Diabetes results from a deficiency of insulin. Proper amounts of chromium may help decrease the requirements for insulin. This important trace mineral may be a factor in reaching and maintaining optimum body weight. It is also important for many body functions.

## COENZYME Q10

The benefits of Coenzyme Q10 have been reported as miraculous. But can there possibly be one nutrient so valuable that it can realistically be called the miracle nutrient? Probably not, but CoQ10 is one of the most important nutrients known to humankind, as it is found in every cell of the body. There are ten different CoQs, but only CoQ10 is found in human tissue.

CoQ10 is an essential nutrient and important antioxidant. It is called a coenzyme because it aids the activity of other enzymes. It is also known as ubiquinone, because it is ubiquitous—it's found in all cells in the body. CoQ10 can be synthesized in the body, but deficiencies are fairly common, as the ability of the body to synthesize CoQ10 decreases with age.

CoQ10 is a primary ingredient inside the mitochondria, where it aids in energy production. It is a catalyst in the production of energy and boosts the biochemical ability to activate cellular energy. Energy is required to perform every function of life: getting up in the morning, walking, talking, and even reading. For this reason alone, it is reasonable to assume that low concentrations could be detrimental to a healthy body. CoQ10 is found in high concentrations in organs that require abundant amounts of energy such as the heart, liver, and the immune system.

CoQ10 is similar to vitamins E and K in its chemical structure. It is also thought to resemble vitamin E in its ability to function as an antioxidant. It has the ability to neutralize free radicals, which cause damage to the cells. It can be synthesized within the body if a proper nutritional base is available. CoQ10 is present in many foods, such as wheat bran, beef heart, spinach, peanuts, and rice. With age, the ability of the body to produce CoQ10 is diminished, which can lead to various serious conditions such as heart disease, gum infections, breast cancer, hypertension, diabetes, and decreased immune function.

Karl Folkers, PhD, a former biochemist at the Institute for Biomedical Research at the University of Texas at Austin, has done extensive research on CoQ10. He feels that many individuals suffering from congestive heart failure or cardiomyopathy are deficient in CoQ10 and could benefit substantially from a supplement. It is interesting to note that Folkers takes a daily supplement of 200 mg of CoQ10 and at the age of eighty-nine is healthy and very active.

CoQ10 may help protect the heart from damage suffered during a heart attack. Some clinical trials have found that CoQ10 can help as a therapy for angina. It may also help reduce tissue damage that occurs during open-heart surgery and may aid with heart transplant patients. The recovery time for individuals undergoing heart surgery was less for those who took CoQ10 than for those who didn't. Patients took it for two weeks before and thirty days following the surgery. They recovered faster, with fewer complications than those who did not take the supplement.

A group of cardiac patients had improvement in health and reduced degeneration from heart disease when taking CoQ10 without the addition of cardiac medications. The same results were found in individuals suffering from angina pectoris. With the addition of CoQ10, angina patients were able to increase exercise and overall health.

Clinical studies done in Japan and the United States have found substantial benefits from adding CoQ10 to the diets of individuals with high blood pressure. One study found significant blood pressure drops in just four to twelve weeks of taking CoQ10. Dr. Philip C. Richardson of the University of Texas in Austin feels that CoQ10 may be the most effective alternate clinical control in treating elevated blood pressure without the use of common drugs and their accompanying side effects.

Along with other antioxidants, CoQ10 helps to protect the immune system by deactivating cell-damaging free radicals. But even more important, CoQ10 has the ability of actually slowing the production of free radicals at the source. This can be beneficial, whether fighting the common cold or a debilitating disease such as cancer. Both animal and human studies have found beneficial effects on the immune system.

Numerous studies have documented the immune-enhancing abilities of CoQ10. Emile G. Bliznakov, MD, a noted researcher on the subject, did his first experiments on CoQ10 involving the immune system. He found that CoQ10 doubled the immune system's ability to protect the body. He also found that CoQ10 protected against chemically induced cancers in animals, causing smaller and fewer tumors, with an increased survival rate. He also found an increase in resistance to viral infections.

AIDS is a disease that may benefit from CoQ10 because of its ability to strengthen the immune system. Karl Folkers reported on research done in 1991. CoQ10 raised the CD4:CD8 ratios of a group of healthy and HIV-positive individuals. CD4 immune cells are responsible for stopping intruders that can cause disease. CD8 cells are supposed to suppress the attack. A higher ratio is thought to help the body in fighting infection. Clinical trials are being done to determine the usefulness of CoQ10 in aiding HIV-positive individuals.

With cancer as a leading cause of death in the United States, research on CoQ10 may help to reduce the incidence of cancer and protect against it. Not only can CoQ10 help stop and prevent tumor growth, it has been shown to help relieve the symptoms of patients undergoing chemotherapy, helping them better tolerate the treatments and enhancing their ability to fight the cancer. Some doctors recommend CoQ10 to their patients undergoing chemotherapy and radiation therapy to help the immune systems of these individuals.

A group of thirty-two breast cancer patients was treated with 90 mg of CoQ10 per day. K. Lockwood, MD, S. Moesgaard, MD, and Karl Folkers conducted the research. After twenty-four months, all of the thirty-two were still alive, six had partial remissions, and all of the tumor sizes had stabilized. One of the patients began taking 390 mg per day, and within three months her tumor had disappeared. Another took 300 mg per day and achieved the same results.

Many diseases are now associated with free-radical damage involved in the aging process, such as heart disease, cancer, diabetes, and Alzheimer's disease. Individuals with these diseases typically have low levels of CoQ10. This nutrient, along with other antioxidants, can help slow the aging process.

## COLOSTRUM

Colostrum passed from a mother to her newborn baby provides some of the most important factors for the immune system. It is produced for approximately the first seventy-two hours of life. All immune factors and growth factors are found in colostrum. These are designed to protect the infant from disease. A newborn does not possess all the basics for immune health. Nature provides for a method of transferring some forms of immunity to the infant. Antibodies are passed through the colostrum, offering protection from specific diseases. Other elements in colostrum have been found to work as immune-system messengers and are known as transfer factors.

The use of bovine colostrum is not a new concept. Ayurvedic physicians in India have used colostrum for health and spiritual benefits. It has also been used in other countries throughout the world. Scandinavian countries make a colostrum pudding to celebrate birth and good health. Evidence is mounting as to the benefits of colostrum.

Research has found that the colostrum in humans and bovine colostrum are virtually identical. Bovine colostrum is not species-specific and can work in humans. The different factors in cows are more potent than human factors. Bovine colostrum can replace the transfer factors and growth factors in humans. Even individuals with lactose intolerance seem to have no trouble ingesting bovine colostrum. After puberty, the body gradually begins to produce less of the immune and growth factors. These factors help to heal the body tissue. Colostrum is the only natural source of these factors.

The optimum time for collection of colostrum is within the first twenty-four hours after birth. This is when the milk contains the highest levels of immune and growth factors. Colostrum should be taken only from cows that are free of hormones, antibiotics, and pesticides. It must be processed without excessive heat to preserve the active components.

Colostrum has been used successfully to help stimulate normal growth and regeneration and repair of muscle, skin collagen, bone, cartilage, and nerve tissue. There is also evidence that colostrum may help to stimulate the body to burn fat for fuel and to build lean muscle mass. It may also help to balance blood sugar levels and maintain blood glucose levels. The immune factors can help to fight viruses, bacteria, fungus, allergens, parasites, and toxic substances. Just about every infection or degenerative disease is preceded by a lowered immune system function. Colostrum contains powerful immune factors. Studies have found that bovine colostrum can help prevent and reduce the severity of infections. It can benefit many conditions, such as arthritis, fibromyalgia, MS, diabetes, cardiovascular disease, cancer, allergies, fatigue, depression, weight loss, AIDS, and Alzheimer's disease.

Colostrum may be one of the most important supplements to hit the shelves. It is a unique combination of natural substances that works on a wide range of ailments. Colostrum factors work together to increase the function of the immune system naturally.

## CONJUGATED LINOLEIC ACID (CLA)

Conjugated linoleic acid is an essential fatty acid important for many body functions. Fats are not all bad; in fact, they are essential for life and serve functions in every cell in the body. The body is able to produce most of the fatty acids necessary for life, except linoleic acid, arachidonic acid, and linolenic acid. Linolenic and arachidonic acid can be made from linoleic acid if it is present in the body. CLA is a form of linoleic acid that is easily assimilated into the body. The best sources of CLA are beef, veal, and dairy products. There is a concern that most individuals are not getting enough CLA in their diets.

This could be due in part to the diets of cattle in the United States. Cows have generally eaten fresh grass as a diet staple. But because of cost and less grazing area, many cattle are fed grains and hay instead of fresh grass. The fresh grass provides more CLA than other food sources. This has led to the belief that there is less CLA in meat than previously thought. This decline in CLA may be a contributing factor in the problem of obesity.

Research has been amazing on this essential fatty acid. CLA has been studied as a protection against some forms of cancer. There was a lower incidence of breast tumors in rats given CLA. The more CLA in the diet, the less the risk of developing tumors. Continuing research has had similar results in preventing other forms of cancer, such as skin and stomach. There seems to be potential in the use of CLA as an anticarcinogenic and antioxidant. This may offer benefit for the immune system as well.

CLA may also be useful in impeding the progression of heart disease. An animal study involving rabbits found that a group fed a diet high in fat and cholesterol but supplemented with CLA had lower levels of LDL cholesterol and triglycerides. The aorta also had less blockage.

It's hard to imagine that fat can actually help to reduce fat, but that appears to be true with CLA. Research done using rats found that those fed CLA had 58 percent less body fat than those not given CLA. The weights of the rats stayed basically the same, but they gained muscle mass while losing fat. Another study involved humans. Half of the group were given CLA, the other group a placebo. The group was followed for three months. At the end of that period, the ones taking the CLA had lost an average of five pounds, along with a 15 to 20 percent drop in body fat. The placebo group had little or no change in either weight or percentage of body fat.

CLA continues to undergo research to validate its usefulness as a natural supplement. Its benefits may be substantial for many individuals.

## CORDYCEPS SINENSIS

Chinese remedies have grown in popularity during the past few years. Reishi, maitake, and shiitake mushrooms are a few of the popular supplements imported from Asia. Another supplement is now making its way into the Western markets. *Cordyceps sinensis* is a Chinese phrase meaning "winter bug, summer herb." This valuable herb is actually a fungus that grows from the carcass of the larva of some insects. It is only found growing naturally in mountain areas above eleven thousand feet. Cordyceps was so rare and expensive that only a few of the most prominent and wealthy individuals were able to use it. It is an extremely expensive process to locate this fungus, but methods have been developed that allow for cultivation in a controlled environment, making it more accessible and cheaper.

As disgusting as this fungus sounds, it is considered extremely valuable in Chinese medicine. There is mounting evidence through research of its value. Historically, it was often recommended as a tonic herb to aid in cases of recovery or weakness due to a prolonged illness, and it still is recommended today. Cordyceps is used to strengthen the kidneys and lungs, improve sex drive, decrease cholesterol and inflammation, aid relaxation, increase blood supply to the brain and heart, ease back and abdominal pain, lessen ringing in the ears and insomnia, reduce menstrual symptoms, and increase immunity.

Cordyceps became recognized by Western nations during the 1993 World Outdoor Track and Field Championship. The Chinese women's national team broke three world records. Questions were raised as to the use of performance-enhancing drugs by these athletes. No drugs were ever detected, but the coach revealed the use of a tonic drink made from cordyceps. It is thought to increase endurance by relaxing the airways.

The benefits of cordyceps do not merely apply to athletes. Remarkable evidence points to this herb for benefiting many different areas of the body. The effects of cordyceps involve the nervous system, respiratory system, immune system, glandular system, liver, kidneys, and heart.

Cordyceps has been found in studies to have a calming effect on the nervous system. Japanese research attributes the calming action to the nucleic acids. Evidence also points to the use of cordyceps in treating impotence. It seems to be able to allow more blood to enter the penis to form an erection. Respiratory ailments may also be helped with cordyceps. It relaxes the trachea and the airways to allow for proper airflow. This may help with lung problems, bronchitis, and especially asthma. A powder form of cordyceps has been used in Chinese medicine to treat heart arrhythmia. The results have been positive. The FDA has approved a component of cordyceps, adenosine, to treat supraventricular arrhythmia.

Other possible benefits include lowering elevated cholesterol levels and stimulating the immune system function by increasing the levels of T cells, leukocytes, and large lymphocytes. This has the potential of protecting the body and helping it fight disease. Cordyceps may also help to lower blood sugar levels in diabetics.

## DEHYDROEPIANDROSTERONE (DHEA)

DHEA is a naturally occurring hormone made in the adrenal glands. It is the most abundant hormone found in the body and is sometimes referred to as the "mother hormone." When the hormone levels are too low or out of sync, the body fails to function properly. Levels of DHEA in the body reach their peak at around twenty-one years of age and then tend to decline over the years. It is a precursor hormone that can be metabolized into other adrenal hormones and acts with other hormones.

Normal levels of DHEA can help to balance the immune system in fighting disease and infection. This protects the body from many serious problems that can occur, such as cancer. The full extent of the benefits of DHEA is not entirely known. But there is evidence that links low levels of DHEA to conditions such as cancer, Alzheimer's disease, arthritis, osteoporosis, chronic fatigue syndrome, diabetes, fertility problems, lupus, rheumatoid arthritis, multiple sclerosis, allergies, PMS, and even weight problems. DHEA is being looked on by some as the single most important factor in maintaining health.

Some research has found that individuals with cancer have lower levels of DHEA than healthy individuals. DHEA has the ability of inhibiting one of the most important enzymes that feed cancer cells. Research has found that DHEA can help with many different types of cancer, such as colon, lung, skin, breast, lymphatic, gastric, prostate, and ovarian. DHEA is thought to aid in retarding the growth of cancer. It blocks some of the enzymes responsible for cancer proliferation. This helps inhibit the activity of the cancer, stopping damage from occurring.

Alzheimer's is a frightening condition associated with loss of memory and senility. Levels of DHEA in Alzheimer's patients have been found to be 48 percent lower than a control group of normal, healthy individuals. DHEA helps to protect the brain cells from damage and deterioration. It is also useful with other senility-type degenerative conditions. DHEA in healthy individuals is plentiful in the brain tissue, which protects against aging and damage.

DHEA is a precursor for cortisol and adrenaline, which are stress hormones. When the body is under stress, DHEA can be depleted because of the effect on the adrenal glands. Chronic stress can lead to lower levels of DHEA, which in turn can be detrimental to health. Prolonged stress can lead to cases of depression. Depression may be helped with the addition of DHEA. Individuals have found favorable results when using DHEA.

Osteoporosis is a condition many women suffer from as they age. DHEA may be an important factor in controlling bone loss. Low levels of DHEA may be a factor in osteoporosis in postmenopausal women. DHEA has also been found to help with the absorption of calcium and the formation of new bone growth.

In addition to concern about bone health, many individuals are concerned about their weight. It is a battle that most face from time to time. DHEA has been found to help burn fat more efficiently, as well as build muscle. Dr. Arthur Schwartz, a researcher at Temple University, has found that DHEA can promote weight loss. Some individuals have found beneficial results with the addition of DHEA even when not altering their diets.

DHEA therapy has been shown to be free of side effects when taken in proper amounts. Some problems with excess amounts in the form of supplements include acne, rapid heartbeat, irritability, and headaches. Most have solved the problem by lowering the amount they are taking.

## ENZYMES

Enzymes are essential for life. Dr. Edward Howell, known as the pioneer of enzyme therapy, said, "Enzymes are substances that make life possible. No mineral, vitamin, or hormone can do any work without enzymes. They are the manual workers that build the body from proteins, carbohydrates, and fats. The body may have the raw building materials, but without the workers, it cannot begin." Enzymes are naturally occurring substances found in the human body, animals, and plants. More than 2,700 enzymes have been identified in the body, and they are constantly in motion. Life involves a series of reactions known as metabolism. Enzymes are involved in making the process work. Enzymes are involved in every individual biochemical function in the human body. Some call them the spark plugs of the body. Enzymes digest food and destroy toxins, viruses, antigens that invade the liver and bloodstream, parasites, and worms, and they help in the destruction of free radicals before cell damage can occur. Without enzymes, the body would deteriorate. Enzymes are responsible for vitamins, minerals, and amino acids being converted into vital neurotransmitters, allowing the body to function properly.

The typical American diet is lacking in enzymes. The only way to get enzymes is from live food or through supplements. A mostly cooked-food diet requires a larger amount of enzymes from the digestive organs. This creates exhaustion and degeneration of the organs. Supplementing with digestive enzymes will help take the stress off the pancreas and the entire system.

Enzymes are divided into two types: digestive enzymes and metabolic enzymes. In the gastrointestinal tract, digestive enzymes help break down food into forms that can be assimilated and utilized by the body. Digestion consumes a lot of energy and needs the assistance of digestive enzymes for proper assimilation of food. Overcooked food destroys enzymes. Foods may be lacking in enzymes due to pesticides, preservatives, pasteurization, and water containing chlorine, which all destroy enzymes. As we age, our bodies manufacture fewer enzymes. The body needs a proper balance of amino acids to manufacture enzymes.

Metabolic enzymes work within the cells to produce energy and detoxification. All bodily functions require metabolic enzymes. They produce the energy required to survive and thrive. Complicated chemical reactions occur and rely on a steady supply of enzymes.

Hydrochloric acid is secreted in the stomach and enzymes are secreted in the small intestine when the body is in a positive state of mind, but when the body is stressed, angry, or tense, enzyme and hydrochloric acid activity is inhibited. The result could be indigestion and malabsorption of nutrients. Chronic disease depletes enzyme reserves. Supplementing with digestive enzymes and eating raw food will build up the enzyme reserves in the body.

Supplemental digestive enzymes should contain protease, which breaks down protein into amino acids. Amylase breaks down starch into sucrose, and lipase's function is in the digestion of fats. Cellulase assists in breaking down cellulose. Enzymes improve digestion and assimilation of food. They help to improve assimilation of vitamins, minerals, amino acids, and essential fatty acids. They help the body break down old encrusted material on the entire digestive system.

Enzymes can be taken after meals to improve digestion. Additional enzymes are needed between meals so they can penetrate into tissues and break down undigested protein that can cause disease. They may help prevent conditions such as cancer, arthritis, and autoimmune diseases. Enzymes affect fibrin, which is associated with the rheumatic diseases. Enzymes will act as scavengers and destroy the protein coatings in the joints and reduce them to a form that can be eliminated by the body. Enzyme levels need to be present at all times to prevent disease and maintain vitality and endurance.

The endocrine system becomes overburdened when cooked food is eaten without raw food or enzymes present. Eating cooked food raises the white blood cell count and overburdens the immune system. A lack of enzymes robs the supply of enzymes needed to maintain metabolism, which can lead to weight gain. An oversecretion of hormones causes exhaustion and depletes the hormone-producing glands.

Antigens, viruses, germs, bacteria, yeast, parasites, and worms can all enter the body through the digestive tract and multiply rapidly when hydrochloric acid and enzymes are lacking. We also breathe in allergens from air pollution, and most antigens, bacteria, viruses, and yeast are protein, so the body needs these protein-digestive enzymes to digest and eliminate them.

Supplemental enzymes are usually necessary because of poor eating habits that deplete the body of its enzyme reserve. Eating too much cooked food, processed food, wrong food combinations, pesticides, preservatives, and additives can cause the destruction of essential enzymes.

## ESSENTIAL FATTY ACIDS

Essential fatty acids, also known as vitamin F or polyunsaturates, must be supplied through the diet because they cannot be synthesized in the body. This is why they are referred to as essential. There are basically three essential fatty acids: linoleic acid, linolenic acid, and arachidonic acid. Linoleic acid is the most vital because linolenic and arachidonic can be converted from linoleic acid. They are needed for cell structure and all body functions. Every cell in the body requires essential fatty acids. They transport the fat-soluble vitamins, A, D, E, and K, in the body.

The essential fatty acids (EFAs) are important for a healthy body. Linoleic acid is the most essential of the fatty acids. Omega-3 fatty acids include EPA (eicosapentaenioic acid) and DHA (docosahexaenoic acid) and are found in marine lipids. Studies have found them to reduce the risk of cardiovascular disease. Omega-6 fatty acids, which include GLA (gamma-linolenic acid), are most often found in plant sources.

The most common forms of omega-3 fatty acids are EPA, DHA, and alpha-linolenic acid, which helps create EPA and DHA. When animals eat plants rich in linolenic acid, they produce omega-3s. The oils of cold-water fish such as salmon, sardines, bluefish, herring, tuna, and mackerel contain omega-3 fatty acids. EPA and DHA are liquid and remain so. This protects the fish by staying fluid even in cold temperatures.

Omega-6 fatty acids are found in the fresh-pressed oils of many raw seeds and nuts. Gamma-linolenic acid is the most common form of omega-6. It has been found to have many health benefits. It helps to facilitate weight loss in overweight persons but not in those who do not need to lose weight. It reduces platelet aggregation. It helps reduce symptoms of depression. It may help to alleviate PMS symptoms.

Essential fatty acids have been found to help with many disorders in the body. They help to reduce blood pressure, aid in arthritis, lower cholesterol and triglyceride levels, reduce inflammation, improve skin disorders such as psoriasis and eczema, and aid

in nerve impulse transmissions, to name a few. Essential fatty acids also help with brain function, learning, and memory.

A lack of EFAs in the diet can cause numerous symptoms such as fatigue, lack of endurance, dry skin, allergies, high blood pressure, angina, aching, frequent colds, digestive problems, dry hair, immune weakness, forgetfulness, depression, and arthritis. The symptoms can be extremely vague and may go unnoticed by health-care providers.

Black currant seed oil is rich in linoleic acid. It provides a rich supply of gamma-linolenic acid and is an excellent source of omega-3 fatty acids.

Borage oil comes from a plant. It is a good source of GLA and helps with PMS, inflammation, heart function, and nail and hair growth.

Salmon oil is high in omega-3 essential fatty acids. It has been found to benefit arthritis, migraines, high cholesterol, bacterial infections, and to thin the blood.

Flaxseed oil is high in EFA content. It contains omega-3 and omega-6 essential fatty acids. It also contains beta-carotene and vitamin E.

Evening primrose oil is a source of linolenic and linoleic acid. The seeds contain GLA and help with low energy, brain and muscle function, cell membranes, multiple sclerosis, PMS, and obesity.

EFAs are so important that deficiencies can be linked to numerous symptoms. They contain superior nutritional support for health and vitality. Many individuals are lacking these essential nutrients that provide support for the immune system and health. These are vital nutrients that the body needs to function.

## GERMANIUM

Germanium is a naturally occurring trace element, like gold and silver. It is considered a trace mineral, but it is also referred to as a semimetal. There is probably no simple difference between a metal and a mineral. But many have become interested in and excited about this amazing product. Little research was done on germanium until 1950.

Germanium is important for many reasons in the body. It helps to improve oxygenation on a cellular level. This is essential for keeping the immune system healthy and in eliminating toxins from the body. Life is dependent on adequate availability of oxygen.

Germanium enables better usage of oxygen on the cellular level.

Germanium has been reported to have many beneficial effects. It has been used to reduce pain. It has been found to help with respiratory diseases to improve oxygen utilization. Evidence has also found germanium to help improve circulation. In cases of Raynaud's disease, it helps improve warmth in the fingers and toes within one half hour. For healthy individuals, warmth has occurred within minutes. Germanium may benefit people suffering from strokes or insufficient oxygen. It also may help to remove or detoxify the body of metal poisoning through its chelating ability. It is recommended for liver disease and arthritis.

Germanium has antiviral and antitumor properties. It was found to slow the progression and spread of tumors, prolonging life. Studies are ongoing in Japan researching the effects of germanium-132, or Ge-132, on different forms of cancer and disease. It may help by increasing the oxygen supply, to which cancer cells are sensitive. They may not be able to survive with oxygen utilization improved. American scientists are also researching this product.

Germanium was first discovered to be beneficial to health by a Japanese scientist, Dr. Kazuhiko Asai. As a chemist, he became interested in germanium extraction from coal. He heard reports that Russians used germanium as a rejuvenator. He studied the germanium in plants. He found that germanium enhanced oxygen utilization in plants and animals. In studies with mice, he found that less oxygen was required to maintain respiration when those tissues were supplemented with germanium.

Germanium may help with many conditions, including cancer, allergies, arthritis, cholesterol, viral infections, and AIDS. It has proven successful in many studies, and its benefits are just beginning to be understood. As more information is made available, undoubtedly germanium will be an important supplement.

## GLUCOSAMINE

Glucosamine is a compound naturally found in the joints of the body. It is formed in the body from glucose. Glucosamine is important as a precursor and stimulant of the construction of proteoglycan synthesis, which is the basis of cartilage. It is also important for the synthesis of substances that make up tendons, ligaments, the respiratory system, and the mucous membranes of the digestive and respiratory tracts.

The normal aging process causes a decline in the amount of glucosamine production. As it is involved in the natural cushioning of the joints, this can lead to damage and pain. When the natural cushion is gone, bone and cartilage may rest against each other, causing deterioration. This can occur in the joints as well as the spinal column.

Glucosamine sulfate is a treatment that has proven effective for osteoarthritis. In fact, some have found it to work better than conventional therapies, because it does more than just mask the pain; it actually aids in rebuilding and stimulating joint repair. It also helps to prevent joint destruction.

Glucosamine sulfate helps heal, relieve pain, reduce inflammation, and improve joint damage without the side effects often associated with drug therapy.

Studies have found that glucosamine metabolism is altered when osteoarthritis is present. Glucosamine supplements have been found to be effective in treating this condition. Trials have found substantial improvement in individuals treated with glucosamine.

There has been little risk, if any, involved with the use of glucosamine in treating osteoarthritis. It appears that glucosamine is very safe, without any known precautions or risks. One study found that glucosamine sulfate may help stimulate the defense mechanisms in the stomach lining. Pain and anti-inflammatory medications often cause stomach problems.

Glucosamine sulfate has been shown to be an important part of treating osteoarthritis. Results showed significant improvement in swelling, pain, and degeneration of joints. Not only is it important for reducing the symptoms involved with osteoarthritis, but it also has been found to actually reverse the degenerative process and induce healing. Glucosamine should be considered as a form of treatment for osteoarthritis.

## GREEN FOODS

Green foods are phyto-foods that usually contain high quantities of chlorophyll, the substance that gives plants their green color. Chlorophyll also allows the plant to utilize sunlight in accessing nutrients from the soil. These plants contain some of the most important nutrients, including vitamins, minerals, bioflavonoids, antioxidants, protein, amino acids, enzymes, and fiber. The high content of nutrients in green foods makes them valuable for keeping the body in optimum health. Green foods include algae, cereal grasses, and legumes.

Green foods are not always green. There are a variety of colors in the green foods category. The greens include spirulina, chlorella, blue-green algae, wheatgrass, barley, alfalfa, broccoli, spinach, parsley, cabbage, rice grass, kale, and celery. Red, yellow, and orange green foods include the tomato, cranberry, cayenne, red and yellow peppers, orange juice, grapefruit, pineapple, brown rice, papaya, and squash. The blue group of greens includes grape skin extract, black cherry, beet juice, and elderberry. Apple pectin, garlic, and onion are included in the white group.

The popularity of green foods has arisen as many individuals concerned about health think they are not getting enough essential nutrients in their diets. Everyone could benefit from the addition of green foods to the diet, including individuals in poor health. Athletes are also in need of extra nutrients. They often put their bodies under stress through intense training. Supplementing with green foods could help with the growth of muscle and bone tissue. Pregnant women, along with the developing fetuses, could use the extra nutrients during the developmental stages.

## GREEN TEA

Green tea has been used for centuries in many Asian cultures for health and vitality. But it has only been in recent years, with research to confirm its effectiveness, that the Western world has recognized the value of green tea. This tea shows promise for healing and preventing disease.

The polyphenols and xanthines found in green tea are the major contributors to the health benefits. Polyphenols are flavonoids that account for the tart flavor of the tea. Polyphenols are antioxidants that help to fight free-radical damage, which is associated with many diseases and conditions.

One of the most promising uses of green tea is in treating and preventing cancer. One study followed nine hundred middle-aged Chinese men and women with esophageal cancer and compared them with fifteen hundred without cancer. Nonsmokers who did not drink alcohol and consumed green tea cut their risk of esophageal cancer by 60 percent. The protection is thought to be due to the antioxidant polyphenols. The polyphenol content in the tea inhibits in vitro and in vivo formation of N-nitrosation by-products, which are cancer-causing compounds. Green tea has also been found to help with other types of cancer. There seems to be a protective effect against colon cancer among green tea drinkers. Studies done on animals have found a preventive effect against tumors of the skin, lung, esophagus, stomach, small intestine, colon, liver, pancreas, and breast.

Green tea consumption may also help to increase longevity. One evaluation of thirty-three hundred Japanese women concluded that the tea does contribute to an increase in life span. It may help by decreasing the incidence of some life-threatening diseases.

Heart disease prevention may be another benefit of drinking green tea. A study in the Netherlands found that over a five-year period, 805 men aged sixty-five to eighty-four had a 58 percent lower risk of dying from a heart attack. The benefits are attributed to the flavonoid content found in the green tea. Lower cholesterol levels may also be associated with the intake of green tea. There was a lower risk of stroke, nearly 70 percent, among men who drank 4.7 cups of green tea per day.

Green tea has also been found to contain antibacterial compounds. They may be effective against a variety of bacteria, including bacillary dysentery, amoebic dysentery, and enteritis. Green tea is also beneficial for wounds, sunburn, acne, athlete's foot, colds, and flu.

Research is beginning to show evidence of the advantages to health in adding green tea to the diet. Chinese and Japanese healers have advocated the use of green tea for centuries. The beverage choice for millions of Asians may help protect against a variety of ailments.

## GRIFFONIA (5-HTP)

Finding a quick fix for obesity has become a national obsession. Prescription drugs have not proven to be safe or effective in the long run, and just about all diets fail. There have been some natural supplements that have been found to have beneficial and safe effects. One of the most promising is griffonia, which is high in 5-hydroxytryptophan and is referred to as 5-HTP.

There has been considerable research on 5-HTP as to its safety and use in weight loss and depression. Serotonin is a neurotransmitter that bridges the gap between neurons. It is essential for many bodily functions and is thought to play a role in depression and obesity. Unlike serotonin alone, it can cross the blood-brain barrier, making it possible for the brain to manufacture more serotonin. Five-HTP may actually help to promote the production of serotonin, making more available. Research has found that increased amounts of 5-HTP can help with weight loss and depression.

One study found that a group of women given 5-HTP ate less than women given a placebo. Weight loss corresponded to the intake of 5-HTP. The women taking it over a five-week period lost an average of three to four pounds. The results have been replicated with other studies on humans. There appears to be a feeling of fullness when eating less.

Low serotonin levels have been linked to depression. Five-HTP may help to improve mood swings and depression. In one study, 5-HTP supplementation was compared to Prozac use. In both cases, there was a 50 percent improvement in depression. But those taking the 5-HTP showed more tolerance for the treatment and had a lower failure rate.

For those suffering from obesity and depression, 5-HTP may help. As a natural supplement, it may help to reduce the appetite and improve moods. It is an alternative to prescription drug therapy, which is known to have adverse side effects.

## MELATONIN

Melatonin is a hormone found naturally in the body. It is secreted by the pineal gland, located in the center of the brain. This gland is very small, about the size of a kernel of corn. The pineal gland is the first gland formed in the body, just three weeks after conception. The pineal gland serves many important functions in the body.

The pineal gland helps to influence the functions of the immune system and the secretion of hormones. This gland takes cues from light and temperature changes to produce the hormone melatonin. Light enters the brain through the eyes to signal the pineal gland. It actually keeps us in sync with daily rhythms. Darkness triggers the production of melatonin, causing drowsiness and helping to set the biological clock. The pineal gland works with other parts of the brain through the secretion of melatonin. It is also thought to be responsible for prompting birds to migrate, dogs to shed their heavy winter coats, animals to store up for the winter, and even some animals to change their color according to the seasons.

Insomniacs were probably the first to try melatonin when it was reported in newspapers across the country. A number of studies have found beneficial results from using melatonin for insomnia. Its effects are especially valuable when melatonin levels are low.

Some people who travel frequently have used melatonin to ease the jet-lag problem. Sleeping pills used to be the choice, but they do not help adjust the body clock. Several studies have found melatonin to help in relieving jet lag. Melatonin has helped many of these people to recover faster when traveling. Shift workers also often have difficulties adjusting the body clock and sleep patterns.

There seems to be protection from melatonin in its ability to neutralize free radicals, protecting the body from damage. It may also help by activating enzymes to heal the damaged cells faster. There are many immune-related conditions that may benefit from melatonin's antioxidant properties, including heart disease, arteriosclerosis, cancer, tumors, Alzheimer's, emphysema, cataracts, aging, and some neurological problems. There seems to be benefit from melatonin in the prevention and inhibition of some forms of cancer, particularly cancers associated with hormone production, such as breast and prostate.

Melatonin is being researched concerning its anti-aging capabilities. Some preliminary research has pointed to improvements in health and longer life span in animal studies. Life was prolonged by about 25 percent in mice treated with melatonin. In other studies, mice in advanced age showed improved health and longevity in comparison to mice not given melatonin. Rodents with their pineal glands removed have shorter life spans.

To really understand the use of melatonin on aging, studies would need to continue for many years, but in some studies, it has been determined that individuals suffering from certain forms of depression had lower levels of melatonin. It has also been shown that children suffering from depression may have lower levels of melatonin. Emotional trauma in childhood or prolonged stress may lead to lower levels of melatonin. Long periods of stress may alter or damage the areas of the brain known to produce melatonin.

Certain foods have been found to contain melatonin. The most abundant source is tall fescue, a grass plant. Other foods high in melatonin include oats, sweet corn, rice, ginger, tomatoes, bananas, and barley. All of these foods are known for their health benefits. Try different ones to see which work best in increasing melatonin in the bloodstream.

Tryptophan, an essential amino acid, can help increase the production of melatonin. Melatonin is derived from tryptophan. As foods containing tryptophan are eaten during the day, the tryptophan is converted into serotonin and then to melatonin in the pineal gland. Levels of melatonin can be increased by eating foods high in tryptophan, such as spirulina, seaweed, soy, cottage cheese, pumpkin seeds, turkey, chicken, tofu, and almonds.

Melatonin appears to be a very versatile and beneficial substance. It has received attention for its ability to induce sleep and fight jet lag, but now there is evidence that it can help improve immune function, reduce stress, lower cholesterol, reduce the risk of heart disease, prevent premature aging, and protect against cancer.

## MSM (METHYLSULFONYLMETHANE)

Methylsulfonylmethane (MSM) is a tasteless, odorless substance crucial to body function and structure. It is a substance found naturally in the body and in all living organisms. MSM is often overlooked as an essential nutrient. Though necessary for life, there may not be adequate amounts of MSM for optimal health in the average diet.

Our knowledge of the importance of MSM has increased through the extensive years of research on dimethylsulfoxide (DMSO) conducted by Dr. Stanley W. Jacob, MD at the Oregon Health Sciences University in Portland, Oregon. He became aware of MSM as a stable metabolite of DMSO. Further research, along with his colleague Robert Herschler, led him to understand the value and benefits of MSM. MSM contains an additional atom of oxygen and is also referred to as dimethyl sulfoxide, or DMSO2. The "S" in DMSO2 is sulfur. DMSO has an odor that is sometimes undesirable, while DMSO2, or MSM, is odorless and colorless, making it more palatable for internal use.

DMSO2 is a derivative of DMSO. Robert Herschler has begun marketing DMSO2 in a crystalline form taken orally or applied to the skin. DMSO2 (or MSM) has wide-ranging benefits similar to DMSO and is in a solid form, making it useful as a nutritional supplement. Research continues but is extremely expensive to conduct. DMSO and MSM are similar chemically, but each has unique functions and characteristics. MSM is found naturally in many foods and can be taken as a supplement with foods or alone. Under the Dietary Supplement Health and Education Act of 1994, MSM can be marketed as a substance for nutritional support of the body's natural structure and function. It is naturally found in the body and foods.

MSM is a safe and natural food derived from seawater. When DMSO is heated, it changes to a crystalline form, DMSO2 or MSM. This form of organic sulfur does not have the unpleasant side effects of some other forms of sulfur, including foul odor and taste, often producing gas and unpleasant body odor.

MSM is a natural source of organic, dietary sulfur. It is found in body fluids and tissues. About half of the body's supply of sulfur is located in the muscles, skin, and bones. The body requires organic sulfur to function properly.

A deficiency of dietary MSM impedes the body's ability to promote cell growth and development. The body continues to produce new cells throughout the day and night. If adequate amounts of MSM are not available, a poor quality of cells may be developed. This, in turn, leaves the body susceptible to many ailments, as it cannot heal itself. Research abounds as to the potential of this powerful nutrient.

MSM has also been found to enhance the availability of vitamin C and other antioxidant nutrients, helping to protect the body from disease. The antioxidants help the immune system function more efficiently, allowing the body to heal itself.

Robert Herschler provides evidence of the benefits of MSM in patent #4616039, entitled "Methylsulfonylmethane in dietary products." He recognizes the use of MSM as a viable source of dietetic sulfur. MSM is important for maintaining good health and healing in both humans and animals. MSM can supply the body with the ingredients to keep the body healthy and strong as it repairs damaged tissue wherever a problem arises. This can help to protect and prevent serious conditions from developing.

Hair and nail growth can be improved with the supplementation of MSM. One of the amino acids, cystine, is found in keratin, a protein found abundantly in the hair and nails. Herschler, in his U.S. patent #4296130, includes the skin and nails as beneficiaries of MSM. This supplement aids in softening the skin and strengthening the nails when applied topically. The MSM compositions may also be administered orally, by injection, or by inhalation. MSM can be used in creams, lotions, or gels to help condition and strengthen the skin and nails.

MSM contains potential benefits for those who suffer from allergies. Individuals found significant relief from taking a supplement of MSM. It may help to reduce the amount of medication some people are required to take to keep their allergies under control. The MSM adds permeability to the cell walls, allowing for prompt removal of the foreign substances.

MSM has been found to be useful in treating interstitial cystitis. S. J. Childs conducted research at the Department of Surgery, University of Alabama–Tuscaloosa. The results of the study found that DMSO2 (MSM) was an effective alternative treatment for interstitial cystitis. There were no side effects associated with the treatment. It was also found to be useful for treating painful bladder syndrome.

Interstitial cystitis in a urinary condition often associated with lupus. Lupus is a serious condition in which the immune system begins to attack its own body tissues, resulting in inflammation, pain, and tissue damage. Any part of the body can be involved, sometimes the entire body. The condition can be active and then go into remission. Natural and nutritional therapies for lupus may help. It has often been hard to treat, requiring aggressive thera-

py. DMSO and MSM have been used to treat this condition successfully.

Snoring, though most often not life-threatening, can be a problem, not only for the one snoring, but for the entire household. MSM may offer some relief. A solution containing MSM can be applied directly to the nostrils within one hour of sleep. In one study, MSM as a 16 percent water solution was put in each nostril of the subjects fifteen minutes before sleep. Treatment was successful for 80 percent of the subjects after one to four days in a trial at the Oregon Health Sciences University conducted by Dr. Stanley W. Jacob. The subjects were treated for ninety days, and none reported any toxic or adverse reactions. MSM may work to keep the nasal passages open. The cells become more permeable and flexible, allowing for clear passage of air and resulting in a reduction in snoring.

Research has been done using both DMSO and MSM in clinical studies involving breast cancer. One study found a longer time in the appearance of mammary tumors in rats with dimethbenzanthracene-induced mammary cancers. D. McCabe and a group of researchers at the Ohio State University College of Medicine studied a group of mice bred to acquire a predisposition for breast cancer when given MSM in their diet and then doses of carcinogenic compounds. The animals were watched for a year. The group given the MSM developed tumors between 100 and 130 days later than the control group. This would be the equivalent of approximately ten years in humans.

Researchers at the Ohio State University College of Medicine injected a carcinogen known to cause colon cancer in rats. The time for the tumors to develop was significantly reduced in the rats given MSM. The group given the MSM developed tumors much later than the control group. The treatment was not associated with the toxicity or weight loss often accompanying chemotherapy and radiation treatments. Further research is warranted as to the benefits of MSM as a chemopreventive agent.

Robert Herschler, in his patent issued on November 27, 1990, claims a reduction in arthritis-induced muscle cramps from the ingestion of MSM. Individuals suffering from arthritis have reported relief from pain, stiffness, and inflammation. A study performed in Russia found similar results. The researchers used a double-blind study method on a group of mice to determine the benefits of MSM on the development of arthritis. It was found that both DMSO and MSM helped to lessen the detrimental changes in the joints that often accompany arthritis. Migraine sufferers have also found relief from severe headache pain.

MSM provides a source of dietary organic sulfur easily assimilated in the body. This is important because MSM provides the tools necessary for the body to create and repair cells. MSM has a broad range of uses for health. MSM helps the body heal on a cellular level, rather than simply masking the symptoms. MSM is a nutritional supplement increasingly understood as helpful for good health.

## NONI (MORINDA CITRIFOLIA)

Noni is an evergreen shrub that is used medically. It is native to tropical areas of Australia, Malaysia, and Polynesia. It has been used for thousands of years for its benefits in healing. Though not well known until recently, noni is emerging as a valuable botanical medicine.

Traditionally, noni was used not only as a medicine but as a food, for clothing, and cloth dyes. Medicinally, it was used for swelling, inflammation, delayed menstruation, coughs, parasites, diarrhea, stomach ailments, gum disease, fever, chest colds, and skin abscesses, to name a few ailments. Polynesians used noni for just about every illness.

Studies support the use of noni to stimulate the immune function, inhibit the growth of some tumors, normalize cellular function, and boost tissue regeneration. Noni possesses a wide variety of medicinal properties. The fruit and leaves have anti-bacterial activity. The roots help to expel mucus. The root contains compounds known to have sedative properties and lower blood pressure. The noni fruit extracts in juice are used for hypertension, painful menstruation, arthritis, gastric ulcers, and depression.

One study found anticancer activity in noni against lung cancer. Mice were used in the research and were artificially exposed to lung carcinoma. Half of the mice given the noni lived more than fifty days, while the ones left untreated lived an average of twelve days. The noni appears to stimulate the immune response to deal with the carcinogen. The component of noni, xeronine, is thought to be involved in normalizing the malignant cell.

Noni may also help to ease joint pain and inflammation due to arthritis. Some researchers think a link to arthritic pain may be an inability to digest proteins, which then can create crystalline deposits in the joints. Noni fruit's ability to improve protein digestion by boosting enzymatic function may help eliminate this problem.

Noni may also work to slow the aging process by stimulating the immune response to destroy free radicals. Noni may help to protect the cells from damage due to pollutants, radiation, and other environmental problems. It may also help in cases of diabetes or other blood sugar disorders. Animal studies have found that noni can help to ease pain and discomfort. Xeronine seems to have analgesic activity.

Traditional uses of noni have brought attention to this powerful botanical. Further research may provide validation of the use of noni for many conditions. The components of noni provide powerful medicinal application.

## PHYTOCHEMICALS

Phytochemicals are substances found in fruits and vegetables that appear to play a role in protecting the body against diseases affecting the immune system, such as cancer. There are hundreds of different phytochemicals, only a few of which have been studied. Many foods contain numerous varieties of these phytochemicals. These compounds interact in complex ways and also overlap in their functions. Many of them are brightly colored and give plants their array of hues.

The difference between phytochemicals and other food components is that they appear to have no actual nutritional value or calories. They don't participate in the normal functions of the body. But they seem to be able to benefit the immune system in fighting disease. New information is appearing rapidly, and it is difficult to keep up with all the data.

"While there's no doubt that diets rich in fruits and vegetables are cancer-protective, much of what we know about individual phytochemicals is still speculative," nutrition researcher Phyllis Bowen, co-director of the University of Illinois's functional foods programs, has been quoted as saying.

Phytochemicals can be classified by different

methods, such as chemical name, food sources, and anticancer action. The following are some of the phytochemicals listed according to their chemical names.

## Indoles

Indoles are probably the most commonly known phytochemical because of their recent popularity. They seem to increase the activity of enzymes that can detoxify carcinogens and may also change the hormone estrogen into a benign form, reducing the risk of breast cancer and other cancers. Scientists think indoles (found in cruciferous vegetables) have the ability to block cancer-causing substances before they enter the cells.

## Allyl Sulfides

The allyl sulfides (found in onions, leeks, and garlic) are credited with boosting the production of an enzyme that may actually aid in excreting carcinogens more efficiently. Some have been found to help inhibit the capacity of tumor cells to reproduce.

## Flavonoids

The flavonoids are often found in vitamin C combinations. They consist of various chemicals commonly found in fruits and vegetables. Flavonoids are considered to be essential in their actions as antioxidants in reducing the risk of cancer. They are able to protect the cells from carcinogens and suppress the malignant changes in cells. Some researchers also believe that they may inhibit the ability of hormones to bind to the cells, limiting cancer development.

## Dithiolthiones

Dithiolthiones, found in cruciferous vegetables, help trigger the production of enzymes that may protect the cell's DNA from being damaged by carcinogens.

## Isoflavones

These are found in soybeans and soy-based products. Studies have found that in countries where soy products are consumed regularly, there is a lower incidence of breast and prostate cancer. This is credited in part to the isoflavones. They act similarly to antioxidants in blocking carcinogens and inhibiting the growth of tumors.

## Lignans

Lignans are found in many foods, especially linseed found in flax. They have antioxidant effects in blocking and inhibiting the cancer cell growth. Flax is high in omega-3 fatty acids, which are thought to help prevent many different immune-related diseases, such as colon cancer and heart disease.

## Limonene

The highest concentration of limonene is found in the rind of citrus fruits. It stimulates the production of certain enzymes known to help eliminate carcinogens. It may also reduce the size of mammary tumors.

## Caffeic Acid

Caffeic acid, found in citrus fruit, has been found to make carcinogens easier to secrete from the body by making them more water-soluble. It may inhibit the formation of carcinogens and suppress the growth of lung and skin tumors.

## Saponins

Saponins are a big group of modified carbohydrates that are found in a large variety of vegetables and herbs. Soybeans have been found to contain eleven different varieties of saponins. Saponins have been researched and found to contain anticancer activity.

Cruciferous vegetables have long been encouraged as part of a healthful diet. The cruciferous vegetables are from the cabbage family and include broccoli, Brussels sprouts, cabbage, cauliflower, collards, kale, radishes, rutabaga, turnips, mustard seed, and watercress. What is the secret ingredient in these cruciferous vegetables that makes them so essential for healing and preventing many ailments, including cancer?

They contain a bounty of cancer-fighting substances, some of which increase the production of enzymes that are responsible for defusing carcinogens and ridding them from the body. The indoles specifically seem to have a profound effect on the metabolism of estrogen by helping the body produce benign forms of the hormone which don't promote some forms of cancer, especially breast cancer.

Various studies have been done researching the effectiveness of indoles. One conducted in 1991 followed twelve individuals for a week as they ate a diet rich in cruciferous vegetables. After the week, there was a 50 percent increase in good estrogen in the blood levels. An article in *Ladies' Home Journal* in July 1994 reported on a study done on one particular indole known as Indole-3 Carbinol. The results seem to indicate that this indole helps change the way in which estrogen breaks down in women's bodies. As this estrogen breaks down, it becomes either harmful or benign. This indole helps in preventing estrogen from becoming harmful and increasing the risk of breast cancer. Another Japanese study reported on a study done with mice. Those exposed to cancer-causing agents and given the indole were much less likely to develop mouth cancer.

Individuals concerned about their health have begun purchasing these cruciferous vegetables in large quantities. And, it seems, with good reason. More than fifty studies conducted in recent years confirm the benefits of this incredible nutrient. These benefits should be taken seriously. The vegetables seem to have the most benefit when eaten raw or lightly steamed. Boiling is known to decrease the nutritional value by half. Supplements are also available containing indoles, which makes getting an abundance in the diet easier.

## PYCNOGENOL

Pycnogenol is a powerful antioxidant that contains a highly bioavailable flavonoid, proanthocyanidin. This is extracted from either pine bark or grapeseed, and both are virtually the same in chemical structure. Pycnogenol is known to be useful in supporting the immune system function and protecting the body from free-radical damage. It is a highly potent free radical scavenger and can improve and protect health.

The proanthocyanidins in pycnogenol have been studied for their remarkable activity. Researchers say these bioflavonoids significantly surpass other known antioxidants in their ability to fight free radicals. Pycnogenol is fifty times more potent than vitamin E, twenty times more potent than vitamin C.

Antioxidants can help to prevent free-radical damage, which is associated with aging and wrinkles. Pycnogenol flavonoids have been found to have an antienzyme effect in preventing the breakdown of collagen and elastin, which help to keep the skin firm and wrinkle-free.

## PYRUVATE

Pyruvate is a naturally occurring substance found in the body and an important component of metabolism. It is actually the end product of the metabolism process. Pyruvate contains carbon, hydrogen, and oxygen. It has been known for many years as a natural and essential part of energy production, though many of its benefits are just beginning to surface.

Pyruvate is a part of the Krebs citric-acid cycle. Glycogen is converted from glucose. Glucose, a form of sugar, breaks down into two molecules of pyruvic acid. The pyruvic acid enters the mitochondria of the cell, aiding in the production of energy. When pyruvic acid is oxidized, it forms acetylcoenzyme. The second step in the process, called the Krebs cycle, results in the release of energy.

Pyruvic acid is not chemically stable by itself. Stabilization is accomplished by combining the pyruvic acid with either calcium, sodium, potassium, magnesium, or zinc, which forms a salt, pyruvate. Calcium is used most often in the manufacturing for stabilization. Pyruvate has only been available commercially for a few months because of the difficulty in manufacturing and stabilizing the product.

Pyruvate is a natural product consumed in the diet on a daily basis. Pyruvate is found in some foods, but generally in small amounts. Red apples contain the most pyruvate, with about 450 mg. Red wine contains approximately 75 mg in a six-ounce glass. Dark beer has about 80 mg per twelve ounces. Cheese also contains pyruvate, but in smaller amounts. It is nearly impossible to get enough in the diet without taking a supplement to promote weight loss or increase physical performance. The amount usually recommended is about 2 to 5 grams per day.

Dr. R. T. Stanko, MD, has done considerable research on pyruvate over the past twenty-five years. He began his research on the ability of pyruvate to increase endurance and athletic performance. But interest in pyruvate as a weight- and fat-loss supplement began with fat reduction seen in animal studies.

Research done by Dr. Stanko in Pittsburgh followed fourteen overweight women to test the effectiveness of pyruvate on fat and weight loss. High doses of pyruvate were given to the women, or a placebo, along with a restricted diet. The group given the pyruvate showed an average of 37 percent greater loss of weight and 48 percent greater fat loss than the placebo group.

Another study conducted in 1994 found weight and fat loss with participants taking a pyruvate supplement. The subjects were given pyruvate in large doses: 22–44 grams. They were also on a low-fat, low-cholesterol diet. There was greater weight and fat loss in the participants taking the pyruvate than those taking the placebo.

Studies conducted at the Montefiore University Hospital in Pittsburgh have found positive results from a supplementation of pyruvate combined with dihydroxyacetone (DHA). Muscular endurance in both arms and legs improved by 20 percent when taking the pyruvate mixture. It increased fatigue time by twenty-three minutes in the arm muscles and thirteen minutes in the leg muscles. These results are certainly significant.

Another study also conducted in Pittsburgh by Dr. Stanko followed the same basic perimeters as the above study on leg endurance. Participants were tested for arm exercise endurance. After the supplementation for seven days and a standard diet, there was a definite increase in arm muscle endurance capacity.

Other possible benefits of pyruvate include the following:

### Free-Radical Prevention

The negative effects of free radicals have been the focus of much research. Free radicals can do damage on a cellular level to influence many immune-related diseases, arthritis, and the aging process. Pyruvate has been studied and found to work as an antioxidant in preventing and inhibiting free-radical damage. The studies have been done on rats but are promising for humans as well.

### Cancer Prevention

Pyruvate may help to slow tumor growth, as seen in one study done on rats implanted with malignant tumors. It can also help with cancer prevention by fighting free-radical damage.

### Heart Disease Prevention

There is some evidence that pyruvate supplementation may help lower bad cholesterol while not affecting the good. This may be a factor in the prevention of heart disease. Pyruvate may also help to strengthen the heart muscle, as it does with other muscles in the body.

It is obvious from some of the research that extremely high doses of pyruvate have been used. And these large amounts (up to 100 grams per day) are highly unreasonable for the average individual, on both the budget and the body. But more recent studies have proven that much smaller doses of pyruvate are also effective. The recommended dosage is 2 to 5 grams per day, according to Dr. Stanko. Larger amounts don't seem to provide better results. But there is little documentation to provide actual evidence on exact amounts needed for benefit.

## SHARK CARTILAGE

Sharks have been referred to as magnificent creatures. They are strong, fast, and disease-resistant. Information on the healthy state of the shark has led some to look further. The shark has an amazingly potent immune system. It has circulating antibodies that attack quickly when an invading element threatens its health. This extremely efficient immune system also works to promote rapid healing and prevention from infection. The cartilage of the shark is thought to be the key to its incredible health. The endoskeleton of the shark is mainly composed of cartilage. Shark cartilage is a combination of proteins and complex carbohydrates called mucopolysaccharides.

During the study of sharks, one anomaly kept reappearing. Sharks have a very low incidence of cancer development. There seem to be certain biochemicals in the shark cartilage that inhibit the growth of tumors, even when sharks are exposed to carcinogens. One study followed sharks for ten years at the Mote Marine Laboratory in Sarasota, Florida. The sharks exposed to high doses of carcinogenic elements never developed tumors. It is thought that the antibodies circulating throughout the shark are able to keep invaders from affecting the immune system.

The shark cartilage as a natural supplement helps to destroy and prevent tumors by preventing the creation of blood vessels that nurture and sustain tumor growth. It seems to actually cut off the tumor blood flow without destroying healthy tissue. This is especially promising considering that radiation and chemotherapy are extremely hard on the body and can destroy healthy as well as cancerous tissue.

One animal study with mice involved giving them melanoma through cancerous skin grafts. Half of the mice were given nothing, while the others were given shark cartilage daily. After three weeks, tumors in the untreated mice had doubled. The group given shark cartilage had experienced a decrease in tumor size.

Mexican studies on human cancer patients have shown positive results. Types of cancer varied, but the results were positive in eight patients followed. Seven of the eight patients had reduction in tumor size of 30 to 100 percent. The best results appear to be with cancers involving solid tumor masses that require a sufficient blood supply through vessels. Typically these types are found in the breast, cervix, pancreas, prostate, or ovaries.

Shark cartilage may also help with arthritis. Studies done on both animals and humans have shown benefits from taking shark cartilage. It appears to work as a natural anti-inflammatory to relieve swelling and ease pain. One doctor in Costa Rica administered shark cartilage to ten patients who were bedridden with severe cases of osteoarthritis. After three weeks of therapy, eight of the ten were able to walk. Shark cartilage may be of benefit to individuals suffering from arthritis pain and inflammation.

There is also evidence of shark cartilage's usefulness in treating skin conditions such as psoriasis. Medical treatment usually consists of corticosteroids and other drug therapies. They do not cure the disease, but they attempt to keep the symptoms under control. Limited studies have found positive results from the use of shark cartilage.

Research continues worldwide to document the use of shark cartilage. There are a considerable number of disorders being investigated for use with shark cartilage, such as eczema, acne, poison oak and ivy, hemorrhoids, colitis, asthma, and gastritis, to name a few. There have been amazing results with use, but it is still a relatively unknown supplement. As research progresses, more information will become available.

## SOY

For the past several years, the spotlight has focused on soy protein for a myriad of beneficial effects. But many individuals have resisted taking the plunge for different reasons. The flavor of soy has not been a staple in the Western world. We are just not used to the taste and texture of many soy products. And most of the soybean production in the United States has traditionally been used to feed animals. But the trend is moving in favor of soy products. The health benefits cannot be denied. In fact, the risk of two of the most dreaded diseases known to man, heart disease and some forms of cancer, can be reduced with an increase of soy protein in the diet.

Soy is an incredible source of valuable nutrients. There are few, if any, plants that compare with the soybean in regard to total nutritional value. Soybeans contain important vitamins and minerals, including calcium, iron, zinc, and B-complex vitamins. Soy provides all of the essential amino acids that are needed by the body to make protein. There are many phytonutrients in soy responsible for its health benefits.

### Phytate

Phytate is found in soybeans and may be a powerful antioxidant in cancer and heart disease prevention. For years, this storage form of phosphorus was thought to be an "antinutrient." Actually, it has in recent years been found to play a role in disease prevention.

### Omega-3

Omega-3 essential fatty acids are a form of fats with multiple healthful properties and are found in soy oil.

### Protease Inhibitor

Protease inhibitor, a phytochemical, used to be considered detrimental to health. Research has found that protease inhibitor can aid in inhibiting cancers of the skin, bladder, colon, lungs, pancreas, mouth, and esophagus. It helps by stopping the action of the specific cancer genes. It also helps protect against the harm caused by radiation and free-radical damage.

### Phytosterols

Phytosterols are similar to cholesterol in plants but not absorbed by humans. Phytosterols compete with dietary cholesterol for absorption in the colon, which aids in less cholesterol being absorbed and more excreted by the body. They are excellent to aid in cancer and ulcer prevention. They go directly to the colon to protect against bile acid damage.

### Saponins

Saponins are naturally occurring substances in soybeans and other foods that aid in reducing the growth and development of colon and melanoma cancer cells.

## Isoflavones

Isoflavones are unique to soybeans. They are similar to estrogen, but less powerful. They aid in the prevention of breast cancer by connecting to estrogen receptors on tissue cells that may become carcinogenic with estrogen. They inhibit certain actions from occurring that can lead to the growth of breast cancer. Asian women and vegetarian women who consume soy have very low incidence of breast cancer. Isoflavones help prevent not only cancer, but also heart disease by lowering cholesterol levels.

Genistein is the main isoflavone in soybeans. It is one of the most powerful flavonoids discovered to date. Clinical studies have found the genistein in soy to be a powerful tool in cancer prevention and treatment. There have been more than two hundred separate research papers written on genistein since 1986. Some consider it to be one of the most powerful anticancer agents. It works by regulating the action of some enzymes that are involved in the cancer process. One of the most amazing aspects of genistein is its ability to change cancer cells to normal cells. It also inhibits the growth of blood vessels that feed the cancer, depriving it of nutrients. Genistein is a powerful antioxidant, aiding in the prevention of free-radical damage known to cause cancer and other disease.

Daidzein is also found in soybeans. A product of the breakdown of daidzein is ipriflavone, which is being investigated for its potential in preventing osteoporosis.

At the First International Symposium on Soy and Chronic Diseases, held in Phoenix in 1994, a paper was presented by Cesare Sirtori, MD, a professor of clinical pharmacology at the University of Milan, discussing the benefits of soy foods in cutting cholesterol. Volunteers with very high levels of cholesterol (353 mg/dl) were recruited for the study. One group continued eating a low-fat diet, while the other added soy to their diets. After a four-week trial period, the group on the diet without soy had the same cholesterol levels, while the group of soy eaters had reduced their cholesterol levels an average of 27 percent. Soy has been found not only to lower LDL

(bad) cholesterol levels, but also to raise HDL (good) cholesterol levels.

James W. Anderson led a team of researchers in analyzing the results of thirty-eight controlled trials to determine the effects of soy protein and a reduction of cholesterol in humans. There were more than 740 individuals involved in the various studies. The average amount of soy consumed was 47 grams per day. The results proved significant. Soy protein added to the diet, rather than animal protein, was found to decrease serum concentrations of total LDL cholesterol and triglycerides. The reduction in LDL cholesterol was the greatest in subjects with the highest initial serum cholesterol concentrations. But even individuals with initial serum cholesterol levels below 200 mg/dl had an estimated decrease of 7.7 percent.

Evidence abounds as to the anticancer potential of soybeans. As mentioned above, soybeans contain at least five known anticarcinogens, including protease inhibitors, phytates, phytosterols, saponins, phenolic acids, and isoflavones. The isoflavones have been found to be effective against breast, lung, colon, prostate, and skin cancers, as well as leukemia.

B. A. Stoll of the oncology department at St. Thomas's Hospital in London studied the anticancer properties of natural isoflavones found in soybeans. Studies have found beneficial results from in vitro tests and research done using rats with carcinogen-induced mammary cancer. There is also thought to be a correlation between the low incidence of breast cancer in Asian women and their consumption of soy products.

One study followed a group of Japanese men eating a low-fat diet rich in soy products, compared to a group of Finnish men. The isoflavone levels in the Japanese men were seven to ten times higher than in the Finnish men. The assumption is that the higher levels of soy in the diet of the Japanese men contribute to lower rates of prostate cancer cell growth.

Soy products may aid in the prevention of osteoporosis. They are an excellent source of the minerals boron and calcium. One study conducted at the University of Texas Health Sciences Center found that volunteers in the study excreted 50 percent less calcium in their urine when they replaced animal products with soy products.

The weak estrogenic activity in soy may benefit in the prevention of osteoporosis. A study done to determine the future problems of osteoporosis in Asian women found that rural populations have a lower risk because of their diets, which are high in protective foods such as bioflavonoids and phyto-estrogen-rich foods such as soybeans.

Soy may help the following:

- Cardiovascular disease
- Ulcers
- Breast cancer
- Prostate cancer
- Osteoporosis
- Diabetes
- Weight control
- Kidney disease
- Fatigue
- Longevity

Soy products may help to enhance health and prevent disease. Recent research only produces more endorsement for this beneficial plant. Individuals in Asian countries have long valued the use of soy for health. Lower rates of heart disease, cancer, osteoporosis, and other problems have caused many to look into lifestyle changes for answers to health concerns. Soy may be a major factor in the future for promoting longevity.

## Soy Products

*Tofu:* Tofu is often used as a meat substitute. It is curdled soymilk pressed into a cake form. It absorbs the flavor of the food it is cooked with.

*Miso:* Miso is a fermented soybean paste, often used for seasoning and in soups.

*Natto:* Natto is a bacterially fermented form of soybean.

*Tempeh:* Tempeh is made from mold-fermented soybeans. It is often pressed into a patty or cake, marinated and grilled or baked.

*Tamari:* Tamari is a naturally fermented soy sauce.

*Soy Flour:* Soy flour is made from ground soybeans. It is very high in protein. It can be combined with other flours to increase protein. Eggs can be replaced in recipes with one tablespoon of soy flour and two tablespoons of water for each egg.

*Soymilk:* Soymilk is made from pureed soybeans in water. It is made to taste similar to milk and can be purchased in a variety of flavors.

*Soy Oil:* Soy oil is extracted from the soybean.

*Soy Sprouts:* Soy sprouts can be added to salads, sandwiches, or other dishes.

*Soy Grits:* Soy grits are left and ground when the oil is extracted.

*Soy Burger:* This is a meat-substitute patty, usually sold frozen at the supermarket.

## Safety of Soy Products

Soy has been used for thousands of years, and such a long history generally means it is safe. There are some individuals, however, who may be sensitive to soy protein, just as some have allergies to eggs, wheat, and dairy products.

# AROMATHERAPY

AROMATHERAPY IS THE PRACTICE of using essential oils to treat various physical and emotional ills. The practice can be traced back thousands of years and is gaining an important place in the worlds of natural healing and traditional medicine. Scientific research is beginning to examine the therapeutic benefits of essential oils, and results are promising as to the benefits of aromatherapy.

Aromatherapy is the practice of using scents to influence moods and pain and to treat and cure minor ailments. The essential oils help to encourage health and bring the body into balance. The theory centers on the fact that the olfactory and emotional centers of the body are connected. By inhaling different aromas, emotional concerns and physical complaints can be eased. This form of natural treatment is related to the use of herbs, but it relies on the benefits of the essential oils of the plants. It is one of a number of therapies involving natural methods.

The nose is responsible for identifying odors, whether good or bad. Smells are related to how we perceive and remember the world and events. Certain odors bring out memories of the past. For this reason, the sense of smell is thought to be involved in the memory function of the brain.

Smell is the first sense that develops in the newborn baby. It is the most acute of all the senses.

There are at least five million cells in the nasal passages linked to smell. Each cell contains receptors that catch the molecules that come in through inhalation. When the aroma is inhaled, the scent goes to the olfactory receptors. The olfactory nerves are the only nerves that go directly to the brain, allowing the individual to smell the aroma.

The olfactory nerves are connected to the limbic system, which is the base for memory, emotions, and sexual arousal, which makes scent an important part of memory and emotions. Scientific studies have established this premise. The limbic system is where scents can trigger emotions and memories and play a part in behavior. Aromatherapy is similar to homeopathy in that the doses are generally given in small amounts. This is thought to be the most effective method of administration. The essential oils are very concentrated and are most effective in small doses.

Essential oils are thought to be able to help with a myriad of complaints. They can strengthen the immune system, reduce aches and pains, relieve stress, increase energy, and promote a feeling of well-being. Aromatherapy is a natural approach to overall health.

Historically, the Egyptians used aromatics in the mummification process and for religious rituals. The oils of choice included myrrh, frankincense, cedarwood, coriander, cypress, juniper, and cassia.

They were probably the first to use aromatherapy as a practice. The Egyptians used oils to honor their leaders, the pharaohs and priests. The rich and royalty often used the oils.

In India, Ayurvedic medical practitioners also used the essential oils in their forms of therapy. Sandalwood was used in religious ceremonies. The aromas were a part of their spiritual lives. Many of the ancient texts suggest the use of coriander, ginger, myrrh, sandalwood, and rose.

The Hebrews, on the other hand, used oils for special purification rituals. After sojourning in Egypt, the Hebrews brought the tradition of essential oils with them to Israel. In the Song of Solomon, spikenard, saffron, calms, cinnamon, frankincense, myrrh, aloes, lily, and camphor are mentioned. Certain oils were reserved for sacred rites and forbidden for individual use. The book of John in the Bible relates the incident in which Mary anointed the feet of Christ with spikenard.

The Greeks considered aromatic plants gifts from the gods. They felt that the plants and oils had significant spiritual value and appeal. They probably gained their knowledge of aromatherapy from the Egyptians. Hippocrates recommended daily soaking in a scented bath and a massage using essential oils to promote longevity.

The Romans used scented oils and perfumes by adding them to their famous baths in Rome and Pompeii. Their knowledge was acquired from the Greeks and used extensively. The tradition of the Roman baths was an important part of their culture. They also used the oils in their homes.

Avicenna, the famous Arabian doctor of the tenth century, was the first to use the process of distillation for essential oils. It is thought by some that the Egyptians had practiced a primitive form of distillation. This was an important development because of the trade industry.

The Europeans learned of aromatherapy from the Crusaders in the Holy Land. This was thought to be the beginning of the famous French perfume industry. The first charter for the French perfumeries was in 1190 AD. This was the beginning of an exciting era. In the Middle Ages, bags of strong-smelling herbs were carried by many to protect themselves from demons and disease. During the years of the plague and other life-threatening ailments, distilled aromatics were in high demand. They were used as antiseptics to protect and heal.

The word *aromatherapy (aromatherapie)* is credited to René-Maurice Gattefosse, a French cosmetic chemist who coined the term around 1936. His theory began with the use of essential oils to help the skin and heal dermatitis. He spent more than fifty years studying the essential oils. These oils can also help with infections and work as a natural antibiotic. He often wrote on aromatherapy and of its therapeutic benefits. Gattefosse is one of the most prominent figures in the history of aromatherapy.

The essential oils are all considered to be highly concentrated natural substances. They are a part of the plant, but also separate from the other compositions of the plant. The essence of the plant is thought to have similar properties to that plant, but it also is more subtle and more connected to emotions. The concentrated oils are used to treat physical, mental, and emotional problems.

The essential oils are found in very small amounts in the bark, petals, leaves, resins, and rinds of plants. They are extracted from the plants by various methods, including pressing, distillation, tapping, and separation using heat. Most of the essential oils are colorless. But some have color, including cinnamon, which has a reddish tone. The essences are found in the plants and give them their characteristic odors. The pure oils are sold in extremely concentrated forms. It may require hundreds of plants to yield only a small amount of the essential oil.

The essential oils are not actually oily. They are more similar in substance to water. They do not feel greasy, and they generally do not stain. They usually evaporate easily when exposed to the air but do not dissolve in water. For this reason, essential oils need to be kept in sealed, colored glass containers to protect them from the air and light.

Everyone can benefit from the use of essential oils, whether you inhale during the day for a quick energy boost or relax in a soothing tub before bedtime. The oils can be used throughout the day to help with stress and increase energy.

The essences are usually applied externally through massage. This is thought to allow the essence to travel through the skin to the body fluids. This permits a slow, gradual absorption in the body. The oils affect different areas of the body through the blood and body fluids. The oil can be applied directly to a wound or through the skin. Massaging is an important part of the process and helps to speed the absorption. Aromatherapy includes massaging the essential oils into the body. This is considered to aid in relieving tension and improving circulation.

Inhalation of the scent is another method of use. Drops of oil can be added to a humidifier or sprayed in the air. A few drops can be put on a cotton pad and inhaled during the day. Smelling the oils has an effect on the mind and body. Inhaling the oils allows them to enter the lungs through the respiratory system. They attach to oxygen molecules that circulate throughout the body. The essential oils are able to work in the body to help heal, relax, and maintain health. Many oils help to strengthen the immune system and boost the immune response.

Some oils are taken internally through the digestion process. They enter the bloodstream in the digestive system and travel throughout the body. This is not used with most of the oils because of their highly concentrated form.

Carrier oils are the oils used to dilute the pure oils. Many different types of vegetables oils are used. Pure essential oils should be mixed with a carrier oil before being applied to the skin. Pure oils are highly concentrated and may cause skin irritation. Only a small amount of the essential oil is required for therapeutic results, and adding a carrier not only makes application easier but also cuts down on cost.

Carrier oils should be odorless, cold-pressed vegetable oils without additives. Some of the most common carrier oils include almond oil, canola oil, grapeseed oil, sesame oil, jojoba oil, olive oil, and sesame oil. Rancid oils should not be used. Most should be refrigerated to retain freshness.

Purity of the essential oils is extremely important to ensure therapeutic results. As always, it is important to only buy products sold by reputable suppliers. Experienced aromatherapists can tell the quality and purity by smelling the product. They can usually identify synthetic versions and lower-quality oils.

There is a difference between pure essential oils and synthetic versions. Aromatherapy relies on the use of the pure product. Synthetic oils do not have the reputation of producing therapeutic results. The whole essential oils are recommended.

When combining essential oils, an entirely new substance is created. This process is important, and it is necessary to use combinations that are balanced and work well together. Some of the more powerful scents may work in combination with a less dominant oil, such as lavender. A very sweet scent may be blended with a citrus oil to lessen the sweetness.

Plant families can be blended together easily. Different flowers, trees, or citrus oils can be found in combinations. Complementary colors can also be combined harmoniously. Blending can be a creative experience in learning and an experiment in what works well together.

Some oils may cause allergic reactions in sensitive individuals. Take caution if you suffer from sensitive skin, and watch for a reaction and then discontinue use. All oils should be kept safely out of the reach of children.

The practice of aromatherapy is fairly new in the United States, but other countries have used this method of healing for thousands of years. In France, aromatic oils are even covered by insurance companies. Memorial Sloan-Kettering Cancer Center in New York City is using the scents to help promote relaxation and relieve anxiety in patients, their families, and staff. A vanilla scent is used to relax patients when they undergo procedures, such as MRIs, that can cause extreme anxiety. The use of fragrances in hospitals has helped to reduce stress and anxiety.

A study done at Duke University by Susan Schiffman, PhD, a professor of psychology, used apricot oil to help obese individuals control their eating. The apricot scent was to help them relax and feel less anxious, which is a common reason for overeating. They all carried a vial of the oil with them and took a sniff when feeling nervous. More than half of the group experienced benefits from the apricot oil. Schiffman also has found beneficial results from using pleasant scents to help women with emotional symptoms related to menopause, such as stress, anxiety, and tension. The scents seem to be able to help release negative emotions and promote positive feelings.

Trygg Engen, a researcher at Brown University, found a link between memory and essential oils. In one study, the memory recall process was at least doubled with the addition of scents from the past. A smell of a scent from the past that hadn't been experienced for many years brought back memories and images.

Robert Tisserand, a British aromatherapist, has researched the effects on brain-wave patterns from the use of scents. While using stimulating aromas such as black pepper and rosemary, the beta brain waves showed increased stimulation. Relaxation was seen in the alpha and theta brain waves when rose, lavender, jasmine, and other calming oils were used.

## ESSENTIAL OILS AND THEIR USES

*Basil Oil:* Basil oil helps to clear and expel mucus, reduce fevers, improve circulation, relieve menstrual cramps, stimulate menstrual flow, fight infection, and relieve depression.

*Bergamot Oil:* Bergamot relaxes muscles and reduces pain. It also helps to fight infection, expel mucus, and calm the nerves, and it aids indigestion. It is also known to encourage new skin tissue growth.

*Cedarwood Oil:* Cedarwood oil is used for the respiratory system to help ease coughs and reduce the discomforts of colds and flu. It works as an expectorant to expel mucus and congestion. It also works to promote urination, as an antiseptic to heal wounds and prevent infection, to ease the pain of arthritis, and to heal skin problems.

*Chamomile Oil:* This oil is refreshing, with a fruity odor. It is used as a general tonic and is soothing on the body and mind. Chamomile oil is often used to relax and relieve stress. It contains anti-inflammatory properties to reduce swelling. It helps to heal skin conditions such as psoriasis, eczema, and sunburn. It helps to prevent infection and speed healing in wounds. It has also been used to ease pain from arthritis, headaches, earaches, and migraines.

*Cinnamon Oil:* This oil is known for its stimulation and warmth properties. It can be mixed with a carrier oil and massaged to increase temperature and promote warmth.

*Clary Sage Oil:* Clary sage oil helps to calm the nervous system and relieve depression. It helps to balance the emotions and is a nervous system tonic. It also helps to relieve muscle pain and spasm.

*Cypress Oil:* Cypress oil can calm the nervous system and relieve stress. It also helps with pain and muscle aches. It can reduce excessive bleeding.

*Eucalyptus Oil:* This is often used with problems associated with colds, allergies, coughs, flu, sinusitis, sore throats, and tonsillitis. It is used for sinus complaints and is effective in relieving congestion and a stuffy nose. It is also considered beneficial in helping alleviate the pain of a sore throat. Eucalyptus oil helps fight infections, whether viral or bacterial. It has been used to relieve pain from headaches and migraines.

*Fennel Oil:* Fennel oil helps to rid the body of toxins. It is also used to help control the appetite, aiding in weight loss. It is sometimes recommended for urinary tract infections. It is used for some female complaints, such as irregular menstrual cycle, PMS, fluid retention, and menopausal symptoms.

*Geranium Oil:* Geranium oil helps with problems such as diarrhea, gallstones, and urinary tract infections. It is also recommended to treat sore throats and tonsillitis.

*Ginger Oil:* Ginger is commonly used for gastrointestinal disorders. It also helps to increase immunity and protect the body from illness. It stimulates circulation and helps to relieve pain.

*Jasmine Oil:* This is used to aid coughs and problems of the female organs. It can be massaged into the lower back to ease the pain from menstrual cramps and induce menstrual flow. Some recommend jasmine oil to soothe the discomforts of menopause. It has been used to help ease the pain of childbirth.

*Juniper Oil:* Juniper oil helps to reduce pain and muscle aches. It increases urination and can stimulate menstrual flow. It can fight infection and water retention.

*Lavender Oil:* English lavender is considered to be the best. It is used to promote a restful sleep. Lavender oil is a versatile oil. It can be used for digestive problems, respiratory disorders, pain and muscle aches, skin disorders, and wounds. It should be used only in small quantities because of its strong aroma.

*Lemon Oil:* Lemon oil is used for respiratory disorders such as bronchitis, coughs, sore throats, and flu and cold symptoms. It contains antibacterial properties. It aids in digestion and strengthens the immune system.

*Myrrh Oil:* Myrrh has been used for thousands of years to boost the immune system, fight infection, and heal when an illness is present. It helps with digestion and stimulates the appetite. Some recommend myrrh for respiratory complaints, fungal infections, healing wounds, menstrual complaints, and skin disorders.

*Orange Oil:* This is thought to aid in relieving tension and relaxing the body. It is used for respiratory problems such as bronchitis. It increases immunity to strengthen the entire body. It is also used to aid in digestion, nervous disorders, diarrhea, obesity, and muscle and joint aches.

*Peppermint Oil:* This essence is used in cases of fever, headache, and to increase energy in the body. It stimulates the nervous system to increase energy and reduce fatigue. It helps with digestion and nausea. It relaxes muscle tension, relieves headaches and migraines, and helps with some skin conditions.

*Rose Oil:* This is probably the most expensive oil. It takes approximately one hundred pounds of petals to extract 1/2 ounce of oil. Aromatherapists recommend this for digestion, coughs, wound healing, congestion, female hormone balance, skin conditions, headaches, and inflammation.

*Rosemary Oil:* This oil is taken from the flowering tops of the plant. It is used for digestion, arthritis, coughs, depression, scalp problems, relaxation, headaches, muscle pain, cardiovascular disorders, respiratory conditions, memory aid, and circulation.

*Rosewood Oil:* Rosewood oil helps to calm the nervous system. It helps ease depression, anxiety, and stress. It fights infection, increases immunity, relieves pain, and can stimulate sexual desire.

*Spearmint Oil:* This is recommended for use with stomach problems. It can aid digestion and help relieve nausea.

*Tea Tree Oil:* Tea tree oil is well known for its antiseptic properties. It is known to kill invaders, whether viral, bacterial, or fungal. It is used to treat acne, burns, cuts, dandruff, respiratory ailments, coughs, urinary tract infections, candidiasis, and eczema.

*Thyme Oil:* Thyme helps to increase immunity and prevent infections. It is used for respiratory conditions such as asthma, bronchitis, tonsillitis, coughs, colds, sinusitis, and sore throats. Thyme helps to heal mouth problems such as sore gums and throat infections. It can help increase energy and reduce fatigue.

# PART 3

# Good Herbs, Good Food, Good Health

# AILMENTS AND HERBAL COMBINATIONS

## ADDICTIONS

Addictions can manifest themselves in many different forms. We can become addicted to television, work, exercise, bodybuilding, gambling, tobacco, alcohol, and other drugs. Anything that monopolizes our time and attention is a potential addiction. The addictions considered here include alcohol, drugs (prescription and over-the-counter), recreational drugs (marijuana, cocaine, heroin, and tobacco), chocolate, sugar, and caffeine. When we depend on one substance to make us feel good, it limits personal freedom. Addictions may be physical or emotional or a combination of both. Addictions are suspected with repeated foods or substances that an individual feels he or she needs each day. Cravings are a symptom of nutritional deficiencies, and an unbalanced diet creates cravings.

Sugar is an underlying basis for most addictions. Children become addicted to sugar when they are fed formula with corn syrup. As children grow, sugar-based cereal, candy, cake, cookies, soda, and foods such as catsup contain sugar. Even fruit juices are concentrated sugars and can damage the pancreas when used in abundance. Sugar gives a false sense of energy. Mental work requires a lot of energy, and sugar gives the body

a boost, but later there is a letdown when another sugar fix is needed.

Addictions are damaging to the brain, nervous system, digestive system, liver, and pancreas, confusing the immune system and creating an autoimmune dysfunction that leaves the body vulnerable to disease. Alcohol and drugs destroy brain cells and weaken the hypothalamus, which controls appetite, and this can lead to cravings or addictions.

Addictions are not easy to admit or to overcome. It's difficult to give up something the body depends on. Giving up the addiction will generally cause pain, either emotional, physical, or both. It can be done when a balance is created in the body. An imbalance of nutrients necessary for normal body functions is one cause of addictions. All addictions are basically the same, because substances become a part of the body cells and create an unhealthy adjustment that needs to be reversed.

Food allergies can be a cause of addictions. Foods that are craved often cause physical or mental reactions. Suspect foods should be removed from the diet for a week and then eaten while watching for a reaction. The pulse test can be a good method for identifying a food allergy. Take the pulse before eating a suspected food and then take it again thirty minutes after eating. If the pulse increases after eating the food, it could indicate an allergy.

Inherited weaknesses can occur when a child is born lacking minerals, vitamins, and essential nutrients. The craving for alcohol can be inherited, and a lack of nutrients can cause cravings of all kinds. Undigested proteins in the blood can irritate the inner organs and cause allergies to occur.

## TYPES OF ADDICTIONS

### Alcohol

Untold misery is afflicted on families, children, and the alcoholic. The liver is affected by excessive alcohol use. Diseases follow, such as cirrhosis of the liver, malabsorption, malnutrition, hypoglycemia, allergies, candida, and leaky gut syndrome. This can lead to allergies, chemical and heavy metal toxicity, and autoimmune diseases.

The liver, colon, kidneys, and blood need to be detoxified and repaired, because cells retain addictive substances. Using herbal formulas will help in the cleansing. Addictive substances take a toll on the nervous and immune system, and they need to be cleaned and repaired.

### Caffeine

This is the most abused substance used by children and adults. It is found in coffee, tea, cola, chocolate, diet pills, headache remedies, and soft drinks. It is dangerous for the unborn child and can cause various birth defects. Caffeine leaches B-complex vitamins and minerals and other vitamins from the body. Caffeine can cause nervous disorders, depression, anxiety, irritability, and insomnia. Caffeine has also been linked to high blood pressure, liver and breast cancer, diabetes, infertility, indigestion, and ulcers. It can also cause adrenal exhaustion, which can lead to hypoglycemia.

### Chocolate

Caffeine is found in chocolate, a popular treat for children and adults. The combination in chocolate of added fat and sugar is very addictive and harmful to the body. Chocolate is the most popular form of caffeine. Many people are addicted to chocolate, and it is a stimulating drug. Dr. Andrew Weil says, "People who regularly consume chocolate-eating binges may not realize they are involved with a drug, but their consumption usually follows the same sort of pattern as with coffee, tea, and cola drinks. Do you know any vanilla freaks or butterscotch freaks?"

### Cocaine

This drug was popular in Europe and the United States in the form of tonics and wine in the late nineteenth century. Cocaine was even added to cola drinks, but it was taken out in the early twentieth century when laws were passed against its use. The abuse of cocaine leads to serious mental, emotional, and physical health problems and a decrease in work productivity. There is a vast black market of cocaine in the United States. It can damage the nervous and immune systems. It depletes the body of vital nutrients and can cause free-radical damage, leading to disease and premature aging.

### Heroin

Intravenous injection of heroin is the most addictive form. It becomes very addictive, to the point that it limits personal freedom. Those addicted spend most of their time thinking about where and when they will get their next fix. It also depletes the body of essential nutrients, especially those that affect the nervous system.

### Marijuana

Marijuana is a drug that can affect the brain for an extended period of time. This can hinder the thinking process. It can also affect memory and the ability to learn. It can cause the same physical problems as tobacco, lung disease, emphysema, and even cancer.

### Nicotine

Nicotine is a legal drug that is very addictive. It is the most common drug, following alcohol and caffeine. It is even more addictive than heroin. It affects the lungs and depletes the body of vitamins A, C, and zinc. It wears down the adrenal glands. It can also cause bone loss because of a loss of essential nutrients.

### Sugar

Sugar depletes the body of enzymes that are necessary for the proper digestion of food. It can cause an imbalance of calcium and promotes bone loss that can lead to osteoporosis. It helps create allergic conditions stemming from poor digestion of food. Sugar weakens the immune system, which can lead to an increase in viral and bacterial infections. Sugar can also damage the kidneys, create a mineral imbalance, lead to other addictions such as alcoholism, and contribute to hypoglycemia. It can weaken the heart, eyes, and gallbladder and cause an acidic stomach.

## EMOTIONAL NEEDS

Addictions are difficult to overcome. It takes more than just willpower to eliminate destructive habits. Nutrition and exercise are very important, but emotional health is vital to conquering addictions. Addictions give us a false sense of well-being and greatly compromise our potential and productivity. I believe that in the case of any addiction, the spiritual component must be addressed in combination with how we react to stress as it affects our mental attitude. Learning to overcome feelings of despair, hopelessness, and rejection rests on our ability to confront the way we react to stressors. By so doing, we recognize the triggers that stimulate our addictive behavior. In other words, we need to confront the hidden causes of our behavior and take responsibility to master our lives. Drug therapy is not always the answer to treating addictions and can often result in an additional drug dependence. We know now that alcoholism can be related to genetic and biochemical disorders; however, the notion of personal accountability must be addressed in settings where professional help is available.

## HERBAL COMBINATIONS
### Herbal Combination #1

The following combination is excellent for sustaining the body when overcoming addictions. It supports the nervous system, regulates vitality, and may help in symptoms that can occur when cleansing the body, such as depression, fatigue, insomnia, and neurosis.

- Bupleurum is a Chinese herb specific for liver stagnation, regulating the liver, emotional and physical imbalances, and creating a sense of relaxation and harmony.
- Perilla helps correct energy imbalances, detoxifies, eases nausea, and helps to relieve bronchitis and asthma.

- *Panax ginseng* is a tonic for the entire body. It helps to reduce fatigue, increase mental power, stimulate the adrenal, pancreas, and pituitary glands, promote sleep, and aid a weak digestive system.
- Hoelen is a useful sedative and tonic, and it helps to improve brain function.
- Licorice increases the function of the liver in eliminating toxins. It also protects the adrenal gland and acts as a demulcent, spasmolytic, and anti-inflammatory.
- Ginger acts as a catalyst in nervine and sedative combinations. It stimulates the digestive system, eases nausea, and acts as a stimulant to increase the effectiveness of other herbs.
- Tang-kuei helps to calm the nerves and relieves muscle spasms. It is a rich source of iron and magnesium that relaxes muscles. It is used to treat anemia, abdominal pain, indigestion, and headaches.
- *Saussaurea lappa* acts as a tonic, increases the production of digestive juices, lowers blood pressure, decreases muscle spasms, and relieves pain.
- Bamboo soothes the nervous system and acts as a tonic. It helps to rejuvenate, helps with bleeding disorders, improves in cases of debility and emaciation, and relieves vomiting.
- *Coptis chinensis* acts as a sedative on the central nervous system, works as an antidepressant, stimulates uterine flow, increases bile flow, and contains anti-inflammatory properties.
- Platycodon glandifiroum works as an expectorant, helps to lower blood sugar levels, and decreases cholesterol in the liver.
- Cyperus rotundus is used for digestive disorders, circulatory problems, female disorders, depression, and emotional complaints.
- Gambir contains astringent properties that make it good for catarrh, chronic diarrhea, and dysentery. It has been used for uterine hemorrhage and leucorrhea.
- Ophiopogon japonicus is used to tone the lungs and nourish the stomach. It helps to relieve coughs and eliminate phlegm. It is a tonic for the lungs, stomach, and heart.

The following herbs are also in this combination: aurantium peel, tryphonium rhizome, zhishi fruit, dang gui root, and liquaticum rhizome.

## Herbal Combination #2

This herbal combination is formulated to remove toxins and waste from the cells and eliminate them from the body. When cells hold on to addictive substances and they are not eliminated, it creates "cell memory cravings." Until the cells are cleansed, the cravings may continue. Fasting, along with herbal combinations, will speed up the process.

- Sarsaparilla purifies the blood and binds endotoxins found in the cells, neutralizes microbes in the bloodstream, and acts as a diaphoretic, allowing the body to sweat and eliminate toxins from the lymph and circulatory system.
- Milk thistle protects the liver and improves liver function. It aids in the regeneration of damaged liver cells.
- Red clover is a great blood purifier used in treating cancer. It helps prevent carcinogenic activity in the cells and blood. It contains antitumor properties.
- Dandelion stimulates the flow of bile to improve liver congestion. It contains diuretic properties similar to the prescription drug furosemide, without the side effects.
- Yellow dock is a blood purifier and contains antibacterial properties. It is a natural antibiotic used to clean and purify the cells and liver. Because it is rich in iron, yellow dock can increase feelings of well-being. It helps to fortify the nervous and immune systems.
- Burdock is a blood cleanser with antifungal action to help remove candida from the blood. It protects the liver against chemicals and inhibits tumor growth.
- Marshmallow is high in mucilage content to form a protective coating in the intestinal tract. It is good for inflammation, pain, and acute diseases. It has a soothing effect on the mucous membranes.
- Fenugreek contains antitumor properties and is effective in lowering cholesterol levels in the blood. It helps with diabetes to reduce urinary glucose levels. It expels waste through the lymphatic system.
- Ginger contains natural antibiotic properties and has been found to inhibit the growth of bacteria. It is useful in nausea, kidney problems, the heart, fevers, vomiting, cramps, and to improve the effectiveness of other herbs.
- Echinacea is a blood purifier to protect against viral infections, tumors, and infectious diseases. It

is effective against candida, as well as viral and bacterial infections such as strep and staph. It also helps to fight chemical toxic poisoning.
- Cascara sagrada works in the large intestine to increase muscular activity, eliminate waste material, replenish the bowel function, and restore tone to the bowel.
- Pepsin helps to break down undigested protein in the cells and blood, protect the intestines from parasites, viruses, and germs, and prevents autointoxication, allergies, and immune-related diseases.
- *Lactobacillus sporogenes* helps prevent the growth of toxic putrefactive bacteria, helps reduce cholesterol buildup, and is a powerful intestinal regulator.

## Other Uses

Acute diseases (colds, flu, fevers), age spots, allergies, ankylosing spondylitis, arthritis, blood purifier, cancer, liver congestion, pancreas, skin infections.

## HEALTHFUL SUGGESTIONS

1. Identify and recognize the addiction. People who give up addictions—whether smoking, alcohol, drugs, sugar, or overeating—have the most success when they make the decision to overcome the problem themselves. People have the ability to give up an abusive habit. Plan a target date for quitting the addiction. Some people change only when the noxious effects become so overwhelming that there is no other way but to change. When people come to realize that they really want to live rather than indulge in drugs, alcohol, food, etc., then a movement in the right direction can occur. Concentrate on the addiction. Take responsibility for personal action. The ability of the human mind to give up a harmful habit should not be ignored.

2. Avoid the substance. Give up the habit, and only quit once. Tapering off is usually not the answer. Do not trade another substance for the one that is eliminated. Changing an alcohol habit for coffee or tobacco overstimulates the endocrine system, giving a false sense of energy, followed by a sudden drop. This can trigger depression, fear, rage, lack of energy, and poor self-confidence. Coffee and tobacco constrict the blood vessels, which can lead to a relaxing substance from drugs or alcohol. Tranquilizers are frequently prescribed for fear and anxiety. These just add to the problem. The easiest way is to give it up

and exchange it for a cleansing and nutritional program to bring back life and vitality.

3. Detoxification is essential. No matter how the program is implemented, there will be a period of withdrawal that will cause unpleasant side effects. It's important to understand before making the change that there will be both mental and physical symptoms of withdrawal. Detoxifying the body is necessary to rid residue from the cells, liver, blood, and colon. Fasting is one of the best ways to improve physical and spiritual well-being. Fasting has been used for thousands of years in almost every culture. Fasting is not recommended for persons with weak hearts, pregnant women, or persons who are sick or weak. Building the body first and then using herbs, such as colon cleansers, can go a long way in ridding the body of the addictive residue in cells. Colonics are beneficial. Skin brushing is also good, because the skin is the largest organ of elimination. Sweating in a sauna can help rid the body of toxins. Lymphatic massage is very beneficial. A liver flush using lemon or lime juice in a cup of water with cayenne pepper and fresh ginger will help. Olive oil will stimulate the liver to detoxify.

4. Exercise is important. It helps maintain heart and lymphatic health. It also helps to release hormones that create a feeling of well-being and helps in the assimilation of minerals.

5. Foods that are beneficial include fresh vegetables, whole grains, tofu, and other soy products. Use fruit sparingly at first, because candida can be involved when the body is depleted of nutrients. Uses juices infrequently and always dilute with pure water. Nutritional imbalance is one reason for addictions or cravings. Cravings occur when the body is lacking essential nutrients.

## HERBS AND SUPPLEMENTS

Single herbs to help rebuild the body include bee pollen, blue-green algae, ginseng, ginkgo, gotu kola, burdock, echinacea, ho-shou-wu, licorice, lobelia, passion flower, skullcap, suma, and valerian.

- Vitamin A is an excellent antioxidant. It helps to prevent free-radical damage, strengthens the immune system, and protects the eyes and lungs from damage. Use both fish oil and beta-carotene in 10,000 to 50,000 units per day.
- B-complex vitamins are needed for the nervous system and brain. They are needed to help rebuild the system. Add vitamins B1, B6, B5, and B12. B5 is needed to assist the adrenal glands to cope with the stress of a cleanse.
- Vitamin C with bioflavonoids protects the immune system and lungs. It is a powerful antioxidant, protecting against free-radical damage. It should be taken throughout the day for detoxification.
- Vitamin E protects the heart and liver from damage. It is a rich antioxidant and strengthens the adrenal glands and immune system. It works best when taken with meals.
- Selenium and zinc help to protect from free-radical damage. Zinc is important for digestion.
- Free-form amino acids are vital for every cell in the body. They are necessary for physical and mental health. They are essential to the biochemistry of the body. A complete amino acid complex in liquid or powder form without added sugar is best. Glutamine and glycine work together to help relieve cravings for addictive substances and help to suppress the appetite. Extra phenylalanine, tyrosine, and methionine help to combat stress, balance emotions, and improve health.
- Essential fatty acids are important because the body is unable to synthesize them. The only way to obtain EFAs is through diet. They help to lower triglyceride levels, eradicate plaque from the walls of the arteries, lower blood pressure, strengthen the cells, and build the immune system. EFAs can be found in flaxseed oil, salmon oil, black currant seed oil, borage oil, and evening primrose oil.
- Digestive enzymes are necessary to break up the undigested protein found in the blood and cells. Taken between meals, they will speed elimination, along with enemas, colonics, and a colon-cleansing formula. Worms, parasites, viruses, and germs all have protein coatings, and enzymes help to digest and eliminate them from the body. Undigested protein in the blood causes allergies and often accompanies addictions. An enzyme deficiency is created when the same substance is eaten often or little raw food is eaten.
- Chromium picolinate is needed to help balance blood sugar levels.
- Gymnema sylvestre helps to curb sugar cravings. It enhances liver and pancreatic function.
- Valerian, lobelia, passion flower, and skullcap can all help with withdrawal symptoms.

• Mineral combinations with extra calcium and magnesium are important.

## ORTHODOX PRESCRIBED MEDICATION

Naltrexone, with the brand name ReVia, is used to treat detoxified former narcotic addicts. It is supposed to help maintain a drug-free state. It is not to be used until detoxification has been accomplished. An overdose could cause seizures or a coma. Side effects include hallucinations, fast heart rate, fainting, breathing difficulties, skin rash, chills, constipation, appetite loss, irritability, insomnia, anxiety, headache, nausea, or vomiting.

# AGING

Lifestyle has a profound effect on how quickly or slowly we age. Premature aging can be a result of a poor diet, drug use, alcohol and tobacco consumption, and when physical and emotional stress are present. It is possible to slow the aging process by implementing dietary changes, using herbs and supplements, and addressing emotional needs. Smoking accelerates the aging process and decreases circulation to the brain and other areas of the body. Alcohol consumption destroys the liver, damages the brain, and leads to malnutrition. Caffeine consumption is implicated in many health problems and tends to accelerate the aging process. Aging should not be something we fear or worry about.

## CAUSES

Brainpower can be diminished because of poor nutrition. The raw materials for feeding the brain cells and neurotransmitters are found in what we consume. Neurotransmitters are the chemicals needed for memory and thinking properly. Supplements are very beneficial for supplying oxygen and nutrients to the brain. Two of the main problems involved with brain-function difficulties are free-radical damage and a lack of oxygen to the brain.

Malnutrition is linked to premature aging. Essential nutrients may not be absorbed or assimilated when there is a lack of digestive enzymes. Eating too much cooked food and not enough raw food diminishes the production of enzymes from the glands, such as the pancreas. One of the most important functions of enzymes is the conversion of vitamins, minerals, and amino acids into vital neurotransmitters, allowing the body to function properly. Enzymes are essential for life; without them, the body's ability to heal and ward off disease is limited. They are considered the "spark plugs" of the body.

The thymus gland shrinks when under stress, and it is the master gland of the immune system. The nutrients that nourish the thymus are essential to longevity and health. The thymus gland is involved in many functions of the immune system. When the thymus gland is healthy, it releases hormones such as thymosin, thymopoeitin, and serum thymic factor. When these levels are low, there is a decrease in the immune system function. The thymus gland needs vitamin A, beta-carotene, C with bioflavonoids, vitamin E, selenium, and zinc. Herbs to enhance thymus function are licorice root, echinacea, ginseng, gotu kola, horsetail, white oak bark, and yucca.

Free-radical damage is another cause of premature aging. Free radicals are in the air, water, and in our food. They are molecules with an unpaired electron, which react like a chemical acid burn to a cell. Rancid oils and grains are common causes of free-radical damage. Cigarette smoking and some drugs are involved with production of free radicals. Packaged food on the grocery shelves is loaded with free radicals. Once grains are ground, they oxidize and cause free radicals to multiply.

Lack of oxygen in the blood and brain increases the chance of premature aging. Low-level exercise helps to increase oxygen in the blood and brain. Ginkgo increases and improves circulation to the brain by increasing the tone and elasticity of the blood vessels. An article in *Herbs for Health*, May/June 1997, reported that elderly patients with memory loss, decreased alertness, and mood swings improved with the addition of ginkgo. CoQ10 is very effective in supplying oxygen to the brain.

Heavy metal poisoning is also linked to premature aging. Aluminum in any form is harmful to the brain. It can be absorbed through the skin, inhaled, or eaten and can be found in food, water, antiperspirants, and antacids, to name a few. When minerals are lacking in the body, heavy metals can accumulate. Daniel Perl, MD, chief of research for the Mt. Sinai Medical Center's department of neuropathology, repeatedly has found the metal aluminum in the brains of deceased Mariana islanders who had been afflicted with Lou Gehrig's disease and Parkinsonism with dementia. In the book *Toxic Metal Syndrome*, it says that researchers found high levels of aluminum in the drinking water and in nineteen common foods grown in Guam and Rota. Low calcium and high aluminum concentrations in the soils, waters, and native foods were strongly suspected.

Autointoxication, faulty digestion, and constipation are some conditions common with the elderly. They are prone to conditions of constipation and hemorrhoids. A lack of fiber in the diet is the main cause. The problem is created when elimination doesn't occur after every meal. A high-fiber diet, including psyllium, is beneficial to correct and prevent these problems. Autointoxication becomes a problem when the feces stay in the colon longer than they should.

## EMOTIONAL NEEDS

As individuals age, it is vital to maintain positive emotional feelings about the aging process itself. Older individuals need to live life to the fullest. In order to do so, they must maximize their physical and emotional health through good nutrition and supplementation. I was interested to learn that in one study of geriatric patients who appeared to be depressed and senile, the real cause of their emotional problems was traced to a deficiency of vitamin B6 and folic acid. Malnutrition can profoundly affect our attitude, and older people often eat poorly. Moreover, older people must deal with the social stigma associated with aging in combination with issues of isolation, loneliness, incapacitation, and unresolved negative feelings. It's hard to grow old naturally. When we add depression or stress, the body is further taxed. In addition, clinical studies have proven that a positive mental attitude improves immune function, which increases our resistance to disease. The elderly need to laugh more, not take life too seriously, think young, and keep the brain active by reading, doing puzzles, enrolling in a class of interest, and doing regular low-impact exercises such as walking or water aerobics. Forgiveness and service are great medicinal healers.

## HERBAL COMBINATIONS
### Herbal Combination #1

This formula is designed to protect the brain against free-radical damage and is an excellent supplement for health and longevity. It helps promote mental acuity and protects against memory loss. A rich anti-aging formula.

- Ginkgo improves short-term memory and strengthens the brain. It helps in fatigue, depression, vertigo, and ear problems, and is popular in Europe for a wide variety of disorders associated with aging. It provides nutrients and oxygen to the head area. It increases circulation in the brain to help prevent strokes from blood clots.
- Huperzine A (from Chinese club moss) is a promising herb for brain dysfunction, Alzheimer's, and aging. Huperzine A boosts the "memory molecule," acetylcholine, which is found to be low in brains with Alzheimer's. This herb blocks the damage that destroys acetylcholine. A natural supplement for preserving the brain.
- Lycopene is an antioxidant and a powerful nutrient to prevent free-radical damage. It is an element found in tomatoes.
- Alpha lipoic acid is a rich antioxidant that helps in the utilization of vitamins C and E and is important in improving memory.
- Phosphatidyl serine, choline, ethanolamine, and inositol are a beneficial blend of nutrients to support neurotransmitters to help improve memory, the nervous system, and brain function. This blend supports the myelin sheath that surrounds the nerves. Choline and inositol are involved in metabolism of fat and cholesterol and fat absorption and utilization. Phosphatidyl helps retain and prevent the gradual loss of memory. It also offers support in cases of Alzheimer's disease and depression.
- *Rhododendron caucasicum* is very rich in antioxidants and more potent than the antioxidant vitamins. It is useful in preventing free-radical damage. It can help prevent and treat health issues such as atherosclerosis, glaucoma, gout, obesity, strokes, heart disease, cancer, and arthritis. A very promising herb.

### Other Uses

Tonic for the brain, Parkinson's disease, senility, memory loss, helping to prevent aging.

## Herbal Combination #2

This combination is rich in antioxidants and acts as an antifungal, anti-inflammatory, antiviral, and antibiotic. It will strengthen the immune system. A rich combination to slow the aging process.

It contains mangosteen fruit juice, wolfberry lycium fruit, sea buckthorn, red grapes, grapeseeds, raspberries, blueberries, apple, and green tea extract.

## Other Uses

Great for inflammatory diseases such as cancer, arthritis, diabetes, and Alzheimer's. These combinations will protect the immune system and prevent diseases. These formulas are designed for individuals over fifty.

## HEALTHFUL SUGGESTIONS

1. Maintain a moderate weight. Most elderly who live long, healthy lives seldom have weight problems. Learn your body type and eat accordingly.

2. Stay active and walk often to maintain the blood and circulation.

3. Most of those who live a long life seldom rely on drugs. One man who lived to be 101 never took drugs and had clarity of mind until his death. He never drank, smoked, or used caffeine, and he was active growing a garden until he was ninety-five years old.

4. Avoid stress. When angry or upset, rather than confrontation or shouting, go for a long walk.

5. Those who live long usually have strong spiritual beliefs and use prayer or meditation in their lives.

6. Avoid becoming bored. Keep the mind active and find young friends to visit and help to keep thinking and feeling young.

7. Autointoxication is a real threat for the aging. Poor eating habits, along with pollution, addictions, heavy metals, and rancid food can all contribute to lazy bowel function and to leaky gut syndrome. The tiny blood capillaries that nourish the small and large colon as well as the stomach can pick up these poisons and transfer them into the bloodstream. This is called autointoxication and can affect all parts of the body. Keeping the colon and blood clean is very vital in maintaining a healthy body free from diseases that plague the aged.

8. Avoid eating when angry, upset, or under stress. Avoid overeating, chew food well, and eat raw food for the enzyme content. Drink purified water to avoid chlorine and cancer-causing chemicals. Chlorine increases the aging process.

9. The pineal gland is considered the youthful gland. It loses functional ability as we age. It calcifies, shrinks, and loses the ability to produce the hormone melatonin. This hormone helps produce a restful sleep and prevents immune impairment. A proper diet and supplements will help regulate hormonal balance.

10. Eat natural food that will nourish and rebuild the cells. High-quality protein and amino acids found in tofu and soy are very beneficial. Brown rice and millet are beneficial for the elderly. Carrots and citrus fruits are rich in vitamin C, bioflavonoids, B-complex, and inositol. Onions, garlic, and shallots are rich in sulfur, protecting against free-radical damage, helping to reduce blood clumping, and aiding in slowing brain degeneration.

11. Spinach and kale contain the carotenoid lutein, which strengthens capillaries and protects against macular degeneration. Broccoli, cabbage, and Brussels sprouts contain cruciferous phytonutrients that protect against chemicals that can cause cancer.

12. The following foods contain nucleic acid, which protects against aging: asparagus, beets, bran, buckwheat, chickpeas, honey, kidney beans, lentils, lima beans, millet, navy beans, nuts, almonds, sardines, salmon, soybeans, split peas, vegetables (steamed and fresh), and green leafy vegetables. These foods help regulate metabolism and cell structure and promote enzyme production and hormone balance. Plain yogurt is also beneficial. Berries contain phytonutrients that protect the immune system. Beans, grains, nuts, and seeds all help protect against toxins.

## HERBS AND SUPPLEMENTS

Single herbs that help reduce the effects of aging: use bilberry to protect the eyes and ears; licorice to help the adrenal gland; ginseng and ginkgo for circulation and as a brain booster; pau d'arco to protect the liver and blood; cayenne to nourish the veins; chaste tree for women and pygeum for men; milk thistle to rejuvenate the liver; echinacea to boost the immune system; and deer antler velvet.

• Antioxidants such as vitamins A, C, E, selenium, manganese, and zinc protect against free-radical damage, radiation damage, autoimmune diseases, and chemicals that cause cancer.

- The B-complex vitamins protect against senility and many chemicals that disrupt the immune system.
- L-carnitine acts as an antioxidant. All of the amino acids are beneficial. A supplement or a protein drink containing all the amino acids would assure that the body is supplied with all the protein building blocks.
- Grapeseed extract is a potent bioflavonoid that is beneficial for the circulatory system.
- Coenzyme Q10 is an antioxidant used to strengthen the heart, increase energy, and supply oxygen to the brain.
- Quercetin is a bioflavonoid with antioxidant properties.
- Progesterone is very beneficial for women and should be used in a natural cream that is absorbed efficiently. It can reverse and prevent osteoporosis, improve cholesterol function, and prevent water retention and other symptoms that often accompany PMS and menopause.
- Soy products contain phytochemicals, "isoflavones," that protect the hormone system against cancer.
- DHEA is short for dehydroepiandrosterone and is one of the most crucial hormones produced by the adrenal glands. It plays a vital role in preventing disease. It enhances immunity, increases estrogen in women and testosterone in men to youthful levels, lowers cholesterol, boosts endurance, and inhibits diseases associated with aging.
- Glucosamine formulas help repair and rebuild damaged cartilage, reduce inflammation and pain in joints, and reduce swelling.
- Digestive enzymes and hydrochloric acid supplements are very beneficial to ensure that food is digested and assimilated properly. This will help prevent leaky gut syndrome and undigested protein, toxins, viruses, germs, bacteria, parasites, and worms from entering the bloodstream and causing problems.
- Essential fatty acids found in flaxseed, borage, or evening primrose oils are beneficial in lowering blood pressure, repairing damaged cell membranes, and constructing new ones. They also help strengthen cell and capillary structures, prevent abnormal blood clotting, and prevent clots from forming. They assist in the manufacture of cholesterol while at the same time removing excess cholesterol from the blood. They nourish the glands and hormones and increase the rate at which the body burns fat.
- Lecithin builds endurance and contains eight known growth factors to speed up the regeneration and repair process, including prostaglandins, fatty acids, prohormones, minerals, glucosamine, and chondroitin sulfate.

## ORTHODOX PRESCRIBED MEDICATION

The elderly are living longer but are not necessarily healthier. A large majority of the older generation have ailments such as high blood pressure, arthritis, heart problems, and brain dysfunction, as well as many other diseases. The elderly have a decreased ability for the kidneys and liver to process toxins and drugs, increasing the risk of reactions to more than one drug, as well as kidney and liver damage.

# ALLERGIES

There are dozens of ailments that occur as a result of allergic reactions. Millions of Americans suffer from one type of allergy or another, and there are many ailments that stem from these allergies. For example, hyperactivity in children, as well as adults,

---

**THE HERBS HAD REALLY HELPED HIM**

Hugh had to be helped into Juanita's health food store. He was accompanied by a woman who had to drive him as well as take care of him. The woman told Juanita that Hugh had Alzheimer's disease and wanted something that might help him. They bought six bottles of a combination of ginkgo and gotu kola. It was weeks later that he came into Juanita's store again. This time, Hugh came in by himself and had driven the car alone. He bought another six bottles of ginkgo and gotu kola. He told Juanita that the herbs had really helped him.

has been linked to allergies in some cases. Crohn's disease, arthritis, various types of headaches, depression, asthma, and upper respiratory infections have all been shown to have allergies as a possible source.

The common effects of allergies we usually think of are sinus infections, eczema, sneezing, runny nose, itchy and watery eyes, nasal congestion, and swelling of the mouth or throat. But the effect of allergies on the brain and other tissues of the body may contribute to autoimmune and nervous disorders as well. For instance, some schizophrenics have shown improvement when placed on a wheat-free or dairy-free diet, only to relapse when those substances are reintroduced in their diet. Undigested protein or partially digested foods can enter the blood as foreign proteins and cause allergic reactions that directly affect the brain.

Allergic reactions are most often manifested with the following foods: wheat and gluten products (e.g., rye, oats, triticale, barley, corn), dairy products (cream cheese, milk, cheese), yeast, coffee, tea, chocolate, peanuts, beef, poultry, eggs, or citrus products. The Solanacea family of plants, such as tomatoes, green and red peppers, eggplants, and potatoes, may also cause problems.

The causes of allergies are due to an internal imbalance and a weakened immune system created by the food we eat, the air we breathe, or the chemicals we come in contact with. Leaky gut syndrome can affect susceptibility to allergies, as can substances that irritate the stomach and colon membranes, such as antibiotics, sugar, alcohol, viruses, germs, bacteria, and a poor diet high in sugar, caffeine, and drugs. The mucous membranes become more permeable with irritations, and large particles of partially digested food can enter the bloodstream and travel to other areas of the body, causing irritations and allergic reactions.

Before allergic reactions develop, catarrh of the stomach is present, due to overeating, eating certain types of foods in the wrong combinations, and eating too many rich foods. Protein acids, starch acids, and acids from overconsumption of fried foods and rancid oils build up in the body. By creating irritations and inflammations of the stomach lining, these acids can lead to chronic gastric fermentation. The gas from this fermentation is passed directly by the stomach and also builds up in the lungs and other parts of the body. Conditions such as hay fever are primarily caused by the irritations from gas elimination—toxic gas that is generated in the stomach.

Allergies, then, are symptoms that signal the body is attempting to eliminate toxins. These toxins cause inflammation and irritation of the mucous membranes and the underlying tissues. When these secretions are suppressed by drugs and overeating, they become thick and hardened membranes as the tissues decompose and ulcerate. There is no difference between a cold, hay fever, asthma, bronchitis, or any other allergy except in the degree of complications. When the stomach is kept in constant turmoil with foods beyond the body's needs, allergies develop. This overstimulates the stomach and creates a toxic state in the blood and may then cause the nervous system to be oversensitive.

Any dust, pollen, perfumes, chemical, or whatever causes the allergy will continue until steps are taken to help nature eliminate the toxic buildup and cleanse the system. A clean body will not cause allergic reactions. It is the condition of the body that causes allergies. When the body is clean, there will be no allergies, no matter what irritant is inhaled or eaten.

Although under normal conditions the toxic substances can be eliminated, when leaky gut syndrome occurs, parasites, bacteria, fungi, toxins, fats, undigested protein, and other foreign matter not normally absorbed can enter the bloodstream. This can put an enormous strain on the liver and colon to detoxify and eliminate these substances from the body. The enlarged spaces in the gut wall also allow for the entrance of larger-than-normal protein molecules. These proteins are not completely broken down, so the immune system recognizes them as foreign matter and makes antibodies to fight them. When these antibodies are produced, the body begins to recognize relatively common foods or other substances as detrimental, and this leads to allergic reactions.

An inflammatory response may occur even when the food or substance is next consumed. If the inflammation occurs in a joint, rheumatoid arthritis may result. If the antibodies attack the gut lining, various gastrointestinal problems can develop, such as Crohn's disease or colitis. Some cases of asthma are thought to be related to leaky gut syndrome because the inflammatory conditions that arise after ingesting a certain food may trigger the asthma. Other associated problems include migraines, eczema, and autoimmune diseases. It is easy to see how this antibody response can produce symptoms in just about any organ or area of the body.

## EMOTIONAL NEEDS

Fear of the future may be a cause. It is essential to face the future with optimism and confidence. Emotions and fears need to be vocalized and discussed to reach the attitude that one can plan and help in future events.

## HERBAL COMBINATIONS
### Herbal Combination #1

This formula is excellent for allergies. It helps clean, heal, and repair the mucous membranes. It will help repair leaky gut syndrome, one of the main causes of allergies. Poor digestion and assimilation of vital nutrients are involved with allergies, and the herbs in this formula will help improve digestion and assimilation.

- Boneset has antiseptic and antiviral properties, strengthens the stomach and spleen, promotes sweating to help in cold and flu, and promotes the production of interferon.
- Fenugreek has antiseptic properties, dissolves hardened mucus, and rids the lungs and bronchial tubes of mucus and phlegm. It helps expel waste through the lymphatic system. Clinical studies have shown that the seeds have antidiabetic effects.
- Horseradish has antibiotic properties and is a strong stimulant to clear the lungs and nasal passages of infections. It is beneficial to stimulate digestion, metabolism, and kidney function.
- Mullein relieves pain, relaxes the body, and controls coughs, cramps, and spasms. It loosens mucus from the respiratory and lymphatic systems. It is a great herb for treating tuberculosis, as well as other lung problems.
- Fennel expels phlegm from the throat, eliminates toxins from the body, and purifies the blood. It aids digestion, colic, and other stomach complaints. It contains essential oils similar in composition to catnip and peppermint.

### Herbal Combination #2

This formula is excellent for relaxing the lungs and bronchial tubes for better healing, and it contains natural expectorant properties, antibiotic properties, decongestant properties, antifungal properties, and blood cleansers.

- Burdock is a blood purifier, contains antibiotic and antifungal properties, and is also used for cleansing and healing. It contains cleansing properties for the glands, intestines, and stomach.
- Goldenseal has antibiotic properties for fighting infections, both bacterial and viral. It has been found to kill toxic bacteria in the intestinal tract and parasites, such as giardiasis, commonly found in many streams in the United States.
- Parsley is rich in minerals and vitamins, has a tonic effect on the body, and increases resistance to infections. It contains cleansing and healing properties.
- Althea relaxes the bronchial tubes, removes mucus from the lungs, and has soothing and healing properties.
- Chinese ephedra contains bronchodilating properties and relieves congestion from allergies, colds, flu, bronchitis, and asthma. It has protecting properties for the lungs. It is a natural energy booster.
- Capsicum disinfects, stops bleeding, contains decongestant properties, and increases circulation.
- Horehound is a natural expectorant, tonic, and diuretic. It helps clean the liver with glandular imbalance. It is good for coughs and lung problems.
- Yerba santa contains decongestant properties, purifies the blood, and stimulates digestive secretions.
- Orange peel strengthens the lungs and bronchials and helps in inflammation and drainage.

### Other Uses

Asthma, mucus buildup, colds, hay fever, bronchitis, sinus infections, and upper respiratory infections.

## HEALTHFUL SUGGESTIONS

1. There is a food allergy test that can help determine if a particular food causes allergic reactions. It is called a pulse test. The pulse is taken before eating the suspected food. Make sure you are relaxed; a normal reading should be between fifty-two and seventy beats a minute. Take the test again about thirty minutes after eating the suspected food. If the pulse has increased more than ten beats per minute, elim-

inate the food for a month and then retake the pulse test. The important part of eliminating allergic foods is to give the body a chance to heal. Once the body heals during the time without the irritant food and repairs itself, the previously allergic food may not cause a reaction anymore. The problem occurs when eating the same foods all the time and neglecting to eat a variety of healthful food types.

2. The colon and digestive systems need to be cleansed and healed. A congested colon is the main reason diseases are manifested. A high-fiber diet, a lower bowel cleanser, and liver and blood cleansers are also important. Psyllium is important and is high in fiber to clean the pockets of the colon. Lower bowel cleansers that contain cascara sagrada, buckthorn, licorice, ginger, barberry, couch grass, red clover, and capsicum will help gradually clean, rebuild, and nourish the colon.

3. The adrenal glands protect against allergies. The adrenal cortex destroys white blood cells and thus inhibits inflammation, while a hormone called aldosterone fights stress and prevents fatigue. Certain nutrients are required in order for the adrenals to produce hormones. When these nutrients are undersupplied for long periods of time, the adrenals atrophy and must be rebuilt. Potassium is essential to strengthen the adrenals, and magnesium is called the antistress mineral. It assists in the absorption of calcium, phosphorus, sodium, potassium, and B-complex, as well as vitamins C and E. It is an activator of enzymes that use protein and vitamins. Protein is essential for the adrenals; therefore, eat more grains, beans, millet, brown rice, and soy foods (i.e., tofu and tofu drinks), along with fresh vegetables. B vitamins are also necessary for the general health of the adrenals and can effectively guard against allergic reactions. Pantothenic acid, a B-complex vitamin, is directly related to the production of natural cortisone. The requirements for the B-complex vitamins increase when the body is under stress, rapid growth, illness, or exposure to toxins, which include pollens, dust, and airborne irritants.

4. The liver needs to be cleansed and nourished. The liver's job is to detoxify poisonous and irritating materials, even those produced by the body. The liver produces an enzyme called histaminase, and when the liver is congested with fats or accumulated toxins, it cannot produce this enzyme. A good liver cleanser should contain some of the following principal herbs: burdock, milk thistle, astragalus, echinacea, pau d'arco, myrrh, chlorella or other greens, licorice, yellow dock, and schizandra. Assisting herbs could include red beet root, parsley, gentian, horsetail, blue vervain, wild yam, goldenseal, and liverwort. Transporting herbs should contain one or more of the following: lobelia, ginger, prickly ash, goldenrod, capsicum, or fennel.

5. The digestive system can be one of the main causes of allergies. Undigested protein and starch can enter the bloodstream and cause allergies anywhere in the body. Protein digestive aids and food enzymes will help in digesting food left in the intestines. Changing the diet is essential. Stay away from additives, artificial food coloring or flavors, chemically grown food, processed and rancid oils, refined flour, and sugar products. Stay away from stimulants, such as alcohol, coffee, tea, or soft drinks. Eliminate sugar from the diet—it is involved in more problems in the body than any other single product. These foods overstimulate the adrenals, lower resistance, and deplete energy.

6. The nervous system is closely linked to the immune system. The nervous system controls and coordinates all of the functions of the body, including that of the pituitary gland. This master gland helps with the entire endocrine network. Nervine herbs will help rebuild and nourish the nervous system. They include skullcap, chamomile, valerian, passion flower, kava kava, catnip, and hops.

7. Interactions to certain types of food mixed together could be a problem. For example, eating meat and starches together could cause fermentation and irritation to the lining of the digestive system. Food combining may be helpful. Sugar and starches together can cause fermentation. Meat takes longer to digest than fruit, so mixing them could cause irritation.

8. Juice fasting would be beneficial. Juices such as carrot, celery, parsley, and fresh ginger are helpful. Always dilute the juices by half with pure water, because concentrated juices can be taxing on the pancreas.

9. Kale, carrots, celery, and garlic are also very nourishing for this ailment.

10. Use kamut (a type of wheat) instead of wheat. Kamut is organically grown and is found to cause

fewer allergic reactions than ordinary wheat. It is high in protein and unsaturated fat and contains less gluten. Use it in thermos cooking, stews, soups, and cook as a cereal. Millet is a useful grain that is high in protein. As an alkaline cereal that is rich in calcium and magnesium, it is very easy to digest. Use brown rice, whole oats, and buckwheat.

11. Eat sprouts, almonds, beans, raw nuts, peas, sesame seeds, green leafy vegetables, root vegetables, yellow fruits, and vegetables. Use garlic, onions, and shallots in stews, soups, rice dishes, and grain stews. Also add lentils, split peas, and wild rice.

## HERBS AND SUPPLEMENTS
Single herbs that help with allergies are burdock, cayenne, echinacea, ginger, goldenseal, kelp, licorice, lobelia, pau d'arco, and saffron.

- Antioxidants such as vitamins A, C with bioflavonoids, E, grapeseed extract, selenium, and zinc protect cells from damage. They prevent oxidation, protecting the immune and nervous systems.
- Bee pollen can build immunity by acting as a barrier against inhaled pollens. Always start with small amounts and gradually increase the dose. It is rich in nutrients and amino acids, and it is very nourishing.
- Essential fatty acids found in flaxseed, borage, and evening primrose oils help the body produce anti-inflammatory substances to protect the cells from damage.
- Fiber supplements with herbs and psyllium help heal the digestive system and colon and prevent constipation.
- Acidophilus is used to restore friendly bacteria in the digestive system and prevent candida and other problems.
- B-complex vitamins are essential for vitality, mental energy, and health of the nervous system. Vitamin B6 and B2 are vital in formation of antibodies.
- Vitamin C and pantothenic acid are crucial in the production of adrenal hormones, which give the system an antiallergenic protection. A balanced mineral supplement will help eliminate allergies. Magnesium, selenium, and zinc are vital for the immune system. A deficiency of magnesium is seen in individuals with allergies. Digestive enzymes and hydrochloric acid are necessary to

**HER ALLERGIES ARE ALMOST COMPLETELY GONE**

Maureen used to have severe allergies, and despite the desensitization shots for seven years and her medication, she had constant sinus infections and one bout of pneumonia. For two years straight, she took a long list of antibiotics to which she was resistant and still had severe sinus infections. After taking combination #2 for allergies for three days, not only had the congestion eased but the infection was also gone, and she has not had a recurrence of the sinus infection in almost seven years. She continues to alternate #2 with a combination containing the following: marshmallow, mullein, slippery elm, lobelia, Chinese ephedra, passion flower, catnip, and senega. She also uses marshmallow and fenugreek and singles like mullein, goldenseal, and echinacea, but #2 is her mainstay. Her allergies are almost completely gone, and she continues to improve.

break up undigested protein and food in the bloodstream so the body can eliminate them. Use after meals to assure food is digested and assimilated. Use between meals to break down undigested food in the bloodstream.

## ORTHODOX PRESCRIBED MEDICATION
Prednisone is the medication most often prescribed for allergies. It is used for allergic and inflammatory responses. It is beneficial in the short-term control of chronic inflammatory conditions. What this type of drug does is stop the secretions and prevent the body from eliminating the toxins that eventually become solidified and create chronic conditions. Typical side effects of these types of drugs include cataracts, depression, a susceptibility to infections, stomach upset, water retention, depletion of calcium, indigestion, stomach pain, and ulcers.

# ALZHEIMER'S DISEASE

Alzheimer's is a devastating disease that affects not only the patient but families as well. It brings heartache, discomfort, frustration, and hopelessness to those involved. New light and beliefs are being shed on diseases affecting the nervous system and brain. Many of these disorders can be prevented, delayed, or controlled with nutritional supplements. The brain suffers when nutrients are lacking, especially minerals and antioxidants. The brain is very susceptible to environmental toxins as well as nutritional deficiencies. It is also sensitive to toxins created in the body from an unhealthy colon. An unhealthy bloodstream can carry toxins to the brain and nervous system and increase brain damage.

Symptoms could include depression, agitation, withdrawal, insomnia, irritability, memory loss, personality change, and senility. Symptoms may be misleading—many drugs prescribed for the elderly can cause confusion and memory loss. Such drugs include antidepressants, statins, corticosteroids, barbiturates, tranquilizers, and sleeping pills.

There are two types of dementia. One is primary, which comes on gradually, without apparent cause. Secondary dementia comes on suddenly from brain injury, surgical procedures, medications, or diabetic coma and is usually reversible. Alzheimer's is primary dementia that shows up in the brain as tangled clumps of nerve fibers and patches of disintegrated nerves in the brain. Alzheimer's disease is characterized by progressive degeneration of the brain, memory, and nervous system. Studies indicate that high aluminum concentrations in the brain tissue may be one causative factor. Another may be the diminished activity of the neurotransmitter acetylcholine, which assists neurotransmitter communication.

## EMOTIONAL NEEDS

Alzheimer's could be related to one's inability to deal with life. Anger can affect the brain along with a feeling that there is no hope left in the world. I believe that in some people life becomes a burden and the willingness to accept changes and go forward becomes a hopeless situation, therefore reverting back to childhood. Having someone take care of you seems an appealing way out.

## HERBAL COMBINATIONS
### Herbal Combination #1

This formula is rich in antioxidants to prevent cell damage, and includes chelating agents to detoxify the body of heavy metals, air pollution, as well as other toxins.

- N-acetyl cystine (NAC) is an amino acid that protects liver from toxin damage, treats infections, lowers cholesterol, and builds the immune system.
- Cilantro relieves inflammation and promotes healing.
- Vitamin B6 is necessary for the production of serotonin and other neurotransmitters.
- Apple pectin contains soluble fiber, absorbs toxins, and eliminates them from the body. Apple pectin is also healing and soothing.
- Sodium alginate protects against heavy metal poisoning and prevents the body from absorbing toxic radioactive material.
- Kelp algae is rich in minerals, fights cancer, cellulite, and constipation.
- L-Methionine protects the liver from fat accumulation, slows the aging process, keeps kidneys healthy, controls cell formation, and is rich in sulfur, which regulates nerve impulses.
- Alpha lipoic acid protects against heavy metal poisoning and free-radical damage, and is also a potent antioxidant.
- Magnesium citrate protects the heart from damage, and helps to maintain healthy blood pressure when taken with calcium and potassium.

### Herbal Combination #2

This formula is a must for the elderly, especially Alzheimer's patients. It protects the circulatory system and is rich in minerals to help eliminate heavy metals from the body. The nutrients nourish and protect the body from toxins and stressful situations.

Herbal combination #2 contains vitamins A, C, D, E, B1, B2, niacin, B6, folic acid, B12, biotin, and pantothenic acid. It contains the following minerals: calcium, iron, phosphorus, iodine, magnesium, zinc, selenium, copper, manganese, chromium, potassium, PABA, inositol, coenzyme Q10, l-Cystine (HCI), l-Methionine. This formula also contains citrus bioflavonoids, rutin, adrenal substance, spleen substance, thymus substance, codliver oil, ginkgo leaf, and hawthorn berries.

### Herbal Combinations #3

This formula protects the brain from free-radical damage. It contains nutrients and herbs that stimulate and nourish the brain. This combination also stimulates the neurotransmitter acetylcholine, which is involved in memory, mental acuity, nerve function, and alertness.

Herbal combination #3 contains Ginkgo biloba, huperzine A, phosphatidyl serine, choline, ethanolamine, and inositol. It also contains *Rhododendron caucasicum*, lycopene, and alpha lipoic acid.

### Other Uses

Attention deficit hyperactivity disorder (ADHD) and attention deficit disorder (ADD), autoimmune diseases, cholesterol buildup, chronic fatigue syndrome, heavy metal poisoning, and airborne toxins.

### HEALTHFUL SUGGESTIONS

1. Purified water is essential to prevent accumulation of toxins. Most tap water contains aluminum and other heavy metals because of acid rain in our soil that leeches into drinking-water sources. Reverse-osmosis water treatment is efficient and has been proven effective in eliminating heavy metals and hard minerals from tap water. At the beginning of a cleansing or fast, distilled water is beneficial because it acts like a magnet and leaches out toxins.

2. Fresh vegetable juices are cleansing and healing. They help flush out toxin and supply vitamins, minerals, and enzymes. The best juices are carrot, celery, parsley, spinach with ginger and garlic, wheatgrass juice, liquid chlorophyll drinks. A rich antioxidant berry drink with blueberries, chokeberries, raspberries, blackberries, and cranberries is also very cleansing and healing.

3. Avoid aluminum cookware and aluminum foil. Avoid baking potatoes as well as vegetables in foil. Avoid any food lined in foil.

# ANEMIA

Anemia is not considered a disease, but can be a symptom of many diseases. It can be a sign of cancer, arthritis, infections, hemorrhoids, liver damage, thyroid disorders, and dietary deficiencies. There are several kinds of anemia. The most common is iron deficiency anemia. There is also folic acid and B12 deficiency anemia. Less common are copper deficiency anemia and sickle-cell anemia, which is common in African Americans.

Pernicious anemia is caused by vitamin B12 deficiency. This disorder is when persons cannot absorb any form of vitamin B12 from the gastrointestinal tract. This can cause depression, lack of energy, fatigue, indigestion, irritability, immune function disorder causing colds and infections. Other symptoms are forgetfulness, headaches, poor concentration, and weakness. See a physician if you are experiencing any of these symptoms.

One of the main causes as we get older is the lack of assimilating iron and other minerals. Scientific experiments have found that in fatal cases of pernicious anemia, a large amount of iron was driven out of the blood (out of circulation), and had settled in the spleen. This revealed that iron was not in short supply and was not being utilized. The importance of making sure that there is enough hydrochloric acid in the body to assimilate minerals is vital.

Iron is necessary to produce red blood cells. Women who have heavy menstrual periods and do not get enough iron in their diets, or the ability to properly absorb iron, may have insufficient levels of either red blood cells or hemoglobin, the oxygen-carrying protein in red blood cells. This causes weakness and fatigue.

### EMOTIONAL NEEDS

Anemia could be linked to the lack of joy in one's life. Life becomes a burden, and the problem may be due to a fear of living life fully. There may be a need to realize that it is all right to experience joy, and that we need to know that humankind is created to experience joy.

### HERBAL COMBINATIONS
### Herbal Combination #1

This formula is rich in iron and minerals, which are necessary for the body to carry oxygen to the cells where it is combined with glucose for energy production. It acts as a blood purifier and blood builder. It is a natural form of plant iron and minerals for easily assimilation.

- Red beet cleans and stimulates the liver and spleen.
- Yellow dock is high in natural iron, blood purifier, and blood builder.
- Red raspberry is rich in iron and nutrients to strengthen the body.
- Chickweed cleanses and purifies the blood. Helps dissolve the plaque in the blood vessels and fatty substances in the system.
- Burdock is a blood purifier; promotes kidney function to help clear the blood of harmful acids.
- Nettle is rich in iron, which is vital in circulation and helpful in lowering high blood pressure. It is rich in chlorophyll, silicon, and potassium.
- Mullein is rich in iron and is a great painkiller and helps induce sleep. It has a calming effect on all inflamed and irritated nerves.

### Herbal Combination #2

This Chinese formula is designed to strengthen the blood, liver, and circulatory system. It helps aid the body of symptoms associated with anemia, such as depression, weakness, and lack of energy.

It contains: Dang qui root, ganoderma plant, lycium fruit, peony root, bupleurum root, cornus fruit, curcuma root, salvia root, achyranthes root, alisma rhizome, astragalus root, atrachlodes rhizome, ho shou wu root, ligusticum rhizome, liqustrum root, cyperus rhizome, and *Panax ginseng* root.

### HEALTHFUL SUGGESTIONS

1. Foods to help nourish and build the blood are whole grains, such as wheat, millet, brown rice, amaranth, yellow cornmeal, kamut, whole oats, quinoa, spelt, and teff. Blackstrap molasses and dried apricots are rich in iron, as are peaches, prunes, sunflower seeds, sesame seeds, egg yolks, fish, sprouts, beets, yams, squash, plums, potatoes (with skins), red cabbage, and beets. Enjoy all natural food, with fresh green salads, lightly steamed vegetables, and fresh fruit.

2. Avoid alcohol, coffee, cola drinks, white flour products, fried foods, excess fats and starches, excess protein, refined sugar, food preservatives and additives, canned foods, and pasteurized milk.

3. Fresh vegetable juices that are beneficial for anemia include: parsley, carrot, celery, and beet greens. Another iron-rich juice drink is carrots, celery, garlic, and parsley. Wheatgrass juice is blood cleansing and building. Chlorophyll builds the blood.

4. Lemon juice squeezed in a cup of warm water with ginger will stimulate gastric juices for better digestion and assimilation.

### HERBS AND SUPPLEMENTS

Single herbs include yellow dock (40 percent iron) and dandelion (helps the liver assimilate iron), alfalfa, kelp, dong quai, and watercress. Also good are barberry, black walnut, burdock, cayenne, chaparral, echinacea, garlic, gentian, ginger, hawthorn, lobelia, red clover, and sarsaparilla.

B-complex vitamins including adequate amounts of B6, B12, and folic acid, and PABA, pantothenic acid, and vitamin C with bioflavonoid—all in assimilation of iron. Vitamin E carries oxygen to the cells.

Antioxidants protect against free-radical damage, radiation damage, autoimmune diseases, and chemicals that may deplete the body of nutrients for healthy blood. They are vitamins A, C, E, selenium, and zinc, also grapeseed extract, lutein, and coenzyme Q10.

### ORTHODOX PRESCRIBED MEDICATION

Treatment includes replacing lost iron. Most iron tablets contain ferrous iron sulfate, iron gluconate, or polysaccharide iron. It takes three to six weeks for the supplements to work. The intestine's ability to absorb iron is limited, so higher doses are prescribed and this can cause indigestion and constipation.

# ANOREXIA NERVOSA AND BULIMIA

Anorexia nervosa and bulimia are eating disorders where thinness and weight loss become an obsession. Starvation and malnutrition may cause distorted thinking patterns, which can lead to a personality change. This condition usually begins during the teen years, when peer pressure can cause feelings of inadequacy and poor self-esteem. Anorexia is a disorder mainly seen in young girls. They feel they can never be thin enough. One-third of those with severe cases of anorexia die. Bulimia is characterized by binge eating and vomiting or using cathartics or diuretics.

Starvation and purging are dangerous and will bring long-lasting health problems, coma, or death. Vomiting often leads to a deterioration of the stomach and esophageal linings, an increase in cavities, gum disease, loss of enamel on teeth—even to the point of losing teeth. It flushes essential minerals from the body that are necessary for proper metabolism and physical and mental health.

In cases of anorexia and bulimia, all food becomes an obsession and brings on suppressed desires, needs, and emotions. These are addictions in which self-induced vomiting and laxatives used after eating or bingeing help rid the body of overwhelming cravings for food. There is also an attempt to deceive family and friends about eating habits. Once a girl starts to lose weight, she is praised. This often encourages the problem.

These addictions can lead to a lower metabolism, making it more and more difficult to lose weight. This causes feelings of failure and a loss of willpower and may ultimately lead to more bouts with bulimia and anorexia. When in a state of dieting or starvation, the body produces endorphins that chemically stimulate a natural high to ease suffering. This feeling also encourages dieting or anorexia. The brain of eating disorder victims can be disturbed and may shrink in mass. Also, the body begins to cannibalize itself. Muscle mass is depleted and heart muscle atrophy can occur.

## EMOTIONAL NEEDS

Eating disorders have been linked to a number of emotional problems, such as a lack of self-esteem or feelings of rejection that characterize certain personality types. Acceptance by family members and friends is also an important consideration. Studies tell us that often, people with eating disorders are perfectionists who feel out of control; therefore, by restricting their eating, they achieve a form of control that gives them a sense of well-being. Naturally, our society's preoccupation with thinness and our constant positive reinforcement of weight loss contributes to the problem. Moreover, it is vital to realize that anyone who is anorexic will also be suffering from malnutrition, which can profoundly impact mental and emotional health.

## HERBAL COMBINATIONS
### Herbal Combination #1
This combination helps strengthen the glands, especially the adrenal glands. It cleans and protects the liver, pancreas, and the digestive system.

- Licorice supplies energy to the body when recovering from illness and acts as a stimulant to the adrenal glands. It helps counteract stress.
- Dandelion purifies the blood and stimulates the liver to detoxify. It promotes healthy circulation, strengthens weak arteries, and restores balance in those who have suffered from severe vomiting.
- Safflower is a popular remedy for jaundice, sluggish liver, and gallbladder problems. It has the ability to remove hard phlegm from the system. It clears the lungs and helps in pulmonary tuberculosis.
- Horseradish contains antibiotic action, which is recommended for respiratory and urinary infections. It acts as a stimulant for digestion, metabolism, and kidney function.

## HEALTHFUL SUGGESTIONS

1. Compulsive eating is a food addiction, and allergies may be a cause. Look in the sections under addictions and allergies to identify a possible problem. A nutritional imbalance can cause a loss of appetite and taste. If allergies are involved, avoiding that substance can enable eating without physical or psychological ill effects.

2. Avoid all processed food, caffeine, alcohol, tobacco, white sugar, and white flour products. There is little nourishment in processed foods. They could be rancid and cause free-radical damage. Avoid all sweets, because they are addictive and deplete minerals and vitamins from the body. This loss includes the B-complex vitamins, which are essential for mental health.

3. Education on the importance of good nutrition must be stressed. Foods high in minerals should be eaten. Millet is an excellent food, easy to digest, alkaline, and rich in calcium, magnesium, and other minerals. Brown rice, almonds, whole grains, molasses, egg yolks, green leafy vegetables, apricots, and black figs are all rich in vitamins and minerals.

4. Juice drinks are beneficial for supplying concentrated minerals and increasing the appetite. Always dilute juices. If hypoglycemia is involved, dilute juices

to one ounce of juice to ten ounces of pure water. Pure juices can be hard on the pancreas and cause digestive problems. Ginger, carrot, parsley, and garlic are high in zinc. Lemon juice in water is an appetite stimulant and can help clean the liver of toxins.

## HERBS AND SUPPLEMENTS

All minerals are essential for the cells and organs. A zinc deficiency contributes to anorexia and bulimia. A deficiency also alters the sense of taste and produces appetite problems. A loss of minerals, especially zinc, potassium, and magnesium, can put stress on the heart and other organs. When depleted through vomiting, low levels of copper can cause many body dysfunctions.

- Amino acid supplements will help provide protein and nutrients to the body and mind. They help restore normal function to the metabolic connection of the brain. A healthy mind will be able to overcome obsessive behavior. Extra phenylalanine, tyrosine, and methionine will help improve emotional health. Glutamic acid is important for the brain.
- Plant digestive enzymes will assure the food eaten is properly digested and assimilated.
- Acidophilus is essential for restoring friendly bacteria to the intestines. It also helps in digestion and assimilation of nutrients.
- Aloe vera is beneficial for healing the digestive tract.
- Chlorophyll helps to build the blood and increase appetite. It supplies essential nutrients for the body. A liquid vitamin and mineral supplement is easy for the body to assimilate and digest.
- Essential fatty acids will help restore health to the glandular system. Some include evening primrose oil, borage oil, flaxseed oil, salmon oil, and black currant oil.
- Kelp is rich in minerals. A combination of kelp, dulse, alfalfa, licorice, dandelion, and yellow dock is rich in nutrients.
- A nervine herbal formula is helpful for emotional stability. Nervine herbs include hops, valerian, skullcap, white willow, passion flower, and St. John's wort.
- An herbal brain formula with *Ginkgo biloba*, gotu kola, suma, bee pollen, ginseng, and capsicum will increase circulation to the brain.
- B-complex vitamins help in eliminating toxins from the liver, improving digestion, and strengthening the nerves. A deficiency is often seen with addictions.
- Antioxidants are important to prevent free-radical damage to the brain and cells. Vitamins C with bioflavonoids, A, E, selenium, zinc, and grapeseed extract are beneficial.

## ORTHODOX PRESCRIBED MEDICATION

Antidepressants are usually prescribed by some psychiatrists. Dr. Peter R. Breggin, in his book *Toxic Psychiatry*, states, "Nowadays biopsychiatrists attempt to make drugs, usually antidepressants, the standard therapy. They also try to conjure up biochemical causes; but there's no meaningful evidence to back them up, and it seems fruitless and misleading to seek genetic and biochemical explanations for a problem that has appeared so recently in a social context that would seem to make it almost inevitable."

Prozac is often prescribed for those suffering from anorexia. Serious, sometimes fatal reactions occur when Prozac is used in combination with other antidepressant drugs such as Nardil, Parnate, and Marplan. Common side effects are agitation, bronchitis, chills, diarrhea, dizziness, drowsiness, and fatigue. There may also be weight gain, tremors, insomnia, nausea, and weakness. More serious side effects include inflammation of the esophagus, gums, stomach lining, tongue, and vagina. There could even be convulsions, difficulty in swallowing, vision problems, irrational ideas, irregular heartbeat, and exaggerated feelings of well-being that may inhibit the healing process.

# ANXIETY, PANIC ATTACKS, AND PHOBIAS

Anxiety, often triggered by extreme stress, can result in fear or panic attacks. People with phobias are often overwhelmed by mental, physical, and emotional stress and cannot control anxiety. Women in particular experience anxieties that can surface as their bodies go through physical changes with menstruation, pregnancy, and menopause. Also, they often carry a great deal of responsibility, which can increase their risk of anxiety and its symptoms.

Excess estrogen may be one of the main reasons that women have more incidents of intense anxiety than men do. Excess estrogen builds up in the body, and when the liver and colon cannot eliminate it properly, it backs up into the blood and can reach the brain and cause anxiety and other problems.

Symptoms of anxiety include dizziness, feelings of unreality or disassociation, confusion, a floating sensation, and feelings of claustrophobia when around crowds. Anxiety, panic attacks, and phobias are directly related to the health of the nervous system. Nervous system disorders can be related to a toxic colon. It creates autointoxication that can poison the body. This causes irritants to wear down the nervous system and brain. Sugar, soda pop, chocolate, white flour products, and meat all take a toll on the body. These products contain no beneficial nutrients. In fact, they pull essential nutrients out of the body, and if not replaced, this lack will cause irritation and imbalance in the nervous system.

## EMOTIONAL NEEDS

Along with body stresses, emotions can stimulate anxiety, especially during periods of trauma or high stress. Feelings of hopelessness or loss of control contribute to anxiety levels and attacks. Stress levels can get so high that panic attacks are the only way the physical body and the mind can deal with overwhelming life events. Sometimes anxiety can be affected by physical factors such as low blood sugar (hypoglycemia) and can surface as fear or agitation.

## HERBAL COMBINATIONS
### Herbal Combination #1

This formula is designed to strengthen and rebuild the nervous system. When the nervous system is affected, the immune system does not function properly. They both work together to keep the body strong and healthy. The nervous system transmits all sensory input, sound, sight, taste, smell, and touch to the brain and controls the workings of the organs. Causes of disorders can include lack of proper nutrition, organic disorders, overwork, worry, noisy surroundings, and physical problems.

- Black cohosh contains alkaloid properties for the nervous system.
- Capsicum distributes other herbs to needed parts of the body. It increases blood circulation and eliminates toxins.
- Valerian is relaxing and can be used for nervous tension, as a pain reliever, and as a remedy for nervous disorders.
- Ginger enhances the effectiveness of other herbs, relaxes the stomach, and works with capsicum to relieve congestion.
- White willow is a natural pain reliever, a sedative for the nerves, and a healer for the digestive tract.
- Devil's claw is a blood cleanser and pain reliever, as well as containing anti-inflammatory properties.
- Hops has sedative properties and makes an excellent relaxant. It contains B vitamins for nerves.
- Wood betony, when used with other herbs, is a natural tranquilizer for adults and a mild sedative for children.

### Herbal Combination #2

This formula is designed to relax the nerves and rebuild nervous disorders. It contains high amounts of B-complex vitamins, calcium, magnesium, potassium, iron, and zinc, as well as other nutrients.

- Chamomile is a soothing sedative with no harmful effects and can be used for children with colds or colic and to induce sleep. It helps with stomach cramps.
- Passion flower helps soothe and relax the nervous system, and it is useful for agitation, unrest, and exhaustion. It has been found to help individuals who want to wean themselves from synthetic sleeping pills and tranquilizers.
- Hops contains rich sedative powers and is considered one of the best nervine herbs for overcoming insomnia, alleviating nervous tension, and promoting a restful sleep.
- Fennel is a good digestive, diuretic, and nerve stabilizer. It is used as a sedative for small children and acts as an anticonvulsive and mild pain reliever.
- Marshmallow relaxes the bronchial tubes and is soothing and healing for lung ailments. It contains anti-inflammatory and anti-irritant properties. It also helps with gastrointestinal problems.
- Feverfew is a natural remedy for pain and is considered excellent for severe headaches. It works

gradually and with a gentle action that allows the body to heal itself.

### Other Uses

Convulsions, headaches, hyperactivity, hysteria, insomnia, nervous breakdown, and as a relaxant for the nerves.

## HEALTHFUL SUGGESTIONS

1. Look for body stressors, such as candida, food allergies, trace mineral deficiencies, hypoglycemia, or female-related problems. Controlled studies at Yale University and the National Institute of Mental Health showed that the amount of caffeine in eight cups of coffee and caffeine drinks significantly increased anxiety in fifteen of twenty-one panic-prone patients. The researchers theorized that caffeine blocks the function of adenosine, a substance that lessens the firing of nerve cells in certain brain areas.

2. Try following a hypoglycemia diet. Hypoglycemia is very common in those who have panic attacks. Changing to a diet conducive to treating hypoglycemia has helped many people. This condition is usually precipitated by a diet high in sugar and refined carbohydrates. It calls for eliminating sugar, caffeine, white flour products, and red meat while introducing more vegetables, grains, sprouts, beans, brown rice, millet, raw almonds, raw seeds, herbal relaxing teas, and pure water to the diet. Stay away from fruit juice for a while, and always use a little juice with a lot of water until the body becomes balanced again. Small amounts of fruit are fine. Hypoglycemia can bring on symptoms of fatigue, depression, anxiety, irritability, confusion, and mood swings.

3. Drugs are not the answer to panic attacks or anxiety. They may provide relief at first, but the body builds up a tolerance to any drug. Actually, drugs can increase life's problems. It is hard to think clearly under the influence of tranquilizers; they only interfere with the healing process of the body.

4. Panic attacks, anxiety, and phobias are real; they are very frightening to those who experience them. The problem needs to be faced. Proper nutrition can help heal the body and overcome these feelings. Changing eating habits and adding supplements will help heal the brain and nervous system.

## HERBS AND SUPPLEMENTS

Single herbs include gotu kola (brain food), dong quai (tranquilizing on the nerves), chamomile (rich in calcium), skullcap (rebuilds the nerves), hops (sedative properties), kava (mild sedative for panic attacks), passion flower (soothing to the nerves), ginkgo (stimulates brain function), suma (increases oxygen supply to the brain), and licorice root (nourishes adrenal glands and helps the liver eliminate excess estrogen). Alfalfa, kelp, horsetail, and oatstraw are particularly rich in minerals.

- Free-form amino acids can be supplemented to the diet. They are easily absorbed and beneficial for health. Whole grains in the diet will help the body produce and supply natural serotonin and melatonin to the brain. It is well known that tryptophan is a precursor to the neurotransmitter serotonin, which relieves anxiety by soothing the nerves and increasing relaxation.

- Glycine is another amino acid that may be lacking in individuals suffering from anxiety. It helps control motor functions. A deficiency may result in disorienting feelings and quick, jerky movements.

- Taurine is needed in large amounts in the central nervous system.

- Glutamine, another amino acid, has been shown to help sustain mental ability and helps in mental and emotional illness.

- Dl-phenylalanine (DLPA) is a nutritional amino acid that helps with chronic pain and depression.

- L-tyrosine is an amino acid that helps with depression, memory loss, and mental alertness.

- Digestive enzymes are very beneficial in neurological disorders. Enzymes will help break down the toxins causing irritation to the nervous system.

- B-complex vitamins are essential for healing the nervous system. Extra B12 and B6 will speed healing.

- Antioxidants including A, beta-carotene, C, E, selenium, and zinc, are essential for preventing free-radical damage to the brain and nervous system.

- A multimineral supplement is essential, since all minerals are necessary for a healthy nervous system. They function by regulating the muscular and nervous systems.

- Magnesium levels that are low have been seen in those with severe stress problems. It is the relaxant of the body.

- Lecithin is high in choline and inositol, which are necessary for the health of the nerve sheath.
- Essential fatty acids contain properties to reduce tension and anxiety. They help stimulate prostaglandins, which relax muscles.

## ORTHODOX PRESCRIBED MEDICATION

Alprazolam, brand name Xanax, is commonly prescribed for anxiety and panic disorders. It can be habit-forming with prolonged use, and it can cause impairment of mental function even with therapeutic doses. It can cause drowsiness and light-headedness. It could impair liver and kidney function. Allergic reaction may occur, causing hives or a rash. Headaches, dizziness, fatigue, blurred vision, dry mouth, nausea, vomiting, or constipation may also occur.

# ARTHRITIS AND RELATED CONDITIONS

This section will cover arthritis and related conditions, such as bursitis, gout, rheumatism, and ankylosing spondylitis. The two most common forms of arthritis are osteoarthritis and rheumatoid arthritis. Osteoarthritis is known as degenerative joint disease. It involves the cartilage that covers the ends of the bones wearing away and deteriorating. There can also be formation of bone spurs in the joints. The cartilage is a gel-like substance and acts as a shock absorber. This process of wearing away the cartilage causes inflammation, pain, deformity, and inability to move the joints. All diseases related to arthritis are characterized by inflammation of the joints. They can be caused by excessive calcium deposits that cause spurs or deposits of crystallized uric acid in the joints that irritate and cause pain.

Research indicates that many arthritic conditions can be allergy-related. Rheumatoid arthritis is a chronic inflammatory disorder causing stiffness, deformity, and pain to joints and muscles. It is an autoimmune disease where the body attacks itself. It can affect the lungs, blood vessels, spleen, skin, and muscles. Early signs can be fatigue, muscular aches and pains, stiffness in the joints, and swelling.

Gout is an arthritis-like metabolic disorder that increases concentration of uric acid in biological fluids. The uric acid becomes crystallized and is deposited in joints, tendons, the kidneys, and other tissues, causing inflammation, swelling, and damage. Gout is most often found in individuals who are obese, prone to high blood pressure, diabetic, or have a record of cardiovascular disease. Some medicines such as diuretics may impair the ability of the kidneys to excrete uric acid, which will build up in the joints.

In bursitis, also called tennis elbow, the elbows become sore and tender, and moving them is difficult and painful. It can also affect the shoulders, hips, or lower knees. If bursitis becomes severe and prolonged, some scar tissue can form and decrease joint mobility. Bursitis is an inflammation of the bursa, the fluid-filled sac located close to joints and between tendons and bones. Persons who lay tile for a living can get bursitis from long periods of kneeling.

Ankylosing spondylitis is an autoimmune disease that leads to arthritis. The body's immune system attacks the tissues lining the joints. Toxins accumulate in the joints, especially uric acid, which is a byproduct of meat. The toxins form crystals and can cause inflammation and pain in the joints. Stress and tension can cause pain and stiffness.

Arthritis and related conditions can be caused or aggravated by autointoxication, constipation, stagnation of blood, and lack of blood supply to the joints, lymphatics, and the nervous system. It could also be caused by infections, autoimmune disorders, bacterium, rich diet, excessive meat intake, white flour, and sugar products. A poor diet and stress can predispose one to these conditions. Allergies can be one cause of arthritis and related diseases. The symptoms of arthritis can be increased with foods and substances of the nightshade family. Tobacco is from the nightshade family, along with tomatoes, potatoes, eggplant, and green and red peppers. They interfere with collagen repair. Stress causes the destruction of protein, which is necessary before ACTH 9, a natural cortisone, can be produced. Arthritis usually means that calcium is out of solution and settles in the joints or other parts of the skeletal system.

## EMOTIONAL NEEDS

Rheumatoid arthritis and other joint conditions that are categorized as autoimmune diseases may be linked to emotional factors. For example, some studies have found that people who have experienced periods of high emotional stress or negativity can be susceptible to immune system dysfunction that can surface in the form of arthritis or related conditions.

## HERBAL COMBINATIONS
### Herbal Combination #1
The following formula is excellent for restoring cartilage and tissue in and around the joints. It contains nutrients to replace and restore healthy bones, cartilage, and tissues. It is very rich in vitamins and minerals. It has soothing, relaxing, and cleansing properties to help restore balance.

- Bromelain helps with tension, pain, inflammation, and swelling.
- Yucca is a cleansing agent and precursor to synthetic cortisone.
- Alfalfa contains alkaloids for pain and nutrients for body strength and works as a diuretic.
- Black cohosh relieves pain and irritation and relaxes and tones the body.
- Yarrow acts as a blood cleanser and soothes the mucous membranes. It helps regulate liver function.
- Capsicum is a stimulant and helps equalize circulation. It is a catalyst for other herbs.
- Burdock reduces swelling and deposits within joints and knuckles.
- Hydrangea acts like cortisone with cleansing power and helps prevent deposits in joints. It is rich in minerals to help build joints.
- Horsetail is rich in silica, necessary for strong bones and cartilage. It furnishes needed minerals.
- Catnip has relaxing properties, which are necessary for the body to heal, and is also rich in vitamins and minerals.
- Valerian is a safe herbal sedative useful in pain relief formulas. It is rich in magnesium, potassium, copper, and zinc.
- White willow is a natural sedative to relieve pain and contains cleansing properties.
- Slippery elm helps rebuild tissues and glands, eliminate toxins, heal joints, and aid in the digestion and utilization of nutrients.
- Sarsaparilla increases circulation to joints, balances hormones, and provides minerals for healthy joints and bones.

- Celery seed is an acid neutralizer and has a stimulating effect on the kidneys, producing an increased flow of urine. It is rich in vitamins A, B, and C, calcium, potassium, phosphorus, sodium, and iron.

### Herbal Combination #2
This combination is very beneficial for arthritis and related diseases. It is excellent for inflammation, which is seen as a cause of many diseases such as cancer and obesity. It contains glucosamine, MSM, chondroitin, and devil's claw.

### Other Uses
Ankylosing spondylitis, blood cleansing, calcification, neuritis, bursitis, gout, and rheumatism.

## HEALTHFUL SUGGESTIONS
1. Check for food allergies by taking the pulse test listed under the allergy section. Try an elimination diet for a week, avoiding the foods that you eat most often. If foods are the cause, you may notice that arthritic symptoms will ease after eliminating that food. The symptoms will reappear when you eat the allergic food again. A basic alkaline diet is good, because with these diseases the body becomes acidic, and the cartilage in the joints begins to dissolve because of acid in the blood.

2. Drink distilled water. Water helps the body's own joint lubricant—synovial fluid. Distilled water acts like a magnet and is considered a natural chelating agent to the deposits in the joints. Drinking more water will help the natural treatments to work better.

3. Essential fatty acids are vital for joint and cartilage health. Oils that have been heated can cause inflammation. The EFAs help to prevent inflammation. The best oils are flaxseed, borage, primrose, and salmon. Eating more fish and less beef will help improve joint health. Salmon is an excellent way to supply more EFAs in the diet.

4. Herbal therapy would be beneficial to treat the skeletal, muscular, circulatory, glandular, and nervous systems. There are herbs and supplements that can rebuild the systems of the body. Cleansing herbs are necessary to eliminate toxins. The three most important are the colon, blood, and liver cleansers. A formula containing psyllium and other herbs would be excellent for providing fiber to the digestive system.

## "I WILL BE ON HERBS FOR AS LONG AS I LIVE"

Gail became ill early in 1990 and went to the family doctor. He started out putting her on nonsteroid anti-inflammatory drugs for her joint pain. After she had stomach problems, he had her go to a rheumatologist and the tests began! At first, the doctor thought she had lupus or rheumatoid, and he put her on more nonsteroidal anti-inflammatory medications. However, the pain did not dissipate, so then she went on steroids. The doctors had to keep a close eye on her because of the side effects of Plaquenil—which can even cause blindness.

She tried this for about six months and was having health problems. At this point, the doctors decided it was rheumatoid arthritis. Then they put her on methotrexate, a powerful chemotherapy agent. She didn't know what it was and what side effects were involved, and by the time she did, she was very ill.

Her body had no resistance to anything, and she caught whatever was around—colds, flu, etc. She was in bed most of the time, very ill, and was in a lot of pain from the bottom of her feet to the top of her head. She was on this for three years. The side effects include damage to the kidneys and liver, loss of hair, mouth ulcers, dark blotches on the skin, internal bleeding, and so forth. She had to have her blood tested every two weeks because of the serious side effects. Then she reached a point where the methotrexate was not relieving the pain anymore, and she was put on gold shots. She was taking these shots every week with blood work for about two months. Then she went every two weeks and then every three weeks with blood work for about two months. Then she went once a month with blood work.

At this point, she met D. W., who had knowledge of herbs. He suggested that she use aloe vera and pycnogenols along with an herbal combination like #1. At first she was taking herbs and getting the gold shots at the same time. For the first time in a while, she started to feel pretty good, but every time she got the gold shot, she felt bad for a few days. She decided to stop the gold shots, and within five weeks, she felt better than she had in six years. She took 1 to 2 ounces of pure concentrate, whole-leaf aloe vera in the morning and evening, with ten pycnogenol during the day. She also took the above formula #1, barley grass juice capsules, glucosamine sulfate, and a relaxing formula. She also takes omega-3 fish oil.

She used to do things around the house for about an hour, and then she would have to rest for two hours before she could do anything else. She was always depressed, overweight because of the drugs, and in constant pain, and she didn't like herself at all. But after starting on an herbal and nutritional program, she felt great. She is losing weight and starting to feel good about herself and can go all day without a nap. The pain is almost gone; when she takes aloe vera, the pain goes away in a very short time. She says, "I thank my Creator every day for supplying herbs, and I thank those who helped me, and I will be on herbs for as lo

5. Exercise and weight control are beneficial to protect against joint and muscular pain. Being overweight increases stress on the joints. Light exercise can help limber the joints without putting stress on the joints. Weight-lifting exercises are beneficial, as well as walking. Add extra antioxidant supplements to neutralize free radicals when exercising strenuously. There is evidence that exercise produces extra free radicals.

## HERBS AND SUPPLEMENTS

Herbal sleep formulas or occasional use of melatonin to induce a deep sleep will help to promote a restful sleep when pain is involved in arthritis.

- Goat's whey powder is an excellent mineral food for the digestive system, glands, and ligaments. It purifies the blood, aids digestion, counteracts acidosis, and is a blood builder.
- Anti-inflammatory herbs are feverfew, devil's claw, turmeric, skullcap, curcumin, boswellia, white willow bark, black cohosh, sarsaparilla, and guaiacum.
- Glucosamine sulfate is natural and safe to use. It improves symptoms and boosts tissue regeneration. It works to protect cartilage in the joints. It is easily absorbed and nontoxic.

- Digestive enzymes help enhance digestion and assimilation and decrease inflammation.
- Hydrochloric acid is essential to digest proteins and destroy toxins such as viruses, bacteria, germs, worms, and parasites.
- Antioxidants such as vitamin A and C with bioflavonoids act as natural anti-inflammatory agents. Vitamin E, selenium, and zinc help to fight free-radical damage, which is implicated in arthritis and related diseases.
- Calcium and magnesium help in rebuilding joints, bones, and cartilage. Herbal calcium is very important, containing alfalfa, marshmallow, plantain, horsetail, oatstraw, wheatgrass, and hops.
- Essential fatty acids help in healing joints. Use flaxseed, borage, black currant, evening primrose, and salmon oils. Improvement is seen in arthritis with essential fatty acids. They also strengthen the glands and boost the immune system.
- Boron, silicon, and trace minerals are important for bone health. A supplement with boron is important, but the main source is found in fruits and vegetables. Silicon is found in horsetail, oatstraw, and in herbal calcium formulas.
- B-complex vitamins are important, with extra B5, B6, and B12. A good B12 supplement that dissolves under the tongue is assimilated faster. B vitamins are necessary for energy, brain function, and nerve health.
- CoQ10 and germanium provide oxygen to the blood for repairing and healing connective tissues and cartilage.
- Chlorophyll products contain vitamin K and assist in mineral assimilation in the bones. They are also cleansing and nourishing for the blood.
- Lecithin protects the myelin sheath surrounding the nerves and prevents nerve damage.
- Superoxide dismutase (SOD) is an antioxidant that protects against free-radical damage to the joints.
- Grapeseed extract is a powerful anti-inflammatory and free radical scavenger that protects against further damage to the joints.
- Capsicum cream can help affected joints to speed circulation and relieve pain.
- Foods can act as natural anti-inflammatory agents. Examples include fruits and vegetables, grains, legumes, garlic, onions, and shallots.
- Sulfur is needed in repairing bone, cartilage, and connective tissues. It is found in garlic, onions, and shallots.
- Juice drinks could include carrots, celery, spinach, garlic, and ginger.

## ORTHODOX PRESCRIBED MEDICATION

Methotrexate is one of the many drugs prescribed for rheumatoid arthritis. Others are corticosteroids, gold injections, and salicylates, sometimes used in combination with drugs such as methotrexate. Methotrexate is an immunosuppressive drug and is very powerful. Side effects include severe depression of the bone marrow, liver damage, ulceration of the mouth and intestine, and birth defects. Avoid alcohol and salicylates during methotrexate therapy. The following drugs can aggravate active or latent arthritis: iron dextran, isoniazid and pyrazinamide (in combination), and oral contraceptives.

# ASTHMA

It is estimated that more than fifteen million Americans, both children and adults, have asthma. It is becoming a real health hazard. Asthma is a chronic, usually allergic, condition that causes difficulty in breathing. This is a condition where there is inflammation that constricts the bronchial tubes leading to the lungs and causes spasms and tightening of the bronchial tubes, which reduces the airflow in and out of the lungs. Breathing becomes difficult and can cause panic. Symptoms are shortness of breath, coughing, wheezing, and a tight feeling in the chest.

There are two types of asthma: extrinsic and intrinsic. Extrinsic asthma is caused by allergic reactions to house mites, dust, animal fur, cigarette smoke, feathers, molds, certain drugs such as aspirin, or food additives such as monosodium glutamate. Certain foods can cause reactions, such as milk products, wheat, sugar, or other food. Intrinsic asthma is caused by genetics, infections, pollutants, and stress and is connected to heart trouble or kidney diseases and improves only when the heart and kidneys are treated. Asthma is also seen as an adrenal dysfunction and can be helped by nourishing the adrenals. Very cold air should be avoided, as it can cause a reaction.

Asthma can occur as young as three years of age or younger. More than half of children with asthma will outgrow it. Asthma is considered an incurable disease; however, attacks can be relieved or avoided with treatment. Treating acute diseases naturally will help prevent chronic diseases such as asthma. Asthma is also seen as a result of vaccinations.

In *Nature Has a Remedy*, Dr. Bernard Jensen, DC, says, "Much of the ill health in adults has its beginning in childhood. Colds and children's diseases such as mumps, measles, discharges of the ears and nose, etc., should be taken care of by natural methods. We should remember that body cleanliness, correct foods, normal activities, and a happy environment, with plenty of love, will prevent most of the ill health found in children. Even with inherent weaknesses they will, if properly cared for, become healthy adults and escape most of the ills of childhood."

In *Power Healing*, Dr. Leo Galland, MD, says, "Asthma is treated with drugs that block bronchial spasm (bronchodilators) and drugs that block bronchial inflammation (chiefly, cortisone). There is considerable evidence that the conventional, disease-based treatment approach to asthma actually contributes to its increasing severity and mortality. . . . The increasing severity of asthma produced by bronchodilation makes sense if one understands that asthma is not a disease, it is a protective response to environmental toxicity." He goes on to say, "Bronchodilators are useful for the emergency relief of breathlessness; the regular use of them causes deterioration in lung function, and increases the risk of death. Respiratory therapists, who are exposed to airborne bronchodilator sprays as part of their work, develop asthma at a rate almost five times greater than expected, after entering their profession." He says that occupational exposure to bronchodilators actually creates asthma.

## EMOTIONAL NEEDS

Resolving emotions from suppressed sadness has been shown to help, along with diet. The inability to cry and release these emotions can also be a cause. Smothering love can create the inability to breathe for oneself. The overprotection of children can cause asthma in childhood.

## HERBAL COMBINATIONS
### Herbal Combination #1

- Fenugreek is excellent for dissolving hard mucus and ridding the lungs and bronchial tubes of mucus and phlegm. It helps expel waste through the lymphatic system and contains antiseptic properties.
- Boneset has antiseptic and antiviral properties, strengthens the stomach and spleen, promotes sweating to help in colds and flu, and promotes the production of interferon.
- Horseradish has antibiotic properties and is a strong stimulant to clear the lungs and nasal passages of infections. It is beneficial to stimulate digestion, metabolism, and kidney function.
- Mullein relieves pain, relaxes the body, and controls coughs, cramps, and spasms. It loosens mucus from the respiratory and lymphatic systems. It is a great herb for treating tuberculosis, as well as other lung problems.
- Fennel expels phlegm from the throat, eliminates toxins from the body, and purifies the blood. It aids digestion, colic, and other stomach complaints. It contains essential oils similar in composition to catnip and peppermint.

### Herbal Combination #2

This is an excellent combination from India. These herbs are specific for the respiratory system, helping in asthma, bronchitis, colds, congestion, pneumonia, and allergies such as hay fever.

It contains the following herbs: *Zingiber officinale* (ginger), *Glycyrrhiza glabra* (licorice), *Adhatoda vasica, Verbascum thapsus, Alpina galanga, Clerodendrum indicum, Inula racemosa, Myrica nagi, Phyllanthus emblica, Hedychium spicatum, Picrorhiza kurroa, Pimpinella anisum, Pistacia integerrima, Ocimum sanctum, Tylopora asthmatica, Abies webbina, Elettaria cardamomum,* and *Ferula assafoetida.*

### Herbal Combination #3

This is a Chinese herbal combination for the lungs and bronchials. It is a natural diuretic, expectorant, and decongestant. It is specific for asthma and bronchitis.

It contains *Fructus aurantia immaturi*, citrus peel, pinellia rhizome, hoelen plant, bamboo sap, fritillaria bulb, bupleurum root, inula flower, xingren, magnolia bark, morus root bark, ophiopogon root, ginger rhizome, schizandra fruit, and licorice root.

### Other Uses

Allergies, colds, ear and eye infections, respiratory infections, and congestion of the bronchial, lungs, and lymphatic systems.

### HEALTHFUL SUGGESTIONS

l. The first line of defense is to strengthen the lungs as well as the entire body. Air pollution and chemicals in our food and water are not going to vanish. Fine particulate matter (toxins in the air) suppress the body's immune system and may even cause cancer. We need to strengthen our immune systems, lungs, livers, colons, and whole bodies. It is easier to prevent than to cure the disease. Deep and proper breathing is essential to keep the lungs clean.

2. The home needs to be clean and free from dust, bacteria, molds, and other toxins. Many people take off their shoes and keep them in the hallway. This prevents dust, dirt, and toxins from getting embedded in the carpets and rugs. An air purifier is an excellent way to clean the inside air.

3. The digestive system needs to be nourished and cleansed. A congested colon is the main cause of diseases. A high-fiber diet, a lower bowel cleanser, a liver cleanser, and blood cleansers are very important. Psyllium is important to clean the pockets of the colon. Lower bowel cleansers nourish, clean, and feed the colon. An excellent lower bowel cleanser contains cascara sagrada bark, buckthorn bark, licorice root, turkey rhubarb root, ginger root, capsicum fruit, couch grass herb, Oregon grape root, and red clover tops.

4. Reduce exposure to tobacco smoke, perfumes, car exhaust, household cleansers, molds, and animal dander. Ventilation in the home will help combat mold growth. Dust mites are everywhere, especially in bed clothing. Encase mattresses and pillows in airtight covers to prevent mite infestation.

5. Avoid MSG (monosodium glutamate). Several years ago it was removed from baby food because of brain damage in infants. It is still widely used and should be avoided. If it causes damage to infants, what is it doing to the major population? It is widely used in restaurants. It is disguised as "autolyzed yeast," "hydrolyzed yeast," "vegetable powder," or "natural flavors." Other additives to avoid are sulfites, BHA, BHT, and tartrazine (yellow dye #5). They all can create an allergic reaction and increase asthma attacks.

6. A vegetarian diet is very helpful, making sure there is adequate protein, which is abundant in seeds, nuts, grains, potatoes, vegetables, and herbs. Brown rice and millet are high in protein. Juice fasting will help eliminate toxins and clean the lungs. Beneficial juices are carrot, celery, parsley, and fresh ginger. Garlic and onion soup will dissolve mucus. Avoid sugar and white flour products.

### HERBS AND SUPPLEMENTS

Single herbs to help with asthma are fenugreek (dissolves hard mucus, protects against infections), licorice (acts as a natural corticosteroid, feeds the adrenals), slippery elm (helps to alleviate inflammation of the mucous membranes), marshmallow (helps to soothe and relax irritated bronchiole tubes), and lobelia (helps to relax and clear airways of mucus).

- Pantothenic acid (B5) is vital in the production of adrenal hormones, which give the system an antiallergenic protection. It protects against stress. Balanced B vitamins are essential.

- Antioxidants fight free-radical damage to protect the cells in the lungs, immune system, and nervous system. They are found in vitamins A, C with bioflavonoids, E, selenium, zinc, grapeseed extract, and pine bark. They enhance the lungs.

- Bee pollen can build immunity by acting as a barrier against inhaled pollens. Always start with small amounts and gradually increase the dose. It is rich in nutrients and amino acids.

- Essential fatty acids found in fish, flaxseed, borage, and evening primrose oils help the body produce anti-inflammatory substances to protect the cells from damage.

- Digestive enzymes and hydrochloric acid are necessary to break up undigested protein and food in the bloodstream so the body can eliminate them. Use between meals to break down undigested food in the bloodstream. Use after meals to assure food is digested and assimilated.

## ORTHODOX PRESCRIBED MEDICATION

Corticosteroids are widely used and are effective at reducing asthma symptoms. If taken for long periods, they may result in poor wound healing, stunted growth in children, loss of calcium from the bones, stomach bleeding, premature cataracts, elevated blood sugar levels, hunger, weight gain, and mental problems.

# ATTENTION DEFICIT HYPERACTIVITY DISORDER (ADHD)

ADHD has had many labels associated with it, such as hyperactivity, learning disabilities, dyslexia, and now we have another label—at-risk children. At first some psychiatrists thought hyperactivity was a brain disease. When a physical brain disease could not be found, they changed the label to a minimal brain disease. When no evidence of a minimal brain disease could be found, the profession transformed the concept into minimal brain dysfunction. When no minimal brain dysfunction could be demonstrated, the label became attention deficit hyperactivity disorder. Biochemical imbalance is the key phrase, but there is no more evidence for that than there is for actual brain disease.

In his book *Toxic Psychiatry*, Peter R. Breggin, MD, a psychiatrist, explains, "It is currently fashionable to treat approximately one-third of all elementary school boys as an abnormal population because they are fidgety, inattentive, and unamenable to adult control. How many children get stuck with one or another label is not known, but it surely runs into the millions." Robert S. Mendelsohn, MD, a pediatrician for more than thirty-five years, made this statement: "Originally, behavior-controlling drugs were used to treat only the most severe cases of mental illness. But today, drugs such as Dexedrine and Ritalin are being used on more than one million children throughout the United States, on the basis of often flimsy diagnostic criteria or hyperactivity and minimal brain damage. But there is no single diagnostic test that will identify a child as hyperactive or any of the twenty-one other names assigned to this syndrome. All a doctor has to go on is a list of inconclusive tests and the educated guess of an expert."

Dr. Mendelsohn goes on to say, "One school in Texas took advantage of this ambiguity and diagnosed 40 percent of its students as minimally brain damaged in a year when government money was available to treat that syndrome. Two years later, this money was no longer available, but funds for treating children with language learning disabilities were floating around. Suddenly, the minimally brain damaged students disappeared, and 35 percent of the children were diagnosed as having language learning disabilities."

Dr. Mendelsohn was very honest and outspoken and further said, "You can expect your doctor to cast a covetous eye on your kids. Educators who don't like unruly pupils have, with the willing help of doctors and psychologists, broadened the definition of hyperactivity to include a substantial percentage of those in the country who are under age twenty-one. As a consequence, for the comfort and convenience of teachers and parents, millions of normally lively kids have been drugged with Ritalin and turned into virtual zombies by its effects."

Hyperactivity is commonly related to children, but adults often suffer with it. Some nutritionists believe that hypoglycemia in adults is an extension of hyperactivity in children. Many adults cannot cope with life's problems and take tranquilizers and drugs that only complicate the underlying cause. It is felt that adults who suffer from ADHD are so common that it puts a stress on families that can lead to divorce, marital difficulties, and even child abuse.

Symptoms of ADHD in children are an inability to sit still, fidgetiness, short attention span, and running instead of walking. They are usually getting into everything and talking constantly in a loud voice. They are impulsive, act before thinking, and forget easily. They have trouble following instructions and are often moody, irritated, and indifferent when disciplined. They throw temper tantrums and are determined to get their way.

Symptoms in adults can be trouble concentrating, difficulty sticking to tasks until finished, impulsive spending, always being in a hurry, blurting out things that are regretted later, trouble sitting still, and difficulty relaxing. Other symptoms include mood swings, low self-esteem, short temper, and a tendency toward addictive substances such as alcohol, drugs, or food. Compulsive behavior and fear of not being in control of their lives are also factors. The symptoms of childhood ADHD don't usually disappear but take on a different aspect. Adults can usually control or hide their symptoms more easily than children can.

To find the underlying cause or causes, consider the diet, lazy colon (the brain and nervous system are very sensitive to toxins), emotional stress, and allergies. Allergies are often involved in hyperactive children and adults. A deficiency in the B vitamins can cause mood changes and depression. White sugar requires B vitamins in order to be metabolized in the body. A high-sugar diet depletes this essential group of nutrients so critical to mental and emotional health. Allergies to milk, wheat, chocolate, oranges, yeast, food additives, and antibiotics are the most common.

Guylaine Lanctot, MD, in her book *The Medical Mafia*, says that one of the neurological disorders from the complications associated with vaccinations is hyperactive children. Behavior problems such as hyperactivity and learning disabilities have increased in the past fifty years. When children are vaccinated, supplements of vitamins A and C are important to boost the immune system to prevent complications.

## EMOTIONAL NEEDS

I strongly believe that when you are dealing with children's disorders, whether physical or emotional, the value of expressing love through physical contact cannot be overestimated. For example, when a child's emotional needs are not met, the frustration he or she feels can be manifested in a number of different ways. While we know that ADHD is caused by a variety of factors and one single cause is evident, providing the child with reassuring love and security through touching and positive reinforcement can be very therapeutic. I have heard of many instances where a dysfunctional child who was failing in school was turned around by a teacher who openly gave him or her special attention to foster greater self-worth. Children who were unresponsive and afraid have been able to improve

their grades and class behavior as a result of a caring teacher who was not afraid to bond with the student.

## HERBAL COMBINATIONS
### Herbal Combination #1

The following combination provides nutritional support for the brain and nervous systems. It helps to relieve anxiety and promote relaxation. It provides food for the brain and helps calm the mind. This formula is rich in B vitamins, which are essential for healthy nerves and brain. It also contains bee pollen, found to be effective in children with ADHD. The nervine herbs found in this formula are important to support the nervous system and the brain.

- Schizandra boosts the immune and nervous systems. It strengthens the lungs and improves digestion. It stimulates the heart and circulation. It is rich in nutrients, especially vitamins A and C.
- Complex vitamins are essential for the nervous system. Vitamin B1 has been used successfully with the emotionally disturbed to treat irritability, depression, fear, and non-cooperation. B2 is valuable in fatigue, depression, hysteria, and anemia. B3 is essential for brain metabolism, and it helps reduce tension, fatigue, depression, and insomnia. B6 is good for stress, insomnia, water retention, and the glands. A B12 deficiency can cause severe psychotic symptoms that may vary in severity from mild disorders of mood, mental slowness, and memory defect to severe psychotic disorders. Pantothenic acid is an antidepressant vitamin. It improves the body's ability to withstand stressful conditions. It reduces anxiety and promotes sleep. Folic acid works on the nervous system and also on the highest center of the brain and helps in depression. Biotin helps to promote good mental health and energy and alleviate insomnia.
- Choline and inositol are components of lecithin and work together for nourishing and strengthening the brain and nervous system. They help relieve anxiety and insomnia and prevent dizziness.
- Vitamin C with bioflavonoids increases nutrient absorption, protects the immune system, strengthens capillaries, and helps prevent many diseases.
- Bee pollen is rich in protein, with all the essential amino acids. It is high in B-complex vitamins and

is said to contain every substance needed to maintain life. It is excellent for the nervous system and hormonal system.

- Wheat germ is rich in fiber and protein. It is very nutritious, with a high content of B vitamins.
- Valerian root is one of the best nervine herbs to build up the nervous system in a short period of time. It is very soothing and calming on the nervous system. It is healing for stomach problems. Hops has strong sedative powers but is safe. It is cleansing for the blood and helps to alleviate nervous tension and promote a restful sleep.
- Skullcap is a stimulating herb. It aids in rebuilding and strengthening the spinal cord and nervous system. It is an excellent antispasmodic agent for restlessness, tremors, spasms, twitching of muscles, and hypertension.

### Other Uses
Addictions, autoimmune diseases, nervous disorders, and a B vitamin deficiency.

### Herbal Combination #2
This combination provides nutrients for the brain. It is in a powder form for easy assimilation. It protects the brain from toxins. It helps in nervous disorders, is helpful in clear thinking, and will benefit children with ADHD as well as individuals with Alzheimer's. It contains vitamins B1, B2, B6, B12, niacin, pantothenic acid, folic acid, biotin, flaxseed powder, DMAE, lemon balm, bacopa, ginkgo, grapeseed extract, natural raspberry flavor, grape skin extract, citric acid, lohan fruit concentrate, eleuthero, malic acid, stevia leaf extract, choline, and inositol. This combination also comes in capsule form.

### Herbal Combination #3
This combination is excellent to help remove heavy metals from the body, especially in the brain, which is seen as one cause of brain dysfunction. It contains nutrients that bind with heavy metals and eliminate them from the body. It contains cilantro, N-acetyl-cystine, apple pectin, sodium alginate, kelp algae, L-methionine, alpha lipoic acid, magnesium, and pyridoxal-5-phosphate.

Another excellent herbal combination for the nerves is #1 under addictions. Another formula for ADHD used to build up the nerves, muscles, and tissues contains the following: white willow, black cohosh, capsicum, valerian, ginger, hops, wood betony, and devil's claw.

## HEALTHFUL SUGGESTIONS
1. The brain needs constant nutrition to maintain its ability to function properly. Changes in behavior occur when the brain lacks oxygen, nutrients, and antioxidants. Free radicals damage brain cells.

2. Allergies can be a contributing factor. Faulty digestion can cause allergies. It can start early—when babies are given cereal before they have teeth, the ability to chew properly, and the proper enzymes to digest starches. The enzymes needed to digest cereals are found in the saliva, usually produced when chewing. Faulty digestion allows toxins to enter the bloodstream and irritates the intestines, organs, and tissues. Allergies are often involved, and taking a pulse test when eating suspect foods could be beneficial. Take the pulse before eating the suspected food and then again thirty minutes later. If it has increased, an allergy may be involved.

3. Environmental toxins, including lead, cadmium, pesticides, additives, and food coloring, act as toxins in the intestines. If there are not enough minerals, vitamins, and nutritional foods, the toxins accumulate in the body.

4. Candida and leaky gut syndrome can be a factor in the development of ADHD. The health of the intestines determines the health of the rest of the body and its ability to heal. The intestines are responsible for the absorption of nutrients. They are also responsible for the elimination of toxins and waste material from the system. If candida takes over from years of sweets, antibiotics, and prednisone use, as well as toxins from molds or fungus, a variety of undiagnosable symptoms may occur. Candida produces an enzyme called thiaminase, which breaks down and destroys thiamine (B1) before it even gets absorbed. Thiamine is crucial in the body's ability to produce energy.

5. Parasites and worms may be common when digestion is faulty. When the wrong diet is eaten, hydrochloric acid can be lacking, allowing parasites, worms, viruses, bacteria, and germs to flourish.

6. A young child's brain, nervous system, immune system, glandular system, and organs are still developing and are more vulnerable than an adult's to

environmental factors. Children are more susceptible to toxins and carcinogens than adults. Children eat more food relative to their body weight, so they receive greater exposure to pesticides from the food they eat than adults.

7. Lead poisoning is suspected in ADHD, and actually affects almost everyone, especially those low in minerals. Children are very vulnerable because they absorb up to 50 percent of ingested lead, whereas adults only absorb 5 to 10 percent.

8. Tofu and soymilk added to the diet help provide protein for the body. Tofu can be added to many foods, such as mashed potatoes, eggs, macaroni and cheese, spaghetti, and soups. Legumes and beans used regularly help eliminate heavy metals.

9. Fiber-rich foods help eliminate toxins and heavy metals. Use more whole grains in soups and cereals. Grains and vegetable soups are excellent because of the rich mineral content necessary to eliminate and prevent heavy metal poisoning. Millet, brown rice, and cornmeal are very nourishing for the brain.

10. Raw vegetables and salads are nourishing. Fruit is cleansing and provides energy when children are taken off sugar. Sunflower seeds, almonds, sprouts, green leafy vegetables, broccoli, cabbage, Brussels sprouts are beneficial. Six to eight servings of vegetables a day can help strengthen the body and brain.

## HERBS AND SUPPLEMENTS

Bee pollen helps protect against and detoxify the body from lead poisoning and toxins. Always start with a few grains and increase slowly. It has been shown to help in some children suffering from ADHD.

- Burdock helps to clean the blood.
- Gotu kola helps to strengthen the brain and improve memory.
- Hops are relaxing and strengthening for the nervous system.
- Dulse and algin found in kelp are natural chelating agents. Pectin also contains chelating properties. Pectin is found under the skin of apples and other fruit.
- Garlic, onions, and shallots contain properties to counteract lead and toxins.
- Lecithin repairs and protects the myelin sheath of nerve fibers. It helps to detoxify poisons in the body. It is very nourishing for the nerves and the brain.
- Amino acids, such as methionine and cystine, contain sulfur properties to detoxify and eliminate toxins and heavy metals.
- Chlorophyll supplements protect against heavy metal poisoning and toxins.
- Vitamin A and other antioxidants, such as vitamins E, C, selenium, and zinc, help neutralize toxins and metal poisoning. They also help prevent free-radical damage, which has a profound effect on the brain. Grape seed extract acts as an antioxidant.
- CoQ10 and other oxygen-providing nutrients help the brain and prevent damage to the brain and nervous system.
- Calcium and magnesium with vitamin D speed recovery from toxins and metal poisoning.
- B6 helps zinc enter the brain. Zinc is vital to prevent heavy metal poisoning.

### ANDY BEGAN READING

Andy's speech development was delayed, and his parents felt that his development was slow. When preparing him for school, his pediatrician sent Andy for some tests at the local school to see if he was capable of handling a regular kindergarten class. His parents found out his ability in expressing himself was that of a three-year-old. The parents took Andy to a children's hospital in Boston for a neurological assessment. Andy was labeled as a learning-disabled child, but the doctor wouldn't put him on Ritalin because he was not as bad as other children. Andy's teacher told the parents that he would not read until he was nine. She actually called Andy's pediatrician to request a prescription for Ritalin. The doctor said no! In the meantime, Andy's mother met a natural food distributor who told her she could help Andy with herbs. He was put on the previous formula along with gotu kola and lecithin. The following year, Andy began reading, not at nine years of age but at six. His mother was very thankful for learning about herbs and those people who helped her.

- Essential fatty acids, such as flaxseed oil, primrose oil, borage oil, and blackcurrant, help produce prostaglandins for positive nerve and immune response.

## ORTHODOX PRESCRIBED MEDICATION

There are presently about four million children taking mind-altering drugs like Ritalin. Side effects include sadness, depression, loss of energy, social problems, emotional difficulties, growth suppression in small children, tics, skin rashes, nausea, headaches, and stomach irritations. Long-term abuse can lead to tolerance and mental dependence with varying degrees of abnormal behavior. Other common side effects are insomnia and nervousness. It almost seems as if children are seen as having a deficiency of Ritalin. Children who take mind- and behavior-altering drugs seem to be more centered, better able to stay focused on their studies, less aggressive, and easier to handle. These changes benefit the parents and teachers. Drugs such as Ritalin, Adderal, and Dexedrine are commonly prescribed. These drugs are stimulants and pose a risk of abuse. Ritalin has properties similar to cocaine, and there is evidence that children taking Ritalin will be at risk of abusing drugs as adults.

# BLADDER AND KIDNEY PROBLEMS

The urinary tract includes the two kidneys and the bladder. The kidneys filter waste material and excess water from the blood down into the bladder, a bag that stores eight to sixteen ounces of urine. The kidneys filter all of the blood molecules, which regulate water, glucose, carbonates, sodium, chlorides, potassium, sulfate, calcium, phosphate, and urea. Urea is the waste product to be eliminated in the urine. All other substances are crucial to normal body function. The kidneys also regulate the acid/alkaline balance. The kidneys are like a filtering system for the body and can become plugged up like a strainer with toxic buildup. When the kidneys are congested with toxins and mucus, irritation to the kidneys can occur and cause infections or kidney stones.

Kidney stones develop when crystals are formed and stick together and continue to grow. A lack of water and too much acid food can cause kidney stones and bladder infections. Symptoms of infections are cloudy, dark-colored, or scanty urine, continuous dull pain in the lower abdomen or lower back, burning sensation during urination, feeling the need for frequent urination, chills, and fever. Frequent urination can be a symptom of diabetes. Kidney problems can cause pain in the lower back.

Infections and inflammations are fairly common, especially in the bladder and urethra. Cystitis is the name for infections in this area. They are usually caused by bacteria but can be caused by chemical irritants in soaps, bubble bath, talcum powder, perfumes, or vaginal deodorants. These can cause inflammation in the urethra. Sexual intercourse can also cause cystitis by bruising the urethra, introducing infection-causing bacteria, and starting the inflammation process. Yeast overgrowth can also cause cystitis. Infections can cause incontinence. In *The Ultimate Healing System*, Donald LePore, ND, explains, "Many doctors believe that a high calcium intake will cause kidney problems. This is partly true, because if there is not enough magnesium to work with the calcium, there will be problems. So, instead of limiting a person's calcium intake (except at the very beginning of the problem), the best thing for you to do is to administer magnesium, which is the controller of calcium, in order to dissolve kidney stones and calcification."

## HERBAL COMBINATIONS
### Herbal Combination #1
This first formula is to help with bladder and kidney infections, neutralize acids, clean the urinary tract, and strengthen the entire system.

- Juniper berries clear mucus in the bladder and kidneys, strengthen nerves, and heal infection. They are high in vitamin C.
- Parsley is high in potassium, which gives muscle tone to the bladder and increases the flow of urine.
- Uva ursi is beneficial for bladder and kidney infections and strengthen and tones the urinary tract.
- Dandelion is very nourishing, neutralizes uric acid, and opens urinary passages.
- Chamomile is a tonic, soothes the nerves, and helps elimination through the kidneys.

### Herbal Combination #2

This formula protects the urinary tract against infections and contains all the nutrients necessary to strengthen the urinary system. It contains the following: potassium, magnesium, asparagus, dandelion, parsley, cornsilk, watermelon seed, dong quai, horsetail, hydrangea, eleuthero, uva ursi, and schizandra.

### Herbal Combination #3

This combination strengthens the immune system and has antioxidant, antiviral, and anticancer properties. It contains colostrum, beta-glucan, arabinogalactan, reishi mushroom, maitake mushroom, and cordyceps.

### Other Uses

Healing urinary tract and protecting against infections and autoimmune diseases.

### HEALTHFUL SUGGESTIONS

1. Juice fasting will help cleanse the kidneys and bladder. Liquid chlorophyll will purify the blood. Drink pure apple juice. Unsweetened cranberry juice or cranberry capsules contain properties that prevent bacteria from adhering to the walls of the bladder. Green drinks will cleanse and heal. Drink lots of pure water to flush out the kidneys and bladder. A half lemon or lime in a cup of warm water is beneficial.

2. Colon cleansing is beneficial. A toxic colon is very common when infections are present in the body. Lower bowel cleansers, herbal laxative teas, or colonics will help clean the bowel.

3. Eat a high-fiber diet. Constipation can cause irritations from a toxin buildup in the blood. Consume dairy products sparingly; they will produce an acid condition. Use whole grains such as whole oats, barley, buckwheat, kamut (an organic wheat), millet, brown rice, amaranth, quinoa, spelt, and teff. Use yellow cornmeal, which is good for the bowels.

4. Blood cleansers can be very beneficial. Vegetable broths contain minerals for healthy kidneys. Change to a low-meat diet. A high-protein diet can lead to calcium accumulation in the kidneys, which may cause kidney stones. Excess protein is broken down by the liver and kidneys, so it would be best to not overwork these organs. A good protein source would be free-form amino acids for easier assimilation.

5. Avoid carbonated beverages, black tea, coffee, alcohol, caffeine drinks, and sugar products. These items may cause an inflammation of the membranes lining the kidneys.

### HERBS AND SUPPLEMENTS

- Cranberry juice powder in capsule form helps prevent bacteria from adhering to the walls of the bladder. It aids in preventing and healing infections.
- Garlic is one of nature's antibiotics but does not destroy the body's normal flora. It has a rejuvenating effect on all body functions. Garlic stimulates the lymphatic system to cleanse the body of toxins.
- Echinacea stimulates the immune system and increases the body's ability to resist infections. It helps remove toxins from the blood.
- Goldenseal contains hydrastine, which acts like an antibiotic. It is a very healing and soothing herb for the mucous membranes. It can help with kidney problems.
- Hydrangea is considered useful for preventing kidney stones from forming. It helps relieve pain when the formations pass through the ureters from the kidney to the bladder.
- Juniper berries are excellent for clearing the blood of uric acid that is retained in the system. This plant helps eliminate yeast infections as well as kidney infections. It also helps to counteract urine retention, kidney stones, pain, bladder discharges, and uric acid buildup.
- Parsley is very effective for the kidneys, bladder, stomach, liver, and gallbladder. It is a great preventive herb and is especially useful when combined with marshmallow. It has a tonic effect on the entire urinary tract and should be used as a preventive aid in kidney infections. It is a very effective diuretic.
- Uva ursi strengthens and tones the urinary tract. It is especially beneficial for bladder and kidney infections. It increases the flow of urine and is useful for inflammatory diseases of the urinary tract, including cystitis.
- Potassium is essential for the urinary tract. The following combination contains herbs that are rich in potassium. It contains elemental potassium, kelp, dipotassium phosphate, alfalfa, dulse, white cabbage leaf, horseradish root, and horsetail.

- Lecithin provides choline. A deficiency of choline has been found to lead to kidney damage.
- Vitamins A and C protect against bladder infections and disease. Vitamin C with bioflavonoids helps prevent the accumulation of toxins in the bladder.
- Magnesium and B6 prevent kidney stones. Chlorophyll cleans and nourishes the kidneys and bladder.

- Acidophilus helps prevent infections.
- Transfer factors found in colostrum are very effective in preventing and helping to heal from acute diseases. Key supplements will help ensure the health of the urinary system.

## ORTHODOX PRESCRIBED MEDICATION

Antibiotics are usually prescribed for kidney and bladder infections. Penicillin is often prescribed for nephritis, or kidney infections. Side effects can include hives, itching, rash, wheezing, diarrhea, nausea, vomiting, blood in urine, excess light-colored urine, and swelling of face and ankles. Antibiotics are a major cause of recurring infections. When antibiotics are prescribed, harmful bacteria have a new opportunity to become resistant. Death from infectious diseases has risen 58 percent worldwide. Most of the deaths are caused by infections in the lungs and the blood that are resistant to antibiotics. Use acidophilus when taking antibiotics. Always wait until the drug is finished, because the drug can interfere with the good bacteria.

# CANCER

Cancer is a severe disorder of the immune system where the cell replication process malfunctions, causing cells to mutate, reproduce rapidly, and invade other organs and tissues. This is known as a malignancy. The basic causes of cancer are environmental, dietary, hereditary, and stress factors that allow normal cells to get out of control. Cancer is a risk for everyone, because we live in an imperfect environment and the body and mind are often under stress. Air pollution, pesticides, food additives, and drugs all contribute to the degree of health we can maintain at any one time. If these chemicals are not eliminated, they accumulate and damage the genetic structure.

Cancer used to be very rare in the United States and was considered a disease of old age. Forty years ago, one in twenty individuals came down with cancer. Now one in three individuals is expected to get cancer. Cancer is found among all ages, including infants. The factors that may contribute to this increase include overeating, depletion of nutrients in the soil, modern food processing, radiation, environmental toxins, and sedentary lifestyles. We are exposed to thousands of carcinogenic substances each day.

There is alarming evidence that chemicals can mimic estrogen in the body, which creates havoc and harm. Lee Davis has argued for more than fifteen years that man-made chemicals can act like hormones in the body, mimicking estrogen or blocking testosterone. These chemicals are found in pesticides used on crops and lawns, some cosmetics, plastic bottles, and dioxin, a bleach found in toilet paper and other paper products.

Diet plays an integral part in the development of cancer. Sugar turns to fat in the liver, and high fat consumption has been linked to breast cancer. Toxins are stored in animal fats, and women who consume a lot of dairy products and meats and eat very little fiber and vegetables are at the highest risk. Since fat is a repository for toxins and women's breasts are comprised mostly of fatty tissues, toxins—including bad estrogen—can accumulate there, raising cancer risks.

In addition, children are more vulnerable to pesticide exposure than an older population. Their organs are developing and their immune systems are not fully developed. Because of their small size, they take in more chemicals per pound of body weight than adults do. A study conducted at the University of Southern California School of Medicine and at the University of North Carolina found children who ate hot dogs once a week doubled their chances of developing brain tumors. Children who consume twelve or more hot dogs a month have nine times the risk of contracting childhood leukemia. The nitrites, chemical preservatives added to hot dogs and other cured meats, seem to be one strong culprit. The body converts nitrites to chemical compounds called nitrosamines. Foods that have these preservatives include bacon, sausage, salami, bologna, and corned beef.

Another suspected contributing factor for cancer, reported in a 1997 issue of the *Journal of the American Medical Association*, is contaminated polio vaccines, given routinely three or four decades ago. Between 1955 and 1963, large batches of polio vaccine were inadvertently contaminated with a monkey virus called simian virus 40 (SV40), which was found to cause cancer in laboratory animals.

Scientists thought then that there was no risk to humans. But recently researchers discovered evidence of SV40 in tissue samples from people stricken with rare childhood brain tumors, as well as bone and abdominal cancers.

## EMOTIONAL NEEDS

How a person deals with stressors will inevitably affect the immune system and resistance to illness. Many recent studies have shown that those with weakened immune systems are more susceptible to serious sickness and disease. For example, one study reveals that women with breast cancer had a greater incidence of emotional trauma—usually five to ten years prior to the onset of the cancer. For those who have cancer, feelings of despair or hopelessness are common and can worsen their condition. Giving emotional support to cancer patients can only improve their physical condition.

## HERBAL COMBINATIONS
### Herbal Combination #1

This formula is well known for its ability to clean the blood and increase the enzyme function of the body. It strengthens the immune system and hormone function so the body can heal itself.

- Burdock prevents inorganic minerals from accumulating in the joints. It is a great blood and lymphatic cleanser, balances hormones, and prevents mineral deposits in joints.
- Slippery elm has cleansing and healing properties. Slippery elm is soothing and healing for the mucous membranes, neutralizes acids in the blood, and nourishes while healing.
- Sheep sorrel can destroy growths in the body. Sheep sorrel is beneficial in eliminating toxins, cleaning the urinary tract, and purifying the blood.
- Turkish rhubarb cleans and nourishes the intestines and blood, neutralizes acids, and is good for liver problems.

### Other Uses

Blood purifier, eczema, liver problems, pancreas, age spots, arthritis, boils, canker sores, erysipelas, infections, jaundice, lymph glands, ringworm, spleen tumors, uric acid buildup, psoriasis, rheumatism, sugar diabetes, undulant fever, venereal disease.

## Herbal Combination #2

This is an excellent formula for cleansing the blood and neutralizing acids. It helps clean and nourish the liver and works as a tonic and antiseptic. It contains nourishing properties while healing.

- Gentian gives strength to the system, tones the stomach, and cleans the blood.
- Irish moss is high in minerals, gives strength to the system, and soothes tissues of the lungs and kidneys.
- Goldenseal has a cleansing action, kills parasites, and strengthens the digestive system.
- Fenugreek dissolves hardened mucus, kills infections, and is rich in vitamins and minerals.
- Safflower clears cholesterol, eliminates gastric disorders, and supports the adrenal glands.
- Myrrh heals the colon and stomach, speeds healing, and stimulates blood flow.
- Yellow dock purifies the blood, stimulates digestion, and improves liver function.
- Black walnut burns up excess toxins in the system and kills parasites and worms.
- Dandelion gives nourishment to the body, destroys acids in the blood, and eliminates toxins.
- Chickweed helps curb appetite, dissolves plaque in the blood vessels, and strengthens the stomach and bowels.
- Catnip is a sedative to the nerves, rids the body of bacteria, and relieves fatigue.
- Cyani is a stimulating tonic for the body and antiseptic to the blood.
- Parthenium contains blood and lymphatic cleansing properties similar to echinacea. It is a natural diuretic and cleans the bladder and kidneys.
- Cascara sagrada cleans and restores bowel function and helps eliminate built-up material on the colon walls.
- Slippery elm contains nourishing and healing properties, cleansing and restoring the intestinal tract.
- Uva ursi heals and strengthens the urinary tract. It contains antiseptic properties to heal infections.
- Oregon grape root is a blood cleanser, stimulates the liver, and aids in the assimilation of nutrients. It is a tonic for all the glands.

### Other Uses

Arthritis, colon, constipation, pain, parasites, skin problems, toxic wastes, tumors, and worms.

## HEALTHFUL SUGGESTIONS

1. Seek out an alternative medical doctor who is willing to treat the whole person and not just the symptoms. Work with a doctor who has a regimen in cleansing, supplements, and the importance of emotional needs. Take a good look at the lifestyle you have been leading and be willing to change. One study found that 88 percent of spontaneous remissions of cancer involved a significant dietary change, mainly toward vegetarianism.

2. Remember that healing can take place at many levels, including physical, emotional, mental, and spiritual. Just learning you have cancer can feel like a death sentence, placing stress on the physical body and causing depression and anxiety. There is always hope, which is a positive attribute, no matter what the diagnosis.

3. Cancer can be brought on by rich and denatured food and environmental toxins, but also by mixing certain foods, such as sweets with breads, meats with carbohydrates, pancakes with syrup, fruits with milk, and other combinations that cause intestinal fermentation, which supplies food for viruses, yeasts, fungi, and carcinogenesis. Proper digestion needs enzymes—not fermentation. Dr. Otto Warburg, a Nobel Prize winner in medicine, is quoted in a book by Paul Pitchford as saying that "a prime cause of cancer is the replacement of the respiration of oxygen in normal body cells by fermentation of sugar."

4. Avoid hormones found in beef, chicken, milk, cheese, and other dairy products. These synthetic hormones, even in small amounts, can accumulate and cause cancer. Antibiotics found in animal products can also weaken the immune system and cause cancer.

5. Natural cleansing therapy is necessary to clean the colon, liver, and blood. The colon is the first area to clean. In *Iridology*, Dr. Bernard Jensen agrees that all sick people have bowel trouble, are tired and worn out, and they are laden with toxins. He says, "Proper bowel function is an essential precondition for staying healthy, and if ill, to overcome sickness and disease. The sewer system must work properly or the body remains soaking in its own putrid waste, encouraging the disease process and forever eluding health-building and vitality-producing forces."

6. Enemas and colonics are very beneficial, especially for serious chronic conditions and stubborn

constipation. Coffee enemas can help stimulate the liver to eliminate toxins.

7. Combinations #1 and #2 in this section are excellent to neutralize acids in the blood and to eliminate them through the colon, along with a colon cleanser.

8. A liver cleanse is important. When toxins and tumors are broken down and the body repairs and rebuilds itself, toxic wastes are released from the cells, which can make a person ill. An herbal liver formula will help clean and rebuild.

9. A lower bowel cleanser is very important to help clean and loosen encrusted material from the colon walls. Look for a lower bowel cleanser that has the following main herbs: cascara sagrada, butternut bark, rhubarb, and burdock. Assisting herbs are fenugreek, couch grass, red clover, slippery elm, licorice, kelp, Irish moss, blue-green algae or other chlorophyll sources, and goldenseal. Transporting herbs are lobelia, fennel, ginger, and peppermint.

10. An herbal fiber formula is essential to help pull out toxins from the colon pockets and prevent further buildup on the colon walls. An excellent fiber formula contains both soluble and insoluble fiber. The insoluble fiber passes through the system without dissolving in water. Its bulk helps make digestion cleaner and faster. Soluble fiber dissolves in water and may help lower blood cholesterol levels. The National Cancer Institute has recommended that people eat at least 20 to 35 grams of fiber each day. A good supplement could contain psyllium hulls, apple fiber, oat bran, guar gum, acacia gum, concentrated cruciferous vegetables, turmeric, and bioflavonoids.

11. Phytonutrients help protect against disease by strengthening the immune system, fighting cell oxidation, and detoxifying the body. Phytonutrients found in broccoli and cauliflower detoxify the liver.

12. Carotenoids are found in red/orange fruits and vegetables and work as antioxidants. Lutein, lignans, flavonoids, polyphenols, terpenes, amino acids, and peptides are phytonutrients found in foods such as garlic, onions, shallots, cauliflower, cabbage, turnips, dark leafy vegetables, and sweet potatoes. Beans, peas, soybeans, and legumes contain protease inhibitors that destroy enzymes that can cause the spread of cancer. Indoles found in mustard greens, broccoli, cauliflower, and cabbage destroy bad estrogen. Carotene found in carrots, sweet potatoes, yams, pumpkins, squash, kale, broccoli, and cantaloupe neutralizes free radicals, enhances the immune system, and may reverse precancerous conditions.

13. In interviewing cancer patients and viewing their lifestyle patterns, the following should be watched, especially when all conditions are present: low thyroid, overproductive adrenals, overproduction of insulin, lack of sleep, stress, and high blood pressure.

## HERBS AND SUPPLEMENTS

Single herbs that stimulate the production of interferon include chlorophyll, astragalus, sea vegetables (i.e., kelp, dulse, and blue-green algae), ginkgo, milk thistle, pau d'arco, schizandra, Siberian ginseng, suma, wheatgrass juice, dong quai, echinacea, red raspberry, ho-shou-wu, germanium, bilberry, and garlic.

- Interferon is an immune booster, produced naturally in the body when proper nutrients are avail-

### BENEFITS WITH DIGESTIVE ENZYMES

All five children in Mary's family seem to have inherited their father's stomach. Cancer surgery resulted in 95 percent of her father's stomach being removed twenty-five years ago. Long before anyone knew her father had any stomach problems, he relied on Tums and Alka-Seltzer to make it through the day and night without the typical symptoms of gastroesophageal reflux disease. The children also used the same medication for their stomach ailments. When Mary learned about the importance of absorbing nutrients in food, she started taking digestive food enzymes, papaya, and mint. As a wonderful side benefit, Mary found that when she took these supplements, she no longer needed the Alka-Seltzer that kept her from vomiting her dinner several times per week. Two of her sisters no longer need their prescriptions for stomach problems and say they go nowhere without taking papaya and mint. They believe that these supplements helped to prevent them from getting cancer like their father.

able. It counteracts viruses, germs, and cancer. Interferon helps regulate immune cells by increasing the production of fighting T cells.

- Antioxidants are important to help prevent free-radical damage that can lead to cancer.
- Vitamin A and beta-carotene are beneficial to protect the lungs and play an important role in the formation of healthy epithelial tissue, which is found in the skin, glands, mucous membranes, organs, and the entire digestive system.
- Vitamin E is an antioxidant and free radical scavenger; it works with selenium to help protect the cells. Vitamin E also protects vitamin A and C from oxidation and helps increase the level of superoxide dismutase, a powerful free radical scavenger produced naturally in the body.
- Vitamin C and bioflavonoids work together as antioxidants, to prevent cancer and strengthen the immune system. They help destroy viruses and bacteria.
- B-complex helps maintain normal cell division and cell function and protects the liver against bad estrogen and other toxins.
- Coenzyme Q10 and germanium help to enhance cellular oxygenation and stimulate the immune system.
- Grapeseed extract is a powerful antioxidant to protect the cells from damage.
- Essential fatty acids, such as evening primrose and borage oils, have demonstrated the ability to inhibit the growth of cancer, especially breast cancer.
- Isoflavones found in soy products (i.e., soymilk and tofu) help balance hormones in humans. Isoflavones inhibit estrogen receptors and may destroy cancer cells. Isoflavone supplements are also available.

## ORTHODOX PRESCRIBED MEDICATION

Tamoxifen is used as a breast cancer therapy and has been reported to cause liver damage, increased occurrence of uterine cancer, severe increase in tumor or bone pain, thromophlebitis, pulmonary embolism, eye changes, corneal opacities, and retinal injury. Megestrol acetate is used in advanced breast and endometrial cancers. It can cause Cushing's syndrome, a hormone disorder of abnormally high blood corticosteroid levels, adrenal suppression, nausea,

dizziness, and vomiting. Cyclophosphamide is used in the treatment of various forms of cancer, such as malignant lymphomas, multiple myeloma, leukemia, and cancers of the breast and ovaries. Possible side effects could be bone marrow depression, fever, chills, sore throat, fatigue, weakness, abnormal bleeding, or bruising. Also, it can cause liver and kidney damage, jaundice, severe inflammation of the bladder, and drug-induced damage of heart and lung tissue. Possible delayed effects include development of other types of cancer. Cyclo-phosphamide is one of the most used chemotherapy drugs and comes from mustard gas. Cisplastin is made of the heavy metal platinum and can cause nerve and kidney damage, hear-

### GAIL HAS NEVER FELT SO GOOD

After many tests at three different hospitals and four blood transfusions, the doctors discovered that Gail had colon cancer and cancer of the lymph nodes. She was too sick to figure out what to do next, so she agreed to have her ascending colon removed. She thought that would be the end of it, but the next thing she knew the doctor wanted to give her chemotherapy, and she was told she only had a 40 percent chance to survive for five years with the chemotherapy and 25 percent chance without it. She was told that she would be back in the hospital within the year to have the remaining colon removed. In the meantime, she was given a pill that was a dewormer for sheep, although her doctor previously told her she had no parasites. Friends told her that because of her high red meat intake, she had parasites.

She told her doctor that she would not take chemotherapy or the dewormer pill. Instead, she immediately started to change her diet—no more meat. She took a parasite cleanse and combinations #1 and #2. She also took chlorophyll, suma, vitamin C, and beta-carotene.

Gail has never felt so good. She has more energy than she has ever had. When she went back to the doctor and had tests run on her colon and blood, they couldn't find the cancer. She is very glad she used an alternative, natural method of healing herself.

ing loss, and seizures. It can cause irreversible loss of motor function, bone marrow suppression, anemia, and blindness.

# CANDIDA

Candida is a parasite that thrives in warm-blooded animals. It is scientifically classified as a fungus and can cause thrush and vaginal infections as well as spread to any part of the body that is weakened. The overgrowth of the fungus *Candida albicans* is known as candidiasis. It debilitates the immune system, and to get it under control, a person must adhere to a strict dietary regimen.

Candida multiplies and develops toxins that circulate in the bloodstream and cause all kinds of symptoms and illnesses. It causes chemical reactions in the body and can produce false estrogen, making the body think it has enough so that estrogen production slows down. It also deceives the body into thinking it has more than enough thyroxine, a thyroid hormone. These results can cause menstrual irregularities and hypothyroid problems. It has been called "the drunk disease," in which the yeast cells, in an overgrowth state, cause production within the body of acetaldehyde and/or alcohol. This production of excessive amounts of alcohol within the body causes even the nondrinker to become drunk. Food can be converted to alcohol in the intestinal tract when starches and sugars are mixed together under the right conditions.

Candida can flourish for a number of reasons, all involving a weakened immune system. The overuse of antibiotics is a serious concern and may be a major factor. Antibiotics are also found in beef, chicken, and dairy products. A high-sugar diet encourages the candida growth. Nutritional deficiencies, birth control pills, steroid hormones, and many drugs weaken the immune system and set the stage for candida growth. Antibiotics are often prescribed even when the infection is viral; this does nothing to kill the virus and only ends up destroying our body's beneficial bacteria. The chlorine added to drinking water upsets the normal bacterial flora of the intestines. Any one thing that disturbs the normal bacterial flora of the intestine can cause candida overgrowth.

The human body was not designed to process large quantities of sugar. Refined sugar and carbohydrates impair the immune system by inhibiting the ability to assimilate nutrients. The overgrowth of candida will not occur overnight. The immune system does not drop significantly in a short period of time. Weakening of the immune system will occur over a period of time due to a number of factors listed above. If you are aware of your body and what it needs to maintain a state of health, candida should not be a problem.

Symptoms can involve many different areas of the body. In the digestive system, there can be bloating, gas, cramps, food allergies, diarrhea, or constipation. In the nervous system, problems can include fatigue, anxiety, depression, memory loss, mood swings, insomnia, or mental confusion. In children, it causes autism, hyperactivity, or learning disabilities. There can also be problems of the skin such as hives, eczema, acne, infections under the nails, and excessive sweating. The urinary tract may also be a problem, with recurrent bladder infections in women. Women may also suffer vaginal infections or PMS symptoms, such as cramps, cravings, water retention, or loss of interest in sex. Men may suffer from chronic anal or rectal itching, prostatitis, impotence, or genital rashes. Other symptoms are fatigue, bad breath, sore throat, chronic infections, thyroid problems, migraine headaches, digestive disorders, depression, feeling disoriented, panic attacks, swollen glands, constipation, or indigestion.

## HERBAL COMBINATIONS
### Herbal Combination #1
This formula is designed to kill and expel parasites, worms, and fungus, and heal and soothe the digestive tract.

- Caprylic acid is a fatty acid found in coconuts and palm oil and is shown to have antifungal properties. It is harmless to friendly gut flora and has the ability to kill both forms of candida, the yeast kind and the invasive mycelial form. It is easily absorbed by the intestinal tract cells. It stops the growth and heals the intestines.
- Elecampane is a natural fungicide, vermifuge, and bactericide. It cleans the liver and digestive organs, helps dissolve mucoid matter, and is rich in inulin, which is healing for the digestive system.

- Black walnut is well known for its ability to expel worms and parasites. It provides oxygen to the blood. It also works to eliminate excessive toxins and fatty materials from the system.
- Red raspberry leaves help in nausea, help prevent hemorrhage, are rich in vitamins and minerals, and help in canker sores, colds, fevers, and flu.

### Other Uses
Parasites, worms, pinworms, fungal infections, and immune system.

### HEALTHFUL SUGGESTIONS
1. Eliminate the foods upon which the fungi thrive. They are sugar, white flour products, yeast breads, wine, beer, fruit juices, cheeses, mushrooms, and vinegar products. Limit fruit to small amounts until the yeast infection is under control. Limit meat and dairy products that have been given antibiotic shots, because this could prolong the healing process. Even eggs can be a problem, so only consume small amounts. Be aware of food combining. It used to be thought that a balanced diet was one that included many different foods at one meal, but actually that is an unbalanced meal. Too many different foods at one time can cause poor absorption, improper digestion, fermentation in the colon, heartburn, gas, and formation of toxins. Simple preparation of food will assure proper digestion, assimilation, and elimination. When proteins and starches are eaten at the same meal, they are in a concentrated form and do not assimilate well together. This is because proteins require an acid medium for digestion, and carbohydrates (starches and sugars) need an alkaline medium for this purpose. An improper combination upsets the digestive system and can cause gas and bloating and a lethargic feeling.

2. Hydrochloric acid and pancreatic enzymes help to prevent yeast overgrowth. Most people are lacking in enzymes, especially when they eat cooked food and only small amounts of raw food. Hydrochloric acid kills worms, parasites, viruses, germs, and bacteria. If hydrochloric acid is lacking, candida can thrive in warm-blooded animals. There are organic glandular pork, lamb, or beef pancreatic enzymes that may benefit some, and others may do well on plant-derived enzymes, which are made from the fungal antigens Aspergillus oryzae. Some are made from herbs and natural products that need to be looked into to see which works the best. Avoid antacids; they eliminate the hydrochloric acid that destroys and prevents fungal infestations. Use natural antacids, such as papaya supplements.

3. Allergies could be a problem. It could be food, molds, or pollen. Eliminate wheat and dairy products first, because they are the most common causes of food allergies. Then look into other allergies, and eliminate one food at a time, taking the pulse test for verification (where you take your pulse thirty minutes before you eat the food, then again thirty minutes after eating the suspected food). There are many foods, preservatives, and additives, such as MSG, that people have reactions to. Reactions can come days after eating the suspected food. Carolee Bateson Koch, DC, ND, in her excellent book *Allergies, Disease in Disguise*, says, "Candida can exist in two forms. The form that is normally seen in the colon is the sugar fermenting or actively reproducing state. In this form it is noninvasive. It does not migrate to other tissues. However, when it changes into its fungal form, it is able to penetrate the cells of the intestine and infiltrate other tissues of the body. In this invasive form, candida is thought to grow mycelia, which are thread-like structures that can penetrate cells and extract nutrients. This can lead to what is called a leaky gut syndrome."

4. Parasites are overlooked by some doctors and are probably more common in the United States than previously suspected. Parasitic infection damages the tissues and the immune system. Giardia is becoming very common in the United States. Giardia is a hard-walled, protein cyst that can get into water and food. These protein-coated organisms are even resistant to chlorine found in the water supplies. These creatures deplete the immune system and can lead to allergies and leaky gut syndrome and can cause all kinds of symptoms.

5. Detoxification is necessary to clean the body of toxins. Colon, parasite, blood, and liver cleanses using herbs are excellent. *The Natural Guide to Colon Health* offers beneficial information on cleanses. Cleansing slowly will gradually clean and nourish the body. Begin to change the diet at the same time. A fast can begin with one meal at a time. If a person is weak, fasting is not advisable; rather, strengthen the body first.

6. Increase fiber in the diet. Psyllium can be taken with a lot of water. Use grains if there is no allergy involved. Use beans, fish, raw and steamed vegetables, and sprouts. Some good grains are millet, brown rice, quinoa, amaranth, spelt, and kamut. Also use yogurt without sugar or fruit added. Use acidophilus, and take on an empty stomach for best results.

7. Consider natural alternatives instead of antifungal drugs. Some doctors are becoming dissatisfied with antifungal drugs such as nystatin. Many are turning toward natural therapies such as acidophilus.

## HERBS AND SUPPLEMENTS

Garlic is a natural antibiotic that helps kill off bad bacteria and fungus; use two cloves daily. Roasting it in the oven with olive oil and spreading it on crackers can be very tasty.

- Pau d'arco contains natural antifungal and antitumor properties, protects the liver, and is beneficial for controlling yeast and molds. It is especially beneficial for *Candida albicans*, a common fungus that some doctors suspect is the underlying cause of allergies to food, chemicals, and molds, as well as disorders of the immune system.
- Acidophilus is very important for supplying the friendly bacteria that are missing when fungal infections take over.
- Caprylic acid is an antifungal fatty acid. It is compared to the antifungal drug nystatin but without the side effects. Look for formulas containing caprylic acid and other products that fight yeast infections.
- Essential fatty acids found in salmon oil, borage, evening primrose oil, black currant, and especially flaxseed oil have strong antifungal properties.
- Pancreatic digestive enzymes help to control fungal growth in the gastrointestinal tract.
- Grapeseed extract is rich in active bioflavonoids and has potent antioxidant properties that neutralize harmful free radicals that can damage tissue and contribute to diseases such as brain dysfunctions, nervous system disorders, and heart disease.
- Coenzyme Q10 and germanium help in overall health and prevent damage to the cells.
- Hydrochloric acid is important for digestion and assimilation, as well as preventing candida overgrowth. A supplement may be necessary if the body is not producing enough.

## THIS BEGAN HER HEALING PROCESS

Karen's health problems started when she had a car accident that dislocated both her arms, right hip, and her right jaw, as well as tearing the ligaments in the jaw. She also had herniated disks in her neck and lower back. She was being cared for by an orthopedic surgeon, a neurologist, a neurosurgeon, an internist, a dentist, an orthodontist, a urologist, a physical therapist, a massage therapist, a chiropractor, and an allergist. After being hospitalized several times, it was discovered that she had a compressed fracture from the accident as well. This went on for a year and a half.

Karen was treated by doctors with muscle relaxants, narcotic pain relievers, sleeping pills, corticosteroids, trigger point injections (from which she went into anaphylactic shock), heat, ice, deep electrical impulses, and finally a TENS unit to block the pain signal to the brain. She had MRIs, CAT scans, X-rays, body scans, diskgrams, electrical muscle testing several times, and much more. She was even in physical therapy three to four times per week for up to six hours at one time, yet she was not getting better.

Karen is a preacher and has a lot of faith. She had prayed continuously, but one night as she cried out in desperation to the Lord to heal her, she said, "Take me home or give me an answer to help my body." After that she felt impressed to get out her Bible and read Genesis, Chapter One. In verse twenty-nine she read, "And God said, behold, I have given you every herb bearing seed, which is upon the face of all the earth, and every tree, in the which is the fruit of a tree yielding seed; to you it shall be for meat." Being a clergywoman, she took this word very seriously. She continued to pray. The word *lobelia* kept entering her mind. She started reading books on nutrition and herbs. She read that lobelia was a major herb that was absorbed better when taken with mullein, one being a catalyst for the other, and both having been used historically for medicinal properties they contained.

Karen had a friend named Pat who told her several times that she needed to get on herbs. After taking lobelia and mullein for one week, she didn't have to take her muscle relaxants, pain pills, sleeping pills, and her five allergy shots per week. The lobelia and mullein relieved the pain, relaxed the muscles, reducing her time in therapy, and cleared up the congestion in her respiratory system.

Karen's body had become so compromised from all the medications that she developed severe candidiasis. She started taking a natural flora formula, a caprylic acid combination #1, and pau d'arco. This got her off the nystatin powder she had been taking for four years with no real freedom from the candida. The herbs have taken care of the problem.

Doctors and the medical field ended up costing her more than one hundred thousand dollars. It took only prayer and one week of herbs to have her up on her feet without excruciating pain. This began her healing process and the telling and retelling of her story as she travels all over the United States and Europe with her ministry

- Glutamic acid and herbal bitters such as goldenseal help dissolve fungal infections.
- Antioxidants such as vitamins A, C with bioflavonoids, E, selenium, and zinc are beneficial for strengthening the immune system. Vitamin C and selenium in high doses have antifungal properties.
- Fiber supplements containing psyllium help clean and regulate colon function. A high-fiber diet is important to prevent bacteria and other harmful toxins from getting into the bloodstream.

## ORTHODOX PRESCRIBED MEDICATION

The drug most often used is nystatin, an antifungal for superficial candidiasis. Topical amphotericin B is effective for candida of the skin and nails, and so is gentian violet, which is also effective for thrush and vaginal infections but is rarely used because it stains the skin. Clotrimazole and miconazole are used in mucous membrane and vaginal infections. Treatment for systemic infection consists of I.V. amphotericin B, flucotosine, or both. Lotrimin is used to treat candida fungal infections in the vagina and fungal skin infections. Side effects may include blistering, burning, hives, irritated skin, itching, peeling, reddened skin, stinging, and swelling due to fluid retention. It is strong and should not be used during the first trimester of pregnancy or by nursing mothers.

# CARDIOVASCULAR DISORDERS

Heart disease, stroke, and related disorders kill more Americans than all other causes of death combined. Heart attacks will strike and kill more than sixty thousand Americans this year and affect more than one hundred thousand. The disease can be in an advanced stage before symptoms even arise. Cardiovascular problems occur when the heart's blood vessels narrow and limit oxygen supply to the heart. This oxygen limitation deprives the blood supply to the heart and can cause chest pains, known as angina pectoris. Hardening of the arteries, or arteriosclerosis, is an abnormal thickening and loss of elasticity of the arterial walls. When the coronary arteries that supply oxygen and nutrients to the heart muscle close up, the flow of blood is cut off completely, and a heart attack occurs, causing damage to the heart muscle. It is also called myocardial infarction. Pressure in the chest, which can extend to the shoulders, arm, neck, or jaw, can be a symptom of a heart attack. Other symptoms are shortness of breath, dizziness, anxiety, fainting, nausea, or loss of speech. Hypertension can lead to heart disorders.

A poor diet is the main cause of cardiovascular disease. Eating too much meat, saturated fats, fried foods, coffee, tobacco, alcohol, and not enough fiber foods, vegetables, fruit, grains, and beans is a contributing factor. A lack of exercise deprives the heart of a sufficient supply of oxygen; a lack of fiber causes fatty deposits in the arteries. A bad diet will invite bacteria and viruses, as well as parasites and worms, to invade the heart and cause infection.

Anxiety, nervousness, and stress can also lead to heart problems, especially when the diet is neglected. Thyroid problems have also been linked to heart problems. Fast living without proper rest and relaxation can put stress on the cardiovascular system. Primary causes of congestive heart failure are hypertension, coronary heart disease, valvular heart disease, congenital heart disease, diabetes, emphysema, and myocarditis.

## EMOTIONAL NEEDS

For some time, we have known that certain personality types are more prone to heart disease. Type A personalities, characterized by perfectionism, intolerance, impatience, etc., may be at higher risk for atherosclerosis. Managing stress and learning to relax are vital to maintaining a healthy cardiovascular system.

## HERBAL COMBINATIONS
### Herbal Combination #1

This is an excellent formula to clean, strengthen, and rebuild the circulatory system. It will help nourish and detoxify the body. It acts as an antioxidant to prevent free-radical damage. Free radicals attack blood vessels, causing blood platelets to clump together, resulting in heart and artery diseases. Free radicals can attack brain cells, causing senility and memory loss. They attack the immune cells and depress the immune system. They can damage the eyes and ears. The vitamins, minerals, amino acids, glandulars, and herbs act as chelating agents to clean the blood. Vitamin A and beta-carotene have antioxidant properties, helping to prevent blindness, slow the aging process, and enhance the immune system.

- B-complex vitamins, including thiamine (B1), riboflavin (B2), niacinamide (B3), pantothenic acid (B5), pyroxidine (B6), folic acid (B9), and cyanocobalamin (B12), help to metabolize fats, proteins, and carbohydrates and improve circulation. B vitamins are utilized as coenzymes in almost all parts of the body. They are essential for healthy nerves, skin, hair, eyes, liver, and mouth. They are also necessary for gastrointestinal health. They provide energy and a feeling of well-being.
- Vitamin C and bioflavonoids work synergistically with antioxidants vitamins A and E. Vitamin C inactivates a variety of viruses, bacteria, and germs. It protects against respiratory infections and is important for the adrenal glands. It is essential for the growth and repair of tissues in all parts of the body. It repairs bone and cartilage. It also helps prevent high blood pressure and atherosclerosis, which can lead to heart attacks and strokes.
- Vitamin E is another vital antioxidant. It helps to prevent cardiovascular disease and cancer. It is needed and utilized by all of the tissues of the body. Vitamin E has been used for conditions such as cataracts, muscular and neuromuscular disease, and in lung, liver, heart, and blood diseases.

- Coenzyme Q10 is a powerful antioxidant that protects the heart and veins from cardiovascular disease. It provides oxygen for the blood to increase stamina and boost energy. It will strengthen the immune system and help normalize blood pressure.
- Free amino acids contain L-cystine and L-methionine, which are chelating amino acids. The free-form amino acids act as chelating agents to eliminate toxic metals from the body. Amino acids are essential for every cell of the body, especially because they help to repair damaged cells.
- Glandular tissue from an animal gland, when used in small amounts, can be picked up by the bloodstream to support and normalize the corresponding glands in humans. It works with amino acids to stimulate and nourish the body and clean the cardiovascular system.
- Ginkgo aids in arterial blood flow, senility, vertigo, tinnitus, depression, memory, and intermittent claudication. It supplies oxygen and nutrition to the brain cells. It can help prevent strokes and increase blood circulation. Because of increased blood circulation, it will help with ear conditions, improve blood flow to the retina, and aid in preventing muscular degeneration.
- Hawthorn berry extract has been found to help dilate blood vessels, resulting in reduced peripheral resistance. It strengthens the heart, lowers blood pressure, and has been found useful in reducing cholesterol and preventing cholesterol deposits. It is known to improve conditions such as arteriosclerosis, angina, heart murmurs, heart valve defects, and cardiac weakness.
- Mineral content includes calcium, magnesium, iodine, manganese, chromium, copper, iron, selenium, and zinc. These minerals are essential for healthy veins. Minerals act as coenzymes and work with vitamins to improve circulatory health.

### Herbal Combination #2

This combination protects against free-radical damage, aids circulation, and helps with cardiovascular diseases. It helps get oxygen to the brain. It contains red clover extract, hawthorn berry extract, capsicum, ginkgo concentrate, folic acid, vitamins B6 and B12, and choline bitartrate.

## Other Uses

Blood cleanser, arteriosclerosis, arthritis, autoimmune diseases, cholesterol, circulatory problems, heart diseases, heavy metal poisoning, and stroke.

## HEALTHFUL SUGGESTIONS

1. The first step would be to change your diet and lifestyle. Stop smoking—tobacco constricts the blood vessels. Limit or stop using caffeine and alcohol products. Avoid drugs if possible, because they only increase the risk of side effects. Eliminate harmful fats, because they raise cholesterol levels, thicken the blood, and interfere with the metabolism of essential fatty acids. Cleansing the blood, liver, and colon is very important to eliminate toxins, viruses, parasites, and whatever interferes with the health of the veins. Some doctors see constipation as the main cause. Constipating foods and drinks are cheese, meat, fried food, white flour, sugar products, dairy products, carbonated drinks, alcohol, and coffee.

2. Go on a cleansing diet. Just changing the diet is the beginning of a blood and cell cleansing. Use herbal colon, blood, and liver cleansers to help neutralize acids in the body and eliminate them. Blood purification is the ultimate of all herbal therapies. When the blood is purified and toxins and acids neutralized, the body can heal itself from disease. The blood and lymph systems carry a multitude of toxins that have accumulated from chemicals, drugs, toxic metals, and poor eating habits.

3. Eat as many raw fruits and vegetables as possible. This preserves the enzymes and nutrients. The bloodstream, liver, kidneys, spleen, pancreas, and immune system depend on these enzymes. There are only two ways to get these necessary enzymes: raw foods and supplements. Enzymes are destroyed in cooking. In other words, if your food is canned, pasteurized, baked, roasted, stewed, or fried, it is devoid of all enzymes. All processed food is devoid of enzymes. Processed food also has rancid oils that cause free-radical damage that can damage the heart, brain, and circulatory system.

4. Add fiber to your diet. Sources of soluble fiber can significantly reduce your risk of developing heart disease. These include dried beans of all types, lentils, split peas, oat bran, rice bran, barley, psyllium, gums, and pectins. Soy fiber is also beneficial in preventing arterial disease. Fiber delays the emptying of stomach contents, which results in less fat absorption. It speeds the transit time, which prevents the absorption of bad fats.

5. Watch your weight. Being overweight increases the risk of developing cardiovascular diseases. The traditional American way of eating has given us an unhealthful appetite for damaging food. We cannot even call it food, for what we eat doesn't begin to satisfy the body's need for nutrition. If it did, our appetites would not be out of control. Changing eating habits is the only permanent way to keep our weight under control.

6. Exercise is very important. Exercise provides oxygen to the blood to prevent heart problems. Even mild exercise three times a week is very helpful. It stimulates the lymphatic flow and blood circulation, which increases the blood flow to the brain and all areas of the body. It can help release hormones that actually make you feel good. Exercise can help relieve built-up anxiety and stress in the body. It can help increase energy and an overall sense of well-being.

## HERBS AND SUPPLEMENTS

Coenzyme Q10 and germanium are powerful antioxidants that work to strengthens veins and provide oxygen for the cells. They strengthen the immune system's ability to clear invading organisms from the blood. They also protect against chemically induced cancer with fewer tumors.

- Germanium has antiviral and anticancer properties and can relieve pain almost instantly in some cases.
- Magnesium and calcium are essential nutrients that work together to improve heart function. The heart is a muscle and needs magnesium to function properly. Research has shown that magnesium can lower blood pressure and help individuals suffering from angina.
- L-carnitine dissolves fatty deposits in the heart and veins. It increases oxygen levels in the blood.
- Ginkgo is a powerful antioxidant and tonic for the brain and blood vessels. It is used in arterial insufficiency, ischemic heart disease, memory loss, tinnitus, and high blood pressure.
- Antioxidants are very important. Vitamins A, beta-carotene, C with bioflavonoids, E, selenium, and

zinc are powerful nutrients used to fight free-radical damage and restore cells. They repair damage caused by oxidation and lipid peroxidation.

- Grape seed extract contains flavonoids that help to reduce the risk of heart disease and cancer. It is a very potent antioxidant that neutralizes harmful free radicals and can help prevent heart attacks, aging, cancer, and immune system disorders.
- Garlic is a natural antibiotic, helps to eliminate toxins from the veins, and is very good for the heart. It also helps to lower cholesterol in the veins.
- Lecithin reduces lipid particles in blood, helps to prevent atherosclerosis, converts fat into energy, and dissolves fatty deposits. It has been used to help in Alzheimer's disease, Parkinson's disease, dementia, and memory loss.
- Essential fatty acids help reduce serum cholesterol levels, dissolve plaque from arterial walls, prevent abnormal blood clotting, lower blood pressure, and have helped in cardiovascular disease.
- Hawthorn berry extract dilates the blood vessels, resulting in reduced peripheral resistance. It also lowers blood pressure and prevents cholesterol deposits. It feeds and strengthens the heart and is used as a cardiac tonic. It improves circulation, fatigue, cholesterol, insomnia, and high blood pressure.
- B-complex vitamins help in the metabolism of carbohydrates, fats, and proteins. They protect

against mental and physical stress. They also enhance the immune system.

- Suma is a powerful herb that enhances energy and promotes longevity. It is considered a tonic for the entire body and helps combat anemia, cholesterol, diabetes, fatigue, and stress while strengthening the immune system.
- Psyllium is high in fiber to help eliminate cholesterol from the veins. It helps to keep the colon clean.
- Red yeast rice is beneficial for lowering cholesterol and maintaining levels within the normal range. It provides nutrition for the circulatory system.

## ORTHODOX PRESCRIBED MEDICATION

Drugs used to treat heart failure are digitalis, diuretics, vasodilators, calcium channel–blocking drugs, and ACE inhibitors. Digoxin is a stimulant in congestive heart failure. Side effects could be headaches, drowsiness, lethargy, confusion, changes in vision, loss of appetite, nausea, hallucinations, disorientation, and heart rhythm disturbances. Captopril treats all degrees of high blood pressure. Side effects can be dizziness, fainting, light-headedness, bone marrow depression, fatigue, weakness, abnormal bleeding, or bruising.

---

**HERBS AND VITAMINS HELP THE BODY TO HEAL ITSELF**

Ora owned a health food store, and one day her cousin came and purchased some of combination #1. He told her he hoped it would help his brother. He also purchased some for his sister and another relative. After the brother had consumed one bottle of this product, Ora found the brother standing outside her shop before she opened up one morning. When he requested another bottle, she questioned him regarding his problem. He immediately rolled up his pant leg and showed her a sore that would not heal until he started taking this formula. He also stated that the doctor was planning to amputate his foot. Thanks to his brother's taking him the product, his leg has healed, and he did not have to have any surgery.

---

**SHE WAS ABLE TO DISCONTINUE ALL MEDICATION**

Maureen learned about herbs after developing a heart irregularity called premature ventricular contraction. Without the three prescriptions she was taking, her heart skipped every third beat. After taking a ginkgo and hawthorn combination for twenty-four hours, she felt better than she had in months. She was able to discontinue all medications without even the slightest irregularity. She later alternated other supplements like hawthorn berries, capsicum, CoQ10, and lecithin. Eventually she needed no supplements for the circulatory system and is grateful to not have a heart irregularity anymore.

# CARPAL TUNNEL SYNDROME

Carpal tunnel is the most common nerve entrapment syndrome. It is a condition that occurs when the median nerve that runs through the carpal tunnel opening in the wrist gets pinched or pressured due to constant repetitive motions. It is seen in workers who perform repetitive tasks, such as painters, carpenters, typesetters, meat cutters, assembly-line workers, musicians, computer workers, and grocery store clerks. People with these types of occupations tend to put a lot of stress on the wrist, which can create pressure on the nerve by overworking the tendons and can cause inflammation and swelling. Carpal tunnel syndrome usually develops over months or years and is the result of continued repetition of movements of the hands or wrists. Women who knit or crochet often may develop this problem.

There is some evidence to support the idea that a change in female sex hormones, which occurs during menopause, may cause an accumulation of fluid or fatty material with subsequent swelling in the wrists. Also, chronic pain in any joint could be related to arthritis. Dr. Arnold Fox believes a low-fat diet will help because fatty deposits in the wrist seem to be one of the main causes. He has seen patients respond to diet change, but as always, prevention is more important in dealing with this syndrome.

Carpal tunnel syndrome can cause numbness or tingling sensations in the thumb or other fingers, such as the middle or index fingers. The loss of dexterity and the inability to perform tasks relating to job performance are serious problems. Weakness in the hand muscles appears to be most severe at night. The pain will become so severe that it will awaken the sufferer. Treatment usually consists of wearing braces or splints at night to keep the wrist from bending.

## HERBAL COMBINATIONS
### Herbal Combination #1
This formula helps to rebuild and heal bones, flesh, and cartilage. It helps to remove toxins and morbid matter from the body. It stops infection, heals, and reduces inflammation. It also contains relaxing properties for faster healing. It contains herbs that are natural sources of calcium and other important minerals.

- Alfalfa is well known for its rich content of vitamins, minerals, proteins, fats, and is a rich source of chlorophyll. It has been researched and found to help lower cholesterol, and it contains antibacterial and antifungal properties. It is used to help remedy poisoning, infections, water retention, muscle spasms, cramps, and digestive problems.
- Marshmallow is rich in vitamin A, zinc, and calcium, which aid in the formation of bones, flesh, and cartilage. It also helps with inflammation and infections and builds the immune system.
- Horsetail is rich in silicon, which is vital in calcium absorption. Silicon has been found to be essential for healing bones and keeping the arteries clean. It is also found to help with bleeding, urinary and prostate disorders, bed-wetting, skin problems, and lung disease.
- Oatstraw is a powerful stimulant and is rich in nutrients to strengthen bones, flesh, and cartilage. It contains antiseptic properties and is an excellent tonic for the whole body. Oatstraw can help with physical fatigue, nervous conditions, depression, and colds.
- Hops is best known for its sedative action and as one of the best nervine herbs. The lupulin found in hops is a sedative and hypnotic drug. It acts as a stimulant to the glands and muscles of the stomach in calming the hyperexcitability of the gastric nerves. It is also used for its antibiotic properties, which are beneficial for sore throats, bronchitis, infections, high fevers, delirium, toothaches, earaches, and pain.
- Plantain is known for easing pain and healing problems in the lower intestinal tract. It will neutralize stomach acids and normalize all stomach secretions. The herb is known to neutralize poisons. It helps with inflammation and swelling. It is rich in calcium and trace minerals.
- Wheatgrass is a rich source of vitamins and minerals. It is high in B vitamins, calcium, iron, and essential fatty acids. It is very high in the amino acids necessary for every function of the body.

**Herbal Combination #2**
Use Herbal Combination #1 under addictions.

**Other Uses**
Any ailment of the body, aches, allergies, arteriosclerosis, arthritis, blood clotting, bursitis, charley horses, colds, colitis, convulsions, cramps, female problems, flu, fractures, gout, headaches, heart palpitations, high blood pressure, hormonal imbalance, hypoglycemia, infections, insomnia, menstrual cramps, pain, nerves, rheumatism, ulcers, varicose veins, water retention, wounds.

## HEALTHFUL SUGGESTIONS

1. Change to a low-fat diet, which inhibits fatty deposits. Use good oils, such as olive oil, in salads and cooking. Foods to emphasize are millet, brown rice, whole grains, lentils, sunflower seeds, salmon, tuna, avocados, fresh fruits, and vegetables, along with some turkey and chicken.

2. Use a typewriter or computer keyboard specifically designed for resting the hands. Change the position of your hands when typing, crocheting, knitting, or using tools to increase and improve circulation.

3. If your job involves repetitive movement, take a break from the activity every thirty to forty minutes. This will help prevent constant pressure for long periods.

4. Avoid beef and pork. Replace them with tofu, soymilk, and soy products for high protein substitution. Soy is also beneficial to prevent cancer cell growth.

5. Eliminate foods from the nightshade family, because they can cause irritation in some people with arthritis or other related diseases. These foods include potatoes, tomatoes, eggplant, green peppers, and tobacco. The solanine in these foods can be neutralized if steamed with miso and parsley or seaweeds.

## HERBS AND SUPPLEMENTS

Glucosamine sulfate has been found to be very beneficial in relieving pain and inflammation in the joints, bones, and flesh. It helps in repairing damaged joints. It is safe and can be used for long periods of time.

- Vitamin B6, 100 mg, along with the complete B-complex vitamins, will help. There is evidence that severe B6 deficiency is seen as a major cofactor in the development of CTS. Repetitive movement aggravates the CTS, but it may not develop without a B6 deficiency.

- Bromelain reduces inflammation, pain, and swelling, and may be a natural treatment for the joint pain and swelling found with carpal tunnel syndrome and arthritic conditions.

- *Ginkgo biloba* provides oxygen in the blood and improves circulation to affected areas. It improves electrical transmission in nerves supplying nutrition to the brain cells. It is a powerful antioxidant to help prevent free-radical damage.

- Essential fatty acids help with inflammations, are necessary for thyroid and adrenal function, strengthen the immune system, and promote healthy blood, nerves, and arteries. They are vital in the transport and breakdown of cholesterol.

- Stress formula #1 found under Attention Deficit Hyperactivity Disorder contains the B vitamins and herbal nervines to help build up the nervous and immune systems.

- Lecithin reduces lipid particles in blood, converts fat into energy, dissolves fatty deposits, and nourishes the nervous system.

- Garlic is a natural antibiotic and analgesic and helps to prevent free-radical damage.

- Willow bark contains salicin, which is an anti-inflammatory and works like aspirin to reduce pain.

- Devil's claw is a natural analgesic and anti-inflammatory. It has been compared to cortisone but has none of the side effects associated with steroids.

- Yucca is a precursor to synthetic cortisone and excellent in controlling swelling and irritation.

- Burdock cleanses, heals, and prevents minerals from depositing in the joints. It helps to reduce joint swelling.

## ORTHODOX PRESCRIBED MEDICATION

Ascriptin is often prescribed for pain and inflammation. It contains aspirin, aluminum hydroxide, calcium carbonate, and magnesium hydroxide. Side effects are stomach irritation, bleeding or ulceration, decreased number of white blood cells and platelets, hemolytic anemia, and possible hearing loss. Indocin and Meclomen are often prescribed for pain and inflammation. Side effects are gastrointestinal pain,

<table>
<tr><td>

**QUICK RELIEF FROM CTS**

Betty's daughter Angie developed carpal tunnel syndrome. She was in severe pain in her wrist and elbow. She had been showing signs of carpal tunnel for some time, but one day it was so bad she couldn't move or lift with her arm. She went to the doctor, and he told her to keep her hand and arm immobile and made an appointment for her with a specialist. So when Angie came home from her first doctor appointment, she and her mother decided that they would try herbs and massage to heal the nerves.

The following is what they used: large amounts of the herbal calcium formula above, aloe vera, bifidophilus, vitamin B6 (three a day), capsicum gel, palm rub and back rub, and chlorophyll liquid. The palm rub was done daily as often as needed. They rubbed from the center of the palm to the fatty tissue of the thumb using a circular motion, going all the way back to the wrist. This was done several times until the pain subsided. Angie eliminated junk food and cut down on red meat and acid-forming foods.

Angie had an appointment with the specialist after they started this treatment, and he feels that she is healing very well. Angie has been able to go back to her regular activities and has done it in less than a month. She is continuing with the program for another month to ensure good nerve health. They feel it would take about three months to heal from carpal tunnel.

</td></tr>
</table>

ulceration, bleeding, possible liver and kidney damage, fluid retention, bone marrow depression, mental depression, and confusion.

# CELIAC DISEASE AND RELATED CONDITIONS

Celiac disease involves a severe intolerance to gluten. It is seen in both children and adults. It is a relative-ly uncommon disorder that can result from a genetic weakness or from environmental factors. One theory is that ingesting gluten may trigger a preexisting immunologic response in a genetically susceptible person. Another theory is that a person with celiac disease may have an enzyme defect that causes an inability to digest gluten. This results in tissue toxicity as well as damage and weakness to the surface membranes of the small bowel. Other causes could be intestinal ailments, changes in intestinal bacteria, drugs or laxatives, and intestinal surgery. This leads to abnormal changes in the lining of the small intestine and impairs absorption of nutrients.

Symptoms of celiac disease may include diarrhea, large and frequently foul-smelling stools that float, anemia, skin rash, nausea, abdominal distention due to flatulence, stomach cramps, weakness, and weight loss. It is also seen as a malabsorption syndrome. Breast-fed babies rarely get celiac disease. Usually the first solid foods introduced to babies are cereals. Babies cannot digest cereals, because the enzyme needed to digest grains is found in the saliva and chewing is necessary. This can irritate the delicate lining of the small intestine, causing it to become damaged and lose the ability to absorb essential nutrients.

## HERBAL COMBINATIONS
### Herbal Combination #1

These herbs help to heal and restore proper function to the stomach, small intestine, and pancreas. Since the villi of the small intestine may be impaired, restoring these is important for the assimilation of nutrients and to prevent malnutrition.

- Goldenseal is soothing and healing to the mucous membranes of the digestive system. It is beneficial in destroying bacteria, viruses, and other toxins in the intestines.
- Juniper berries contain diuretic and antiseptic properties. They work as a blood purifier and help with digestive problems.
- Uva ursi contains antiseptic and antibacterial properties. It helps with yeast infections. It helps to strengthen the kidneys and bladder.
- Cedar berries help restore function to the pancreas with their antibacterial properties.
- Mullein is soothing and healing for the intestinal system, works as a mild diuretic, and eliminates

mucus from the digestive tract. It is beneficial for the small intestine.

- Yarrow is relaxing and healing to the digestive system. It benefits the liver, bladder, and kidneys.
- Slippery elm bark contains mucilage and is rich in essential minerals. It is healing for the gastrointestinal tract.
- Capsicum heals peptic ulcers as well as inflammation in the intestines, arrests bleeding, and soothes and heals the intestines.
- Dandelion is a tonic and stimulant to the liver and intestines. It increases the bile flow and balances indigestion.
- Marshmallow is high in mucilage, which is healing and soothing to the digestive system. It contains vitamins and minerals essential for celiac disease.
- Nettle contains alkaloids that neutralize uric acid. It is rich in iron and chlorophyll to clean and nourish the blood. It is rich in protein, vitamins, and minerals.
- White oak bark is healing and cleansing for inflamed areas and mucous membranes. It contains calcium, manganese, and zinc. It is valuable and nourishes the body.
- Licorice root is healing and relaxing to the system. It contains an expectorant and anti-inflammatory properties. It also helps to strengthen the adrenal glands.
- Garlic bulb is nature's antibiotic. It stimulates cell growth and is a health-builder and disease preventive. Garlic stimulates the lymphatic system to throw off waste materials. It opens the blood vessels and reduces blood pressure.

## Herbal Combination #2

This combination aids in the digestive process, soothing and calming the digestive tract. It contains chamomile flowers, marshmallow root, plantain herb, rose hips, slippery elm bark, and bugleweed herb.

## Other Uses

Blood sugar problems, liver, gallbladder, glucose intolerance, kidneys, pancreas, and spleen.

## HEALTHFUL SUGGESTIONS

1. Eliminate gluten foods such as wheat, barley, and rye grains. Good health can be maintained by eliminating gluten products and giving the small intestines a chance to heal. Read labels to make sure foods do not contain gluten products.

2. Use rice, millet, oats, soybeans, buckwheat, quinoa, and amaranth, which do not contain gluten. Use tofu and soymilk, because they are rich in protein and will help heal the intestines. Spelt is high in protein and is a water-soluble fiber that dissolves easily and allows for assimilation of vital nutrients. Kamut, a type of organic wheat, is rich in protein. It could be tried in small amounts to make sure the body can tolerate it.

3. Strengthen and nourish the spleen and pancreas. Chinese physicians believe that the inability to digest any healthful food is due to a weak spleen, pancreas, or liver. This condition may show symptoms of a lack of energy and the inability to digest food.

4. Foods to heal are carrots, apricots, sweet potatoes, sprouts, fertile eggs, yellow fruits and vegetables, tofu, soymilk, almond milk, legumes, green leafy vegetables, sunflower seeds, berries, avocados, and potatoes.

5. Allergies could be a problem. Some foods are irritating to the gut lining, such as sugar, coffee, tea, rancid oils, and wheat products. Eliminate foods that may be a problem to give the stomach lining time to heal. Celiac causes irritation to the lining of the small intestine and causes food to enter the bloodstream and may lead to allergies.

## HERBS AND SUPPLEMENTS

Single herbs to help include alfalfa, burdock, dandelion, kelp, papaya, saffron, slippery elm, and yellow dock.

- Turmeric has been found as effective as cortisone in reducing inflammation, without the side effects. It is used in Native American medicine. Turmeric kills bacteria, counteracts toxins in the blood, and cleans and improves liver function. Recent studies have found turmeric to have liver-protective properties similar to milk thistle.
- Pancreatic digestive enzymes are necessary to heal the pancreas and clean the undigested protein from the blood and cells.
- Essential fatty acids are healing and nourishing. Use flaxseed, borage, black currant, evening primrose, and salmon oil. They nourish the glands and cells.
- Blue-green algae and chlorophyll supply nutrients

and clean the blood and glands. They help to rebuild a damaged pancreas.

- Free-form amino acids are easily assimilated by the body for healing and nourishing the glands and entire body.
- Acidophilus is necessary to provide friendly bacteria in the intestines.
- Multivitamin and multimineral supplements will help to provide the body with essential nutrients. A supplement is necessary because of malabsorption problems associated with celiac disease.
- Vitamins A and E may be deficient because of the body's inability to absorb fat. B vitamins, vitamin C, and iron can help because they are quickly depleted with cases of diarrhea.
- All minerals must be supplemented, especially calcium and magnesium.
- Use flaxseed and fenugreek seeds steeped in pure water for about twenty minutes and let sit for another twenty minutes. Add fresh ginger and licorice root. This combination is very healing for the mucous membranes.
- Nettle leaf tea encourages the renewal of intestinal villi.
- Lactase supplements may help if levels are low. Adults with celiac disease have been found to be low due to a reduction in epithelial cells and alterations in their function.

## ORTHODOX PRESCRIBED MEDICATION

Prednisone, a steroid, is recommended to reduce inflammation. Side effects could include hives, faintness, indigestion, nausea, vomiting, constipation, diarrhea, headaches, dizziness, and heartbeat irregularities.

# CHEMICAL IMBALANCE

A chemical imbalance is not a disease in itself, but is any condition that alters the normal pattern of chemical reaction in the body. This can take place prior to an illness. Depletion of nutrients experienced in bulimia can create a chemical imbalance in the body. Many women and children are being diagnosed as having a chemical imbalance in the brain. It is seen as an illness that needs antidepressants in

order to replace the natural chemicals that have reached low levels in the body. Drugs only cover up the symptoms; they will not give lasting results.

Many times nutrition is the answer to a chemical imbalance. In order to change the imbalances of the body, get rid of symptoms, and help the body heal itself, you need to supply the body with the necessary nutrients. Correct food, including vitamins, minerals, and herbs, will help the body heal itself. The brain is the seat of emotions and is another organ in the body, requiring proper nourishment (as does any other body organ).

Individuals with a chemical imbalance usually need more nutrients than the average person, or they are not assimilating their nutrients. Because the brain is extremely sensitive, it can suffer even when the body seems strong in other areas; consequently, this condition will alter the functions of neurotransmitters. There are three major neurotransmitters that appear to have a profound effect on the brain: acetylcholine, serotonin, and epinephrine. These are made in the body, but they require dietary biochemical precursors. What we lack in our diet causes an imbalance in these neurotransmitters. Although the kinds of nutrients needed by all humans are the same, some people have a much larger requirement for certain vitamins and minerals in order to recover from their illness.

Symptoms are emotional disturbances, deep depression, confusion, irritability, forgetfulness, and the inability to cope with everyday problems. Evaluating nutritional requirements is necessary in order to understand what the body needs in the case of a chemical imbalance. A healthy liver is essential for a healthy brain, as the liver is responsible for regulating hormones. It helps eliminate estradiol, the unfavorable type of estrogen. If estradiol is allowed to enter the bloodstream, it can travel to the brain and cause depression and bizarre mental manifestations. The one natural source to help chemical reactions in the brain is wholesome food. Intestinal toxemia cannot be overlooked in cases of depression, mental illness, or other types of brain dysfunction.

In the early twentieth century, many medical doctors diagnosed toxemia (self-poisoning) as the major cause of illness. Dr. Henry A. Cotton, a physician involved with performing autopsies on mentally ill patients, found that every body he examined had a colon with one or more problems. Colon problems result in bacterial poisons that eventually act on the nerve supply of the abdominal organs and cause spastic colitis. They also contribute to the atrophy of the bowel walls, resulting in delayed motility, constipation, and stasis. The ileocecal valve soon ceases to function normally and ileal stasis follows.

## HERBAL COMBINATIONS
### Herbal Combination #1

This formula is rich in vitamins, minerals, and herbs that will help maintain the body's nutritional balance. Usually, an imbalance is caused by a lack of nutrients or the inability to assimilate them properly. These supplements are proven necessary for a healthy body.

- Vitamin A is necessary for the healthy formation of the epithelial tissues, which are found almost everywhere in the body. They are found in glands, skin, the mucous membranes, and the respiratory, gastrointestinal, and genitourinary tracts. This vitamin helps to prevent free-radical damage and protects the immune system.
- Beta carotene is converted to vitamin A by the liver. It is an important antioxidant. It is stored in the liver and is used whenever needed.
- Thiamine, B1, is important for the nervous system. Disorders of the nervous system are often associated with a thiamine deficiency. It plays a vital role in the metabolism of carbohydrates in the body. It helps in protecting against illness and helps decrease oxidation of fats in the body.
- Riboflavin, B2, aids in the metabolism of carbohydrates, fats, and proteins. Riboflavin also is involved in the production of hydrochloric acid for proper digestion of protein.
- Niacinamide, B3, is essential for proper circulation and healthy skin and assists in the metabolism of fats, carbohydrates, and protein. It helps strengthen the nervous system.
- Pantothenic acid, B5, assists the adrenal gland in the production of steroids and cortisone. It also converts nutrients into energy. It has been found helpful in treating depression and anxiety.
- Pyridoxine, B6, is necessary for the nervous system, normal brain function, and synthesis of DNA and RNA. It is vital for the production of

hydrochloric acid and the absorption of fats and proteins. It helps in the assimilation of nutrients.
- Cyanocobalamin, B12, is involved in the health and production of the myelin sheath covering the nerves. It is beneficial in many physical and emotional functions, such as confusion, moodiness, memory loss, depression, and psychosis. Studies have shown low levels of B12 in the blood of dementia patients. It aids cell formation and cellular longevity.
- Vitamin C is an excellent antioxidant and works synergistically with vitamin E. It enhances immunity, healthy gums, tissue growth and repair, and adrenal gland function. It promotes wound healing and is vital for the formation of collagen.
- Vitamin D is necessary for calcium and phosphorus absorption and utilization. It helps in the development of bones and teeth. It aids in the prevention of osteoporosis and enhances immunity.
- Vitamin E is an antioxidant and helps prevent cancer and cardiovascular diseases. It improves circulation and tissue repair, reduces blood pressure, and protects against cataracts.
- Biotin maintains strength of the fingernails and contributes to healthy skin and hair. It is beneficial in preventing and treating nervous system disorders. It is useful for disorientation, sleep disorders, memory failure, restless leg syndrome, and tremors.
- Choline is a vital nutrient for optimum nerve function. It is needed for nerve transmission, liver function, and gallbladder regulation. It helps to enhance memory and brain function and prevents fatty deposits in the liver.
- Inositol, along with choline, works in lecithin formation and metabolism of fat and cholesterol. It prevents hardening of the arteries.
- Para-aminobenzoic acid, PABA, is necessary for the metabolism of protein. It is an antioxidant that acts as a coenzyme in the breakdown and utilization of protein.
- Chromium activates many enzymes involved in the metabolism of glucose and the synthesis of proteins. A deficiency is seen in the formation of cataracts, atherosclerosis, and high blood fats. Individuals suffering from diabetes and hypoglycemia may be deficient in this nutrient.
- Copper helps the body absorb and use iron to syn-

thesize hemoglobin. It is also needed for the myelin sheath covering the nerves and for energy production. Copper helps with the formation of bone, collagen, and red blood cells. An early sign of deficiency is osteoporosis.

- Iron is essential for a healthy immune system, energy production, and enzyme function. It helps oxygenate red blood cells and helps form hemoglobin. It is an essential mineral for healthy blood.
- Iodine is necessary for a healthy thyroid gland. It is involved in the metabolism of fat and assists in physical and mental development.
- Selenium is an antioxidant mineral that works with vitamin E to aid production of antibodies. It protects against free-radical damage.
- Calcium is essential for strong bones and teeth, muscle growth, and maintenance of blood pressure. It is vital for nervous disorders, along with magnesium.
- Magnesium assists in calcium and potassium absorption and helps with the metabolism of carbohydrates and other minerals. It also is beneficial for depression, muscle weakness, dizziness, and high blood pressure.
- Manganese is necessary for normal bone growth and reproduction. It is required for the proper function of the nerves and is a component of the enzyme superoxide dismutase (SOD). It prevents free-radical damage and protects against aging processes and cell damage that may lead to cancer.
- Potassium is essential in maintaining the fluid balance in the cells and is used to convert glucose into glycogen for storage. It is used for nerve transmission, muscle contraction, and hormone secretion.
- Zinc is an antioxidant and protects the liver from chemical damage. Low levels are linked with complications during pregnancy, miscarriage, and birth defects. Zinc also helps to heal wounds.

This combination also contains lutein, lycopene, silicon dioxide, alfalfa aerial parts, asparagus stem, broccoli flowers, cabbage leaves, hesperidin, lemon bioflavonoids, rutin, rose hips concentrate, and kelp leaves and stems.

### Herbal Combination #2

Another excellent formula to help restore balance to the body is #1 found under Attention Deficit Hyperactivity Disorder.

### Other Uses

Addictions, autoimmune diseases, nervous disorders, vitamin B deficiency, and malnutrition.

## HEALTHFUL SUGGESTIONS

1. Taking control of one's own health is important. Realize that the health of the body is really up to the individual. Research and study will help you understand how the body works and what it needs to heal itself.

2. Correct nutrition will play an important role in recovering from any illness. Eating whole grains, fruits, and vegetables, instead of refined products, is helpful. Whole grains help the body make melatonin and serotonin in the brain. They help calm the mind. Cooking whole grains in a slow cooker or in a thermos overnight is one way to retain the B-complex vitamins and enzymes. Enzymes are essential for every function of the body. Mixing rye, whole oats, whole wheat, buckwheat, and kamut together and adding almonds and a few currants or dates makes a delicious breakfast.

3. Adding more raw food to the diet helps the body heal. Raw juices provide concentrated nutrients that will heal the body faster. Many people have gone on raw juice diets and healed themselves from heart disease, cancer, and many other diseases. These types of diets work simply because they give the body what it needs to recover. Juices full of minerals are kale, carrot, celery, garlic, parsley, spinach, carrot, and beet greens. Always dilute fruit juices, because they can overtax the pancreas.

4. Exercise increases circulation and helps the body in the healing process. It provides oxygen, the most critical nutrient for the health of the body. Oxygen metabolizes our food and turns it into energy. Oxygen can also destroy or neutralize free radicals.

## HERBS AND SUPPLEMENTS

Single herbs to help with chemical imbalance include alfalfa, kelp, yellow dock, passion flower, hops, skullcap, chamomile, valerian, kava, and St. John's wort. They are high in minerals and vitamins and help stimulate serotonin production in the brain. They will help strengthen the nervous system and brain.

- Valerian is a natural sedative to help regulate nervous disorders.

- St. John's wort is considered one of the best herbs for mood swings. It has helped in mild to moderate depression and in insomnia, helplessness, sadness, and exhaustion.
- Ginkgo provides oxygen to the brain, helps improve chemical imbalances, increases mental function, and helps in mental depression.
- Gotu kola, ginkgo, and suma stimulate brain function and provide oxygen and nutrients to the brain and nervous system.
- Melatonin can be taken to normalize sleep patterns. It should not be taken for long periods. Melatonin is a natural hormone, so when it is used occasionally, your body should have no trouble excreting any excess.
- Amino acid supplements are needed to help the healing of the mind. Diet alone may not provide this important brain stimulant. They should be taken on an empty stomach. Amino acids encourage production of the neurotransmitter epinephrine, which stimulates the brain and increases metabolism.
- Digestive enzymes are necessary for preventing autoimmune diseases. Lack of enzymes prevents cooked food from being properly digested. Enzyme supplements will help heal the body and break down undigested food in the cells and blood.
- Lecithin contains choline and inositol, which boost the neurotransmitter acetylcholine, needed to stimulate memory and learning.
- B-complex vitamins are essential to enhance brain neurotransmitters. B vitamins also boost acetylcholine levels in the brain.
- Vitamins A, D, C, and E help protect the body from free-radical damage. Free radicals are one cause of brain and nervous disorders. These vitamins work with minerals to balance body chemistry.
- Essential fatty acids include flaxseed oil, evening primrose oil, borage oil, salmon oil, and black currant oil. These are required for normal development of the brain and nervous system. They help make a group of chemicals in the body called prostaglandins, hormone-like chemicals that regulate many functions and activities of the body.
- Multimineral supplements are necessary for balancing body chemistry. Calcium, magnesium, and chromium deficiency can lead to depression.

- Blue-green algae, chlorophyll, spirulina, and chlorella are rich in protein. They are also rich in vitamins and minerals and are easily digested. They help nourish and clean the blood.
- Bee pollen is rich in protein and B vitamins, especially B12. It is very important in overcoming depression and imbalances in the body.

## ORTHODOX PRESCRIBED MEDICATION

Tricyclic antidepressants such as Elavil, Tofranil, and Pamelor and selective serotonin reuptake inhibitors such as Prozac and Paxil are often prescribed for depression and chemical imbalances. Tofranil has dozens of side effects, but the most common are nervousness, sleep disorders, stomach and intestinal problems, and tiredness. It is a drug that can be fatal when taken in high enough amounts. It should never be taken with alcohol.

# CHEMICAL POISONING

This has been named multiple chemical sensitivity (MCS) syndrome and environmental illness syndrome. These are real conditions and not all in the mind, as some doctors tell their patients. They usually say, "You will just have to live with it." Dr. Sherry Rogers, MD, who suffered from devastating environmental sensitivities, says that you do not have to learn to live with it. She explains her dramatic recovery and now is helping others understand this destructive and real disease. In her book, *The E.I. Syndrome, An Rx for Environmental Illness*, she says she has helped many people recover from chemical poisoning.

The number of toxic chemicals in our environment is increasing every year. The waste material generated by industry is improperly disposed of and ends up in the drinking water, open fields, and in the air we breathe and will eventually end up in our bodies. More than six thousand chemicals are in commercial use, with another thousand new ones added every year. In addition to these chemicals, we have radiation, petrochemicals, industrial waste, medical and street drugs, and pesticides and herbicides that end up in our food and are very dangerous to the human body. The combination of two or three chemicals that disrupt hormone function in humans is far more powerful than one chemical alone. Dioxins are among the most toxic chemicals known to man and are linked to birth defects and cancer. They are emitted by municipal and industrial incinerators.

Dioxins are also used in many household goods, such as toilet paper, face tissues, tampons, paper towels, milk cartons, juice cartons, coffee filters, tea bags, paper plates and cups, the packaging of TV dinners, and other foods. Dioxin is developed by a chlorine bleaching process and is found in our environment in the air and water. It is only one of the chemicals suspected in immune suppression disorders, liver congestion, cancer, and birth defects.

The Gulf War syndrome is seen as having a devastating effect on soldiers, not because of one toxin, but because of a combination of several. The vaccines administered to the soldiers suppressed the part of the immune system, Th1, which combats viruses and cancers. The Th2 part of the immune system, which ordinarily reacts mildly to pollen or house dust mites, became hypersensitive to outside irritants. This caused the soldiers to become vulnerable to common diseases and to experience highly allergic reactions to what are normally harmless substances. This created new diseases that caused birth defects and autoimmune diseases.

In a special issue of *What Doctors Don't Tell You* on chemical sensitivities, Dr. Zane R. Gard stated that he believes exposure to chemicals leads to autoimmune diseases, such as lupus. He gave an example of an area in Arizona where they have had twenty-five to thirty years of trichloroethylene-type products getting into the water supply. For a population of this size, there should have been only one or two cases of lupus, but they had eighteen. He sees patients with muscular aches, muscle weakness, joint pain, swelling, or early arthritis. In analyzing them, he usually found volatile or aromatic hydrocarbons. These are found in closed buildings with new carpet and poor ventilation, and they poison people. Diseases from chemical poisoning can lead to autoimmune diseases such as lupus, arthritis, scleroderma, Sjögren's syndrome, polymyositis, ankylosing spondylitis, bacteremia (a condition in which bacteria invade the bloodstream), cancer, Epstein-Barr, multiple sclerosis,

tuberculosis (which is increasing in the United States and in South America), glandular problems, intestinal disorders, depression, headaches, fatigue, and eye problems. Symptoms can be chronic problems such as headaches, sinusitis, and nasal cavity inflammation.

## EMOTIONAL NEEDS

Anytime the body is chemically poisoned, the mind is also affected. Consequently, because toxic chemicals can damage the nervous system, behavior may be altered. Symptoms such as depression or other mental changes may be seen.

## HERBAL COMBINATIONS
### Herbal Combination #1

This is a lower bowel formula. It is an excellent combination of herbs to help clean, nourish, and strengthen the bowels. This is considered a natural therapy that will help clean the colon and help the body eliminate toxic chemicals.

- Cascara sagrada restores tone to a relaxed bowel and cleans and nourishes; it also rebuilds a lazy colon. It is a natural laxative without side effects and is non-habit-forming.
- Buckthorn stimulates the bile, is good for constipation, and is calming on the gastrointestinal tract.
- Oregon grape is an excellent blood cleanser, tonic for all glands, and rich in minerals.
- Turkey rhubarb strengthens the intestinal tract, tones the bowels, cleans and heals the entire intestinal tract, and has natural laxative properties.
- Ginger is an internal stimulant, holds herbs together, settles the stomach, and prevents stomach cramps.
- Licorice is a mild laxative, supplies energy, is beneficial for the liver, and eliminates toxins.
- Red clover is a powerful blood cleanser, fights infections, and is high in iron and minerals.
- Capsicum stimulates the bowels, is an internal cleanser, and increases the power of other herbs.
- Couch grass contains antibiotic properties, works as a tonic, cleans the urinary tract, and is a mild diuretic.

## HERBAL COMBINATION #2

This is a Chinese liver formula and is excellent for cleaning and nourishing the liver and the nervous system. It is considered a natural antidepressant and digestive aid. This combination assists the lower bowel formula in cleaning the liver and eliminating toxic chemicals from the blood.

- Bupleurum contains antibacterial properties, is an alterative, detoxifies the liver, promotes bile secretions from the liver, and relieves depression.
- Peony is a natural detoxifier, sedative, and tonic, and when combined with licorice, it can treat diseases of the liver and purify and nourish the blood. It has antibacterial, antifungal, antiviral, and anti-inflammatory properties. It also improves memory.
- Pinella is another Chinese herb used to treat nausea, cancer, bronchitis, dyspepsia, chest pain, and rheumatism.
- Cinnamon is used for indigestion and flatulence and contains antiviral, antibacterial, and antifungal properties.
- Dang gui is a blood tonic, sedative, analgesic, and emmenagogue. It cleans the liver and veins.
- Fushen is a natural diuretic and cardiotonic. It also lowers blood sugar levels and is a natural tranquilizer.
- Zhishi soothes, calms and relaxes tensions, and is a natural expectorant, stomachic, and nervine. It increases circulation and strengthens the heart muscle.
- Scute is a liver tonic and is beneficial for viral hepatitis, nephritis, and jaundice. It has antibacterial properties and is effective against the influenza virus. Scute helps eliminate toxic material.
- Atractylodes has a calming effect and is an appetite stimulant, diuretic, and diaphoric. It is useful for diarrhea, edema, chronic gastritis, nausea, and jaundice.
- *Panax ginseng* strengthens the entire body and enhances memory, stamina, and immune function. It protects the liver from the harmful effect of drugs, alcohol, and toxic chemicals.
- Ginger relaxes the stomach, works as a stimulant, and contains anti-inflammatory properties. Ginger also contains antioxidant properties and increases the effectiveness of other herbs. It has been found to lower cholesterol and promote bile secretions from the liver.
- Licorice protects against chemical damage to the liver, cleans the liver, provides energy, soothes the

intestinal tract, works as an adrenal agent, and is a mild laxative.

## Herbal Combination #3

Another herbal combination that is essential to help clean the body is #2 under cancer. It is very important to help clean the blood and cells of chemical toxin accumulations.

## Other Uses

Age spots, anemia, arthritis, blood purifier, boils, cancer, canker sores, colon, constipation, infections, jaundice, liver, lymph glands, pancreas, poison ivy/oak, rheumatism, scurvy, skin problems, spleen, diabetes, tonsillitis, tumors, undulant fever, uric acid buildup, and venereal diseases.

## HEALTHFUL SUGGESTIONS

1. Realize that toxic chemicals are dangerous and can affect the body, especially young babies and children. Become aware of chemicals in the air, food, and water and discover ways of protecting the body with nutrients. The soil is not only depleted of vital minerals but is contaminated with chemicals to make the food grow faster and prevent diseases to the crops.

2. Chemical toxins contribute to the prevalence of autoimmune diseases. ADHD is common among schoolchildren. Nervous system disorders are common, and antidepressant drugs are prescribed at the highest rate in history. Toxic chemicals can accumulate in the body when little or no supplements of vitamins and minerals are taken. Some chemicals may take years to accumulate.

3. Read labels on food you purchase. Avoid foods labeled irradiated or electronically pasteurized. Watch for preservatives; they can accumulate and cause problems. Avoid packaged foods, because they may be rancid and can cause free-radical damage to the brain and nervous system, as well as other organs of the body.

4. Don't depend on government protection. The powerful industrial world has enormous vested interests and little interest in individual health problems. Take charge of your own health.

5. Fasting is very beneficial, but don't go on a water or all-juice fast. When releasing toxins, heavy metals, or chemicals from the body, they can enter the bloodstream too fast and can cause serious reactions.

6. Change the diet. A diet high in meat and fat accumulates in the fatty tissues. A change of diet is the first step in cleansing. Use fresh vegetable juices, such as carrot, celery, parsley, spinach, garlic, and fresh ginger. But also use millet, brown rice, and steamed vegetables. Use tofu products and soymilk in place of dairy products. Choose organically grown food if you can get it. Use distilled water while cleansing; it acts like a chelating agent. Avoid meat, dairy products, white sugar, and white flour products. Meat and dairy products contain antibiotics and hormones that will further deplete the immune system.

7. Chemical poisoning can put a stress on the body and cause strain and depletion of the body systems. It has a very negative effect on the glandular system. One of the main causes of accumulation of chemical toxins is a lazy colon. The toxins themselves can cause constipation, and due to slow elimination, metabolic by-products and waste material accumulate. These toxic materials can cause fermentation and rancid free radicals that can recirculate into the bloodstream. Since the bloodstream goes to every part of the body and cells, these toxic materials can cause intoxication with many symptoms, such as depression, mental confusion, irritability, fatigue, and allergies.

8. Foods that help eliminate chemical toxins from the body include beans, grains, and vegetables (including garlic, shallots, watercress, and artichokes), and pineapple. Others that can help are soy products, goat's whey, seeds, grains, and olive oil.

## HERBS AND SUPPLEMENTS

Single herbs to help chemical poisoning include burdock, cascara sagrada, dandelion, echinacea, Oregon grape, pau d'arco, red clover, sarsaparilla, alfalfa, aloe vera, angelica, comfrey, goldenseal, gotu kola, marshmallow, dong quai, ginseng, ho-shou-wu, and uva ursi.

- Free-form amino acids with extra sulfur can help, including the amino acids l-cystine and l-methionine, which protect against chemical toxins.
- Multivitamin and multimineral supplements are essential. They help prevent toxins and heavy metals from accumulating in the body.
- Kelp, wheatgrass juice, chlorophyll, and blue-green algae attach to any toxic chemicals and harmlessly carry them out of the body.
- Psyllium is an excellent fiber to pick up toxins and prevent them from entering the bloodstream.

- B-complex vitamins, with extra B6 and B12, help the liver detoxify bad estrogen and other toxins. They help with symptoms such as anxiety, depression, nervousness, and poor memory.
- Essential fatty acids, found in flaxseed, borage, evening primrose, and black currant oils, protect the body, veins, and heart from toxic buildup.
- Grapeseed extract is a powerful antioxidant to prevent damage from free radicals.
- Coenzyme Q10 and germanium provide oxygen to the cells to prevent damage and the accumulation of toxins in the blood and tissues.
- Ginkgo protects against DNA damage. Radiation emits free radicals, which can cause chromosome damage, birth defects, and cancer.

## MEAT WRAPPER SYNDROME

After Joyce spent years of wrapping meat with film made from polyvinyl chloride, which was cut by a hot wire as she wrapped, she would start feeling dizzy every afternoon. She finally went through a series of tests and was told she had an enlarged liver, low-grade fever, and a high white blood cell count. She also had low blood sugar because the liver had so much to do with glucose storage. She also had two large, dark liver spots on the side of her face. This was about twenty years ago, and the doctors told her then that there was nothing wrong with her.

She discovered that she wasn't the only meat wrapper to get sick. It was called "meat wrapper syndrome," and when it became known what the cause was, the markets finally changed the hot cutting wire to a cool, Teflon-coated rod that didn't get coated with the plastic and smoke. Breathing these chemicals is what caused her problems.

She was introduced to herbs and started taking the following formula to help balance her glands: licorice root, safflower, dandelion, and horseradish. She took this formula faithfully for six months and realized that she was free from all the problems she had. Today she takes her herbs, vitamins, and minerals, and she no longer has liver spots on her face.

## CHARLIE'S ANGELS FOR HEALTHY NERVES

Charlie grew up in Montana and felt he was very strong and full of energy. He thought he was an iron man and his health was not any concern. In the 1970s, he became a house painter, along with owning a paint store and fishing shop. He didn't realize the effect it would have on his health. After a few years, his health really slipped, and he spent most nights in the bathroom coughing up fluid and blood. He developed asthma, along with numerous other symptoms. He had constant headaches, raw lungs, and loss of taste and smell. Parts of his body went numb, and he had violent mood swings. He became so toxic that his feet were draining, and he had to soak his socks loose at the end of the day. Everyone was telling him how much his personality had changed.

Charlie's older sister, Sharon, sold herbs and lived in South Dakota. She was very alarmed and was constantly sending him products and begging him to take them. At the time, Charlie could see no value in taking them, and as his situation worsened, he attempted suicide.

Charlie went to a chemical dependency center and was turned away because he was too suicidal. He was sent to a psychiatrist, who put him on antidepressants and then sleeping pills. He continued to paint, and with the medication, his life grew worse and very confusing. After he had a near head-on accident while driving because of the new medication, he was put in another chemical center and put on more antidepressants. The medical profession did seventeen thousand dollars in testing and said counseling would fix him right up. After leaving the center, he became worse and even more suicidal. He had pushed his body to the point that it would literally go no more. His neurologist told him that he couldn't get better and to quit hoping for more—he was lucky he was alive.

In desperation, a friend took him on a plane to see his sister, and she, along with others, put him on a detox and health program. When he returned to Montana two and a half months later, his friends were shocked. The local newspaper ran a front-page article. It was then he decided that he wanted to warn and help others with chemical poisoning.

He was very shocked at how toxins develop from occupation, environment, and drugs. His health is excellent now, and he is so excited to have his life back again. He says that words can't express how hopeless he felt and how the herbs enhanced his quality of life when the drugs only increased his ill health.

The detox program included formulas #1 and #2. He took a formula for blood sugar. He took vitamins and minerals, and now he has three special supplements he takes every day and calls them Charlie's Angels: herbal calcium formula, passion flower, and B-complex. These all help him rebuild and maintain healthy nerves.

- Antioxidant vitamins and minerals protect against free-radical damage. Vitamin A, beta-carotene, and vitamin C with bioflavonoids protect the body from the effects of toxins and eliminate them. Vitamin E, selenium, and zinc are important antioxidants.
- Calcium and magnesium prevent the accumulation of lead and other toxins in the body tissues.
- Milk thistle and pau d'arco protect the liver from damage, clean the blood, and repair liver damage.
- Aloe vera and lecithin repair the myelin sheath of the nerves, which is affected by chemical poisoning. They also protect against the effects of radiation.

# CHILDHOOD DISEASES

Childhood diseases include chicken pox, measles, mumps, rubella (German measles), rheumatic fever, scarlet fever, and whooping cough. Childhood diseases are the body's way of cleansing and healing from inherited or acquired weaknesses. This is a natural process the body provides for eliminating accumulated poisons from the system.

There are natural laws that all acute diseases are the same in nature and purpose and that they run stages of inflammation. These five stages are necessary for cleansing the body. When childhood diseases are not treated naturally and are suppressed with drugs and eating heavy food, the body stores them in the cells and organs, which eventually builds into chronic diseases.

Childhood diseases are an opportunity for the body to cleanse as well as strengthen the immune system. In a June 29, 1996, article in *The Lancet*, researchers from Southampton General Hospital in England reported that measles may well prevent allergies in the future and that having measles is good for the body; in other words, measles makes healthier children.

Germs and viruses are nature's scavengers and can live only on weak cells, toxins in the body, and accumulated mucus. If a child has a strong body, he or she will not get childhood diseases. But when children have access to sugar and dairy products daily and do not have access to natural, wholesome food, the body weakens, inviting germs to feed off the toxins. Sugar is a major culprit in a weakened American diet; it leaches the body of nutrients that are vital for health, which in turn weakens the immune system.

Any childhood disease can have serious complications. The danger is small for strong and healthy children. Be alert for warning signs: high fevers, extreme listlessness, delirium, breathing problems, or extreme pain anywhere in the body. Meningitis is a complication of childhood diseases. It causes inflammation and swelling of the meninges, the tissues around the brain. It causes vomiting, nausea, drowsiness, and aches in the neck or head. A medical practitioner should be contacted immediately if symptoms are severe.

## EMOTIONAL NEEDS

A child is developing mentally, emotionally, and spiritually, and the physical body is developing and eliminating accumulated toxins. When the toxins are suppressed, this slows the growth of the physical body, which can interfere with the emotional level of a child's growth. When childhood diseases are treated naturally, this strengthens all the aspects of a child's life.

## HERBAL COMBINATIONS

### Herbal Combination #1

This combination is excellent for children. It is in powder form, which can be put in water and easily assimilated. This combination helps with inflammation, provides nutrition, and is rich in antioxidants for protecting the cells against free-radical damage.

- Vitamin C is an excellent remedy for childhood diseases to help heal and strengthen the body. It is a rich antioxidant and helps eliminate toxins from the cells.
- Stevia and fructose are natural sweeteners to improve the taste of the drink.
- Chokeberry fruit, blueberry fruit, raspberry fruit, blackberry fruit, and cranberry fruit are rich in antioxidants to clean and nourish the system. They are easily digested and assimilated. They help eliminate toxins from the stomach and colon. The symptoms in childhood diseases eliminate and squeeze toxins and mucous into the stomach, where it can be eliminated from the system. Liquids help the healing process.

### Herbal Combination #2

This herbal formula cleans the blood and liver and protects against invading germs and viruses. It has diuretic and laxative properties. It contains burdock root, pau d'arco bark, red clover tops, sarsaparilla root, yellow dock root, dandelion root, buckthorn bark, cascara sagrada bark, peach bark, yarrow flowers, Oregon grape root, and prickly ash bark.

### Herbal Combination #3

This formula is an all-around herbal combination to help with the following symptoms: allergies, coughs, congestion, ear and eye infections, gland problems, respiratory congestion, other infections, and indigestion. This formula comes in a liquid form that is easier for young children to ingest. It also comes in capsules. It contains boneset, horseradish, mullein, fennel, fenugreek, glycerin, and water.

## HEALTHFUL SUGGESTIONS

1. Childhood diseases should be taken seriously and treated naturally. Keep the child warm and dry. Spend quiet, relaxed time with the child, reading quietly and protecting him or her from overstimulation. Complications can follow childhood diseases if

they are not treated properly. Vegetable broths will help, and use plenty of pure water. For fever, sponging with cool water will help bring it down. Avoid bright light. Be alert for warning signs such as high fever, delirium, listlessness, chest pains, and breathing difficulties.

2. During chicken pox, avoid aspirin because of its known implications in causing Reyes syndrome. Measles can lead to complications such as pneumonia and other lung, ear, and eye infections. Mumps is a contagious viral infection and can spread to the ovaries, pancreas, testicles, and nervous system. Rheumatic fever is a strep infection that can affect the brain, heart, and joints. Scarlet fever is a strep infection with sore throat, swollen lymph glands, and cough. Scarlatina is a mild form of scarlet fever.

3. Homeopathic remedies are beneficial for acute diseases. There are homeopathic medicines for symptoms such as fevers, coughs, inflammation, colds, distress, nervous system, sore throat, pain, and many others.

4. Cleansing the colon and blood purification will help eliminate the toxins. The body is trying to eliminate toxins by dumping them into the stomach, so it is helpful not to eat acid-causing foods. Use juices diluted with pure water and broths using potatoes, carrots, celery, onions, and garlic.

## HERBS AND SUPPLEMENTS

Catnip acts as a sedative on the nervous system. It is useful for many symptoms of childhood diseases, including fevers, convulsions, and insomnia. Catnip is good for restlessness, colic, and as a painkiller, especially for small children and infants.

- Chamomile acts as a soothing sedative and is useful for small babies and children for colds, stomach trouble, and colitis.
- Echinacea is excellent for cleansing the blood and improving lymphatic drainage and is a natural antibiotic. It stimulates the immune system, increasing the body's ability to resist infections.
- Elderflower is an alterative, blood purifier, and cell cleanser. It contains constituents that act as sedatives and pain relievers. It works as an expectorant and has anti-catarrhal and anti-inflammatory properties. It is an excellent remedy for childhood diseases.

- Garlic is nature's antibiotic and will help prevent and heal diseases. It is effective against bacteria. It stimulates the lymphatic system to throw off waste materials, opens the blood vessels, and reduces blood pressure in hypertensive patients.
- Ginger is an excellent herb for the respiratory system and is good for symptoms of childhood diseases such as pain, headaches, congestion, and sore throat. It is excellent for upset stomach and indigestion. It is used in combination with other herbs to enhance their effectiveness.
- B-complex vitamins help the liver detoxify toxins. They help with symptoms such as anxiety, depression, nervousness, and poor memory.
- Essential fatty acids found in flaxseed, borage, fish, evening primrose, and black currant oils protect the body, veins, and heart from toxic buildup.
- Grapeseed extract is a powerful antioxidant to prevent damage from free radicals.
- Antioxidant vitamins and minerals protect against free-radical damage. Vitamins A and C, and beta-carotene with bioflavonoids protect the body from free-radical damage. Vitamin E, selenium, and zinc are vital in protecting against germs and viruses.
- Calcium and magnesium help prevent accumulation of lead and other toxins in the body tissues. They also are nutrients for the heart and bones.

Other single herbs that help are goldenseal, lobelia, mullein, pau d'arco, peppermint, rose hips, slippery elm, and yarrow.

## ORTHODOX PRESCRIBED MEDICATION

Aspirin and Tylenol are usually prescribed for symptoms of childhood diseases. Aspirin is an anti-inflammatory and pain reliever to reduce fever and relieve aches and pains. Side effects of aspirin may include heartburn, nausea, vomiting, bleeding, and stomach ulcers. Tylenol may cause an allergic reaction such as rash, hives, swelling, or difficulty breathing.

# CHRONIC FATIGUE SYNDROME

Chronic fatigue syndrome (CFS) affects about two million people in the United States. More than 85 percent of CFS sufferers are women, usually between the ages of thirty and fifty. But men also suffer from CFS. CFS has been linked to the Epstein-Barr virus, a member of the herpes virus that causes mononucleosis. It's disguised as a low-grade kind of flu that comes and goes as it sees fit. It leaves you chronically run-down and susceptible to illness and many other symptoms that were never a problem before. The long-term symptoms of this virus include extreme fatigue, low stamina, muscle weakness, body aches and pains, swelling of lymph glands in the neck, low-grade fever, flu-like symptoms of chills and fever, sore throat and tongue, headaches, nausea, poor concentration, memory loss, and depression.

The symptoms of CFS resemble many other viral infections, and many individuals with CFS are treated for depression instead of getting to the real cause. Since it is hard to pinpoint the real problem, it is often treated as if the person is a hypochondriac. Most routine tests do not detect any problem.

Research in *What Doctors Don't Tell You* of January 1996 that investigated chronic fatigue and post-polio syndrome showed that the virus that most often triggers chronic fatigue syndrome is closely related to the one that causes polio. It almost seems to be an alternative to polio. Some researchers say that CFS is just another form of polio that has appeared with the use of polio vaccinations. It is estimated that one in every five hundred Americans may have CFS, according to the Centers for Disease Control.

Stress has been implicated as a possible cause, because people with high stress levels seem more prone to develop the disease. Other causes that have been linked to this disorder are mercury poisoning from amalgam fillings, hypoglycemia, anemia, hypothyroidism, sleep apnea, food and chemical allergies, weak adrenal function, parasitic infections, amino acid deficiencies, and *Candida albicans* infections. Candida is a fungus that can prevent the body from utilizing sugars properly by blocking the body's energy production and causing extreme fatigue.

## EMOTIONAL NEEDS

Grief, despair, and other emotional triggers have been linked to increased CFS vulnerability because of the effects of emotional stress on the immune system and the lifestyle changes that often accompany these emotions—like changes in exercise and diet, for instance. People who take on more than they can handle or who deny themselves regular sleep and regenerative activities are more vulnerable to developing CFS. CFS sufferers should make their emotional stresses a priority, so they can direct their energies toward the task of physical healing after they have resolved emotional issues. After their health is restored, preventive measures—like developing constructive ways of dealing with emotional strain—will help reduce the risk of relapse.

## HERBAL COMBINATIONS
### Herbal Combination #1

*Cordyceps sinensis* is a natural Chinese supplement that provides nutrients for relieving fatigue and improving endurance. It helps increase blood supply to the heart and brain. It also helps to increase the production of superoxide dismutase (SOD). In China, it has traditionally been used for the nervous system. It contains a high amount of L-tryptophan and helps strengthen the kidneys and liver.

### Herbal Combination #2

The herbs in this formula help restore energy to the system. It is an excellent combination of herbs to feed and nourish the entire system. It provides nourishment for the adrenals (licorice) and for the thyroid (kelp). It contains bee pollen to nourish and supply energy to the body. It contains barley grass to nourish and clean the blood. It contains schizandra, which is an adaptogen herb that increases the energy supply of cells in the brain, muscles, liver, kidneys, glands, nerves, and in the entire body. It also contains gotu kola, eleuthero, yellow dock, rose hips, and capsicum. This combination of herbs will rebuild the blood, liver, and digestive system.

## HEALTHFUL SUGGESTIONS

1. Exercise is very helpful, and even mild exercise will increase stamina and oxygenate cells. Exercise also helps to improve sleep. Exercise and massage, in combination with elevation of limbs, are believed to stimulate the lymphatic system, which can help strengthen the immune system.

2. Allergies can be involved with CFS. Look into food allergies, chemicals, and heavy metals, and eliminate them. Anytime there is inflammation any-

where in the body accompanied by pain, swelling, heat, and redness, allergies can be suspected. Most people have a few limited foods they eat or like best. Daily consumption of a few specific foods can stress the enzyme systems of the body, making it difficult to handle that certain food. The loss of essential enzymes puts a stress on the body and weakens the immune system.

3. Candida is usually involved when the immune system is weak. A candida diet would help restore natural flora to the system. This fungus can prevent the body from utilizing sugars properly, blocking the body's energy production and causing extreme fatigue. Use acidophilus on an empty stomach to help restore the friendly bacteria. Eat unsweetened yogurt.

4. Look into leaky gut syndrome, which allows germs, viruses, bacteria, worms, and parasites to flourish. This weakens the immune system and the nervous system and causes diseases such as CFS to weaken the body. If the lining of the intestinal tract becomes more permeable than normal, it can lead to serious health concerns. The large spaces that develop between the cells of the gut wall allow toxic material to enter the bloodstream. Under normal conditions these toxic substances could be eliminated, but when leaky gut syndrome occurs, parasites, bacteria, fungi, toxins, fats, and other foreign matter not normally absorbed enter the bloodstream. These microbes can put an enormous strain on the liver and lessen its ability to detoxify.

5. If candida is involved, eliminate sugar, alcohol, mushrooms and all fungi, molds, and yeast in any form, as well as any fermented foods such as sauerkraut, soy sauce, all dry-roasted nuts, potato chips, soda pop, bacon, salt pork, lunch meats, and cheeses of all kinds. Foods that support the immune system include brown rice, millet, whole grains (buckwheat, whole oats, rye, and yellow cornmeal), fresh fruits and vegetables, sprouts, seeds, nut milks, and vegetable juices diluted with pure water. Cleansing the body with lemon water, chlorophyll, and vegetable broths will help heal and strengthen the body.

## HERBS AND SUPPLEMENTS

Single herbs to help include echinacea, garlic, goldenseal, pau d'arco, red clover, burdock, cat's claw, and milk thistle.

- St. John's wort can be a natural alternative to drugs. It contains properties that have positive effects on depression, insomnia, and anxiety attacks. Natural products take longer but have positive effects. Treatment with St. John's wort for mild to moderate depression is as effective as synthetic antidepressants, without side effects.

- Kava kava is generally considered an important herb for insomnia and other nervous conditions, as well as being beneficial for pain relief. It is unlike synthetic drugs, as it does not seem to lose effectiveness over time.

- Glucosamine sulfate with magnesium is very beneficial for chronic fatigue. It helps repair joints and connective tissue. It treats the origin and cause of the disease and acts as a healing agent and a pain reliever. It provides some of the same benefits as anti-inflammatory drugs in controlling pain and inflammation. It actually contributes to the repair of joints that have deteriorated.

- Magnesium is essential to protect the muscles. When under stress, hormones are secreted that initiate a number of different biochemical processes. Magnesium is taken out of muscle cells and replaces calcium. The muscles lose too much magnesium and become more rigid, stiff, and sore.

- Antioxidants are very important to prevent free-radical damage. Vitamin A increases resistance to infection and protects against pollution, cancer, and viral infections. Vitamin E prevents the oxidized state in which cancer cells thrive. It deactivates the free radicals that promote cellular damage, leading to malignancy. Vitamin C with bioflavonoids can activate white blood cells to fight against foreign substances and increase the production of interferon—the body's antivirus protein.

- Grapeseed extract is an antioxidant that acts as a potent free-radical scavenger. Other antioxidants are turmeric, suma, ginkgo, CoQ10, cystine, glutathione, phytochemicals, pycnogenol, selenium, and zinc.

- B-complex vitamins are vital to protect the nervous system, prevent fatigue, and increase resistance to disease. Take extra B12 to prevent anemia and increase energy. B6 helps in the absorption of B12 and in the production of hydrochloric acid. It also helps in depression.

- A multivitamin and mineral supplement is important and necessary for all functions of the body. They are essential for enzyme function. All vitamins and minerals work together.
- Selenium and zinc protect against cancer, but they are lost in food processing. Zinc is also vital for the immune system. It produces histamine that dilates capillaries so that the blood that is carrying the fighting white blood cells can hurry to the scene of an infection and foreign matter in the body.
- Acidophilus improves digestion, combats yeast infections, and helps the body manufacture B vitamins in the intestinal tract.
- Chlorophyll and blue-green algae help the body produce interferon for restoring health.
- Coenzyme Q10 and germanium help oxygenate the cells to promote a healthy immune system and supply oxygen to the blood and brain.
- Essential fatty acids such as evening primrose oil, flaxseed oil, and salmon oil help the body balance glandular function and improve vitality.
- Digestive enzymes are important keys to proper assimilation of nutrients to feed the cells, tissues, and organs of the body.
- Free-form amino acids are easily digested proteins that help heal cells, nourish the body, and increase stamina.

## ORTHODOX PRESCRIBED MEDICATION

CFS is often misdiagnosed as depression or hypochondria. The symptoms are often treated with antibiotics, which will have no effect if it is caused by the Epstein-Barr virus. The most prescribed drugs are the antidepressants. Widely prescribed drugs for depression are fluoxetine (Prozac), paroxetine (Paxil), and sertraline (Zoloft). These drugs inhibit the reuptake of serotonin and allow more of it to remain in the system for longer periods. Most people who suffer from depression have low levels of serotonin in the brain. These drugs are being prescribed for many ailments in both adults and children. The long-term effects of these drugs have not been established. Side effects are insomnia, anxiety, dizziness, nervousness, fatigue, nausea, stomach discomfort, constipation, or diarrhea. Withdrawal symptoms can usually be avoided if a person gradually stops medication over a period of weeks, depending on your doctor's advice, but withdrawal symptoms can include headache, fatigue, and mental confusion.

### IN FACT, HE FELT NORMAL AGAIN

Dan had been plagued with chronic fatigue syndrome for thirty-five years. He had tried many natural supplements that concerned friends had recommended but did not feel long-term benefits. He heard of an herbal company that was going to market cordyceps, and he had never heard of it, even though he was an herbalist. After obtaining a bottle, he took eight capsules the first day and felt remarkably better that day! In fact, he felt normal again. It was indeed a miracle to him.

Not wanting to be deceived and to counter the possible placebo effect, he stopped taking it a few days later and noted that the good effects remained—in other words, some rather stable progress had been made for the first time. He resumed taking cordyceps and continued to improve, each time in proportion to how much he took. The only negative side effect was an increase in vivid dreams occasionally.

# COLDS, FLU, AND FEVERS

Colds are very contagious and easily transmitted at home, school, or work. The common cold brings about inflammation of the mucous membranes of the respiratory passages caused by viruses. It is the body's way of trying to get rid of toxins and poisons built up in the body. An acute catarrh infection can cause chills, scratchy throat, sneezing, backaches, cough, stuffy nose, and headache. Colds, flu, and fevers are part of nature's eliminative process—a safety valve that gives the body a chance for natural healing and recovery. If drugs are used to suppress flu or cold symptoms, the elimination process is inhibited and toxins remain in the body. As long as we continue to suppress the natural process of elimination, the toxic material begins to settle in the organs of the body and can eventually create what we call chronic disease, such as arthritis, diabetes, or asthma, among others.

Modern medical science's theory is to kill the germ and cure the disease. Drug therapies have been developed to suppress the acute disease, but this often complicates the condition or throws it deeper into the organs, causing a chronic disease later. All acute diseases are based on nature's law. Scientists all around the world have been seeking a cure to eliminate the common cold. They will never find a cure for acute diseases, for the diseases are the cure.

Colds are caused by respiratory viruses. One of the most common is the rhinovirus and is spread through hand-to-mouth contact. Symptoms may appear two or three days after being exposed. A runny nose and nasal blockage are more common in colds. A strong immune system can help protect against serious symptoms.

The flu is caused by influenza viruses. This can last as long as three or four weeks, with coughs lingering longer. Aches and pains accompany the flu, as well as a cough, headache, fevers, and a feeling of weakness. The influenza virus causes an infection in the respiratory tract, and a cough and high fever are common. Fevers are the body's way of burning off an infection, and it is part of the cure.

## EMOTIONAL NEEDS

Scientists are discovering that people who experience high stress in the workplace may be more at risk for developing colds and flu. Obviously, immune defenses are impacted by mental stress; in fact, feelings of anger, resentment, and anxiety can actually inhibit T-cell function vital for fighting viral invaders.

## HERBAL COMBINATIONS

There are several herbal formulas that are well known to help relieve the symptoms of the flu, colds, and fevers, and many help to strengthen the immune system, which in turn helps rid the body completely of the condition. For instance, fenugreek and thyme help decongest the sinuses, and garlic is a powerful antibiotic. The following combinations help the body heal itself naturally.

### Herbal Combination #1

This formula is especially beneficial for providing a natural antibiotic to stop infections, heal the mucous membranes, and help with nausea, chills, and fevers.

- Rose hips is rich in vitamin C, well known for fighting colds. It helps inflamed ears, eyes, nose, and throat.
- Chamomile works on inflammations in the ears, eyes, nose, and throat and acts as a mild sedative to relax and calm.
- Slippery elm removes mucus from the system and soothes and nourishes the lungs in cases of colds and coughs.
- Yarrow purifies the blood of waste material and is effective for fevers.
- Capsicum is a natural stimulant to warm the system, help lower fevers, and increase the effectiveness of other herbs.
- Goldenseal is a natural antibiotic. It helps stop infection and heals mucous membranes.
- Myrrh gum contains antiseptic properties and is used as a tonic to stimulate lungs and bronchials.
- Peppermint is excellent for nausea, chills, and cleaning and strengthening the system.
- Sage is good for excessive mucus discharge, fevers, and the lungs.
- Lemongrass is used as an antifever herb for flu, colds, and fevers. It is high in vitamin C.

### Herbal Combination #2

This is very useful for symptoms of colds and flu. It helps the body eliminate toxins and heal at the same time. It is high in sulfur, which helps eliminate toxins.

- Boneset is excellent for the flu and colds. It stimulates the liver to eliminate toxins and strengthens the stomach and spleen.
- Fenugreek dissolves and softens built-up mucus in the body, contains antiseptic properties, and dissolves cholesterol. It soothes and nourishes during colds, flu, and fevers.
- Horseradish contains antibiotic and strong stimulant properties to clear nasal passages and clear infections. It is rich in vitamin C, sulfur, and potassium, which help to heal the body in the case of colds, flu, and fevers.
- Mullein relieves pain and relaxes the body, loosens mucus to be eliminated by the body, and soothes

and nourishes the lungs. It is high in iron, sulfur, magnesium, and potassium to balance the body.

- Fennel contains anticonvulsive and pain-relieving properties, eliminates mucus, soothes the nerves, helps in digestion, and eases coughs and bronchitis.

### Herbal Combination #3

This combination helps relieve symptoms of colds and flu. It helps with circulation, liver, and nerves. It provides energy, kills germs, and helps in weakness. It contains elderberry, reishi mushroom, and astragalus.

### Other Uses

Bronchitis, childhood diseases, ear infections, fevers, flu, general infections, mucus, tonsillitis, and viral infections.

### HEALTHFUL SUGGESTIONS

1. Natural methods create a positive effect on the health of the whole body. If drugs are the method chosen to treat acute disease, the body is hindered in its ability to eliminate the toxins and they remain in the body, usually in the weakest part.

2. Treat fevers naturally; it speeds up the body's healing process. The heart beats faster and the liver increases its activity (destroying more toxins), the kidneys excrete more acids to clean the blood, the glandular system produces more hormones for normal body function, and the body cells produce more interferon to fight illness.

3. Cleansing the colon and blood purification will help eliminate the toxins. Because the body is trying to eliminate toxins by dumping them into the stomach, it is helpful to not eat. When eating during colds, flu, and fevers, the healing and cleansing has to stop so that food can digest. Use herbal teas and citrus juices for cleansing the body. Drink a lot of pure water. Rest is necessary for healing.

4. Homeopathic remedies are beneficial for acute diseases. There are homeopathic medicines for symptoms such as fevers, coughs, inflammation, colds, distress, nervous system, sore throat, pain, and many others.

5. Deep breathing is positive because it pumps oxygen into the system. This will help repair and heal tissues. Take a deep breath through the nose, hold it, and then exhale through the mouth. Deep breathing is important to clean the cells.

6. If your body is weak, eat alkaline foods, such as fruits and vegetables, almond milk, and millet in soups. Use lots of vegetables in soups with millet and drink the broth, which is rich in minerals.

### HERBS AND SUPPLEMENTS

Single herbs to help with colds and flu include alfalfa and mint tea, aloe vera, capsicum, fenugreek, garlic, ginger (settles the stomach), goldenseal, kelp (provides minerals and heals), licorice, lobelia, marshmallow, mullein, passion flower, red raspberry, rose hips, and slippery elm (for coughs and to heal the throat).

- Echinacea will help strengthen the immune system and fight infection. Echinacea activates white blood cells, stimulates immune function, and neutralizes harmful enzymes. It is useful for the prevention and treatment of colds and flu.
- Astragalus is a well-known Chinese tonic and adaptogen. It boosts the immune system and fights viruses, bacteria, and inflammation.
- Aloe vera is very healing and soothing, and it prevents adhesions.
- Transfer factor found in colostrum strengthens the immune system. There are no side effects, and it is beneficial for colds, flu, and fevers.
- Elderberry in tea or syrup will help fight infections, heal, and help eliminate symptoms.
- Garlic promotes expectoration to help cough up mucus. Mash fresh, uncooked garlic into food to receive the best benefits. It is also a natural antibiotic.
- Licorice root contains glycyrrhizin, which inhibits the growth of viruses, germs, and bacteria. It also promotes interferon and activates white blood cells.
- Ephedra clears up congestion and relaxes the airways. It is also a stimulant for the central nervous system.
- Feverfew is used for fevers, inflammation, and pain.
- Ginger is beneficial for colds and flu. It helps relieve pain and nausea.
- Vitamin A and beta-carotene help heal infections. Take high amounts for a few days.
- Vitamin C with bioflavonoids fights infection, increases resistance, and heals capillaries.

## ORTHODOX PRESCRIBED MEDICATION

Antihistamines, cough suppressants, and pain remedies are usually prescribed for colds, flu, and fevers. These interfere with the body's natural healing powers. All antihistamines have potential side effects. Terfenadine, Seldane, astemizole, and Hismanal were pulled off the market because they can cause a very rare and potentially fatal heart arrhythmia. Most antihistamines cause drowsiness and should not be combined with alcohol or antianxiety drugs such as Librium, Valium, or Xanax. Side effects can be water retention, dermatitis, asthma, lupus-like symptoms, rash, or even life-threatening anaphylaxis. These cold and flu suppressant drugs can coat the throat to suppress a cough but will clog the cilia hairs, thus preventing the healing process. If the cilia hairs are clogged too often, it will interfere with the digestion process and cause serious diseases such as celiac disease.

## THE TWO COMBINATIONS WORK EVERY TIME

Renée woke up one morning with a runny nose and watery eyes. When this happens, she can expect to be in bed with a severe cold within eight hours, even though she would start popping cold medicine at the first sign. If she didn't go to bed immediately, she could expect to be on antibiotics for as much as the next four months.

She was desperate not to get sick because she was expected to go out of town to a college basketball game with friends. Then she remembered a friend had told her about the benefits of herbs just a few days before. Her friend suggested she take the Chinese formula #1 and the combination for infections containing the following herbs: parthenium, goldenseal, yarrow, and capsicum. Parthenium is a blood cleanser, excellent for infections, and it cleans the liver and kidneys. Goldenseal is a natural antibiotic, kills poisons in the system, reduces swellings, and is valuable for all catarrh conditions. Yarrow is a blood cleanser, opens pores to permit perspiration, eliminates impurities, and reduces fevers. Capsicum reduces dilated blood vessels in chronic congestion and is a stimulant and disinfectant.

She took the first dose at noon. By 3 p.m. when they got to the game, she felt fine. All her symptoms were gone. She was ecstatic. She continued the herbs for three days. She was so happy that she wasn't going to spend the next week in bed and the next few months on antibiotics. Now, anytime Renée gets the symptoms, she knows just what to do. The two combinations work every time.

## CHRISTIE'S SYMPTOMS WERE GONE

Christie lay in bed; her fever had reached 104 degrees Fahrenheit. Her little body shivered. "Mommy, please help me, I feel so sick," she said. Barbara didn't know what else to do for her. Her two sons had just gotten over whatever it was that was causing Christie to feel so bad. Deep inside herself, Barbara knew that there was an answer somewhere. The doctors in town said it was just another bug going around, and it would have to run its course.

A friend introduced Barbara to a person who knew about herbs. She explained to her some of the products that would help her children to fight infections and viruses and build up their immune systems. Christie was put on a program using combinations #1, #2, and #3. Within a matter of a few hours, all of Christie's symptoms were gone. By that evening she was up and playing. Barbara said, "Since that day, I knew that I had something to give my children—the gift of good health. All the things in this world I could buy for them or even teach them does not compare to giving them days and years without sickness and disease. Each day I hear of people who are feeling better than they have in years, or of people changing their lifestyles for better health."

# COLITIS AND ULCERATIVE COLITIS

Colitis is an inflammation of the colon that causes loose and watery stools (often containing mucus), diarrhea, and bleeding from the rectum. There can be alternate constipation and diarrhea, incomplete emptying of the bowels, and pain. Inflammatory diseases of the colon, such as ulcerative colitis, amoebic colitis, and bacillary dysentery, may also be problems. In the early stages there are abdominal cramps or pain. Instead of being absorbed by the body, water and minerals are rapidly expelled through the lower digestive tract, which can cause dehydration or anemia. Other symptoms are indigestion, headaches, fatigue, and distension. It is a disease of the large intestine and affects an estimated 250,000 people in the United States.

There are different types of colitis that can be mild or serious. Inflammation of the small intestine, such as enteritis and ileitis, is associated with colitis. In severe cases there can be anemia, weight loss, fever, and a tender, bloated stomach. Colitis can also be an allergic reaction, most likely caused by leaky gut syndrome. This causes the intestinal tract to become irritated from certain foods, drugs, or drinks that allow undigested food to enter the bloodstream and cause an allergic reaction in the colon.

## EMOTIONAL NEEDS

It is not uncommon to find that some people suffering from colitis may be internalizing stress or anxiety. For these people, the colon seems particularly vulnerable to feelings of anxiety. Much in the same way that some people experience neck or back problems when stressed, people with colitis often find that symptoms such as chronic diarrhea, constipation, cramping, etc., are directly related to their emotional state. These negative feelings directly impact bowel function; therefore, those with colitis need to recognize how they react to stress and learn to diffuse it through exercise, massage, and meditation.

## HERBAL COMBINATIONS

### Herbal Combination #1

This formula has been designed to soothe, heal, and eliminate impurities in the intestines. It has relaxing, antibacterial, and antifungal properties.

- Marshmallow contains mucilage that aids the bowels and is very healing and soothing.
- Slippery elm soothes, draws out impurities, heals, and acts as a buffer against irritations. It is also very nourishing because of its high protein content.
- Ginger helps hold together all herbs, relieves gas, and settles the stomach.
- Wild yam relaxes the muscles of the stomach and acts as a sedative on the bowels. Healing is beneficial when the body is relaxed.
- Dong quai stimulates the production of interferon to help fight infections. It contains antibacterial and antifungal properties, purifies the blood, and improves circulation.
- Lobelia removes obstructions from any part of the body. It is a powerful relaxant that helps the body heal.

### Other Uses

Indigestion, irritable colon, diarrhea, intestinal mucus, bowel problems, stomach upset.

### Herbal Combination #2

This formula benefits the entire gastrointestinal tract. It supplies nutrients for a healthy colon. It strengthens and heals the stomach, nourishes and cleans the intestines, stimulates bile function, and improves liver health. It dissolves and eliminates mucus from the intestinal tract. It contains nutrients for proper digestion and assimilation. It contains betaine, HCL, pepsin, pancreatin, and bile salts for the upper gastrointestinal system.

- Psyllium hulls, kelp, and chlorophyll clean and nourish the lower bowels.
- Vitamins C, E, A (beta-carotene), selenium, and zinc help prevent free-radical damage. They nourish the intestines and heal damage from leaky gut syndrome.
- Algin, cascara sagrada, bentonite clay, apple pectin, marshmallow root, parthenium root, charcoal, ginger, sodium, copper, and chlorophyll are all very important for cleaning and healing the small and large intestines.

### Other Uses

Autoimmune diseases, acute diseases, high blood pressure, heart problems, diabetes, cancer, and all chronic diseases. It helps in acute diseases because it can help nature clean the toxins, viruses, parasites, and worms from the body.

### HEALTHFUL SUGGESTIONS

1. Allergies can be involved in colitis. Dairy products and gluten-containing grains, such as wheat, rye, and barley, may be a problem. There are other foods that may trigger adverse reactions. Additives, pesticides, herbicides, and many other toxins can increase risk of colitis.

2. Candida can be another problem. It can lead to bowel and other problems. The fungus produces toxins irritating to the digestive tract. A diet eliminating the foods common to yeast overgrowth would help in colitis.

3. Avoid over-the-counter laxatives, sugar, and other refined carbohydrates. Also, insufficient chewing of food can cause problems. Avoid fried food, condiments, and excessive amounts of dairy products, chocolate, and caffeine drinks. Avoid smoking, fumes, chemical sprays, and toxic food additives.

4. Use demulcent herbs as a cleaning therapy. Enemas or colonics may help to clean the bowels. Use mild food until healing takes place. Nervine herbal therapy can speed healing. A change in diet and lifestyle will eventually stabilize peristaltic movements and remove irritation.

5. A few days of fasting using carrot juice and demulcent herbal teas, such as mullein, comfrey, and slippery elm, are healing. Eat steamed carrots, potatoes, sweet potatoes, squash, avocados, eggplant, bananas, grated fresh apples, pears, and peaches.

Apricots are high in iron. Add psyllium to liquids; they are healing for the colon.

### HERBS AND SUPPLEMENTS

Single herbs that can help are aloe vera, alfalfa, dandelion, garlic, hops, kelp, lobelia, marshmallow, myrrh, papaya, pau d'arco, psyllium, skullcap, slippery elm, and yellow dock.

- Essential fatty acids and gamma linolenic acid reduce inflammation by increasing production of prostaglandin. Flaxseed, borage, evening primrose, and salmon oil are all good.
- Demulcent herbs such as comfrey, marshmallow, and slippery elm soothe and heal the lining of the digestive system.
- Licorice root tea or deglycerinized licorice is healing for the intestines.
- Chlorophyll is soothing and healing for the intestines.
- Psyllium seeds are cleansing for the digestive tract.
- Acidophilus protects the body from bad bacteria. It should be used when cleansing the colon. Acidophilus will help in the digestion of food. Take on an empty stomach for best results.
- An amino acid combination helps restore proper function to the bowels. L-glutamine is essential for the regeneration of the lining in the intestinal tract. It also helps reduce water loss and controls diarrhea. Histidine and glycine promote natural secretions of stomach acid and also increase saliva production in the mouth. Amino acids are healing and will digest and assimilate properly.
- Digestive enzymes are very important to break down protein. Lipase breaks down fat, amylase breaks down starch, and cellulase assists in breaking down cellulose. Digestive enzymes will also clean the blood and cells of protein lodged in the body. Viruses, germs, bacteria, parasites, and worms all have protein coatings, and enzymes help eliminate these.
- Hydrochloric acid is necessary to break down protein into amino acids for proper digestion. It destroys bacteria, germs, viruses, parasites, and worms. It is essential for life and the only acid our body produces. It breaks down food to prevent undigested waste residue from entering the bloodstream and causing toxins to damage the cells.

- Essential fatty acids, found in flaxseed, evening primrose, borage, black currant, and salmon oil, are essential for every function of the body. They work with vitamin E to help prevent heart attacks and strokes.
- Antioxidants provide valuable nutrients. Vitamins A, beta-carotene, C with bioflavonoids, E, selenium, and zinc are all beneficial. Antioxidants are very important for healing the digestive system, preventing free radicals from invading the cells, supplying oxygen, and carrying nutrients needed to support the mucous membrane linings. They may also help prevent leaky gut syndrome.
- B-complex vitamins help eliminate toxins in the liver. They are essential for balancing and eliminating bad estrogen from the liver. They are needed for nervous system disorders and depression.
- Blue-green algae and chlorophyll increase oxygen utilization, provide nutrients, and protect against viral diseases.

---

**THE BENEFITS OF COMBINATION #1**

Darlene had ulcerative colitis, and the doctors wanted to do a colostomy on her when she was twenty-eight. She responded well to combination #1, slippery elm, and a lot of acidophilus.

---

**"GOD DESIGNED OUR BODIES TO RUN ON FOOD! HERBS ARE FOOD!"**

Carolyn developed spastic colitis when she was a senior in high school. Twenty years later doctors said that she had breast cancer, for which their only answer was a radical mastectomy, twenty cobalt treatments, and six months of chemotherapy. She said she didn't know she had a choice, and felt panic. She lived through all that, then developed real colon trouble. She went back to her doctor and told him that she was sick and tired of being sick and tired, was there any cure for this spastic colitis? He told her that there was not, go home and learn to live with it.

She went to a health food store and was fortunate to overhear a woman with the same problems she had. She said she took psyllium seeds and a special formula to clean the blood. She tried it and digested her first raw apple in twenty years. She canceled her last mammogram and hasn't been back to a doctor for anything since, and that was nearly seventeen years ago. She says, "God designed our bodies to run on food! Herbs are food!"

---

- Indoles increase the activity of enzymes, destroy toxins, and may also change the hormone estrogen into a benign form. They have the ability to block cancer-causing substances before they enter the cells. They are also found in cruciferous vegetables. However, supplements are stronger.
- Cat's claw is an excellent herb that helps to cleanse the entire intestinal tract. It contains anti-inflammatory properties that are vital for treating diseases such as arthritis and allergies. Some believe it has antiviral and immune-enhancing activity more effective than both echinacea and pau d'arco.

## ORTHODOX PRESCRIBED MEDICATION

Azulfidine is an anti-inflammatory medication prescribed for ulcerative colitis. It is prescribed to decrease severe attacks of ulcerative colitis. Side effects include diarrhea, dizziness, headache, itching, loss of appetite, nausea, sunlight sensitivity, rash, vomiting, aching of joints and muscles, difficulty in swallowing, pale skin, unexplained sore throat, fever, unusual bleeding, bruising, unusual fatigue/weakness, and yellowing of the eyes or skin. Drugs that can cause intestinal diseases are Alka-Seltzer, effervescent antacid and pain reliever, Anturane capsules, Bayer aspirin, Bufferin, Ceptaz, Cuprimine capsules, Feldene, Fortaz, Llosone liquid, Lamprene capsules, Pancrease MT capsules, Prepidil gel, Retrovir capsules, Ticlid tablets, and Vascor, just to name a few.

# CONSTIPATION, TOXIC BUILDUP

Constipation is probably the least understood condition of the body and the most common problem. More than 90 percent of human ailments begin with a congested colon. Even if an individual eliminates three times a day, there could still be a problem with constipation.

A lack of dietary fiber is one of the main causes. The average American ingests white flour and white sugar products, a diet high in meat and fried food, with very little raw vegetables and fruit, and little or no whole grains. With this type of diet, there will be problems in the bowel area. A congested colon will balloon and create pockets and weaken the walls of the colon, allowing bacterial toxins to enter the bloodstream.

Intestinal toxemia or autointoxication is produced by the decomposition of protein in the intestinal tract. In normal digestion, the protein molecules are broken down into twenty amino acids. The amino acids are nontoxic; however, under the influence of bacterial growth they are capable of producing amine, which is highly poisonous and found in a toxic colon. A congested colon causes the poisons to be reabsorbed into the bloodstream and settle in the weakest areas of the body, eventually leading to chronic diseases. These toxins back up into the veins, arteries, lymphatic system, and cells.

There are many types of poisons that can be found in a toxic colon. Some of these are ammonia, agamatine, butyric acid, botulin, cadaverin, cresol, histidine, indican, phenol, skatol, and muscarine. Some of these poisons are highly active and can produce detrimental effects, even in small quantities. In many cases, these toxins can seep out into the bloodstream and poison the rest of the body. Poisons from the colon weaken and stress the heart, irritate the lungs, cause foul breath, settle in the joints and cause pain and stiffness, and cause blemishes, paleness, psoriasis, liver spots, wrinkles, and other facial problems. If the poisons settle in the muscles, they can cause weakness and terrible fatigue and can lead to chronic diseases.

Diarrhea can be a form of constipation. Dr. John Christopher explains that diarrhea occurs when the intestinal tract is clogged and that diarrhea can be caused by an irritation in the colon. Chronic diarrhea is caused when the irritating substance is glued to the walls of the colon and cannot be eliminated. A lower bowel herbal formula will gradually peel off the hardened crust on the colon walls. Not all types of diarrhea are related to constipation. The following can cause diarrhea: food poisoning, parasites, flu, colds, anxiety and conditions (e.g., Crohn's disease), ulcerative colitis, diverticular disease, irritable bowel syndrome, or cancer of the large intestine.

Normal laxatives on the market are harmful and habit-forming. They work against nature and pull liquids and minerals from the body, creating more damage in the long run. Lower bowel herbal formulas are excellent in assisting nature to clean, nourish, rebuild, and restore the bowel's normal function. Herbs work on the root of the problem. With a cleansing diet and then adding raw vegetables and fruit, brown rice, and whole grains, the bowels can be restored to normal function.

Most people have dried fecal matter stored in the colon, preventing food from being properly digested and assimilated. Because of this, many people eat more food than the body requires, trying to get sufficient nutrition, and yet they are still hungry. It may take months to restore the lower bowel area, but by using herbs, food will assimilate better. A person can be sustained on less food with more energy and vitality.

In 1929, Dr. Arbuthnot Lane, a well-respected English physician and colon specialist, made the dramatic statement that constipation was the cause of all the ills of civilization. Dr. Lane had worked for years as a surgeon who continually dealt with bowel problems. His hands-on experience in repeatedly removing sections of diseased bowels provided him with impressive data and a firsthand look at the profound role of the colon in overall health. One of the most striking correlations he discovered was between a malfunctioning colon and seemingly unrelated diseases. He noticed this particular phenomenon when some of his patients, who were recovering from colonic surgery, experienced remarkable cures in other parts of their bodies that had no apparent connection to the colon.

One young boy had suffered from such serious arthritis for several years that at the time of his colon surgery, he was confined to a wheelchair. Six months after the colon surgery, he experienced a complete recovery from the arthritis. A female patient who had suffered with goiter showed signs of remission within six months of her colonic surgery. Dr. Lane was intrigued and subsequently discovered a long list of diseases, ranging from tuberculosis to rheumatism, which were cured when certain diseased sections of the bowel were removed. He found that specific areas of the colon affected certain body organs. Dr. Lane was so impressed with the notion that a toxic bowel could determine the health of other body systems that he completely changed his methods of medical treatment. He spent the last twenty-five years of his life teaching people how to care for the colon through proper nutrition, thereby avoiding the risk of bowel surgery.

He emphasized the importance of transit time, or how long waste material is retained in the colon. The lower end of the intestine is the size that requires emptying every six hours, but by habit, we retain its contents twenty-four hours. The result is ulcers, cancer and other diseases, and symptoms like an enlarged abdomen, discomfort, headaches, depression, anxiety, irritability, fatigue, exhaustion, indigestion, gas, insomnia and frequent waking up in the night, overweight, malnutrition, glandular imbalance, lower back pain, and skin, hair, and nail problems. The main cause is lack of fiber in the diet, which slows the elimination of fecal matter, allowing toxins to infect colon pockets. Adhesions can be a cause of constipation due to infected mucous membranes of the bowel wall. Other causes include a stretched colon from overload of food contents; ileocecal valve incompetence, which allows bowel content to reenter the small intestine and damage organs, joints, nerves, and the immune system; and lack of exercise, especially in the abdominal area.

Poor posture can interfere with the voluntary and reflex contractions of the important muscles necessary for normal elimination. Constipation causes hemorrhoids, and hemorrhoids cause spasms or tightness of the anal muscle and prevent normal bowel elimination. Weak bowel muscles can become paralyzed and prevent complete emptying of the bowels. This allows toxins from the fecal matter to irritate the mucous membranes and produce chronic catarrh, infections, adhesions, and even cancer. Lack of liquids causes dehydration, which creates hard fecal matter and prevents normal elimination. Lack of water is usually the cause. Lack of hydrochloric acid and digestive enzymes can eventually lead to constipation and autointoxication.

The lack of fiber and eating large amounts of mucus-forming food causes the body to produce excess amounts of mucus to protect the intestines from absorbing toxins. This mucus medium develops and slows the transit time through the colon walls. This causes the contents to remain in the colon longer than they should. Moisture is pulled from the contents and becomes packed together and hardens on the intestinal walls. If a lot of fat and white flour products are eaten, it causes a glue-like substance to stick to the colon walls. As this glue-like material hardens, it builds up on the colon walls layer after layer and becomes rubbery and hard. The pockets of the colon collect this hard material because it has a strong adherence that does not allow it to pass from the body with the daily bowel eliminations.

When cooked food is eaten, the T cells come to the rescue, because they recognize food without enzymes as a foreign invader. This puts a burden on the immune system, eventually weakening it. Mucus is also formed to protect the body from poisons. If cooked and processed food is eaten day after day without raw food and fiber, the contents eventually build up on the colon walls like rings around a tree. This causes the immune system to become overworked and creates a medium for germs, viruses, parasites, and worms to invade the body. Autoimmune diseases develop, because the immune system is confused and overworked and begins to attack the body. We have overstimulated and overworked the immune and digestive systems, and they can no longer protect us.

## HERBAL COMBINATIONS
### Herbal Combination #1
This formula is excellent to help clean, nourish, and restore natural function to the bowels.

- Cascara sagrada restores tone to a relaxed bowel and cleans and nourishes the colon.
- Buckthorn stimulates the bile, relieves constipation, and is calming on the gastrointestinal tract.

- Oregon grape stimulates liver function and aids in the assimilation of nutrients, as well as being an excellent blood cleanser.
- Licorice milk laxative supplies energy and is beneficial to the liver.
- Capsicum stimulates the bowels, is an internal cleanser, and increases the power of all the other herbs taken.
- Ginger is an internal stimulant, holds herbs together, settles the stomach, and relaxes the colon.
- Couch grass is a natural antibiotic and tonic, cleans the urinary tract, and acts as a mild diuretic.
- Red clover cleans mucus from the system and fights infection, and is high in iron and minerals.
- Turkey rhubarb strengthens the intestinal tract, tones the bowels, cleans and heals the entire intestinal tract, and has natural laxative properties.

### Herbal Combination #2

- Cascara sagrada stimulates the gall bladder and adrenal glands and helps with liver problems.
- Turkey rhubarb root reduces blood pressure and inflammations, and it is good for chronic diarrhea.
- Dong quai is a natural bowel relaxant and lubricant, has antibiotic properties, and cleans and purifies the blood.
- Goldenseal is a strong antibiotic, relieves inflammations, strengthens the liver, and contains healing properties.
- Capsicum increases blood circulation and distributes herbs throughout the system.
- Ginger binds other herbs together, helps with intestinal gas, and is soothing to the nervous system.
- Fennel relieves gas, colic, and cramps, as well as nourishing the system.
- Red raspberry is good for stomach problems and strengthens the system in addition to supplying valuable nutrients.
- Oregon grape stimulates liver function and aids in the assimilation of nutrients, as well as being an excellent blood cleanser.
- Lobelia removes obstruction in the system, acts as an expectorant, and relieves spasms.

### Other Uses

Bad breath, bowel discomforts, cleansing, colitis, colon, croup, diarrhea, intestinal mucus, parasites, acute diseases, and chronic diseases.

## HEALTHFUL SUGGESTIONS

1. Lifestyle changes need to be made. Eliminate alcohol, tobacco, carbonated drinks, white flour and sugar products, and greasy food. Increase dietary fiber and raw foods and reduce meat and fat. This will decrease the accumulation of bad bacteria while building and protecting the immune system.

2. Exercise is important, especially for the abdominal area. Jumping on a mini-trampoline and walking are good exercises. Using a rowing machine and doing squatting exercises will strengthen the abdomen and intestinal system. Also, remember that it is important to use the restroom as soon as the urge arises.

3. Learn to listen to the inner body and eat only when hungry. Avoid eating when emotionally upset. Learn to combine foods that digest well together. Combining meat and sugar and starch will cause fermentation and create an alcohol substance in the stomach and intestines. Learn about your own body and your particular weaknesses and what nutrients will build and maintain physical, emotional, and mental health.

4. Eliminate over-the-counter laxatives, because they interfere with the proper absorption of sodium and with potassium balance in the large intestine. Laxatives pull water and minerals from the body.

5. Add more whole grains, such as whole wheat, whole oats, brown rice, millet, kamut, buckwheat, yellow cornmeal (polenta dishes are delicious), amaranth, quinoa, and spelt. Whole grains provide fiber, the fatty acids, and B vitamins and minerals when in their whole state. Cooking in a slow cooker or thermos overnight is very nutritional. Chew food longer to assure enzyme activity and to help prevent constipation. Chewing longer satisfies hunger and prevents indigestion.

6. Juice fasting for one to three days will start a cleansing of the bowels. Good juice combinations are carrot, celery, parsley and garlic or cabbage, and ginger. Wheatgrass juice is cleansing for the colon and blood. Some have benefited from a wheatgrass and garlic enema to speed colon cleansing.

7. A liver flush is very beneficial with all the toxins in water, food, and air. First thing in the morning, mix one cup of warm water, the juice of one lime or lemon, one capsule ginger or one teaspoon fresh ginger, and one teaspoon pure olive oil in a blender.

> **IN NO TIME SHE WAS FREE OF HER MEDICATION**
>
> Anna was plagued with sinusitis, bronchitis, hemorrhoids, and varicose veins most of her life. She had no idea it was due to constipation. She discovered the formula #1, and within weeks she started feeling better. In no time she was free of her medication for bronchitis and sinusitis, and her hemorrhoids and varicose veins were gone. She also suffered from skin rashes so bad she would at times get blood poisoning. She never had a skin problem again once she cleaned her colon and kept it clean. She changed her diet, eliminated milk, and used herbs for cleansing the blood and liver. She started using more grains, vegetables, fruit, nuts, seeds, and herbs, and ate less meat, white sugar, and white flour products.

This will clean and stimulate liver function. A psyllium herbal formula is beneficial for cleansing deep into the pockets of the colon. A flaxseed tea is also helpful for the colon. Soak a tablespoon of flaxseed in a pint of pure water overnight. Mix in blender, strain, and drink a cup twice a day. Plain yogurt, made from live culture, is very nourishing for the bowels. It provides friendly bacteria in the bowels and builds immunity to disease.

### HERBS AND SUPPLEMENTS

Single herbs to help with constipation include aloe vera, alfalfa, barberry, buckthorn, burdock, cascara sagrada, fenugreek, licorice, and psyllium.

- Psyllium hull herbal formulas work very well. Drink first thing in the morning with a lot of water. Psyllium should be taken with a full glass of water or it could plug up the intestines. Add more fiber to the diet.
- Acidophilus is used to protect the body from bad bacteria. It is necessary to use when cleansing the colon. It also helps in the digestion of food.
- Blue-green algae neutralizes toxins in the blood, nourishes the body, increases oxygen utilization, and protects against viral diseases.
- Indoles increase the activity of enzymes, destroy toxins, and may also change the hormone estrogen into a benign form. They have the ability to block cancer-causing substances before they enter the cells. They are also found in cruciferous vegetables.
- Essential fatty acids, found in flaxseed, evening primrose, borage, black currant, and salmon oils, are essential for every function of the body. They work with vitamin E to help prevent heart attacks and strokes.
- Hydrochloric acid is necessary to break down protein into amino acids for proper digestion. It destroys bacteria, germs, viruses, parasites, and worms. It is essential for life, and the only acid our body produces. It breaks down food to prevent undigested waste residue from entering the bloodstream and causing toxins to damage the cells.
- Digestive enzymes are needed to help break down any undigested food in the transverse colon, where putrefaction occurs when food remains too long in that area. They improve elimination and neutralize the odor in stools.
- Amino acids help restore proper function to the bowels. Histidine and glycine promote natural secretions of stomach acid and also increase saliva production in the mouth. Amino acids are healing and will digest and assimilate properly. B-complex vitamins help regulate and eliminate toxins in the liver. They are especially essential for balancing and eliminating bad estrogen from the liver. They are also needed for nervous system disorders and depression.

### ORTHODOX PRESCRIBED MEDICATION

Saline laxatives, such as Epsom salts or milk of magnesia, draw water and electrolytes and can alter the body's fluid and electrolyte balance. Mineral oil is sometimes recommended but can leach out vitamins A, D, and E. Any artificial laxatives, if used too often, can cause a dependence and create a lazy bowel syndrome. Drugs that can cause constipation are diuretics, antidepressants, antihistamines, painkillers, or tranquilizers.

# CROHN'S DISEASE

Approximately two million Americans suffer from Crohn's disease and ulcerative colitis. These are among diseases referred to as inflammatory bowel disease (IBD). This disease is becoming more and more common, which is significant, because if it is left untreated, it can lead to cancer. Crohn's disease is an inflammation of any portion of the gastrointestinal tract and extends through all layers of the intestinal wall. Symptoms are diarrhea, abdominal pain, rectal bleeding, anemia, weight loss, abdominal infections, and low stress tolerance.

Doctors are puzzled as to the cause of this sickness. However, there is speculation by some in the medical profession that it is related to allergies, other immune disorders, or an overburdened lymphatic system. Medical professionals generally treat Crohn's disease with steroids and antibiotics. When medical therapy is not effective, surgical removal of the diseased area may be necessary. Crohn's disease is an autoimmune disorder. The digestive tract is overtaxed with the constant eating of cooked food without enzymes to break it down. The body becomes so toxic from many years of toxic buildup from medications and poor eating habits that the immune system becomes confused. It then attacks the toxic tissues and begins to destroy them, thinking they are foreign organisms. Another cause or result is parasite infestation, which further debilitates the immune system.

## HERBAL COMBINATIONS
### Herbal Combination #1
This formula is very rich in soluble fiber, with more than eight times that of oat bran. It provides necessary bulk to clean the pockets of the colon, heal, and prevent a buildup of toxic material.

- Psyllium is an excellent intestinal cleanser. It does not irritate the mucous membranes of the intestines but strengthens the tissues and restores tone. It lubricates and heals the intestines and colon.
- Hibiscus flower is an antispasmodic and nervine herb, relaxing for the intestines.
- Licorice root helps reduce inflammation of the intestinal tract, counteract stress, and supply energy to the body.

### Herbal Combination #2
This combination helps clean, heal, and rebuild the intestinal system. It contains chamomile, marshmallow, plantain, rose hips, slippery elm, and buglewood.

## Other Uses
Constipation, colon blockage, diverticulitis, colitis, gonorrhea, dysentery, intestinal tract, ulcers, urinary tract.

## HEALTHFUL SUGGESTIONS
1. Eliminate mucus-producing foods such as refined pastries, partially digested meats, dairy products, junk food, pork, chocolate, alcohol, caffeine, and tobacco. These products contribute to the slime on which the microbes thrive. They are also void of live enzymes to speed the healing of the digestive system.

2. Look into allergies that can irritate the gut lining and cause leaky gut syndrome. The most common allergic foods are cheese, dairy products, wheat, chocolate, coffee, eggs, citrus (usually not tree-ripened), tea, corn, barley, oats, and rye. It is usually the food that is eaten every day. The body may become used to one type of food, and over time it begins to irritate the mucous membranes.

3. Digestive problems are one cause of an irritable gut lining. The lack of hydrochloric acid and pepsin in the stomach may lead to disorders. Inadequate secretions of digestive enzymes by the pancreas can also be a problem. Undigested food remnants irritate the lower digestive tract and cause leaky gut syndrome, which can lead to many other diseases.

4. A cleansing program is necessary to clean and repair the damage that has been done to the intestines. Eliminate parasites by taking a lower bowel formula, blood cleanser, and liver cleanser. These steps will enable the body to begin the job of repairing the damage. The body will heal itself, given the proper tools.

5. Juice fasting will take the burden off the digestive system and supply nutrients to the GI tract. Carrot, cabbage, parsley, and ginger taken together will heal. Always dilute the juices so as to not overburden the pancreas. A juice combination of carrot, celery, endive, and garlic is healing. Vegetable soups are healing, as they are rich in minerals. No healing can take place without minerals. An herbal mineral drink, high in potassium, will heal the mucous membranes. Potassium is essential for good digestion. Use garlic and ginger in soups; they will heal and kill parasites. Millet is easy to digest and is healing and high in minerals, especially calcium and magnesium, and is also high in protein. Cook grains

and vegetables in a thermos overnight using pure water and drink the juice; it is rich in enzymes for healing. Well-tolerated foods are brown rice, millet, sweet potatoes, winter squash, non-citrus fruits, and yellow and green vegetables.

6. Watch food combining. It is important, because foods such as sweets combined with meat or grains can cause fermentation and irritation. Eat meat or grains with vegetables. Eat fruit alone; it digests quickly, and if you eat it with meat or carbohydrates it causes fermentation.

## HERBS AND SUPPLEMENTS

Single herbs that can help with Crohn's disease include aloe vera (healing and prevents adhesions), alfalfa (provides minerals and vitamins), dandelion (cleans liver), garlic, hops, kelp, lobelia, marshmallow, myrrh, papaya, psyllium, skullcap (repairs nerves), slippery elm (food for the colon), and yellow dock (rich in iron).

- Aloe vera juice heals inflammation, enhances digestion, cleans the colon, and heals adhesions.
- Acidophilus heals, helps the body digest food, and protects it from bad bacteria.
- Blue-green algae and chlorophyll are rich in minerals and are cleansing and healing for the digestive tract.
- Wheatgrass is also healing.
- Slippery elm is healing and nourishing for the digestive tract. It is soothing while restoring normal function.
- Goldenseal and capsicum are excellent for healing internal bleeding and inflammation.
- Licorice root contains antiviral properties and is healing for the digestive tract.
- Germanium and CoQ10 fortify the immune system and aid in healing damaged tissues due to their oxygenation properties.
- Essential fatty acids, including flaxseed, borage, evening primrose, and salmon oils, are healing and nourishing for the digestive tract.
- Cat's claw cleans the intestinal system and contains anti-inflammatory and healing properties.
- Red clover herbal formulas clean and heal the blood and digestive tract. They should contain red clover, buckthorn, burdock, echinacea, licorice, prickly ash, and sheep sorrel.
- Nervine formulas will strengthen the nervous system. Formulas usually include herbs like passion flower, skullcap, hops, valerian, kava, wild yam, and St. John's wort.
- Olive leaf extract supports the immune system to fight diseases, strengthens the circulatory system, and protects against free-radical damage.
- Colloidal silver acts as a natural antiseptic and disinfectant and helps in colds, flu, and childhood diseases. It is used for dysentery and infections in the body.
- Colostrum strengthens the immune system to fight infections and diseases.

## ORTHODOX PRESCRIBED MEDICATION

Zoloft is prescribed for those who are depressed as a result of Crohn's disease. It is chemically similar to Prozac. Common side effects are confusion, diarrhea or loose stools, dizziness, dry mouth, fatigue, headache, increased sweating, indigestion, insomnia, nausea, sleepiness, and tremors. Less-common side effects may include abdominal pain, abnormal hair growth, abnormal skin odor, acne, agitation, altered taste, chest pain, constipation, difficulty breathing or walking or swallowing, fainting, earache, enlarged abdomen, and eye pain, with one hundred more side effects listed.

# CYSTIC FIBROSIS

Cystic fibrosis is considered a genetic disorder, a recessive genetic trait that has to be carried by both parents in order to have an afflicted child. It is the most common fatal genetic disease of Caucasian children. The disease is usually diagnosed early when a child is a newborn, but it can also develop in children, adolescents, and young adults. Cystic fibrosis is a generalized dysfunction of the exocrine and endocrine systems. It especially affects mucus-secreting glands, such as the pancreas and sweat glands. There is an accumulation of mucus, which for some reason is not easily removed from the body. When mucus is in the body, it invites germs, viruses, parasites, and worms, which cause many more problems. The gastrointestinal effects of cystic fibrosis occur mainly in the intestines, pancreas, and liver. One of the earliest such symptoms is meconium ileus. The newborn with cystic fibrosis doesn't excrete meconium, a dark-green mucilaginous material found in the intestines at birth. The child then develops symptoms of intestinal obstruction, such as abdominal distention, vomiting, constipation, diarrhea, dehydration, and electrolyte imbalance. Eventually, obstructions of the pancreatic ducts and resulting deficiency of protease, amylase, and lipase prevent the conversion and absorption of fat and protein in the intestinal tract.

The undigested food is then excreted in frequent, bulky, foul-smelling, and pale stools with a high fat content. Without proper bowel function, constipation can eventually develop. The inability of the body to absorb nutrients produces poor weight gain, a ravenous appetite, sallow skin, and distended abdomen. The inability to absorb fats produces deficiencies of the fat-soluble vitamins (A, E, K, and essential fatty acids), leading to clotting problems and retarded bone growth.

## HERBAL COMBINATIONS
### Herbal Combination #1
- Marshmallow heals and soothes lung tissues and eliminates toxins. It heals the irritations associated with diarrhea and dysentery.
- Fenugreek softens and dissolves hardened mucus, expels phlegm and mucus, and kills infections. It also helps to expel toxic waste through the lymphatic system.

### Herbal Combination #2
This formula soothes and heals the digestive system for better digestion and assimilation. It helps heal the small and large intestines. It contains pau d'arco, cloves, inula racemosa, licorice (deglycyrrhized), capsicum, and lecithin.

## HEALTHFUL SUGGESTIONS
1. A cleansing and healing of the small intestine is needed to repair the damage that has been done. The damage could be caused by viruses, germs, parasites, or worms. Blood cleansers, with red clover combinations, and lower bowel cleansers will help the body eliminate and heal itself. A congested colon can balloon and cause a dysfunction of the ileocecal valve, which allows toxic poisons to enter the small intestine and cause irritations. Children can be born with a toxic colon.

## HE'S A PICTURE OF HEALTH, DESPITE HIS SCARY START IN LIFE
When Dusty was born, there seemed to be nothing out of the ordinary, except his mother, Rhonda, knew something was wrong. There was a raspy, clicking sound in the baby's chest. There was projectile vomiting of what should be perfect food for a newborn, mother's milk. Constant trips to the pediatrician were fruitless. Finally Rhonda's persistence paid off. A sweat test was performed at a children's hospital. A sweat test analyzes the perspiration of babies suspected of having cystic fibrosis, since the disease causes a high salt content from the perspiration. At three months old Dusty was diagnosed with cystic fibrosis.

The mucous membranes in the lungs of children with cystic fibrosis produce a thick mucus, blocking lung passages and causing bacterial infections. Malnutrition is common because of a lack of digestive enzymes caused by the disease. Primary medical treatment is as follows: a pancreatic enzyme that helps digest food to prevent malnutrition, beating on the child's back to break up mucus, antibiotic therapy, and extra calories in the diet to help prevent malnutrition.

Rhonda felt the prognosis was very bleak for the traditional therapies. She had recently experienced a health crisis of her own and had sought a natural alternative to colostomy surgery. Her efforts had been rewarded with generally improved health and avoidance of the surgery that would have drastically changed her life at the age of twenty-one. Rhonda read everything she could find in regard to alternative approaches to cystic fibrosis. Along with prayer and a belief in natural healing, she decided on the following: raw goat's milk, which has the enzymes necessary for digestion and appears to be a more nutritious choice than cow's milk.

Dusty was now able to keep his bottles down. Lobelia extract is an herb often used for mucus in the lungs. Two drops were placed in each bottle, and the extract was rubbed into his chest. Black walnut was used, because cystic fibrosis has been linked to parasites. This herb is used for intestinal parasites (five to six drops in each bottle). Lower bowel formula in extract form was used because of the impaired digestion that translated into only weekly eliminations.

The thought of having to deal with a dirty diaper once a week may be appealing to parents, but it is disastrous to the health of the baby! One-half dropper twice a day was used for this extreme case. Capsicum (cayenne pepper) extract was also used, one drop per bottle. Cayenne is often used to increase circulation, to clear lung problems, and to make other herbs more effective. Pau d'arco extract was used for its powerful antibiotic capabilities. Five to six drops were used in each bottle. Castor oil packs were placed on Dusty's abdomen to encourage elimination.

Warm water enemas were used to aid elimination. The small bulb aspirator given by the hospital for the new baby was used with petroleum jelly for insertion. No other food or liquid was given to Dusty for the next six months. At nine months of age, after six months of treatment, he developed a fever of 104 degrees. Based on what Rhonda had read, she was prepared. A healing crisis is inevitable and is a good sign. But sometimes even good signs are frightening. An immediate enema lowered his fever and resulted in the expulsion of parasites only! Eventually the fever returned. The fever continued to return over the span of two days. Each enema produced twenty to thirty parasites. At the end of this period, Dusty was a different infant. He sleeps normally, he is no longer irritable. He is a normal nine-month-old and has begun to thrive. A sweat test at the children's hospital confirmed that there was no sign of cystic fibrosis.

Dusty is now a very healthy sixteen-year-old. He is very athletic and is a member of the track team at school. He's a picture of health, despite his scary start in life. This is all especially amazing since at the age of three, Dusty was taken from his mother in a custody battle. At that point, Dusty's diet became the typical American diet of "pseudo food" and sugar. But the healthy start he got in the first three years of life was enough to impact the last eleven years. Rhonda now helps parents from all over the United States who have children with cystic fibrosis.

2. Allergies can be involved and are created when food is not digested properly. A lack of digestive enzymes causes malnutrition. The pancreas is not able to provide essential enzymes to digest food properly. The pancreas may have parasites, which can lead to a lack of enzymes being produced.

3. A change in diet has helped with improvement in CF patients. Learning what foods are irritating to the intestines and eliminating or reducing them through a rotation diet can help. Use raw juices, always diluted, to help provide enzymes and heal the small intestine. The diet should include raw fruits and vegetables and lightly steamed vegetables. Goat's milk can be very healing for the small intestine and provide all the nutrients a baby needs for at least six months. Introducing grains too early can cause more irritation to the small intestine. Until the baby can chew grains, the needed enzymes are not there to provide proper digestion and assimilation.

4. Digestive enzymes are essential to assure that food is properly digested. They will also help break up any undigested protein in the bloodstream. Parasites, worms, viruses, and germs all have protein coatings that enzymes can destroy. Pancreatin and digestive enzymes should be used with each meal and between meals to break up any undigested protein in the blood.

5. Avoid animal products, processed and cooked food, white sugar, and white flour products.

## HERBS AND SUPPLEMENTS

Single herbs to help with cystic fibrosis include chlorophyll and aloe vera juice, which will help heal and provide nutrients.

- Burdock cleans the blood, and cascara sagrada is a colon cleanser.
- Goldenseal heals and kills parasites.
- Kelp supplies minerals and valuable nutrients.
- Saffron helps digest oils.
- Slippery elm and fenugreek are healing and nourishing.
- Slippery elm and other herbs provide protein and nutrients. They are also helpful in healing the gut.
- Pancreatic enzymes are very effective to improve the digestion of fat and help in breaking up undigested protein in the blood.
- Acidophilus is useful in providing good bacteria in the digestive tract.

- Antioxidants are essential to prevent free-radical damage. They also provide nutrients that can be missing in those with cystic fibrosis.
- Vitamins A, E, and D can be extremely deficient because pancreatic obstruction prevents release of the enzymes necessary for their absorption.
- Free-form amino acids help repair the body from damage caused by diarrhea or constipation.
- B-complex vitamins are poorly absorbed and are needed for healthy intestinal flora. An extract form of B-complex would be better digested.
- Vitamin K or blue-green algae are easily assimilated by the body.
- Essential fatty acids in the form of flaxseed oil are beneficial. They should be used along with vitamin E to protect them from destruction by oxygen.
- Vitamin C with bioflavonoids helps protect against infections.
- Black walnut contains organic iodine and tannins and has antiseptic properties. It kills parasites and worms, stops bleeding, and is excellent for cleaning the blood.
- Colostrum is an immune boost to help infection.
- Cordyceps strengthens the immune system, boosts energy, and helps recovery from extreme exhaustion.

## ORTHODOX PRESCRIBED MEDICATION

Infections are common in cystic fibrosis patients, so antibiotics are prescribed for respiratory infections. They destroy the good bacteria in the intestines, which will cause viruses, germs, parasites, and worms to flourish. Intestinal problems are common when using antibiotics, which creates even more problems with the small intestines. They can even cause colitis or inflammation of the colon. Tetracyclines are often prescribed and can cause allergies, shortness of breath, heart abnormalities, headaches, dizziness, and rashes.

# CYSTS, POLYPS, AND TUMORS

A cyst is a closed sac or pouch with a defined wall that contains fluid, semifluid, or solid material. Polyps are benign, usually soft, grapelike growths. Tumors are a swelling or abnormal growth of tissue having no useful function in the body. Cancer cells are abnormal cells that invade healthy tissues. They travel through the system and deposit themselves in the weakest areas of the body, causing growths or tumors.

Suppressing acute diseases can be the cause of cysts and tumors. Mucus is allowed to accumulate and harden in the body when acute diseases are not allowed to go through the five stages of healing. Suppressing acute diseases during the abatement stage, when excess waste begins to eliminate, will cause the glands to become congested. This can result in lymphatic congestion, glandular secretions, tumors, cysts, polyps, moles, and skin diseases. Decongestants, painkillers, and antihistamines all interfere with the proper cleansing process. If this is repeated over and over, it will cause growths. Other causes are repeated infections and inflammation that leave scar tissue in the area. Allergies, anti-inflammatory drugs, and yellow food coloring (FD&C No. 5) found in food such as hot dogs and margarine may also be triggering agents.

## HERBAL COMBINATIONS
### Herbal Combination #1

This formula helps to detoxify and purify the blood. It helps to repair the liver, kidneys, and pancreas. It also helps in eliminating waste material from the cells. It may increase cellular metabolism by normalizing blood chemistry and strengthen the immune system and T cells by regulating hormonal balance.

- Burdock contains antitumor properties, reduces cell mutations, balances hormones, and activates the pituitary gland. It is a great blood and lymphatic cleanser and neutralizes toxins. It is also beneficial for treating catarrh and stomach ailments.
- Rhubarb cleanses the liver and dissolves tumors. It contains rhein, which helps inhibit the growth of bacteria, parasites, and candida. It has a mild laxative effect, improves digestion, and contains anti-inflammatory properties.
- Slippery elm contains antitumor properties, is a natural antacid, and regulates intestinal flora. It is rich in protein necessary for new cell growth. It is nutritious and heals inflammation and ulcerations in the GI tract. It is healing and soothing to the mucous membranes.

- Sheep sorrel is useful in tissue repair because it is rich in vitamins and minerals. It is soothing and works as a blood purifier, cleans the urinary tract, eliminates toxins, and is rich in calcium.

## Other Uses

Age spots, arthritis, blood purifier, boils, cancer, canker sores, colon, infections, liver, lymph glands, pancreas, skin problems, spleen, diabetes, tonsillitis, tumors, uric acid buildup, venereal disease.

## Herbal Combination #2

- Pau d'arco is a blood cleanser, contains antibacterial properties, protects the liver, and improves assimilation of nutrients. It eliminates fungal infestations.
- Buckthorn is cleansing for the blood, liver, and gallbladder. It is calming and healing to the intestinal tract.
- Peach bark contains healing properties, strengthens the nervous system, and has natural diuretic properties.
- Prickly ash is a great stimulant to remove toxins from the blood and improve circulation.
- Yellow dock is a nutritive tonic very high in iron, and it nourishes the liver and spleen.
- Dandelion helps the liver to detoxify poisons, works as a blood purifier and cleanser, and is rich in vitamins and minerals.
- Burdock is a blood purifier and promotes kidney function to clear the blood of harmful acids.
- Red clover eliminates toxins, is a tonic with valuable minerals and vitamins, and contains high amounts of iron and nutrients.
- Cascara sagrada is a safe laxative. It stimulates the secretions of the digestive system.
- Yarrow opens the pores and purifies the blood.
- Sarsaparilla contains stimulating properties and is noted for increasing the metabolic rate.
- Oregon grape root is a blood purifier and aids in the assimilation of nutrients. It is a tonic for all the glands.

## HEALTHFUL SUGGESTIONS

1. Add more potassium foods, which increase alkalinity and eliminate acid in the body. Potassium is vital to help neutralize acids and toxins. It reduces excessive gastric acidity and intestinal acidity and promotes good health. Potassium foods are almonds, apples, whey powder, potato peeling broth, bitter greens, bananas, beans, whole grains, olives, pecans, rice bran, sunflower seeds, and watercress. Herbs high in potassium are dulse, kelp, Irish moss, sage, red clover, ginger, skullcap, valerian, peach bark, licorice, horsetail, hops, and garlic.

2. Juice fasts will help dissolve growths. Try short fasts to begin with. Always dilute the juices to prevent stress on the pancreas. Try parsley, celery, and

### MARSHA IS SOLD ON THE VALUE OF HERBS

Marsha suffered for years with pain in her right side and took a lot of painkillers. She went to a doctor who performed laparoscopic surgery on her in 1993 for cysts that infested her ovaries. The one that hung from her right ovary was lemon-sized and was connected by a vein that, when she moved, would cut off the blood supply, which was causing all the pain. The doctor removed the ovary and all the cysts. She recovered quickly.

In April 1994 she was told, after her checkup, that the cysts had reappeared and were multiplying and growing fast. She was scheduled for surgery but was concerned that if the cysts recurred after the first surgery, how would a second surgery prevent them from coming back? The first surgery cost eight thousand dollars, so she knew it would cost at least that again.

She told her husband, after leaving the doctor, that it was time to see a friend who sold herbs and had knowledge of their use. She was still unsure that herbs would help. She canceled her surgery and decided to give them a chance. After purchasing formula #2 and taking it faithfully for six weeks, she returned to her doctor and had an internal ultrasound. He told her that he could not find any cysts. She was shocked, because she thought he would say that they were smaller or that there were not as many, but to say that they had disappeared was just a miracle. Needless to say, Marsha is sold on the value of herbs.

carrots, add whey powder, blend and drink while fresh. Parsley, carrots, celery, and garlic juice blended is very rich in potassium.

3. Cleansing the blood with red clover blends, a lot of pure water, and herbal liver cleansers will help loosen and eliminate the cysts and tumors. Colon cleansers will also help get the toxins out of the body.

4. Add oxygen-rich supplements. In the 1920s, Dr. Otto Warburn, a Nobel Prize winner, demonstrated that the metabolism (chemical changes incidental to life and growth) of cancerous tissue differs radically from that of normal tissue. Normal tissue acquires its nourishment from oxidation and usually dies if deprived of oxygen. Whenever the blood supply is poor, such as around or near scars, ulcers, in atrophied organs, injuries, or any place where energy is blocked, malignant tumors can develop. Germanium, CoQ10, ginkgo, and suma are examples of nutrients to supply the blood with oxygen.

5. Eliminate processed foods; they only cause free-radical damage. These foods become rancid quickly and cause oxidation in the body, which increases damage to the cells. Such foods include pancake, cake, and cookie mixes, as well as packaged cookies, chips, doughnuts, or any processed food that has been on the shelf a long time. Once the wheat products have been ground, they start the oxidation process. Rancid oils are very harmful and are found in processed food. Learn to read labels.

6. A change of diet will be the first step in cleansing. Learn to use whole grains. Make food from scratch using a lot of vegetables, and add tofu to mashed potatoes, cream dishes, and soups, sauté in olive oil, and use soy sauce.

## HERBS AND SUPPLEMENTS

Single herbs include aloe vera, burdock, chaparral (cleans and dissolves cysts, polyps, and tumors), dandelion, echinacea (cleans the lymphatics), garlic, goldenseal, kelp, milk thistle, pau d'arco, prickly ash, red clover, suma, and yellow dock.

- Natural interferon supplements can help strengthen the immune system. Interferon is an antiviral protein produced by the white blood cells. It is produced by the body naturally when it is given the proper nutrients. The following nutrients stimulate production of interferon: chlorophyll, astragalus, vitamin C with bioflavonoids, sea vegetables such as kelp and dulse, blue-green algae, ginkgo, milk thistle, pau d'arco, schizandra, Siberian ginseng, suma, wheatgrass juice, dong quai, licorice, echinacea, red raspberry, ho-shou-wu, and germanium.

- Essential fatty acids protect the immune system, help in dissolving growths, and protect against autoimmune diseases. They help to balance body chemistry.

- Vitamins are essential, especially antioxidants like vitamin A, beta-carotene, vitamin E, vitamin C with bioflavonoids, selenium, and zinc. They protect against cellular damage, improve immune function, and protect the mucous membranes.

- Minerals are vital to protecting against growths. There may be a mineral imbalance when tumors, cysts, and polyps develop. Silicon eliminates waste material such as uric acid. It strengthens the connective tissue to ward off growths. Calcium, magnesium, and iron are important. All minerals are essential for protecting the body from disease.

- Chlorophyll and blue-green algae are important for cleansing the blood and supplying nutrients to the system.

- Germanium and CoQ10 promote immune function and supply oxygen to the blood to prevent growths and dissolve them.

- Suma, *Ginkgo biloba*, and gotu kola promote a healthy immune system and increase circulation. Poor circulation is the beginning of many health problems, including cysts and tumors.

- Psyllium and other fiber foods prevent stagnation in the colon and the blood.

- Lecithin helps to regulate metabolism and break down fat and cholesterol. It prevents plaque from adhering to artery walls. It aids in rebuilding tissues in the cells.

- Garlic has been shown to reduce tumors. It is a natural antibiotic that acts on germs and viruses.

- Vitex agnus castus has been known to help with some types of uterine cysts (fibroids) and is beneficial in dissolving hardened mucus (as in cysts and tumors), killing toxins and germs, and strengthening the adrenal glands.

- Echinacea, red clover, and burdock also clean the blood and help dissolve growths.

## ORTHODOX PRESCRIBED MEDICATION

The benign cysts, growths, and tumors are usually harmless. If they become bothersome, they are usually removed surgically.

# DEPRESSION

Depression is the number one public health problem in the United States, and its occurrence is on the rise. One in twenty Americans develops a case of depression serious enough to require professional treatment. Depression is a real concern in our modern society. Approximately three million children suffer from depression. Childhood depression is on the rise and adolescent suicide attempts are escalating. How can a child's life be so bleak that he or she would want to commit suicide?

Rita Elkins, in her book *Depression and Natural Medicine*, says, "Unquestionably, untreated depression can lead to suicide, which is the ninth leading cause of death in this country and the third leading cause in teenagers. Every day, fifteen people between the ages of fifteen and twenty-four kill themselves. For thousands of people, doing away with themselves has become an acceptable method of escape and resolution. Anyone who has entertained the thought of suicide, even if just momentarily, needs help in confronting their depression. Keep in mind that if someone you know has made even the most casual reference to suicide, it should be taken seriously."

Depression was called melancholia in the past. Many doctors found that autointoxication was the main cause of depression and mental problems. The brain is very sensitive to toxins. When the bowels are not kept clean, the toxins enter the blood and travel to the brain. One medical doctor wrote in an article in *Medical Record* in 1937, "No matter how many stools or what their physical character may be, marked retention of toxic or sapremic substances may exist. Many of the most toxic individuals that I have seen have daily and often more frequent bowel movements."

The World Health Organization conducted a survey and found that two hundred million individuals worldwide suffer from depression. Everyone faces depression at one time or another in one form or another. Stressful situations cause depression. Normal depression comes with grief, as in a death, divorce, loss of a job, medical problems, or other stressful situations.

Symptoms can be feelings of hopelessness, finding no joy in life, wanting to sleep all of the time, feeling tired after sleeping all night, experiencing loneliness even when around people, dislike of self and others, and wanting to escape life and problems. Panic attacks and sudden attacks of rage are some symptoms.

Women especially seem to be prone to depression. This is partly due to the immense responsibilities of balancing work and family duties. This can put a big strain on wives and mothers and prevent them from performing everyday tasks that are necessary in raising children and running a household. Strengthening the nervous system with nutritional support can help the body cope with stressors that can precipitate depression.

There are many reasons for depression. Unresolved memories of abuse or a traumatic experience, such as divorce, can trigger feelings of depression. These issues need to be addressed with proper treatment, and counseling may be necessary, but nutrition can go a long way toward healing the mind and emotions. Manic depression, which causes extreme mood swings, can cause a lot of misery for the person suffering from it, as well as for their loved ones. When someone you love or someone you are acquainted with is manifesting symptoms of antisocial behavior, before you make an appointment with a psychiatrist, please examine his or her diet. Is it loaded with artificial additives, white sugar, pastries, soda pop, white flour products, or too much red meat? Remember that meat and dairy products are loaded with hormones, which cause imbalances in the body. Also reduce consumption of caffeine drinks, alcohol, drugs, and tobacco, which put a stress on the physical body and affect the brain.

### EMOTIONAL NEEDS

While we know that many physical factors impact brain chemistry and may contribute to depression, anyone with the disease needs tolerance and understanding from those in their acquaintance. Depressed people will not be cured with pep talks, but rather by knowing that they have the support of loved ones and access to professionals who can help level the brain chemistry disruption or whatever other factors may be causing the problems. Malnutrition and sleeping disorders, common in depressed individuals, can further worsen the mental outlook.

## HERBAL COMBINATIONS

### Herbal Combination #1

This formula nourishes and rebuilds the nervous system and the brain. The nervous system transmits all sensory input, sound, sight, taste, smell, and touch to the brain and controls the workings of the organs. It helps maintain the temperature of the body and blood pressure.

- Black cohosh has a soothing effect on the nervous system and helps to lower blood pressure.
- Capsicum stimulates other herbs to be more effective, increases blood circulation, and helps eliminate toxic wastes.
- Valerian has a sedative effect on the entire system and is a natural remedy for nervous disorders.
- Passion flower relaxes the nerves, is good for strengthening the nervous system, and has natural pain-relieving properties.
- Hops is a general tonic for the nervous system, helps with sleep, and works as a sedative.
- Wood betony cleans impurities from the blood and is an effective sedative.
- Catnip herb helps in fatigue, improves circulation, and has a sedative effect on the nervous system. It is useful for many ailments.

### Herbal Combination #2

This formula helps the body cope with depression and stressful situations. It energizes the body and helps increase needed nutrients to counteract mood swings. It contains *Rhodiola rosea*, *Eleutherococcus senticosus*, Korean ginseng, ashwagandha, rosemary, *Gynostemma pentaphyllum*, and schizandra. It also contains astragalus, Reishi mushroom, suma, and *Ginkgo biloba*. Alfalfa, kelp, chromium, and a fruit and vegetable base provide rich nutrients to nourish the cells.

### Other Uses

Anxiety, convulsions, headaches, hyperactivity, hysteria, insomnia, nervous disorders, nervous break-down, relaxant, restores proper function to the nervous system.

## HEALTHFUL SUGGESTIONS

1. Learn stress management through exercise, which can relieve or eradicate depression symptoms. Learn to manage stress through relaxation, meditation, and massage therapy. There are tapes available on relaxing methods using music.

2. Allergies can put a tremendous stress on the physical body, thereby stressing the nerves. Allergies to molds, dusts, grasses, and pollens can cause depression and mood swings, even bipolar and psychotic disorders. Allergies cause swelling, heat, and pain. When swelling occurs in the brain area, depression may result.

3. A detoxification program will help clean and purify the body so it can digest, assimilate, and eliminate properly. A juice fast, starting slowly, depending on the strength of the body, can be very beneficial. A weak body needs to build, then cleanse. Fresh juice using parsley, carrots, celery, and garlic will help clean and nourish. Always dilute the juices to eliminate stress on the pancreas.

4. A colon cleanse is important. Constipation is the number one cause of depression. Use a lower bowel cleanse and colonics to eliminate the toxins. This will help cleanse, nourish, and restore normal colon elimination. Add more fiber food to the diet. A high-fiber diet, also rich in cruciferous vegetables, is essential for balancing hormone levels. At the turn of the twentieth century, J. A. Stucky, MD, made the observation that the blood is poisoned through absorption of toxic material from the intestinal canal more frequently than from any other source. The overproduction of estrogen in the body has been linked to autointoxication. When the body is loaded with toxins, the liver will be burdened and will not be able to process the excess estrogen. If the intestinal tract is not able to eliminate this estrogen, it is reabsorbed into the bloodstream and carried to various parts of the body, including the brain.

5. Change the diet. A diet change is the first step to cleansing the body. If allergies are the cause, eliminate the irritant and reestablish normal function in the digestive system. When the body is strengthened with proper nutrients, the brain can handle stressful

situations. Whole grains, such as millet, brown rice, whole oats, rye, buckwheat, and whole wheat contain the amino acid tryptophan, which is responsible for producing serotonin and melatonin in the brain. When these neurochemicals are lacking in the brain, it can cause depression of varying degrees. Sugar can deplete the body of B-complex vitamins and minerals, especially calcium and magnesium.

## HERBS AND SUPPLEMENTS

Single herbs to help depression include gotu kola (brain food), kelp (cleans glands and veins), dong quai (tranquilizing on nerves), chamomile (rich in calcium to feed the nerves), skullcap (rebuilds nerves), hops (has sedative properties), passion flower (soothing on the nerves), and ginkgo and suma (stimulate brain function and increase oxygen).

- St. John's wort and kava have been found in European studies to help balance mental health. They have been found effective in treating anxiety and mild to moderate depression.
- Digestive enzymes are very beneficial in neurological disorders. A lack of enzymes can cause nervous system disorders. Enzymes will help break down the toxins causing irritation to the nervous system.
- Amino acid supplements help the healing of the mind. Diet alone may not provide this important brain stimulant. They should be taken on an empty stomach. Amino acids encourage production of the neurotransmitter epinephrine, which stimulates the brain and increases metabolism.
- Vitamins A, D, C, E, selenium, and zinc help protect the body from free-radical damage, which can affect the brain and nervous system. They work with minerals to balance body chemistry.
- Lecithin contains choline and inositol, which boosts the neurotransmitter acetylcholine and is needed to stimulate memory and learning.
- B vitamins also boost acetylcholine levels in the brain. B-complex vitamins are essential to enhance brain neurotransmitters. They help clean bad estrogen from the liver. Supplements will help speed healing of the nerves and brain.
- Essential fatty acids include flaxseed oil, evening primrose oil, borage oil, salmon oil, and black currant oil. These are required for normal development of the brain and nervous system. They help make a group of chemicals in the body called prostaglandins, hormone-like chemicals that regulate many functions and activities of the body.
- Multimineral and multivitamin supplements are necessary for balancing body chemistry and nourishing the brain and nervous system.
- Calcium, magnesium, and chromium deficiency can lead to depression.
- Blue-green algae, chlorophyll, spirulina, and chlorella are rich in protein. They are also rich in vitamins and minerals and are easily digested. They help clean the blood and liver.

- Bee pollen is rich in protein and B-complex vitamins, especially B12. It is very important in overcoming depression and imbalances in the body.
- Gotu kola, ginkgo, and suma stimulate brain function and provide oxygen to the brain. A lack of oxygen is one cause of brain dysfunction.

## ORTHODOX PRESCRIBED MEDICATION

Doctors routinely prescribe drugs to treat depression, such as Prozac, Paxil, Zoloft, Lovan, and Luvox. However, there is much controversy over their merits versus their side effects. The debate surrounding these drugs is that while they raise the level of a certain type of serotonin, they lower another. There is also concern that these drugs act as nervous system stimulants, which can result in altering one's perception of reality and impairing judgment. Despite the conflict enveloping Prozac, many doctors stand by it as a highly effective drug in treating depression. This class of drugs is designed to raise brain levels of serotonin by inhibiting the process of serotonin reuptake, thereby keeping levels elevated in brain cells. This process prevents serotonin from going into the bloodstream. As mentioned earlier, some experts are concerned with this unnatural buildup of serotonin in the brain. They warn against a hormonal cascade effect, which can, in some individuals, prompt bizarre or destructive behavior. Side effects include nervousness, insomnia, drowsiness, fatigue, weakness, tremor, increased sweating, dizziness, anxiety, headache, and loss of appetite in some, weight gain in others. Constipation is another side effect.

# DIABETES

Diabetes is a chronic degenerative disease caused by lack of or resistance to insulin, which is essential for the proper metabolism of blood sugar (glucose). The pancreas, a small pink gland located below and behind the stomach, is an important organ of the human digestive system. It takes part in the digestion of proteins, starches, sugars, and fats. The small islands of glandular tissue that are scattered throughout the pancreas, called the islets of Langerhans, produce insulin. If the pancreas cannot secrete enough insulin, the liver is unable to store the sugar necessary for strengthening the muscles. When the liver can no longer get insulin, the sugar enters the bloodstream, kidneys, and urine and causes diabetes. The main problem with this is the inability of the body to utilize all the sugar that then enters the bloodstream.

Cases of diabetes are increasing—right now more than ten million Americans have this disease, and it is estimated that two out of five do not realize they have diabetes. People with diabetes are up to four times more likely to die from a heart attack and have a greater risk of strokes. Diabetes can also lead to heart and kidney disease, atherosclerosis, hypertension, cataracts, retinal hemorrhage, neuropathy, gangrenous infections of cuts or sores, loss of hearing, blindness, and even death.

Dr. John Harvey Kellogg observed when he X-rayed diabetic patients that their ileocecal valves were usually incompetent. The ileocecal valve protects the small intestine from infection. The regurgitation of the colon contents into the small intestine is estimated to be twenty times faster than in the large colon. Alloxan, a toxin produced in the colon, was injected into animals, and it destroyed the islets of Langerhans in their pancreas. These poisons are found in chlorine in the municipal drinking water and in the bleach used in commercial flour products.

Other causes of diabetes include obesity, stress, pregnancy, and oral contraceptives. Increased levels of estrogen and placental hormones antagonize insulin. Other medications that are known insulin antagonists are thiazide diuretics, adrenal corticosteroids, and phenytoin. A diet high in sugar and white flour products can put extra burden on the pancreas. Parasites are also implicated in diabetes, especially childhood-onset diabetes. This seems very logical, because parasites are known to harbor in the cecum, below the ileocecal valve, and when it is incompetent, the parasites are dumped into the pancreas or other organs. Symptoms can be excessive thirst, excessive urination and hunger, general weakness, skin disorders that do not heal quickly, blurred vision, tingling leg cramps, and dry mouth.

## EMOTIONAL NEEDS

Remember, fluctuations in blood sugar (common with diabetes) can predispose a person to periods of anger, depression, or other emotional symptoms.

Learn to recognize these emotional red flags as possible indicators of low blood sugar due to excess insulin.

## HERBAL COMBINATIONS
### Herbal Combination #1
This formula is designed to help regulate blood sugar, restore proper function of the pancreas, and strengthen and heal the body, particularly the glands. The pancreas gland performs two important functions. It is necessary to produce the pancreatic acid juice used in digestion, and it also produces insulin. Pancreatitis symptoms can be acid indigestion, nausea, pain, and gas. The weakness for diabetes can be inherited, so it is important to strengthen the pancreas gland, digestive system, and colon.

- Goldenseal is a natural insulin, regulates blood sugar, feeds the glands, builds resistance to diseases, and heals and soothes mucous membranes. It also helps in ulcerations and sore eyes.
- Juniper berries are high in natural insulin and help restore the function of the pancreas.
- Uva ursi helps regulate sugar levels and helps alleviate pancreas and urinary disorders.
- Mullein contains antibiotic properties, nourishes the body, and strengthens and calms nerves.
- Yarrow is a blood cleanser, dilates the pores, produces sweating, and removes congestion.
- Garlic stimulates cell growth and activity, rejuvenates body functions, and prevents infections.
- Capsicum helps heal the pancreas and increases and regulates circulation.
- Dandelion increases activity of the pancreas, clears obstructions, and purifies the blood and liver, as well as being a natural tonic.
- Marshmallow is high in vitamin A and minerals and has healing and phlegm-removing properties.
- Cedar berries help regulate blood sugar and protect against bacteria such as *E. coli* and staph infections, as well as candida.

This formula also contains slippery elm bark, nettle herb, white oak bark, and licorice root.

### Herbal Combination #2
This was formulated to nourish and strengthen the glandular system. When one gland is weak, it weakens them all. The vitamins, minerals, and herbs are combined with necessary essential ingredients to stimulate proper hormone production and metabolism.

- Vitamins A, C, E, and zinc protect against free-radical damage. Vitamin A nourishes the thymus gland, as well as all the other glands, to increase size and antibody production.
- Zinc protects the immune system and supports the T cells. Low zinc intake decreases thymus growth.
- Vitamin C with bioflavonoids nourishes and cleans all the glands and protects the immune system.
- Lecithin breaks down fatty deposits and is especially effective on the liver.
- The minerals, especially the trace minerals in the herbs, are vital for glandular health.
- Kelp is rich in iodine and contains all essential minerals.
- Alfalfa is rich in minerals and eliminates uric acid from the body.
- Parsley is a natural diuretic and eliminates toxins such as uric acid.
- Dandelion stimulates bile production and benefits the spleen and pancreas.
- Licorice root strengthens the adrenals, pancreas, and spleen.
- Dong quai helps regulate hormones.
- Schizandra nourishes the nervous system.
- Marshmallow and uva ursi soothe and heal the entire digestive system.

### Herbal Combination #3
This is an ayurvedic formula containing gymnema, which blocks sugar absorption. It contains the following herbs: Momordica charantia, Pterocarpus marsupium, Aegle marmelos, Enicostemma littorale, Andrographis paniculata, Curcuma longa, Syzygium cumini, Azadirachta indica, Picrorhiza kurroa, Trigonella foenum-graecum seed, and Cyperus rotundus. It helps normalize liver and pancreatic function. This combination is beneficial for all the glands and the digestive system.

### Other Uses
Blood sugar problems, gallbladder, hyperglycemia, glucose intolerance, glycosuria, kidney, liver, and spleen.

## HEALTHFUL SUGGESTIONS
1. Digestive enzymes are important for proper digestion. Increasing digestive enzymes and raw foods aids digestion. Cooked food destroys all food

enzymes and forces the body to produce more enzymes, which causes an enlarged pancreas and other digestive organs. All of this wears them down so they cannot function properly. The body has a rich supply of enzyme activity in the saliva and pancreatic juices, but it needs to be replenished, or the organs will break down and cause diseases such as diabetes, hypoglycemia, and obesity, to name a few. Diabetics have been shown to have low levels of the enzyme amylase. Eating more raw food and adding digestive enzymes will take a load off the endocrine glands, especially the pancreas, to increase its healing power.

2. Eliminate sugar, white flour products, fruit juices, greasy and fatty foods (meat, eggs, cheese, excess oil, rancid nuts and seeds), and high-fat foods. They weaken the spleen and pancreas, making insulin less effective, as well as causing damage to the liver. This can lead to an imbalance in the spleen and pancreas, causing pancreatic secretions such as insulin to be less effective. Zoltan P. Rona, MD, says, "Sugar increases the body's loss of chromium, and essential minerals, through the urine and leads directly to glucose intolerance (i.e., diabetes and hypoglycemia). Sugar in moderation for any diabetics is unrealistic, hazardous and perpetuates the disease." Sugar is the modern person's weakness and downfall. It is prevalent in our diets and difficult to avoid. It is found in canned, frozen, and fast foods. Read labels and become familiar with the different forms of sugar: sucrose, dextrose, fructose, high-fructose corn syrup, honey, molasses, and the sugar in milk—even fruit juice is hard on the pancreas. All sugars should be eliminated until the pancreas has a chance to heal. Fructose, the sugar in fruits, and fruit juices provide a steady stream of energy instead of a rush, and some have recommended them for diabetics, but use caution.

3. Allergies can be implicated in an enzyme deficiency, especially those who suffer from chemical and food sensitivities. It is hard sometimes to recognize what is causing the allergies. There is strong evidence that one of the triggers of insulin-dependent diabetes mellitus is an allergy to cow's milk albumin and to wheat gliadin. Allergies weaken the immune system over time and cause disease. An inflammation anywhere in the body is one sign of allergies. If a person eats the same foods over and over, it puts a stress on the body and causes irritations that lead to inflammation.

4. Using only high-quality natural foods is important: whole grains such as buckwheat, millet, barley, brown rice, whole oats, yellow cornmeal, amaranth, kamut, quinoa, spelt, and teff. Eat raw vegetables and fruits. Raw foods stimulate the pancreas to increase insulin production. Sprouted grains can be added to salads and in vegetable casseroles. A high-fiber diet helps to lower blood triglycerides in diabetics and prediabetics. Fiber has the ability to repair faulty sugar metabolism by its complex effects on gastrointestinal function. Protein foods such as yogurt, kefir, tofu, and soy products are helpful. Raw nuts and seeds and avocados are also good. Vegetables such as asparagus, green beans, okra, celery, watercress, parsley, alfalfa, and Jerusalem artichokes are beneficial in a diabetic's diet. Jerusalem artichokes contain a starch that the pancreas can handle. Eat small, frequent meals that will help the pancreas and digestive system to heal. Large meals and overcooked foods overtax the pancreas and cause swelling and inflammation.

5. Cleansing the colon and blood are very important. Use formulas under Constipation, a lower bowel combination. Use blood cleansers, as well as liver cleansers. Add chlorophyll foods and supplements to the diet. Concentrated vegetable juices in large quantities can overstimulate the pancreas. Always dilute juices with pure water.

6. Exercise is very important, because it excretes glucose from the muscle tissue so that sugar is burned up. Overexercising can cause feelings of exhaustion, so start slowly and gradually increase activity.

## HERBS AND SUPPLEMENTS

Single herbs that can help with diabetes include alfalfa, aloe vera, black walnut (kills parasites), buchu, burdock (cleans blood), cedar berries (heal pancreas), cornsilk, dandelion, garlic, gentian, goldenseal (acts as insulin, stops internal bleeding), horsetail, kelp, and psyllium.

- Chromium has been found to be an essential nutrient for the pancreas. It has been found to decrease fasting glucose levels, improve glucose tolerance, lower insulin levels, and decrease total cholesterol and triglyceride levels. Chromium helps the body stabilize blood sugar levels. It is the major mineral involved with insulin production. Some nutritionists believe that many cases of diabetes could actually be a chromium deficiency—induced by eating a lot of refined grains and sugars.

- *Gymnema sylvestre* is a plant from India and has been found very useful for diabetics. It was shown to reduce insulin requirements and improve blood sugar control.
- Antioxidants, including vitamins A, C, E, selenium, and zinc, help oxidative stress caused by excessive glucose and free radicals in diabetics. They help the body store sugar as glycogen and reduce artery complications.
- Vitamin C with bioflavonoids is essential for arterial health. It cleans the veins and strengthens the immune system.
- Chromium, zinc, and manganese will help control blood sugar levels.
- B-complex vitamins help to cut down on insulin intake; they also strengthen and repair the nerves. B vitamins are missing in the average American diet.
- Liquid chlorophyll and blue-green algae increase the utilization of all nutrients and assist in rebuilding a damaged pancreas.
- Magnesium deficiencies are often seen in diabetics and can cause high blood pressure, plaque in the arteries, and other cardiovascular problems. Low magnesium can contribute to insulin resistance and carbohydrate intolerance.
- Essential fatty acids in flaxseed, borage, black currant, evening primrose, and salmon oils all nourish and feed the glands.
- Digestive enzymes are necessary to strengthen the pancreas and clean the undigested protein from the blood and cells.
- Free-form amino acids are essential for healing the glands and nourishing and strengthening the body.
- Cat's claw is useful for diabetes and helps the body get rid of parasites. This remarkable herb has anti-inflammatory, antioxidant, and antimicrobial properties.
- Ginkgo and bilberry provide oxygen to the brain and eye areas to prevent damage to the eyes.
- CoQ10 and germanium provide oxygen in the blood to protect the capillaries and veins.
- L-carnitine helps to dissolve fat in the veins and protects against fat buildup.

**ALTERNATIVE SOLUTIONS**

Juanita developed diabetes and didn't want to go on the medication recommended to her by the medical doctors. She was concerned about her health and was very fortunate to find someone who knew about herbs and natural health. She went on what was called a "bentonite cleanse," using bentonite, cascara sagrada, psyllium, and chlorophyll. She would put this in a juice drink and drink it down. She did this for five days and passed two large tapeworms. She said that she probably had them since she was a child, because her family ate a lot of pork. Since she passed the worms, she has never had any symptoms of diabetes. Juanita also took combination #1, chaparral, a liver cleanse, red clover, and goldenseal to help rebuild the health of her pancreas. She is a grandmother now and is very healthy.

**ORTHODOX PRESCRIBED MEDICATION**

Acarbose (Precose) is one of the newest types of diabetes drugs. It works by slowing the digestion of carbohydrates in the small intestine. The drug works by blocking enzymes that normally break down carbohydrates. Side effects can be stomach and digestive problems such as gas, cramps, and diarrhea. It can impair kidney function and has caused cancerous kidney tumors in rats. It could also cause hypoglycemia or low blood sugar levels, and one should have a source of dextrose on hand to counteract hypoglycemia. This drug is intended to be supplemental therapy to diet and exercise.

# DIVERTICULITIS

Diverticulitis is a common and serious disease of the intestines. It strikes nearly 70 percent of people past the age of seventy. It usually begins with persistent constipation, which can alternate with diarrhea. It can cause nausea, vomiting, abdominal swelling, cramps, and pain. It can even bring a flu-like feeling of chills and fever. Fiber (the indigestible part of food) helps the muscle contractions of the walls of the intestines. It increases peristaltic action to draw food quickly through the alimentary canal. When food moves too slowly through the alimentary canal, the hard elimination and undigested food causes pouches to form on the intestinal wall. These are called diverticula. These pouches become filled with toxic feces, which cause irritation and infections. This is due to poor bowel function and autointoxication. Also, undigested protein can leak through the intestinal wall and cause all kinds of diseases.

Autoimmune diseases are increasing with bowel problems such as leaky gut syndrome. Constipation and a low-fiber diet are the main causes of this problem. Straining from hard stools causes pockets in the colon to form, allowing toxins to accumulate. This can be serious and develop into cancer if left untreated. Diverticulitis is another form of autointoxication. Symptoms are similar to appendicitis, except on the left-hand side. This disease causes malnutrition because of poor digestion and absorption. It causes improper secretion of saliva in the mouth and prevents proper digestion and enzyme processes. Cataracts are formed and hearing is impaired because the organs are starved of nutrition and oxygen.

## HERBAL COMBINATIONS
### Herbal Combination #1
This formula is designed to clean the liver. The liver attempts to eliminate the toxins from the bloodstream. These include fried fats, drugs, preservatives, rancid oils, and pollutants in the food, water, and air. It is important to clean the liver. If the liver is allowed to accumulate poisons, then the blood and body as a whole create a toxic internal environment that will prevent the cleansing process.

- Black cohosh is calming for the nerves, cleansing for the liver and gallbladder, and relaxing for the body to help increase the healing process.
- Red beet is nutritious for the liver, helps correct liver diseases, and restores proper function.
- Dandelion stimulates the liver, detoxifies poisons, and clears liver obstructions.
- Parsley cleans the liver of toxic wastes, tones the body, and is nutritious to build the colon.
- Horsetail is rich in vitamins and minerals, aids in circulation, builds and tones the body, and is a natural diuretic.

- Birch has natural properties for cleansing the blood and has a high content of vitamins and minerals.
- Blessed thistle is a general tonic to the system, stimulates liver bile, and purifies the blood.
- Angelica helps eliminate toxins in the liver and spleen and is a tonic for mental and physical harmony.
- Chamomile destroys toxins in the liver, and has healing properties. It is calming to the nerves, and helps relieve insomnia.
- Gentian stimulates liver function, is high in iron, strengthens the system, and aids in digestion.
- Goldenrod stimulates circulation and kidney function and strengthens the system.
- Yellow dock is an astringent and blood purifier. It is one of the best blood builders in the herb kingdom. It stimulates elimination, improves bile flow, and acts as a laxative.

### Other Uses
Age spots, cleansing, gall bladder, kidneys, pancreas, and spleen.

### Herbal Combination #2
Other herbal combinations that help in diverticulitis are #1 under Colitis, to help heal the intestines, and #2 under Colitis, to help nourish and rebuild colon health. Also, #1 under Constipation for the lower bowel is a blood cleanser and will help eliminate toxins.

## HEALTHFUL SUGGESTIONS
1. Juice fasting is one of the quickest ways to heal the digestive system. Fast for one to three days at a time, depending on the strength of the body. Use carrots, celery, endive, and garlic. Extract the juice and drink it immediately for the best results. Always dilute the juices to prevent stress on the pancreas. Another nutritious combination is carrots, celery, parsley, and cabbage or green peppers.

2. Eat a high-fiber diet and include whole grains, such as whole oats, kamut, millet, brown rice, rye, whole wheat, amaranth, yellow cornmeal, quinoa, spelt, and teff. Buy the whole grains and grind them yourself or have them ground as you use them. Once you open the grains, they oxidize quickly and can cause free-radical damage. Try thermos cooking.

High-fiber foods pass much more smoothly through the intestines, preventing the possibility of developing spasms and hernias. These foods move other food residue along the digestive tract and help prevent infection and inflammation. Another healthful laxative is one tablespoon ground flaxseeds, one teaspoon fenugreek powder, one tablespoon goat's whey powder, and one teaspoon fresh ginger. Mix ingredients in pure water or juice and drink first thing in the morning. It is excellent for the colon.

3. Vegetable soups are healing; they are rich in minerals. Cook the following vegetables and use the broth as stock: cabbage, potatoes with skin, carrots, celery, onions, parsley, garlic, shallots, and ginger. An herbal mineral drink, high in potassium, will heal the mucous membranes. Potassium is essential for good digestion. Add millet and brown rice to the diet. Millet is rich in calcium and magnesium and is easy to digest. Other well-tolerated foods are sweet potatoes, winter squash, non-citrus fruits, and green vegetables.

4. An herbal fiber formula will heal and help clean the pockets of the colon wall. It should contain psyllium husk and other cleansing herbs. Slippery elm is very cleansing, healing, and nourishing to the colon. An excellent formula is psyllium hulls, hibiscus flower, and licorice. It will help clean and speed the healing.

5. Exercise is very important. Use squatting exercises to develop muscles in the colon area. Walking is a very good exercise. Using a trampoline will help build muscle coordination. Massage therapy will also help stimulate and rebuild the colon.

6. Enemas and colonics are very helpful. Dr. Norman Walker stated: "Experience has taught me that no health and healing procedures can be as successful as those which have a series of colon irrigations as the prelude to any health treatment. This makes sense because just so long as there is material in the colon which may be conducive to the generation of poisons in the colon and to the diffusion of such poisons throughout the system, no healing can take place which is not the precursor of a chain reaction of ailments at a future date." Colon therapy with oxygen helps to destroy parasites, worms, bacteria, viruses, germs, and toxins. It has a calming effect on the nervous system. Colon therapy is a gentle washing of the large intestine. Oxygen therapy helps to heal the inflamed tissues in the colon and the cells. Most modern-day colonic machines are equipped with disposable hoses and speculums to ensure cleanliness. Colonics are more effective than enemas. Dr. Norman Walker also said, "One colonic is equivalent to thirty enemas." Acidophilus should always be used after enemas and colonics. This replaces the friendly bacteria for better bowel health.

## HERBS AND SUPPLEMENTS

Single herbs to help with diverticulitis are aloe vera (heals scars and adhesions), alfalfa (rich in minerals), fenugreek (cleans and heals the colon), garlic (a natural antibiotic), glucomannan (cleans the colon), hops (relaxing to the colon), kelp (provides minerals), marshmallow, and papaya (healing).

- Psyllium is very useful in irritations of the bowel, spastic colon, or hemorrhoids. Cholesterol can even be lowered with the use of psyllium. It needs to be taken with a lot of water to prevent obstruction in the colon.
- Lower bowel formulas help to clean, nourish, and rebuild the colon.
- Licorice root tea or deglycerinized licorice is healing for the intestines.
- Chlorophyll is soothing and healing and provides nutrients to the colon.
- Acidophilus is necessary for restoring the friendly bacteria; it also helps in the digestion of food.
- Aloe vera juice is healing, helps to prevent scarring, and aids in healing adhesions.
- Digestive enzymes help the breakdown of undigested proteins in the cells and blood. They will also help speed healing and prevent toxins and food from adhering to the colon walls.
- Antioxidants, vitamins A, C, D, selenium, zinc, CoQ10, and grapeseed extract help to protect from free-radical damage. Vitamin A is healing for a healthy digestive tract. Vitamins C and E help heal and protect the digestive tract.
- Multimineral supplements are necessary for healing and protecting the lining of the entire body.
- B-complex vitamins are necessary for a healthy digestive tract. They feed the nervous system.
- Essential fatty acids protect the cells, nourish the glands, and strengthen the entire body.
- Amino acid supplements help speed the healing of the digestive tract.

- Chlorophyll, blue-green algae, and green drinks help in restoring health to the colon.

## ORTHODOX PRESCRIBED MEDICATION

Saline laxatives such as milk of magnesia, Fleet's, or Epsom salts may alter the body's fluid and electrolyte balance. Lubricants such as mineral oil can decrease the absorption of vitamins A, D, and E. Antibiotics are also prescribed for infections. Antibiotics can worsen the symptoms of colon disease. They upset the bacterial balance within the intestines by killing the healthful bacteria and promoting the harmful ones. Wait until the antibiotic therapy is finished, then take acidophilus to reintroduce the friendly bacteria in the colon.

# ENDOMETRIOSIS

Endometriosis develops when small pockets of the uterus lining grow outside of the uterus into the pelvic cavity. It is a very common disease, and it is estimated that 40 to 50 percent of women who undergo hysterectomies have endometriosis. It can cause irregular bleeding, pain during intercourse and menses, severe pelvic pain, and even infertility. This condition was discovered in 1899 and described in medical journals. In 1920, Dr. J. A. Sampson described the ever-increasing disease as very serious. Dr. Sampson found clumps of brown, sticky tissue and old, clotted blood adhering in unusual places: ovaries, rectal ligaments, intestines, appendix, cervix, bladder, and fallopian tubes. In severe cases, the abdominal organs were glued together and twisted out of place by the contortions of the unusual and strange tissue. Then he discovered that the sticky, clotted tissue was the same as that which lined the normal uterus. It also reacted to the hormonal cycle the same way as the uterine tissue, proliferating when stimulated by estrogens and actually bleeding during menstruation.

When the lining of the uterus, called the endometrium, grows outside the uterine walls and appears in other places and bleeds, it causes cysts, inflammation, scar tissue, and damage to the areas. It seems to appear and disappear according to the hormonal profile of the woman. It is not fully under-stood how the tissue escapes from the uterus in the first place. One theory is that the excess uterine lining is forced upward and out through the fallopian tubes by heavy menstrual contractions. Another theory is that endometrial tissue develops from simple, undifferentiated epithelial cells in the abdomen, like what essentially happens in the female fetus during early pregnancy.

A compromised immune system may be another reason some women get endometriosis and some don't. When the immune system is compromised, the tissues of the uterus are able to spread throughout the pelvic area. It may be considered an autoimmune disease. An immune dysfunction can lead to an imbalance in the uterus and be caused by mucus-forming foods and hormones and antibiotics in meat and dairy products. A diet high in sugar and white flour products contributes to endometriosis. When the immune system is depleted, it will invite imbalances in the body, usually in the weakest areas.

Symptoms can be pelvic pain, low back pain, menstrual cramps, pain at ovulation, infertility, excessive menstrual bleeding, menstrual irregularity, constipation, rectal bleeding, and pain and bleeding with urination. Some of the causes may include constipation, overuse of estrogen-polluted foods such as meat, chicken, and dairy products, use of prescribed estrogen, and obesity. A weakness for endometriosis can be inherited. Stress and lack of nutrients such as B vitamins can contribute to this disease.

## HERBAL COMBINATIONS
### Herbal Combination #1

- White willow is a natural pain reliever, contains antiseptic properties, and is cleansing and healing.
- Valerian is a nerve tonic, promotes relaxation, and relieves headache pain and menstrual pain.
- Wild lettuce helps after-birth pains and is a general pain reliever.
- Capsicum is a stimulant, relaxant, and cleans and nourishes the veins.

### Other Uses

Aches and pains, after-birth pain, cramps, headache, arthritis, menstrual cramps, relaxant, toothache.

## Herbal Combination #2

This is formulated especially for the female reproductive organs and also benefits the glandular system. It is rich in herbs that contain vitamins and minerals that feed and strengthen the female glands.

- Red raspberry strengthens the uterus wall, reduces nausea, prevents hemorrhage, and relieves pain.
- Dong quai nourishes the female glands, strengthens all internal organs and muscles, relaxes the central nervous system and brain, and is healing for bleeding and body injuries.
- Ginger relieves congestion, settles an upset stomach and indigestion, and enhances the function of other herbs.
- Licorice counteracts stress, supplies energy, reduces inflammation, and is healing.
- Black cohosh is a tonic for the central nervous system, a hormone balancer, and neutralizes poisons in the blood.
- Queen of the meadow treats urinary problems, helps with pain, and relieves water retention.
- Blessed thistle is a tonic to help with digestion, blood circulation, and the liver. It helps ease cramps, balances hormones, and supplies oxygen to the brain.
- Marshmallow is soothing and healing for inflammations and pain, a powerful anti-inflammatory and anti-irritant, and healing for growths.

## Other Uses

Hormone imbalance, hot flashes, gland malfunctioning, menstrual problems, morning sickness, sexual impotence, uterus problems.

## HEALTHFUL SUGGESTIONS

1. A colon, blood, and liver cleanse will help rid the body of built-up toxins in the bloodstream and cells. Colon congestion is one of the reasons toxins accumulate in the body. Glue foods such as white flour products and fried, greasy food will adhere to the colon wall and can enter the bloodstream.

2. Fasting with herbal teas, vegetable juices, and alkaline foods will help the body eliminate toxins. Fasting should be done according to the strength of the body. A weak body should first strengthen and build, then fast. Fasting should never be done when a person is already weak. Water fasts are not recommended; they can move toxins too quickly, which can cause serious reactions because of all the toxin in the environment.

3. Avoid animal meat and dairy products that contain hormones and antibiotics. The excess estrogen can lead to endometriosis. Avoid chocolate, coffee, salt, sugar, fried food, and all processed foods, which can cause free-radical damage. They weaken the immune system and aggravate the symptoms.

4. A good diet can help detoxify excessive estrogen and other toxins. Steamed and fresh vegetables are very beneficial. Use fresh salads made from leaf lettuce, cabbage, carrots, broccoli, and other vegetables. Use olive oil and lemon juice for dressing with added garlic, onions, parsley, and vegetable seasoning. Use brown rice, millet, buckwheat, and all whole grains (thermos cooking will retain the enzymes and B-complex vitamins).

5. Exercise is very beneficial to prevent adhesions from adhering to the wall of the uterus and other organs. It also helps to normalize hormone levels by metabolizing fat. Exercise will also help in stress reduction and in controlling menstrual and back pain.

## HERBS AND SUPPLEMENTS

Single herbs to help endometriosis include black cohosh, cramp bark, dong quai, false unicorn, ginseng, gotu kola, kelp, licorice, sarsaparilla, squaw vine, and wild yam.

- White willow bark is very beneficial for pain relief, without side effects of bleeding or ringing in the ears, as aspirin does. A tea would assimilate faster.
- Feverfew has been found effective for migraine headaches without side effects. It has been used to relieve pain other than headaches.
- Digestive enzymes help reduce inflammation and aid in digesting proteins in the bloodstream and cells. They will also prevent digestive problems.
- Soy isoflavone extract balances hormones and prevents cancer growths. Use soy products such as tofu and soymilk to provide plant protein.
- Essential fatty acids, including evening primrose, flaxseed, borage, black currant, and salmon oils, help the body produce anti-inflammatory prostaglandins.
- Vitamins A, C, E, selenium, zinc, and grapeseed extract are powerful antioxidants. Recent research

indicates that free-radical damage is connected to endometriosis.

- Iodine is found in kelp, dulse, salmon, Swiss chard, watercress, and egg yolks (organic). A deficiency in iodine can trigger endometriosis.
- Natural progesterone cream aids in hormonal balance. The cream is absorbed through the skin and goes where it is needed. It works faster than taken internally in capsule form.
- Cruciferous vegetable concentrate supplements help balance hormones and detoxify the bad estrogen in the liver and intestinal tract.
- Chlorophyll and blue-green algae help to clean the blood and supply nutrients to the blood.
- Free-form amino acids are very important for healing the body and providing strength and protein to every cell.
- Pancreatic enzymes and hydrochloric acid help in digestion of food, protect the body from free-radical damage, and eliminate undigested proteins from the blood and cells.
- B-complex vitamins are needed daily and lost quickly when the body is under emotional and physical stress. Extra B12 will help with stress, and B6 with magnesium will reduce symptoms of estrogen overload. The liver is the site of eliminating excess estrogen, and it cannot do it without adequate B vitamins.
- A vitamin supplement is important. Vitamins A and E help heal and protect against scar tissues and aid in hormone imbalance. Vitamin C with bioflavonoids is essential in healing and cleansing the body.

## ORTHODOX PRESCRIBED MEDICATION

Anti-inflammatory agents are prescribed, such as ibuprofen (Advil). Drugs are sometimes recommended to fool the body into thinking it's either pregnant or menopausal. Surgery is also recommended. Ibuprofen is a potent drug with serious side effects. It can cause chronic digestive problems, is related to aspirin, and can cause stomach bleeding, diarrhea, constipation, gas, heartburn, chronic stomach pain, and irritation. When stomach trouble develops, drugs such as Tagamet or Zantac are prescribed. This cuts down on the hydrochloric acid production, which is needed to protect the entire digestive tract.

# ENVIRONMENTAL POISONING

Environmental toxins are a real health hazard. We are constantly exposed to an overwhelming quantity of toxins daily. The U.S. government is spending a lot of money to clean up toxic waste dumps, but they are not the only health hazards. Other health risks include smog, polluted drinking water, acid rain, and chemical toxins. We also have polluted soil, waterways, noxious gases, and contaminants discharged from industrial sources. Herbicides and pesticides are found everywhere, and we are constantly being exposed—residues are found in the blood and urine of people living in both urban and rural areas. They have also been found in mothers' milk. These poisons are capable of causing mutations and cancer.

Radon gas also poses a health threat. It is a radioactive by-product of uranium decay that seeps up from the ground, and is becoming one of the most dangerous sources of radioactivity in the home. It has been found to seep up from the basement, and is often stored in building materials such as cinder blocks and brick and in well-insulated homes, which doesn't allow air to circulate from outside. National Cancer Institute officials report that at least thirty thousand lung cancer deaths are attributable to radon exposure every year.

Lindane (bug bombs) is used in home gardens and on farms for treating seeds and hardwood lumber. Insecticides are also found in animal shampoos, flea collars, shelf paper, and floor wax. They can cause cancer, are toxic to a growing fetus, damage the reproductive organs, and can be particularly harmful to children.

We have food additives, preservatives, artificial colorings, chemicals applied to our fruit to ripen it artificially, and colors to enhance their shelf appeal. Nitrites and nitrates are found in hot dogs and lunchmeat and have been found to cause stomach and brain cancer. We are threatened with electromagnetic radiation, which has been linked to leukemia.

We are bombarded with all kinds of pollution. Radiation poisoning suppresses an already weakened immune system. When you undergo radiation therapy you may experience radiation burns, scarring, fatigue, and a strain on the immune system. Radiation destroys many nutrients in the body. Supplements are vital to strengthen immune function and protect the system from diseases.

Mercury is another health threat. In Europe, "mad as a hatter" was an expression used by men who worked in hat factories who went insane because of mercury used in making felt hats. Mercury accumulates in the system. It causes neurological and behavioral disruptions and affects the immune system by decreasing the production of white blood cells, including T cells, which protect the body by eliminating harmful toxins.

Other environmental toxins are aluminum, cadmium, carbon monoxide, chlorine, copper, fluoride, hexavalent chromium, dioxin, DDT, lead, nitrates and nitrites, nitrogen dioxide, pharmaceuticals, and tobacco smoke.

## HERBAL COMBINATIONS
### Herbal Combination #1
This formula helps the body to eliminate toxins from the liver, kidneys, lungs, bowels, and skin. These environment toxins can accumulate in the body's organs and cause diseases. The following herbs help to nourish, cleanse, and rebuild cells and organs in the body.

- Burdock is known as one of the best blood purifiers and eliminates calcification deposits and removes accumulated acids.
- Dandelion clears obstructions and stimulates the liver to detoxify poisons. It promotes healthy circulation, strengthens weak arteries, and contains protein, vitamins, and minerals.
- Fenugreek has antiseptic properties and kills infections. It softens and dissolves hard mucus in the body, and helps to expel toxic waste through the lymphatic system.
- Ginger relieves congestion, aches and pains, and is used for upset stomach and indigestion. Ginger works with other herbs to enhance their effect.
- Marshmallow is soothing for the lungs as an expectorant. It also heals inflammation and is good for asthma.
- Pepsin is a digestive enzyme that breaks up undigested protein in the bloodstream. Protein coatings are found in germs, parasites, and other toxins in the body.

- Red clover is considered a good dietary supplement to build up the body. It is a useful tonic for the nerves and as a sedative for nervous exhaustion.
- Sarsaparilla is a valuable herb used to balance hormonal secretions. It has stimulating properties that increases the metabolic rate and promotes circulation.
- Yellow dock is one of the best blood builders in the herb kingdom. It stimulates elimination, improves flow of bile, and acts as a laxative. It is rich in digestible plant iron.
- Echinacea stimulates the immune system to increase the body's ability to fight infections. It improves lymphatic drainage, and helps remove toxins from the blood.
- Lactobacillus helps restore natural bacteria in the digestive system.
- Cascara sagrada helps promote natural peristaltic action in the intestines. It increases the secretions of the stomach, liver, and pancreas.
- Milk thistle is effective in restoring impaired liver function, as well as protecting the liver from damage by toxic substances. Milk thistle is an antioxidant that protects against free-radical damage and helps to protect the entire body.

### Herbal Combination #2
This formula is excellent to bind with heavy metals and eliminate them from the body; it cleans, detoxifies, and supplies essential minerals.

It contains cilantro, N-acetyl-cysteine, apple pectin, sodium alginate, kelp, lk-methionine, alpha lipoic acid, magnesium, and pyridoxal-5-phosphate.

Other uses include Alzheimer's disease, brain dysfunction, blood cleanser, among other diseases.

## HEALTHFUL SUGGESTIONS
Whole grains, including wheat, brown rice, millet, barley, oats, corn, buckwheat, rye, and the new (and ancient) grains amaranth, kamut, quinoa, spelt, and teff. Whole grains are rich energy food, and are high in complex carbohydrates, which give the body long-lasting energy. Buckwheat and millet have been found to help eliminate radiation poisoning. They are high in protein and easily digestible.

Whole grains supply vitamins, minerals, carbohydrates and fiber, as well as protein. Whole grains also supply tryptophan, which increases production of the neurotransmitter serotonin, which reduces tension and stress, improves sleep, and increases one's sense of well-being.

Vegetables: Organic vegetables are superior and are free from pesticides, herbicides, and other chemicals that are derived from petrochemical sources and may be carcinogenic. Vegetables are rich in nutrients, especially vitamins and minerals. Kale, mustard greens, collards, and parsley are rich in calcium. They are low in fat, rich in fiber, and easily digestible.

Green vegetables, such as broccoli, Brussels sprouts, and all green leafy vegetables are rich in chlorophyll and help counteract radioactive and environmental poisoning. The following are important: cabbage, alfalfa sprouts and other sprouts, mustard greens, cilantro, collard greens, kale, watercress, carrots, squash, pumpkin, potatoes, sweet potatoes, beets, dark leaf lettuce, onions, and garlic. Avocados are rich in essential fatty acids, vitamins, minerals, and protein.

Legumes and beans are rich in protein, fiber, vitamins, minerals, and carbohydrates. They include black-eyed peas, black beans, soybeans, adzuki, chickpeas, kidney beans, lima beans, lentils, navy beans, pinto beans, split peas, and soybeans. Soy-based foods include tofu, tempeh, soymilk, soy "ice cream," and soy yogurt; they are nutritious and high in protein. Beans are rich in amino acids.

Fruits cleanse the body. Whole fruit is rich in fiber and vitamins and minerals. Apples and bananas contain potassium and pectin. Peaches and apricots contain beta-carotene, iron, and fiber and are rich in antioxidants, pectin, and minerals such as iron.

Fiber is important because it dilutes stool bile acids and reduces the concentration of toxic carcinogenic substances in the colon and eliminates them. Fiber also eliminates excess fat in the body. Fibers such as psyllium, oat bran, and whole grains are excellent. Apple pectin removes lead. It is changed into galacturonic acid (one of nature's cleansing agents) after digestion. This acid combines with lead to form an insoluble metallic salt that cannot be absorbed.

Avoid all food additives and foods that are prepackaged; they become rancid, which causes free-radical damage. Avoid foods that contain preservatives and artificial colorings. Don't smoke and stay away from secondhand smoke. Cigarette smoke is devastating to the lungs and the whole body. Do not smoke around children, especially infants. Numerous cases of sudden infant death syndrome (SIDS) are attributed to secondhand smoke in the home. Avoid sugar and all white flour products. Meat has antibiotics and hormones and fried foods contain rancid oils that can weaken the immune system.

## HERBS AND SUPPLEMENTS

Garlic is rich in sulfur, which attracts metals and eliminates them from the body. Garlic contains germanium and selenium with chelation ability to neutralize heavy metal toxicity.

Herbs containing sulfur are excellent to protect the body from environmental toxins include horseradish, watercress, alfalfa, burdock, dandelion, comfrey, garlic, onions, sarsaparilla, kelp, echinacea, lobelia, mullein, parsley, cayenne, eyebright, nettle, and fennel.

- Ginkgo is a strong antioxidant, free radical scavenger, and increases the flow of nutrients and oxygen to all cells. It improves memory, mental efficiency, and concentration, reduces anxiety, tension, and symptoms of senility and age-related brain disorders.
- Gotu kola is food for the brain and protects the body from toxins. It purifies the blood and helps eliminate fatigue and memory loss.
- Kelp attaches itself to any lead that is present and carries it harmlessly out of the system.
- Coenzyme Q10 protects the immune system, strengthens the body's resistance to stress and disease by making tissues stronger and healthier. It aids in oxygenation within the cells and tissues. It is good for heart disease, aging, cancer, and obesity.
- Chlorophyll is nature's cleanser. It cleanses the bloodstream and eliminates toxins from the bowels.
- Suma contains germanium to protect the immune system. It protects the body from stress, and improves circulation and arthritis. It also balances hormones.
- Algin is a natural extract from kelp and is a concentrated form of nutrients that is very effective in eliminating radioactive strontium 90 from the body. It is also beneficial in eliminating the chemical additives that we ingest daily. Algin grabs hold of the toxic material and excretes it out of the body.

- Zinc and selenium are essential minerals that help to eliminate lead as well as other heavy metals and toxins from the body.
- Nervine herbs are essential to protect the central nervous system and the brain. Nervine herbs include hops, lady's slipper, skullcap, valerian, passion flower, wood betony, chamomile, black cohosh, and lobelia.
- Hydrochloric acid and digestive enzymes are essential nutrients, binding metals and eliminating them from the body, especially when you eat a lot of cooked food.
- Vitamins: A is necessary for the cells to eliminate the toxic metal absorbed from chemicals in food, air, and water. B-complex vitamins protect the immune system and help detoxify the liver. Calcium is an indispensable mineral; it actually penetrates the bones and slowly displaces lead, especially when silicon (found in horsetail) is present. It prevents accumulation of lead from the intestinal tract. The best form of calcium can be found in herbal formulas.
- Oral chelation is a formula with vitamins, minerals, glandulars, amino acids, and herbs used to cleanse the system. These natural nutrients gradually dissolve and eliminate deposits in the arteries. Oral chelation is very effective in ridding the body of high levels of toxic metals.

# EPILEPSY

There are close to one million epileptics in the United States. Although the exact cause is unknown, certain injuries to the head can cause the onset of epilepsy. In two out of three individuals suffering from the disorder, no structural abnormalities or scar tissue is present. In one-third of epileptics, epilepsy is a secondary complication resulting from physical damage to the brain caused by traumatic birth, bacterial meningitis, malaria, rickets, rabies, tetanus, malnutrition, poisoning, cerebral palsy, mental retardation, brain tumors, hydrocephalus, stroke, lack of oxygen, or injury to the head. Aspartame is seen as a cause of some epileptic seizures. The actual epileptic seizure is due to a sudden abnormal and excessive electrical discharge within the brain. In primary epilepsy, the basic cause is unknown, but there is usually a genetic predisposition. Secondary epilepsy can be from a head injury, bacterial meningitis, or malaria; it is often associated with cerebral palsy, mental retardation, brain tumors and cysts, and hydrocephalus. For further information, read about epilepsy in *The Complete Home Health Advisor*, by Rita Elkins.

At the turn of the twentieth century, Henry Lindlahr, MD, had an interesting concept of the cause of epilepsy, hysteria, and St. Vitus dance. He says, "When the drainage system of the nose and the nasopharyngeal cavities has been completely destroyed, the impurities must either travel upward into the brain or downward into the glandular structures of the neck, thence into the bronchi and the tissues of the lungs. If the trend be upward, to the brain, the patient grows nervous and irritable or becomes dull and apathetic. How often is a child reprimanded or even punished for laziness and inattention when it cannot help itself? In many instances the morbid matter affects certain centers in the brain and causes nervous conditions, hysteria, St. Vitus dance, epilepsy, etc. In children the impurities frequently find an outlet through the eardrums in the form of pus-like discharges. This may frequently avert inflammation of the brain, meningitis, imbecility, insanity, or infantile paralysis."

In his book *The Ultimate Healing System*, Donald LePore, ND, states, "We believe that epilepsy is not a disease, but is actually nature's way of getting rid of the deteriorating matter on the brain. The epileptic seizure is like an electrical storm; this is nature's way of giving an electrical charge to correct the malfunction of the brain which sometimes is scar tissue in the area."

Doctors in the past felt that epilepsy was caused by derangement of the digestive organs, injury, suppression of the menses, or impure blood. New evidence in *What Doctors Don't Tell You* shows that vaccines, allergies, or nutritional deficiencies may bring on epileptic seizures, and certain simple dietary changes may control them without drugs.

In his book *A Shot in the Dark*, Dr. Harris L. Coulter says, "Vaccination causes a slight degree of encephalitis in children. Doctors recognize this happens but insist it occurs only once in every 100,000 cases. In my opinion, it happens about once in five.

When you have encephalitis, the child may recover completely, but it may not and may suffer some long-term damage." One of the most common after-effects of seizures is epilepsy.

There is evidence that food allergies or intolerance or even chemical sensitivities may be one of the causes of epilepsy. In *The Complete Guide to Food Allergy and Intolerance*, British physician Dr. Jonathan Brostoff describes a trial involving eighty-eight children, forty of whom underwent a placebo-controlled, double-blind trial. All of the children suffered from migraines, and some had recurrent epileptic fits. Once their allergies had been identified and the offending foods removed, seventy-eight recovered completely from their migraine attacks, but most important, their epilepsy disappeared as well.

## EMOTIONAL NEEDS

Anyone with epilepsy may have to deal with social stigmas associated with seizures. As a result, support and good education on this disease are crucial. Reassurance after a seizure is also a great value in helping dispel feelings of embarrassment.

## HERBAL COMBINATIONS
### Herbal Combination #1

This formula contains an amino acid called GABA (gamma-aminobutyric acid), which stimulates neurotransmitter activity in the brain. This will help calm nervous systems that become overstimulated. This promising formula also contains the amino acids glutamine and taurine, which also play a beneficial role in brain function.

- Spirulina is rich in vitamins, minerals, and nutrients that nourish the brain.
- Passion flower is a calming herb that has been used to treat hyperactive children. It is useful for insomnia, hysteria, and convulsions in children.

### Other Uses

Anxiety, convulsions, headaches, hyperactivity, hysteria, insomnia, nervous breakdown, relaxant, restores nervous system.

## HEALTHFUL SUGGESTIONS

1. Allergies may be a cause. There is evidence that food allergy or chemical sensitivity could be one of the causes of general epilepsy. Allergic epileptic seizures can be precipitated by exposure to certain chemicals. They could include gases, airborne droplets, pesticides, fumes from engines, diesel emissions, solvents, perfumes, drugs, or food additives. Some children were put on a gluten-free diet and improved their epilepsy. Health-care professionals can do tests to see if allergies are involved.

2. Exercise can be very beneficial to keep the brain alert and help counteract the side effects of drug therapy. Exercising on a regular basis is important. Walking, jumping on a trampoline, and weight lifting will strengthen the body and the mind. Fresh air and a sound sleep are important to keep the body and mind in balance.

3. A hair analysis can determine whether or not toxic heavy metal levels are elevated in the body. Heavy metals have an adverse effect on the brain and may be linked to epilepsy.

4. A supervised fast may help rid the body of toxins that weaken the brain area. Using chlorophyll and green drinks will help clean the blood. Juices using carrot, celery, parsley, and garlic are very cleansing. Using lower bowel formulas will also prevent toxins from entering the blood.

5. A high-fiber diet with wholesome food will help nourish the brain and nervous system. The brain is affected by lack of oxygen and free-radical damage. Rancid food is one cause of free radicals. Avoid prepared foods and use only whole grains, and grind them yourself. Once a grain has been ground, it causes oxidation and can cause damage. Avoid white sugar products and salt, because they can stimulate the brain. White flour has bleach, which is damaging to the brain. Thermos cooking of grains, nuts, and seeds helps to retain enzymes, vitamins, and minerals essential for brain nourishment. Soups can also be made in the thermos.

6. Eat regular meals using dark green leafy vegetables, carrots, raw fruits, fresh juices, whole grains, low-fat cheeses, and low-fat meats. Avoid alcohol, caffeine, coffee, tea, chocolate, and artificial sweeteners.

## HERBS AND SUPPLEMENTS

Single herbs to help with epilepsy include black walnut (parasites can cause epilepsy), ginkgo (stimulates brain), gotu kola (brain food), hops (nervous disorders), lady's slipper (strengthens brain function), lobelia (relaxant), passion flower

## HE FEELS AN IMMEDIATE IMPROVEMENT

Stan has had grand mal epilepsy ever since he was nine years old. After decades of strong drug treatment, with his wife's help, he has discovered that by emphasizing certain nutrients and treatments he can function normally on a much lower dose of anticonvulsant drugs. First of all, he and his wife discovered that whenever he is prone to a seizure, he feels a tightening of the muscles at the base of his skull. They had never heard of a correlation between this phenomenon and epilepsy until Dr. John R. Christopher, MH, ND, suggested that a spasm in that area may predispose an epileptic to abnormal brain activity and to rub lobelia extract into those muscles for relaxation. They have done so and have found that he feels an immediate improvement. They always keep lobelia extract on hand.

They have also discovered that low blood sugar seems to play a role in his seizure activity, so it has been very helpful for him to stay away from high-glycemic foods that are low in fiber. They discovered that antiseizure drugs such as Dilantin and Depakote can destroy nutrients such as most of the B vitamins, suggesting that supplementation is vital for anyone taking these medicines.

They have found that eating plenty of raw foods, especially dark green leafy vegetables, supplies plenty of live enzymes, which seem to help promote good brain health. The following nutrient plan is the one they have had the best luck with. They found that after a month of this therapy, they slowly cut down on medication, with several weeks at each new level. They also noticed that the more Stan exercises, the better he feels, and that increased exercise has been linked to decreased seizures. It is important to fortify the body with added nutrients if you exercise and to always get adequate sleep.

By taking these supplements, they have been able to reduce Stan's dosage from nine Depakote pills daily to only four and seem to achieve the same results. Using 400 IU of vitamin E daily helps reduce the incidence of seizures under certain circumstances. He takes chromium for blood sugar control; magnesium to keep his muscles healthy, 500 mg per day; and vitamin D, 200 IU daily. Danish medical studies done on a small scale indicate that when vitamin D supplements were given to epileptics being treated with anticonvulsants, the incidence of seizures was significantly reduced.

Some epileptic medications interfere with the metabolism of vitamin D. B vitamins are important, with extra B6. Anticonvulsant drugs deplete the body of these vitamins. Essential fatty acids are crucial for proper nerve impulse transmission, because the brain is composed of unsaturated fatty acids.

The following amino acids are important for the proper functioning of brain cells. Take on an empty stomach with fruit juice: L-taurine, L-tyrosine, and L-glutamine. Ginkgo helps to stimulate brain function and can boost memory capacity, which may be impaired by anticonvulsant drugs, by helping oxygen levels in the brain. An herbal combination like combination #1 is important to rebuild nerves in the brain and nervous system. Kava contains kavalactones, which have distinct anticonvulsant and muscle relaxant properties and act on the limbic system of the brain, which is the seat of brain activity and contributes to sleep. Passion flower is considered a natural CNS depressant and antispasmodic. This herb contains alkaloids and flavonoids, which have nonaddictive narcotic effects that quiet the brain and promote sleep and relaxation.

They also found the following tips have helped:

- Don't get up too quickly in the morning. Allow your body to slowly adjust to waking up.
- Perform stretching exercises while still in bed and take some deep breaths.
- Do not attempt to blow up balloons. For some epileptics, this activity can precipitate a seizure.
- Some epileptics have used biofeedback and have actually been able to avoid a seizure that they feel coming on through some mental distraction. While this is not recommended alone, its possible value should be explored.
- Take your medication at the same time each day and in the exact prescribed dose.
- Do not become overly fatigued or stressed. Use exercise, biofeedback, and relaxation techniques, including meditation, to relax.
- Be more careful if you have an infectious illness, especially if a fever is present. This type of situation may increase your susceptibility to a seizure.

(nerve relaxant), skullcap, and valerian (brain relaxant).

- Skullcap has been studied in Russia and found to be a tonic, a sedative, and antiepileptic.
- Ginkgo and gotu kola provide oxygen and nutrients to the brain. Hydrochloric acid aids in digestion and the removal of toxic material that interferes with brain function.
- B-complex vitamins are necessary for the nervous system and brain disorders. Extra B3 relieves depression, is a blood cleanser, and dilates blood vessels to increase blood flow to the brain. Extra B6 is essential for the nervous system to prevent brain dysfunction and convulsions. B6, along with calcium, magnesium, and vitamin E, may be useful for epilepsy. B12 is vital for nervous system disorders and relaxing the nerves.
- Magnesium chloride relaxes muscles and nerves. It maintains function of the nerves. Low magnesium may be associated with nervous system disorders. Magnesium works with enzymes to break down sugar stored in the liver to create energy.
- Amino acid supplements with extra L-tyrosine, along with B6 and niacin, help control depression. L-taurine helps in nervous system function and protects the immune system.
- Digestive enzymes help to accelerate the healing process and help to prevent undigested protein in the blood and brain.
- Lecithin rebuilds the nerves and helps protect against damage to the myelin sheath around the nerves.
- Essential fatty acids are important for nervous system function. Flaxseed and salmon oil are very beneficial.
- CoQ10 provides oxygen to the brain to prevent brain dysfunction.

### ORTHODOX PRESCRIBED MEDICATION

Carbamazepine is an anticonvulsant and an antineuralgic, pain syndrome modifier. Brand names include Epitol, Tegretol, or Novo Carbamaz. It is used to relieve pain in tic douloureux or the control of several types of epilepsy. Possible side effects can be dry mouth and throat, constipation, and impaired urination. Other side effects include allergic reactions, fatigue, dizziness, exaggerated hearing, ringing in ears, nausea, indigestion, diarrhea, aching muscles and joints, and leg cramps. Serious side effects could be swelling of lymph glands, low white blood cell count, low levels of thyroid hormones, bone marrow depression, fever, abnormal bleeding, bruising, systemic lupus erythematosus, abnormal heartbeats, liver damage, kidney damage, mental depression, and many more. Drugs that can cause epilepsy or aggravate existing epileptic disorders include amphetamines, antihistamines, chloroquine, cimetidine, cycloserine, monoamine oxidase inhibitors, oral contraceptives, phenothiazines, and tricyclic antidepressants. Women receiving phenytoin (Dilantin) have a strong chance of bearing malformed children. All epileptic drugs can cause birth defects. Babies born with birth defects from this drug are affected with fetal valproate syndrome. It is characterized by distinctive facial features and can include spina bifida, heart disease, cleft lip or palate, limb defects, and genital malformations.

# EYE PROBLEMS

There are more than ten million people in the United States who suffer from severe vision disability, and the medical profession gives them no hope. The drugs prescribed and the surgeries performed offer no relief. Macular degeneration is the leading cause of severe visual loss in the United States and Europe. It usually hits individuals fifty-five years and older. It is associated with hardening of the arteries and hypertension. Many eye specialists feel that clogged blood vessels are big contributors to blindness. The cause is lack of blood, nutrients, and oxygen to the eyes. The small blood vessels become constricted and hardened. Free-radical damage is also a major factor due to a high-meat and high-fat diet. The liver and gallbladder cannot eliminate the excess oils and toxins because of constipation and autointoxication.

Other diseases of the eyes include diabetic retinopathy, optic nerve atrophy, and cataracts. Retinitis pigmentosa, an inherited genetic eye disease, occurs when the retina's nerve elements cause progressive atrophy, clumping of pigment, and finally atrophy of optic disks. Night blindness is one of the first signs. All of these diseases will increase the incidence of blindness by 60 percent in the next forty years.

Common drugs also have an adverse effect on the eyes. Sedative drugs such as tranquilizers and sleeping pills destroy the electrochemical balance, interfering with nerve transmission by putting out foreign energies as well as preventing vital nutrients from entering the eyes. Air pollution, especially tobacco smoke, can cause burning, dry, itchy, irritated, and bloodshot eyes. Eye problems are often an early indication of diseases in the body. Dark circles under the eyes are a sign of allergies, watery and red eyes are a sign of a cold coming on, bulging eyes can indicate a thyroid problem, and yellowing of the eyes is an indication of hepatitis, liver problems, or gallbladder problems. An eye specialist can recognize signs of high blood pressure and diabetes in patients when doing a regular eye examination.

## HERBAL COMBINATIONS
### Herbal Combination #1
Goldenseal is a natural antibiotic for eye infections. It helps to regulate liver function (eyes are related to liver congestion).

- Bayberry is high in vitamin C, kills germs, and stimulates the mucous membranes. It builds resistance to infections and is a tonic for the system.
- Eyebright is healing, stimulates the liver to clean the blood, and relieves eye problems. It contains antiseptic properties that heal eye problems, improve failing vision, and relieve eyestrain.
- Red raspberry is soothing and nourishing and rich in iron, calcium, phosphorus, and manganese. It is effective for sore eyes or colds in the eyes.

### Herbal Combination #2
This formula is excellent for the nervous and circulatory systems. It is food for the brain. This formula heals and protects the myelin sheath, helps in improving memory, and aids in maintaining healthy cholesterol. It contains DHA (docosahexaenoic acid) and EPA (eicosapentaenoic acid), essential fatty acids for normal brain function.

### Other Uses
Air pollution, eyewash, allergies, cataracts, diabetes, eye inflammation, hay fever, itching, and poor vision.

## HEALTHFUL SUGGESTIONS
1. Blood, liver, and colon cleansers are essential and will help clean the veins and capillaries in the eyes. The liver is connected to eye problems, and using milk thistle and other liver herbs would be beneficial. The eyes absorb toxins from the lower bowel, part of a process known as autointoxication or self-poisoning.

2. A natural herbal eyewash will cleanse and stimulate circulation to the eye tissues. Use an eyewash often to prevent the clogging of tiny capillaries and veins.

3. Juices beneficial for eye health are carrots, celery, parsley, and endive. Add garlic or fresh ginger to the juice. Carrot, kale, and ginger is also a good combination.

4. Increase the diet with natural foods such as whole grains, beans, lentils, and split peas, because they are high in nutrients for healthy veins. Add more green salads and raw and lightly steamed vegetables. Add sprouts and use onions, shallots, and garlic in recipes. Use brown rice, millet, yellow cornmeal, raw seeds, and nuts.

5. Avoid smoking, alcohol, and irritations that affect the eyes.

6. Avoid sugar, because it depletes calcium and B vitamins that are essential for eye health. Mineral oil depletes vitamin A. Caffeine has an adverse effect on the ability of the eyes to focus for reading or other close work. Eliminate white sugar and white flour products. Instead of red meat, use fish, lean chicken, and soy-based foods. Drink plenty of pure, fresh water.

## HERBS AND SUPPLEMENTS
Single herbs for eye health include bilberry (strengthens eyes), capsicum (cleans capillaries), eyebright (improves eye health), goldenseal, hops, and passion flower (improves nerves).

- Antioxidants protect against free-radical damage. Free radicals are implicated in eye problems such as cataracts. Studies show that 15,000 IU of vitamin A each day can slow the progression of night blindness and a narrowing of the visual field. Vitamins E, C, selenium, and zinc are important to prevent free-radical damage. CoQ10 and grapeseed extract are powerful antioxidants.
- Bilberry is a rich source of antioxidant and nutrients. It is rich in potassium, vitamins A and C,

**FOREVER GRATEFUL FOR HERBAL PRODUCTS**

Hessie had known for a long time that she had very small cataracts. Her vision was getting increasingly worse. She wanted to be able to see better, so she made an appointment to have her glasses changed. When new glasses didn't help, she asked the doctor what was the matter. He told her that surgery couldn't help and that her vision would get worse, not better. He told her it had to do with the optic nerve, which was cutting off light. Hessie looked up her condition in the medical dictionary and found that a heavy yellow or brown waxy substance was involved. To her, that was similar to cholesterol.

She started on a program to help improve her eyes. She took herbal combination #1 and also took herbal combination #1 under Cardiovascular Disorders. She took vitamins A, D, and beta-carotene with eyebright. She took them faithfully for twenty months. When she went back to the eye doctor, he told her that her eyes were clear enough to get good results from cataract surgery, which was done with wonderful results. She is forever grateful for the herbal products that helped her get her sight back.

iron, magnesium, manganese, phosphorus, potassium, selenium, and zinc. It improves circulation and helps prevent plaque buildup in the blood vessels and capillaries. It improves circulation and blood flow to heal the eye area.

- Eyebright aids in stimulating the liver to clean the blood and veins. It has antiseptic properties that fight infections of the eyes. It has traditionally been used as a remedy for eye problems such as failing vision, inflammation, ulcers, conjunctivitis, and eyestrain.
- Minerals are very important for eye health. They work with vitamins. Prolonged mineral deficiency can result in squinting, distorted visual perception, vertigo, fatigue, headaches, and painful eyes. Zinc is necessary for the transformation of vitamin A. Chromium and zinc protect against

cataracts. Calcium is important to the connective tissue of the eyes.
- Essential fatty acids are important, such as flaxseed, borage, black currant, and salmon oil, and they help protect and nourish the veins and capillaries. They help eliminate bad oils from building up in the body.
- Lecithin helps protect the nerves and brain. It protects against the buildup of fatty material in the veins and capillaries.
- Blue-green algae and chlorophyll are nourishing and healing for the veins. They protect against damage from air pollution.
- The amino acids glutathione and cystine help in protecting the eyes.
- B-complex vitamins are essential for the liver and eye health.

# FIBROMYALGIA SYNDROME

Fibromyalgia (fibrositis) is a common condition, and the incidence is increasing every year. There are more than six million patients diagnosed with this condition in the United States. It is a rheumatic disorder and is often difficult to diagnose. It is a very painful disorder with a collection of symptoms; for that reason, it is referred to as a syndrome. There has been success in using a holistic approach in treating fibromyalgia. Traditional medical forms of treatment have offered little relief.

Chronic fatigue syndrome and fibromyalgia may be closely related. Some believe they are both viral and related to polio vaccinations. Research into chronic fatigue and post-polio syndrome has made the astounding discovery that the virus which most often triggers chronic fatigue is closely related to the one that causes polio (*What Doctors Don't Tell You*, January 1996). Chronic fatigue and fibromyalgia seem to be an alternate polio. Some researchers say that CFS is just another form of polio that has increased with the advent of the polio vaccination. It is estimated that one in every five hundred Americans may have CFS, according to the Centers for Disease Control and Prevention.

Fibromyalgia and CFS are similar in some symptoms. The main difference is the deep musculoskeletal pain in fibromyalgia and the severe fatigue in CFS.

Fibromyalgia is thought to involve brain disturbances causing impaired deep sleep. Depression is common with fibromyalgia and may be a result of faulty serotonin metabolism. Some other symptoms common to fibromyalgia are anxiety, fatigue, depression, exhaustion, irritable bowels, tension or migraine headaches, sleep disturbances, pain in the joints, tension, and low stress tolerance. Although these symptoms are not uncommon in the general population, they are found with much higher frequency in patients with fibromyalgia. There are specific trigger areas of pain in the body that are common to the condition.

Autointoxication and malnutrition are two main causes of the disease. Trying to pinpoint the cause of the disease is often difficult, though, because it seems to be triggered by a number of conditions that start with a susceptibility on the part of the sufferer. The causes appear to be numerous and involve the environment, body, and mind.

Leaky gut syndrome may be involved because of an imbalance in intestinal microorganisms, such as candida, bacteria, and parasites. When the lining of the intestinal tract becomes more permeable than normal, it can lead to serious health concerns. The large spaces that develop between the cells of the gut wall allow toxic material to enter the bloodstream. Under normal conditions, these toxic substances would be eliminated, but when leaky gut syndrome occurs, parasites, bacteria, fungi, toxins, fats, and other foreign matter not normally absorbed enter the bloodstream.

Dr. Allen Tyler of Thorne Research believes that both the central and autonomic nervous systems are involved and that there is a physiological change in the connective tissue. Muscle pain creates physical inactivity, which results in muscle weakness. Weakness in the connective tissues causes severe pain. Long periods of undue stress and emotional disruption appear to be the underlying cause of fatigue, pain, and weakness.

## EMOTIONAL NEEDS
Like chronic fatigue syndrome, fibromyalgia may be related to prolonged periods of emotional stress or depression. While the link is not fully understood, some studies suggest that women with unresolved emotional problems may be more susceptible to this condition.

## HERBAL COMBINATIONS
### Herbal Combination #1
Magnesium is usually deficient in those with fibromyalgia. It is necessary to help use oxygen for muscle energy and to detoxify aluminum, which has been linked to metabolic disturbances.
- Malic acid is effective in eliminating aluminum through the urine and colon. Magnesium and malic acid work together to eliminate toxic amounts of aluminum and other toxins in the body. This reduces the concentration of metals found in the internal organs, tissues, and the brain.

### Herbal Combination #2
This is a nutritional tonic to help the body heal itself and recover from illnesses. It helps in joint health with its anti-inflammatory properties. It is derived from the antler velvet of deer. This formula also contains stevia and lecithin. It comes in a spray form, to put under the tongue.

### Other Uses
Ankylosing spondylitis, arthritis, joint pain, rheumatism, calcification deposits, bursitis, gout, neuritis, and chronic fatigue syndrome.

## HEALTHFUL SUGGESTIONS
1. Eliminate foods and substances that might aggravate the problem, such as tobacco, tomatoes, potatoes, green peppers, and eggplant, which are from the nightshade family and can aggravate the joints. Avoid alcohol, white sugar and white flour products, meat, fatty foods, caffeine, and chocolate, because they can cause imbalances in the body and deplete essential nutrients.

2. Drink plenty of pure distilled water—it helps to clean the joints. Vegetable juices such as celery, carrot, and parsley are beneficial. Always dilute the juices. Eat plenty of green leafy vegetables and lightly steamed vegetables. Use millet, brown rice, whole grains, and soy products, such as tofu. Add more fiber to the diet, such as psyllium herbal formulas. Soy products are rich in protein, calcium, and other minerals.

3. Allergies can be involved, which irritate the intestinal tract. Allergies may be related to food, environmental pollutants, chemicals, molds, dust, or pollens. There can be a connection between allergies and leaky gut syndrome, which can be further aggravated by drugs used for fibromyalgia. The spaces widen between cells in the intestinal lining and cause material to invade the body, such as viruses, germs, and parasites. These particles of food or other irritants pass through the intestinal tract into the bloodstream and cause allergic reactions and weaken the immune system.

4. Parasites and candida may be involved. Some nutrition-oriented physicians have reported success in treating fibromyalgia when parasites and candida were treated and cleared up. Herbal formulas to eliminate parasites and candida may be helpful.

5. Exercise has been shown to be beneficial in reducing the symptoms of fibromyalgia. Low-stress exercises, along with weight lifting, will strengthen the muscles, including the heart. Walking, jumping on a mini trampoline, or using a rowing machine are all beneficial. Decide on an exercise that is right for your body and that you like the best.

## HERBS AND SUPPLEMENTS

Single herbs to help with fibromyalgia include alfalfa, aloe vera, buckthorn, cat's claw, ginger, turmeric, echinacea (cleans glands), horsetail, oatstraw, pau d'arco, red clover, garlic, and goldenseal.

- Glucosamine is very effective in treating inflammation, which helps alleviate pain. It also acts as a free-radical scavenger, preventing more damage to the cells. It helps to rebuild and restore new tissue to repair joints.
- Magnesium and malic acid work together to reduce the severity of symptoms associated with inflammation of the joints. Improvement in symptoms has occurred when using these together.
- Essential fatty acids are beneficial and help reduce inflammation in the joints. Use essential fatty acids, such as cold-pressed flaxseed oil, evening primrose oil, borage oil, and salmon oil. They inhibit prostaglandins that cause pain and swelling. Use vitamin E along with EFAs; they should be taken after a meal.
- Antioxidants found in vitamins A, C, E, selenium, zinc, and grapeseed extract are beneficial. They are powerful antioxidants that help inhibit the inflammatory response and scavenge for free radicals that cause muscle pain or damage.
- Coenzyme Q10 and germanium help to boost oxygen supplies to muscle tissue, which helps in reducing inflammation and pain.
- Digestive enzymes are important keys to proper assimilation and digestion of nutrients to feed the cells, tissues, and organs of the body.
- Free-form amino acids are easily digested proteins that help heal the cells, nourish the body, and improve stamina.
- B-complex vitamins are very important to protect the nervous system, prevent fatigue, and increase resistance to disease. Take extra B6 and B12 to prevent anemia and increase energy. They work together in the absorption and production of hydrochloric acid, help in preventing depression, and aid the liver in eliminating toxins.

## ORTHODOX PRESCRIBED MEDICATION

Acetaminophen (Tylenol) is widely prescribed for pain relief. Anti-inflammatory drugs are usually prescribed, such as Naproxen and Motrin. The advertising suggests that the drugs are harmless. They are potentially dangerous and harmful on the liver. If the liver is sluggish and the colon is congested, medication can be very dangerous. They can also cause low white blood cell count, excessive bleeding, fever, open sores, and jaundice. Antidepressants are often prescribed. They should be used with caution, because they can build up in the liver if used for long periods. Using drugs only covers up the underlying problem. There is a need to get at the source of the problem and find out the cause.

# HEADACHES AND MIGRAINES

Headaches come in many forms—they can be mild, causing only minor discomfort, or severe, such as migraines, which can cause nausea and vomiting. There are allergy headaches, which seem to be caused by an allergy to food, preservatives, or even chemicals, as well as hay fever. Another common headache is a sinus headache; this occurs when the head is saturated with mucus, causing earaches and a sore throat. A stress headache is common to those who work and live under stressful conditions. A toxic headache is one that causes pressure behind the eyes and usually lasts for several days.

In 1932, in *Medical Journal and Record*, a doctor wrote, "Headaches are among the most frequent complaints of human life." Today, headaches are still one of our most common complaints. It is commonly believed that headaches are the price we pay for fast-paced living, but it isn't true. Headaches are as old as recorded history and were as common in primitive societies as they are today. In ancient Melanesian, European, and Mesoamerican societies, it was believed that puncturing the skull (called trephining) to free evil spirits would cure persistent headaches, epilepsy, or insanity. Skulls with trephining punctures go back to the Neolithic and Bronze ages.

An estimated eighty million Americans will suffer from headache pain and about ten million will be afflicted with migraines, and because of this, thirty million pounds of aspirin are consumed each year just in the United States. However, headaches are a symptom, not a disease—they are a result of dietary habits, lifestyle, environment, tension in the neck, shoulders, or back, sinus problems, and, less commonly, from brain tumors.

Migraine headaches develop when an artery in the head dilates. It throbs and the vessel wall expands, causing pain. The spasms that develop can cause dizziness, ringing in the ears, seeing sparks or colors through the eyes, and tingling in the temples. The Chinese see pain as an obstruction of energy flow. Migraines develop when the body is under a great deal of stress or before the menstrual period when energy flow is slowed down.

Migraines in women are often linked to menstrual cycles. During the week before the menstrual cycle, an imbalance of hormones takes place. This puts the liver in the position of detoxification and elimination. The liver has a connection to the eyes. Migraine headaches usually start with changes in the eyes, such as pain behind or above one eye, or vision changes. Headaches seem to be related to toxicity, which causes inflammation of the nervous system and tightens up the muscles, which causes pain.

Autointoxication headaches are the most common and, in the opinion of many health-oriented doctors, originate in the gastrointestinal system. Wrong food combinations, overeating, and junk food will cause fermentation in the intestines and stomach. This causes gas, which enters the blood and causes irritation on the nerves and brain and causes headaches. Pressure in the temples and forehead usually indicates that there are stomach problems. Throbbing pain often results from congestion in the liver, spleen, or digestive tract.

Excess starches and sugars in the diet often cause migraine headaches. If the stomach, colon, and mucous membranes were healthy, allergic reactions to food wouldn't cause headaches. Stress, tension, constipation, sinusitis, head injury, air pollution, poor circulation, and poor respiration are all causes of headaches. Allergies to MSG, chocolate, caffeine, wheat (pesticides), sulfites, sugar, dairy products, and alcohol can also cause headaches. An emotional conflict or anxiety can cause headaches. High blood pressure can cause headaches. Children with headaches often have eye problems, but allergies or emotions could also cause them.

## EMOTIONAL NEEDS

Daily tension and stress may contribute to the onset of chronic headaches. Once again, how stress triggers a migraine is not fully understood, but the link is a valid one. For this reason, staying in touch with indicators that we are reacting to environmental stress, and taking the proper steps to diffuse it, may help avoid the onset of a serious headache.

## HERBAL COMBINATIONS
### Herbal Combination #1

- White willow bark works like aspirin except that it is mild on the stomach with no depressing after-effects. An excellent nerve sedative, it is cleansing and healing.
- Valerian root is an effective and strong nervine, calming, relaxing, and useful for anxiety and insomnia.
- Lettuce leaves are natural sedatives, as well as relaxing and calming to the nerves.
- Capsicum works as a catalyst for other herbs. It is a stimulant to strengthen the blood vessels.

**Other Uses**

Nervous disorders, relieves pain, cramps, reduces tension, relaxes the body, and aids in cases of colds and flu.

## HEALTHFUL SUGGESTIONS

1. Chiropractic treatment has helped many people with chronic headaches. Tension in the jaw, neck, or head can be helped by manipulation of the muscles. A cool cloth on the back of the neck and head will relieve some headaches. Lobelia extract rubbed on the back of the neck will help to relax the muscles.

2. The first step should be a detoxification program. This would include a colon, liver, and blood cleansing. A kidney herbal formula will help eliminate acids from the blood. Use a lower bowel formula and a red clover blend blood cleanser.

3. Exercise is beneficial in a detoxification program. Walking in fresh air will help provide more oxygen to the blood. Get some exercise at least three times a week. A mini trampoline is excellent for the lymphatic system to eliminate toxins from the blood.

4. Change to a natural diet using fresh and steamed vegetables and fresh fruit. Eat whole grains, cooked thermos-style for retention of B vitamins and enzymes. Detoxify the body with fresh vegetable juices, which are healing, and fruit juices for cleansing. Use wheatgrass juice and green drinks. Add beans, fresh salads, seeds, nuts, and sprouts to the diet. Use herbal teas such as chamomile, mint, and ginger with pure water. A magnesium-rich juice drink can be made from carrots, celery, one clove of garlic, parsley, and a bunch of endive.

5. Allergies may be a problem. Start by eliminating the bad foods, such as red meat, sugar, and salt. If you can do this for a month, you will never have the same taste for that food as you did before. Add new foods one at a time. Start with brown rice and millet dishes. They will nourish and strengthen the nerves because of the B vitamins, calcium, and magnesium. Use grain and vegetable soups with onions, garlic, shallots, and a lot of vegetables. They are rich in minerals. Use almonds, which are rich in calcium, protein, and other vital nutrients, and soak them overnight, making them easier to digest. A hypoglycemia diet may be beneficial. Low blood sugar levels can trigger migraines.

## HERBS AND SUPPLEMENTS

- Feverfew has been found to demonstrate effectiveness in reducing the severity and number of migraine headaches.
- White willow bark is an effective pain reliever, especially for headaches and arthritis pain. It can be used as a tea or in capsule form.
- Digestive enzymes help break up the undigested protein in the blood and cells. Use after and in-between meals.
- Hormone-balancing herbal formula should contain black cohosh, licorice, Siberian ginseng, sarsaparilla, squaw vine, blessed thistle, and false unicorn. This will help headaches caused by hormonal imbalance.
- Essential fatty acids are needed for brain function and to help eliminate toxins from the capillaries. Examples include evening primrose oil, borage, salmon oil, flaxseed, and black currant oil.
- Tea tree oil rubbed on the temples helps to relieve headaches.

### A SOLUTION FOR MIGRAINES

Sara had developed migraine headaches, and the vitamins she was taking weren't helping. She went to a foot reflexologist to get some relief, and the reflexologist told Sara that she needed to try some herbs. Sara told the reflexologist that she was taking vitamins and didn't need herbs, but she finally agreed to try some. She took formula #1 found under Addictions and formula #1 found under Allergies. She was surprised to find that her migraines cleared up, plus her stiff and sore neck and shoulders improved considerably. She was so impressed that she started telling everyone she knew who had allergies, headaches, sore shoulders, and depression. The formulas she took are excellent for allergy headaches. Sara also took the following formula: chamomile, passion flower, hops, fennel, marshmallow, and feverfew for her migraines. This formula also provides nutritional support for the nervous system.

- Low levels of magnesium are seen during migraine attacks. Magnesium is the relaxant of the body.

## ORTHODOX PRESCRIBED MEDICATION

Sumatriptan succinate (Imitrex) is prescribed to relieve pain from migraine headaches by constricting the blood vessels in the brain. It has a powerful constricting effect on the heart and blood and can cause fatal heart spasms and possibly lead to a fatal stroke. Heart disease needs to be ruled out if using this drug. It can also cause damage to the eyes. Ergotamine is also used for migraine headaches by constricting the blood vessels of the head. Side effects could be diarrhea, dizziness, or vomiting. It could cause a rise or fall of blood pressure, weak pulse, and even convulsions.

# HEARING LOSS AND RELATED CONDITIONS

Hearing loss, including Ménière's disease and tinnitus, is not a natural process of growing old; instead, it is often caused by poor diet, air pollution, and the side effects of drugs. Environmental noise is also a very serious problem. Young adults are experiencing hearing loss to one degree or another, as well as children and even newborns. One factor causing hearing loss in youth is noise pollution. Ears are not meant to be exposed to loud noises for long periods of time. Nerve damage can result.

Ménière's disease has many symptoms that can affect both ears. Ringing in the ears, loss of hearing, and loss of balance are the most common. Because of balance problems associated with Ménière's disease, nausea and vomiting may occur. Acute attacks can be so severe that an individual may keel over from violent dizziness.

Listening to music through headphones or a headset when the sound is loud enough for someone else to hear could be causing gradual hearing loss. Conductive deafness in an adult is most often caused by earwax blocking the outer ear canal. In children, otitis media (middle ear infection) is caused by a collection of sticky fluid in the middle ear. Sensorineural deafness can be congenital due to an inherited fault in a chromosome, birth injury, or damage to the developing fetus. This may be the result of the mother having rubella or another illness during pregnancy. Sensorineural deafness that develops in later life can be caused by prolonged exposure to loud noise or some drugs (such as streptomycin) or through viral infections.

A bad diet can cause plugged ears. A high-fat diet increases the levels of fats in the blood, which reduces the flow of oxygen and vital nutrients to the ear. White sugar causes the adrenal glands to overreact and constricts tiny blood vessels in the ear. Mucus-forming food can cause an accumulation of waxy and cholesterol material in the head area and especially the ears. The head area requires more nutrition and circulation than any other single body organ. Poor nutrition causes tiny arteries, veins, and capillaries that help support ears and hearing to clog up. This happens over a period of years with gradual clogging of the tubes to the ears. That is one reason why so many elderly people have hearing problems.

Some other causes of hearing loss are fetal damage, trauma at birth, infections, drugs (people have complained of hearing problems after being treated with some drugs), thyroid disease, diabetes, injuries, noise exposure, measles, mumps, chicken pox, bacterial meningitis, nerve deterioration, or malnutrition.

## HERBAL COMBINATIONS
### Herbal Combination #1

This formula is in extract form for quicker assimilation and action. It strengthens the immune and nervous systems. This is useful to help fight infections and all kinds of ear problems such as ear infections, accumulation of wax in the ears, itching ears, and some types of hearing loss. It can also be used for throat infections.

- Black cohosh is a tonic for the central nervous system and heals, loosens, and expels mucus from the bronchial tubes, throat, or ears. It neutralizes poisons in the bloodstream.
- Chickweed is excellent for treating blood toxicity, fevers, and inflammation. It helps dissolve plaque in blood vessels and capillaries leading to the eyes and ears. It acts as an antibiotic in the blood.
- Goldenseal helps to regulate liver function, which is connected to eye and ear problems. It is a natu-

ral antibiotic to stop infections and kill poisons in the body. It is valuable for all catarrh conditions in the sinuses, head, ear, eyes, bronchial tubes, throat, intestines, stomach, or bladder.

- Desert tea strengthens the bronchial tubes and is good for acute diseases. It is a natural treatment for throat, ear, and eye infections.
- Licorice stimulates natural interferon production to fight acute diseases. It counteracts stress and supplies energy to the body. It contains glycosides, which help purge excess fluid from the lungs, throat, and body.
- Valerian has a calming and sedative effect, which is relaxing for anxiety and insomnia. It is also useful in pain-relieving remedies and for its ability to relax muscle spasms. Healing takes place when the body is relaxed.
- Passion flower is used for insomnia, hysteria, hyperactive children and adults, and convulsions. It is good for unrest, agitation, and exhaustion. It is believed that passion flower kills a form of bacteria that causes eye irritations, which can also work on the ears.

## Other Uses
Allergies, bronchitis, colds, flu, eye irritations, loss of equilibrium, hay fever.

## HEALTHFUL SUGGESTIONS

1. Fast and use herbal cleansing formulas such as blood, lower bowel, nerves, kidneys, and digestive enzymes. Juice fasting using carrot, celery, endive, and garlic is beneficial. Alternate with kale, spinach, and ginger. Diet change is the most important thing you can do to help change the inward health.

2. Mucus-forming food is the cause of most hearing problems and ear infections in small children. These infections can build up throughout the years and cause gradual hearing loss and other ear problems. A natural diet high in whole grains, fresh vegetables, fruits, nuts, seeds, sprouts, legumes, and beans will build the immune system. Grape juice and green drinks are high in potassium. Potassium helps prevent autointoxication and a buildup of mucus in the ears. Eat almonds, baked potatoes with skin, apples, apricots (dried), cashews, sunflower seeds, black cherries, broccoli, carrots, dates, dried figs, leafy lettuce, and lentils.

3. Avoid fried foods, white flour, white sugar, and packaged food on the grocery shelves, which can cause free-radical damage because of the rancid oils and grains. Eliminate smoking, alcohol, caffeine, and a high-meat diet. Exposure to cigarette smoke in the household can cause chronic middle ear disease in children, and smoke is dangerous for children who have lung and nasal congestion. Ear damage increases sixfold in children who are exposed to second-hand smoke in their formative years.

4. Regular exercise such as walking, swimming, or jumping on a mini trampoline may help to improve circulation in the head area. According to the February 1991 issue of the *New England Journal of Medicine*, high-impact aerobics may increase the impairment by disrupting transmission of information from the ears to the brain.

5. Strengthen the immune system, and keep it strong. Sensorineural hearing loss, which is one cause of sudden hearing loss, can develop within twenty-four hours and is thought to be the result of viral or other infections. Keeping the immune system strong and the body clean and free from toxins that germs, bacteria, viruses, parasites, and worms thrive on will go a long way in protecting the immune system.

## HERBS AND SUPPLEMENTS
Single herbs that can help prevent hearing loss include black cohosh, black walnut, burdock, echinacea, garlic, ginkgo, gotu kola, hawthorn, hops, kelp, lady's slipper, licorice, lobelia, red clover, suma, and yellow dock.

- Interferon is important to keep the immune system strong. The following nutrients will stimulate production of natural interferon in the body: licorice, chlorophyll, astragalus, vitamin C with bioflavonoids, sea vegetables such as kelp, dulse, and blue-green algae, ginkgo, grapeseed extract, milk thistle, pau d'arco, schizandra, Siberian ginseng, cordyceps, suma, wheatgrass juice, dong quai, echinacea, red raspberry, ho-shou-wu, germanium, and CoQ10.
- Antioxidants are important to prevent damage by free radicals and are vital to protect the ears, eyes, and brain. Vitamin C with bioflavonoids is necessary for healing and health in the small capillaries leading to the head area. Vitamins A, C, E, seleni-

um, zinc, and grapeseed extract are important antioxidants.

- Minerals are very important and work with vitamins to protect the body. Fluid and pressure imbalance in the inner ear may be due to an electrolyte imbalance. Imbalances between sodium and potassium can be triggered by the adrenal gland when under stress. Calcium, magnesium, sodium, and potassium are important minerals, and along with vitamin D, strengthen the bones in the body. Silicon and boron are also important for bone health—even the tiny bones in the ear.
- The B-complex vitamins work with magnesium to provide energy to the body. They are important for nerve health.
- Pantothenic acid is helpful in balancing the adrenal glands. Ménière's disease has been helped by large doses of niacin, along with the other B vitamins. Vitamin B2 helps with dizziness, B6 is necessary for proper function of the central nervous system, B12 helps fight exhaustion and pain in facial muscles and facial nerves. They also help the liver to eliminate toxins from the body. They provide energy necessary for the metabolism of carbohydrates, fats, and proteins.
- Lecithin and vitamin E work together in stimulating circulation in the head area. They help keep the arteries flexible and provide proper oxygen usage by the sensory cells.
- Ginkgo, CoQ10, and germanium are very useful in providing oxygen to the head area. They increase circulation and provide nutrients for better brain function.
- Essential fatty acids found in flaxseed, evening primrose, borage, black currant, and salmon oil help to prevent cholesterol in the veins and capillaries. They strengthen the immune system.
- Chlorophyll and blue-green algae contain antiseptic properties, clean the blood, and inhibit the growth of bacteria, germs, and viruses. They also help to clean and nourish the blood.

## ORTHODOX PRESCRIBED MEDICATION

Antibiotics like gentamycin and streptomycin, some diuretics, aspirin, and aspirin substitutes such as ibuprofen can cause tinnitus. These drugs can cause irritating sounds in the ears or even deafness.

# HEMORRHOIDS AND VARICOSE VEINS

Chronic constipation and a circulatory system weakness cause hemorrhoids and varicose veins. There are external hemorrhoids and internal hemorrhoids. External are easily identifiable and usually more painful. Internal hemorrhoids may be present for years and not cause trouble. They can also appear externally if they become swollen and protrude from the anal ring. Bleeding may be the first sign of internal hemorrhoids. Constant bleeding over a period of time can cause anemia. Liver congestion has been implicated as another cause. These ailments occur as a result of pregnancy, junk-food diet (clogs the circulatory system), lack of exercise, sitting while working, heavy lifting, and obesity. They are also seen in individuals with low-fiber diets. If left untreated, varicose veins can lead to phlebitis, leg ulcers, permanently swollen legs, pulmonary emboli, and even surface leg hemorrhaging.

Varicose veins occur most often in the legs. Weakness in the veins allows blood to accumulate and stretch the capillaries and veins, causing discoloration, tenderness, and sometimes pain. Internal hemorrhoids are varicose veins. Constipation adds excess pressure to the veins, thus interrupting the blood flow toward the heart. Straining the stool blocks off the veins and causes pressure. Symptoms are inflammation, swelling, pain, irritation, and bleeding. Straining at stool distends the veins and cracks the mucous membrane, thus opening up the tendency for infections. Infections result from the retention of fecal matter in the folds of the mucous membranes.

## HERBAL COMBINATIONS
### Herbal Combination #1
This is an excellent combination of nature's fibers to clean the bowels and digestive system. It will absorb toxins and rid them from the body. It will help lower cholesterol, and it is a natural way to restore normal bowel function with the natural fiber.

Psyllium is an excellent colon and intestinal cleanser. It is soothing and healing, strengthens the tissues, and restores tone. It lubricates as well as heals the intestines and colon.

Oat is a natural fiber that is healing and nourishing to the digestive tract. It is well known for lowering cholesterol. It adds bulk and eliminates the toxins from the pockets of the colon.

Apple fiber contains natural pectin that is cleansing and healing for the intestines. These three fibers work together to bring natural function to the colon.

### Herbal Combination #2

This formula will act as an oral chelation therapy to clean the digestive tract and the cells. It helps in chemical poisoning, inflammation of the bowels, diarrhea, and multiple sclerosis. This formula contains psyllium hulls, apple fiber, acacia gum, guar gum, oat bran, and the following vegetables in a concentrated powder form: broccoli, carrot, red beet, rosemary, turmeric root, tomato, cabbage leaf, Chinese cabbage leaf, hesperidin, grapefruit bioflavonoid, and orange bioflavonoid. Drink with a large glass of water to speed proper assimilation.

### Other Uses

Autointoxication, constipation, colitis, digestive tract, irritable bowel syndrome, ulcers, acts as oral chelation, high cholesterol, hemorrhoids, inflammatory bowel diseases.

### HEALTHFUL SUGGESTIONS

1. Colon cleansing will help eliminate the problem and aid the body in proper digestion, assimilation, and elimination. Blood cleansing will help neutralize the acids in the blood and eliminate them. The liver needs to be strengthened using liver cleansers to promote better filtering of toxins. The circulatory system needs to be nourished to strengthen all the veins. When the veins are weak in the legs, they are probably weak all over.

2. Eat a high-fiber diet. A lack of bulk fiber in the diet leads to straining during bowel movements due to the formation of small and hard feces. A high-fiber diet will allow the bowels to move freely three or four times a day and prevent hemorrhoids and varicose veins. Use whole grains such as whole oats, wheat, millet, brown rice, and yellow cornmeal. Cook them in a slow cooker or in a thermos overnight. This will prevent free-radical damage. Use prunes, dates, raw fruits, vegetables, and beans.

3. Use short fasts using green drinks, wheatgrass juice, and pure water. This will help clean and purify the blood. Carrot, celery, endive, and garlic juices will speed the healing. Dilute with pure water. Drink six to eight glasses of pure water daily. Use grain and vegetable broths to strengthen the body while fasting, especially when the body is already tired and weak. Add onions, garlic, shallots, and ginger to the soups; they will help promote blood flow by stimulating circulation and preventing blood clots. Soak figs, raisins, and prunes in pure water; drink the water as well as eating the fruit. Citrus fruits, using the inner skin, will strengthen and heal veins. Okra, rich in silicon and selenium, helps open clogged veins and strengthens capillaries. Buckwheat contains rutin, a bioflavonoid that strengthens the veins and decreases the tendency of the capillaries to break.

4. Exercise—even simple walking—will strengthen the veins and increase circulation. It will also help prevent deposits of clotting blood within the veins. Raw red potatoes or a clove of garlic can be used several times a week as a suppository for hemorrhoids. Sitz baths, continued for several days, will help strengthen the veins. A sitz bath involves using two basins, one with hot water, one with cold. Use the hot basin first and cold second. The warm water relaxes the spasms of the muscles, and the cold tightens the tissues.

5. Avoid refined foods that are void of nutrients and fiber. White flour and sugar products are depleted of nutrients and fiber. They also can cause free-radical damage. Avoid salt, coffee, caffeine, and alcohol.

### HERBS AND SUPPLEMENTS

Single herbs to help hemorrhoids include aloe vera, butcher's broom, cascara sagrada, comfrey, capsicum, goldenseal, horsetail, mullein oil (relieves pain), and white oak bark (strengthens veins).

- Zinc oxide cream is an inexpensive over-the-counter ointment that is good for pain and swelling. Zinc oxide will toughen the skin over the hemorrhoid, which lessens the risk for additional irritation.
- Aloe vera gel soothes and cools the area and promotes healing.
- Witch hazel compresses can speed circulation and help in healing.

- St. John's wort oil can be rubbed on veins.
- Vitamins A and E can be taken internally and rubbed on the legs. They strengthen, heal, and nourish the veins. They are antioxidants and help to prevent free-radical damage.
- Grape seed extract is a powerful antioxidant, and it works to calm inflammation while fortifying blood vessel strength.
- White oak bark taken internally and used as compresses to varicose veins and hemorrhoids will stimulate blood flow and heal.
- Bilberry strengthens the blood vessels and capillaries. It will help heal and prevent hemorrhoids and varicose veins.
- Vitamin C with bioflavonoids feeds and strengthens the fragile capillaries. It tones and heals the veins and capillaries.
- Butcher's broom acts as a vasoconstrictor and contains anti-inflammatory properties.
- Bromelain is an enzyme from the pineapple that helps to prevent the formation of fibrin, a substance that surrounds varicose veins in the rectum or anus. It contains anti-inflammatory properties.
- CoQ10, germanium, ginkgo, and suma provide oxygen and nutrients to the veins. They heal and nourish the veins.
- Essential fatty acids are very healing for the veins and will strengthen and heal hemorrhoids and varicose veins.

## ORTHODOX PRESCRIBED MEDICATION

For hemorrhoids, local anesthetic creams, lotions, or suppositories are recommended. Severe symptoms may need rubber-band ligation, cryosurgery, injection therapy, or surgical removal. For severe cases of varicose veins, surgical removal is an option. Bulging, discolored veins may cause pain and ulcers. The removal is called stripping with a small incision. This is done under general anesthetic.

# HIATAL HERNIA SYNDROME

The hiatus is a small hole in the diaphragm through which the esophagus passes to join the stomach. The term hernia refers to a weakened area of muscle or a severely stretched muscle. A hiatal hernia occurs when the hole in the diaphragm weakens and enlarges, allowing a portion of the stomach to protrude upward through the hole beside the esophagus.

There are three types of hiatal hernia based on their severity, but the sliding hiatal hernia is the most common. A small part of the stomach slides back and forth in and out of the chest cavity through the small hole in the diaphragm. This type causes no problems and rarely any symptoms. Most people don't even know they have the disorder, even though it's estimated to be present in up to 60 percent of the population by age sixty.

Why hiatal hernias happen is not certain, but many natural health advocates feel there is a strong correlation between the incidence of hiatal hernia and diet. A high-fat diet will slow digestion and may cause irritation to the hiatal. Obesity can also be an important factor. Obviously, it takes time for the body to heal, but a change in diet, an increase in exercise, and reduction in stress will help speed the

## LET THE HEALING BEGIN

Jane had fissure surgery on her hemorrhoids that failed, and the fissure began to tear open again. A fissure is a tear in the rectum that begins with hemorrhoids and continues to tear until it is repaired. Jane was in severe pain and was bleeding so much that she needed a feminine pad to protect her clothing. She had large amounts of scar tissue that almost totally prevented her bowel movements. She started on a healing program. She took formula #1 found under Colitis, capsicum, and black currant oil, which are all healing and nourishing to the mucous membranes. Within one and a half weeks she had to return to the doctor for what she believed would be an examination to prepare for another surgery. Instead the surgeon found new pink skin growing over the tear, which meant the healing process had begun. Jane did not have to have surgery for the fissure again. She is very careful with her body to prevent the hemorrhoids from flaring up again.

healing process. Eating small meals in a calm place and chewing thoroughly will also reduce symptoms. A chiropractor may be helpful in manipulating the hiatal hernia back into place.

The medical community recognizes that the cause of hiatal hernia is difficult to determine. It is more common among obese individuals, middle-aged women, and pregnant women. Some believe the condition is due to a congenital abnormality or a trauma to the hiatal area. A hiatal hernia often occurs when there is an increase in intra-abdominal pressure. This could be due to pressure created by straining to move hard feces when constipated.

Symptoms of hiatal hernia center on chronic heartburn and belching. Stomach acid sometimes comes up into the throat, which can cause burning and discomfort in the chest and throat. The tissues in the esophagus can become sore and irritated from the acid. Symptoms include the following: bloating, regurgitation, vomiting, constipation, burning in the upper chest, pressure below the breastbone, heartburn, intestinal gas, nausea, diarrhea, fatigue, allergies, and dizziness.

## HERBAL COMBINATIONS
### Herbal Combination #1
This herbal formula is soothing and healing for the digestive tract. It helps with inflammation and contains herbs that tone and soothe the digestive tract.

- Chamomile contains properties that aid digestion and relieve indigestion, it is relaxing and acts as a sedative, and is excellent for stomach troubles and inflammation.
- Marshmallow is soothing and healing, and it protects and heals inflammations. It is rich in vitamin A, which is healing.
- Plantain helps to neutralize stomach acids and normalize stomach secretions. It also neutralizes poisons.
- Rose hips are rich in vitamins A and C, which are essential for healthy digestive system. They heal and prevent infections in the digestive tract.
- Slippery elm soothes and heals the digestive tract. Rich in vitamins and minerals to strengthen the intestinal system.
- Bugleweed contains compounds that contract tissues of the mucous membranes and reduces fluid discharges. It helps relieve irritation and pain.

### Herbal Combination #2
This herbal formula contains natural ingredients to help neutralize excess acid, and prevent acid reflux from "backwashing" into the esophagus. It helps reduce indigestion while healing and building the digestive tract.

It contains calcium carbonate, alginic acid (from kelp), wintergreen oil, papaya fruit, slippery elm bark, licorice root, and ginger. It also contains a sweetener called xylitol that has powerful antibacterial properties.

### Herbal Combination #3
This herbal formula is a natural tranquilizer that relaxes nervous and muscle tension. Nervous tension can increase the symptoms of hiatal hernia, and this combination will improve and strengthen the digestive system. It contains chamomile, passion flower, hops, fennel, marshmallow, and feverfew.

## HEALTHFUL SUGGESTIONS
1. Use a lower-bowel formula to help clean, nourish, and rebuild the colon and digestive system. Most diseases are caused by a toxic colon. Cleaning the colon will help prevent toxins from entering the bloodstream and cause diseases.

2. Drink plenty of clean, pure water daily. Make sure it's purified. Distilled water is very beneficial when cleansing and healing the body. The juice of half a lemon or lime in a glass of warm water in the morning is cleansing for the liver.

3. Avoid fatty and fried foods and food that causes indigestion. Give the stomach time to heal. Eat more raw food than cooked. Cooked food lacks enzymes and causes irritation to the digestive system. Eat fruit alone, and it will digest quickly. When eaten with cooked food, it can cause fermentation in the stomach and colon.

4. Avoid coffee, tea, alcohol, cola drinks, and smoking. Use herbal teas for healing the digestive tract. Chamomile tea is soothing to the digestive system.

5. Eat a high-fiber diet. Add more grains and use thermos cooking that allows foods to maintain their live enzymes and vitamins and minerals. Millet, an alkaline cereal, is healing and nourishing to the digestive system and is high in protein.

6. Chewing food more thoroughly will improve digestion and assimilation. Food combining would

help heal and nourish the body. Eat less food at meals; instead of eating a whole potato, eat a half. Do not eat when you are upset, and relax and take time at meals.

7. Fasting one day on juices will heal and help the body eliminate toxins. Fresh juices made with carrots, celery, parsley, fresh ginger, and garlic are very cleansing. Drink pure water throughout the day.

8. A chiropractor in some cases can manipulate the hiatal hernia back where it belongs. Drinking two to eight ounces of water and bouncing on the heels twelve times may help jar it into place.

## HERBS AND SUPPLEMENTS

Single herbs for hiatal hernia are alfalfa and aloe vera (healing), capsicum (healing and stimulates circulation), comfrey and pepsin, gentian (healing and strengthens the digestive system), ginger, goldenseal (healing), hops, horsetail, marshmallow, papaya, skullcap, slippery elm (healing and provides protein). Other helpful herbs are black walnut, burdock, echinacea, garlic, hawthorn, yellow dock, and yucca.

- Blue-green algae and chlorophyll increase oxygen utilization, provide nutrients, and protect against viral diseases.
- Essential fatty acids contained in flaxseed, evening primrose oil, borage seed oil, black currant oil, and fish oil are essential for every function of the body. They work with vitamin E to heal the intestines and keep them healthy.
- Licorice root tea or deglycerinized licorice is healing for the intestines.
- MSM is necessary in the body to repair cells and remove toxins. MSM has been found to enhance the availability of vitamin C and other antioxidant nutrients, helping to protect the body from disease. It allows the body to heal itself.
- Lecithin prevents damage to blood and liver cells from oxidation, free radicals, and toxins. Helps the body to process fats better.
- Indoles increase the activity of enzymes, destroy toxins and block cancer-causing substances before they enter the cells. They are found in cruciferous vegetables. However, supplements are stronger.
- Acidophilus protects the body from bad bacteria. It should be used when cleansing the colon. It will help in the digestion of food. Take on an empty stomach for best results.

- Digestive enzymes break down protein. Lipase breaks down fat, amylase breaks down starch, and cellulase assists in breaking down cellulose. They will also clean out the blood and cells of protein lodged anywhere in the body. Viruses, germs, bacteria, parasites, and worms all have protein coatings, and enzymes help to eliminate these.
- Coenzyme Q10 and germanium help the body utilize oxygen. These are considered essential nutrients that boost the biochemical ability to activate cellular energy.

## ORTHODOX PRESCRIBED MEDICATION

Reglan is used to speed food through the intestinal tract; it inhibits digestive enzymes. This means the food is not digesting properly and will cause other problems. Side effects could be fatigue, restlessness, and drowsiness. It is one of those drugs that may cause symptoms similar to those of Parkinson's disease such as rigidity, tremors, or slow movements.

# HIGH BLOOD PRESSURE (HYPERTENSION)

Hypertension is the medical term for high blood pressure. It is called the silent killer and can strike without symptoms. It can cause stroke, heart disease, kidney disease, and even brain damage, along with other problems. It is estimated that close to thirty million Americans have high blood pressure. When the blood pressure gradually rises over months and years, it is particularly dangerous, as it slips by the body's warning signals.

There are two types of pressure: systolic, the top reading, which shows peak pressure when the heart contracts to pump blood, and diastolic, the lower number, which measures the pressure when the heart is resting between beats. Normal blood pressure for adults is from 110/70 to 140/90, borderline hypertension is 140/95 to 160/95, and severely elevated blood pressure is over 180/115.

The most common cause of high blood pressure is arteriosclerosis (hardening of the arteries), where the arteries become narrowed and plug up with fatty deposits because of poor eating habits.

A toxic lymphatic system can be a cause, as can a toxic liver that does not clear out built-up estrogen and other toxins. Heavy metal contamination could be a cause. It was found that people whose hypertension was left untreated had blood cadmium levels three to four times higher than those with normal blood pressure (*Alternative Medicine*, The Burton Goldberg Group, p. 726). A lack of exercise and increased stress, anger, and anxiety play a part in causing high blood pressure. But a diet rich in saturated fats, meats, and refined products and little fresh fruit, vegetables, and fiber from whole grains is usually the cause. Being overweight increases the risk. A genetic background can contribute but is not the main cause. Although symptoms are not always present, some of the symptoms could include dizziness, headache, fatigue, restlessness, difficulty breathing, insomnia, intestinal complaints, and emotional instability.

## HERBAL COMBINATIONS
### Herbal Combination #1
- Garlic helps stabilize blood pressure, purifies the system, stimulates the lymphatic system to throw off toxins, and is rich in minerals and vitamins.
- Capsicum carries the herbs to where they are needed in the body, affects circulation, and increases heart action but not blood pressure. It is said to prevent strokes and heart attacks.
- Parsley is high in minerals like iron, is a natural diuretic, and helps resist infections.
- Ginger enhances the effectiveness of other herbs, removes excess waste, and aids digestion.
- Siberian ginseng stabilizes blood pressure, is a hormone regulator, helps in stress, and improves fatigue and weakness.
- Goldenseal cleans any infections, controls secretions, boosts the glandular system, and regulates liver function.

### Herbal Combination #2
This formula contains powerful herbs to help the body maintain healthy blood pressure levels. The ingredients help protect blood vessels, promote blood flow, and prevent cell damage. This is a rich antioxidant formula. It contains Coleus forskohlii, olive leaf extract, hawthorn berry extract, goldenrod, the amino acid arginine, vitamin E, and grapeseed extract.

### Other Uses
Circulation, colds, flu, infections, low blood pressure, stress, and tension.

## HEALTHFUL SUGGESTIONS
1. A change of diet is necessary. Vegetarians are known to have few problems with high blood pressure, and since a vegetarian diet is high in fiber, leaning toward a high-fiber diet would be beneficial. Studies have confirmed the ability of fiber supplements to reduce blood pressure. Some health practitioners believe that a low-sodium, low-fat, high-fiber diet can be more useful in treating hypertension than any single dietary approach. Nuts such as almonds, potatoes, millet (high in calcium, magnesium, and protein), brown rice, tofu, and soymilk are all high in plant protein, vitamins, and minerals. They are low in saturated fats and salt and rich in fiber. Foods high in potassium are asparagus, avocados, cabbage, potatoes, corn, lima beans, tomatoes, bananas, oranges, grapefruit, prunes, and raisins.

2. Weight loss may be beneficial, even if it means losing only ten pounds. A vegetarian diet, using whole grains and vegetables, is both rich in complex carbohydrates and burns more slowly in the body. Vegetable protein such as beans, lentils, brown rice, millet, potatoes, tofu, and soymilk can replace meat. If meat is eaten, fish such as salmon and chicken breasts are low in fat. Use vegetables such as cabbage, cauliflower, broccoli, Brussels sprouts, and tossed salads using leaf lettuce, tomatoes, celery, and cucumbers. Use olive oil for salads with lemon juice. Olive oil is nourishing for the veins. Use psyllium formulas for fiber. Fiber is an appetite suppressant, swelling to form bulk in the stomach, and prevents the reabsorption of fats. It also helps to clean the veins. Drink at least six to eight glasses of water a day. Replace soda pop or sugar drinks with water.

3. Exercise is important. The best kinds of exercises for a healthy heart are walking, mini trampoline, swimming, bicycling, and aerobics—all of which increase the heart rate and lung activity to bring in more air to increase the oxygen to the muscles and the heart. Even three days a week is very beneficial.

4. Relaxation is important. For some people, stress is one of the main causes of high blood pressure. Relaxation responses can only help in cases when stress is at least a part of the problem. Behavioral

changes are needed with diet and lifestyle and learning to cope with stress. Using the relaxation response can make all changes easier.

## HERBS AND SUPPLEMENTS

Single herbs to help with hypertension include garlic (lowers blood pressure), hawthorn (strengthens the veins), hops (relaxes veins and nerves), passion flower (nerve relaxant), parsley (natural diuretic), pau d'arco (blood cleanser), skullcap (calms the nerves), capsicum (cleans the veins), and echinacea (helps eliminate toxins from the veins).

- Calcium, magnesium, and potassium are needed for strengthening the heart and giving proper tone to blood vessels and arteries. A deficiency is linked to high blood pressure.
- Essential fatty acids contain linolenic and linoleic acid, which are metabolized into prostaglandins, hormone-like substances that expand the veins and arteries, enhancing sodium and water excretion.
- Vitamin C improves blood vessels and capillaries, works as an antioxidant to prevent cellular damage, and helps prevent high blood pressure and hardening of the arteries.
- CoQ10 supplies oxygen to cells and prevents free-radical damage to the veins and arteries.
- Garlic thins the blood, reduces and stabilizes high blood pressure, and cleans the blood.
- Raw pumpkin and sunflower seeds are rich in zinc and other minerals that help to counteract heavy metals in the blood.
- Ginkgo and hawthorn regulate high blood pressure, dilate blood vessels, strengthen the heart, reduce blood pressure, lower cholesterol, and reduce risk of angina attacks.
- Lecithin breaks up cholesterol and allows it to pass through the arterial wall, helping to prevent arteriosclerosis.
- Watermelon cleans the system. The seeds contain cucur-bocitrin, which dilates the capillaries to relieve pressure.
- Vitamins A, C, E, selenium, and zinc are powerful antioxidants to prevent damage to the cells and plaque buildup in the veins.
- Olive leaf contains oleuropein, which dilates coronary blood vessels, regulates heartbeat, and reduces hypertension.

- Butcher's broom has a toning effect on the internal surface of the veins and helps to protect against strokes, varicose veins, and other circulatory problems.
- Bugleweed acts like digitalis in calming the pulse and is excellent for heart diseases whenever irregular heartbeat is involved.

## ORTHODOX PRESCRIBED MEDICATION

Hypertension drugs usually lower high blood pressure, but they treat the symptoms and not the underlying cause. They may also have significant side effects. Diuretics are the most common blood pressure drugs prescribed. They are designed to reduce fluid levels by increasing urination. Diuretics can be dangerous, because the loss of minerals can be very harmful; they eliminate sodium, potassium, magnesium, and calcium, which are essential to proper

### THE BENEFIT OF NATURAL METHODS

Janet is a nurse and has had twenty years of experience in the medical field. She realized that she was in big trouble when her blood pressure read 200/110, with medication. She was bleeding from her nose three to four times a day. She felt a stroke or heart attack was imminent. She knew what was ahead for her if she chose the conventional method of treatment. She turned to God and was led to the natural method of caring for the body. Within weeks of using natural methods, she went off all her medications, her blood pressure was 116/74, and her nosebleeds were gone. She had experienced blockages being dissolved in both the aorta and the carotid arteries. Her stress level was much improved, and she felt better than she had in twenty years. She is so grateful for those who helped her, and she is now spending her time helping others as she has been helped. Janet used the combination #1, combination #I under Cardiovascular Disorders, which feeds and cleans the veins, gotu kola, ginkgo, and hawthorn. She added a formula for the nerves, another to balance hormones and glands, and an allergy formula.

heart function. Numerous studies have shown that people with high blood pressure seem to be deficient in magnesium, so losing more with diuretics can be very harmful. Diuretics can also deplete the B vitamins. Signs of mineral imbalance can be dizziness, dry mouth, weakness, muscle pains or cramps, rapid heartbeat, insomnia, and confusion. Thiazide diuretics are benzthiazide (Exna), indapamide (Lozol), and metolazone (Aquatensen or Enduron). Research has shown that the drug of choice could be hydrochlorothiazide, which decreases the rate of bone mineral loss when taken in low doses of 12.5 mg daily. Always check with your doctor.

# HYPOGLYCEMIA (LOW BLOOD SUGAR)

Hypoglycemia is a glucose metabolism disorder where the pathology is the opposite of diabetes. Hypoglycemia means low blood sugar. "Hypo-" means low and "-glycemia" means sugar. Hypoglycemia is a condition of too little glucose in the blood, often as a result of the pancreas producing too much insulin. The pancreas may overproduce insulin due to a diet high in sugar, white flour products, soda, junk foods, and too much cooked food.

There are two types of hypoglycemia. The first is called reactive hypoglycemia, in which symptoms are experienced thirty minutes to one hour after eating sugar or a meal high in white flour products, which are simple sugars. Simple sugars are found in refined white flour bread, pastries, pasta, refined white rice, and in foods stripped of fiber. The other is called simple hypoglycemia, which occurs hours after fasting or may not occur for four to six hours after eating. Simple sugars are too quickly absorbed by the body, causing blood sugar levels to rise sharply and putting the pancreas under a great deal of stress. The pancreas tries to compensate for the sudden rise in blood sugar levels; therefore, large amounts of insulin are released, causing a sharp fall in blood sugar levels.

Moods may change drastically from happy and energetic to anxious, irritable, tearful, and depressed when hypoglycemia is involved. Mental confusion and phobias can also manifest themselves when hypoglycemia is present, because of the ups and downs in blood sugar that come with hypoglycemia. There is wear and tear on the body that affects the nervous system. The muscles, cells, and the glands may be affected. Hypoglycemia is seen as the first step on the road to chronic degenerative disease because of its devastating effect on the body, especially in the stress-related adrenal glands. The symptoms of hypoglycemia are very subtle.

Individuals suffering from this condition often don't realize that they are acting peculiarly. The way they perceive and react to situations becomes distorted. Common symptoms of hypoglycemia are anxiety, antisocial behavior, confusion, depression, emotional instability, exhaustion, headaches, impatience, inability to cope, intense hunger, phobias, and sugar cravings. Many people with hypoglycemia accept it as their fate because it seems to run in their family, but Dr. Robert Atkins, one of the foremost pioneers in the field of blood sugar disturbance, did not agree. He said, "Without improper nutrition, I don't believe diabetes could develop, even if both parents are diabetic. No one is doomed by heredity to develop diabetes; I also feel that we are not doomed to develop hypoglycemia or many of the diseases plagued by mankind just because our parents have it."

Poor dietary choices are the main cause of hypoglycemia. A diet high in refined foods and excessive sugar exhausts the adrenals. White sugar is not a food; it is a chemical that wears out the glandular system. The adrenals and pancreas are overstressed when refined starches, sugars, and a high-meat diet are consumed. Sugar is an addictive substance, and the low blood sugar state you get from eating it makes the cravings more intense. The food industry has discovered that increasing the sugar content in products increases the amount a person will eat, which will increase sales. Some doctors feel that if hypoglycemia goes untreated for a long period of time, it can develop into diabetes.

The adrenals can become exhausted from the combination of stress, worry, and the toxic accumulation of undigested starches, sugars, proteins, and dairy products. This depletes the cortin hormone and the ability to digest food properly. Alcohol, drugs, cigarettes, caffeine, chemical food additives, deadline pressures, inadequate sleep, etc. can also contribute to this problem. Glandular dysfunction and mineral deficiencies are other causes. Heavy metal poisoning can produce hypoglycemia. Stress will uncover weaknesses and imbalances in various organs of the body. It will affect these weak organs in various ways. A sick colon, for instance, may manifest itself under stress with constipation or diarrhea. Tension will place an undue burden on any weak area of the body and make it more vulnerable to disease.

Hans Selye, an early pioneer in stress research, discovered a relationship between stress and physiological response. This response is a chain reaction that starts in the hypothalamus area of the brain, stimulating the pituitary gland to generate hormones that regulate the endocrine system. The adrenals are part of this endocrine network. The adrenals release the hormone adrenaline and a group of hormones known as corticosteroids. One of these corticosteroids is called hydrocortisone or cortisol. Elevated levels of cortisol suppress the immune system by debilitating the beneficial T cells and reducing the virus-like interferon.

Health author Dr. Michael A. Weiner explains: "A wide range of diseases are associated with elevated cortisol levels, including depression, cancer, hypertension, ulcers, heart attack, diabetes, infections, alcoholism, obesity, arthritis, stroke, psychoses of the aging, skin diseases, Parkinson's disease, multiple sclerosis, myasthenia gravis, and even perhaps Alzheimer's disease. Elevated levels of cortisol are even reported to be a useful predictor of suicide."

## EMOTIONAL NEEDS

Because low blood sugar can initiate dramatic changes in behavior, those with hypoglycemia need to be aware that their actions may be a direct reflection of their condition. Moreover, anyone who must deal with a hypoglycemic individual needs to learn how to recognize these behavioral markers and respond with food support.

## HERBAL COMBINATIONS
### Herbal Combination #1

These formulas are designed to help nourish, clean, and support the glandular system. All glands work together. When one gland is deficient, this puts a strain on all the glands.

- Licorice supplies quick energy to weakened glands and nourishes the adrenals.
- Safflower helps the adrenal glands to produce more adrenaline and encourages the pancreas to manufacture natural insulin.
- Dandelion destroys acids in the blood, helps in anemia, and balances blood in all nutritive salts.
- Horseradish contains antibiotic action and stimulates digestion, metabolism, and kidney function.

### Herbal Combination #2

- Goldenseal regulates blood sugar, controls uterine hemorrhaging, and kills viruses, germs, parasites, and worms. It is healing to the mucous membranes.
- Juniper berries are a natural diuretic and contain antiseptic and antifungal properties. They clean the blood and urinary tract.
- Uva ursi helps to eliminate excess sugar in blood, is a natural antiseptic, and cleans the liver, kidneys, and bladder.
- Cedar berries are healing for the glands, especially the pancreas, and disinfect and heal the urinary tract.
- Mullein soothes and heals the urinary tract, is a pain reliever, and heals inflammation.
- Yarrow strengthens the liver and pancreas, controls bleeding, and heals mucous membranes.
- Garlic is a natural antibiotic, cleans the blood and veins, and destroys parasites that are felt to be one cause of diabetes.
- Slippery elm is very healing and soothing to the mucous membranes. It nourishes the blood and glands, heals the digestive tract, and improves assimilation of nutrients.
- Capsicum heals wounds and prevents bleeding, increases circulation, cleans blood, and improves glandular activity.
- Dandelion is rich in minerals, is a natural diuretic, and cleans and protects the liver and the blood.
- Marshmallow is soothing for the urinary tract and eliminates toxins.
- Nettle is rich in minerals, heals and shrinks tissues, and cleans the blood, lymphatic system, and glands.
- White oak bark contains astringent properties to control and stop bleeding, heals damaged tissues, and strengthens the glands, stomach, and intestines.

• Licorice stimulates interferon production to protect against viral infections and other germs, nourishes the adrenal glands, supports all glands, and is cleansing for the liver.

### Other Uses

Adrenal glands, anemia, energy, liver, pancreas, weakened system.

### HEALTHFUL SUGGESTIONS

1. Allergies may be a problem. It could be food or other substances. Dr. William H. Philpott, author of *Victory Over Diabetes*, noticed allergic reactions to chemicals. He tells of a man with diabetes who reacted very seriously to petrochemical hydrocarbons, found in exhaust fumes from cars, in perfumes, and in fumes from natural gas. An allergy is just a toxic overload. It is estimated that each person takes in five pounds of toxic material each year. The pancreas is responsible for supplying enzymes, and when the enzymes are lacking, it puts stress on the pancreas. Allergies could be a result of a toxin overload. It is only after eliminating a substance that one is allergic to that the symptoms can disappear. Staying off the allergic substance for a month may help the body to heal.

2. Thyroid malfunction may be a cause of low blood sugar. Fluctuations can occur if the thyroid gland is over- or underactive. Check with your doctor.

3. Avoid refined carbohydrates; they put a stress on the pancreas and cause the body to metabolize sugars too quickly. Avoid fruit juices, which also stress the pancreas. Sugar and white flour products are void of nutrients and are classified as refined carbohydrates. Avoid alcohol, tobacco, tea, coffee, and drugs. Some drugs can cause hypoglycemia reactions.

4. Malnutrition is one of the main causes of disease. Deficiencies of chromium, magnesium, potassium, and the B vitamins are associated with an increased tendency for low blood sugar.

5. Missed meals can cause problems. Even small children who miss meals can experience reactions to low blood sugar. Some people should even eat between meals to avoid a reaction.

6. Add more complex carbohydrates such as oats, millet, rye, buckwheat, barley, and the new grains such as amaranth, cornmeal, and kamut (a form of wheat that may not cause allergies). Wheat and dairy

products, when eaten often, can cause low blood sugar reactions. Quinoa, spelt, and teff are grains that may be used. Eat beans, raw nuts, seeds, vegetables, and some fruit. Use soy products, such as tofu and soymilk, as they are high in protein. Individuals with hypoglycemia are often lacking in protein.

### HERBS AND SUPPLEMENTS

Single herbs to aid hypoglycemia include alfalfa (nourishes the glands), black cohosh, cayenne, dandelion, garlic, ginger, gotu kola (stimulates the brain and relieves fatigue), hawthorn (strengthens the heart when under stress), juniper berries, kelp (cleans and nourishes the thyroid), lady's slipper, licorice (strengthens the adrenals and provides energy), lobelia, mullein, parsley, saffron (helps digest oils), skullcap, and uva ursi.

---

### WHAT A CHANGE CAME OVER HER

When Jane's husband got cancer, she had to go back to work. She became very stressed with her job, as well as taking care of her daughter and husband. The financial stress, along with a lack of health insurance to pay for cancer treatments, took its toll on her body. She became so tired that she would sit on a chair and not have the energy to get up. It was so bad that she would sit and cry. She didn't have the energy to cook or clean, but she knew she had to.

She checked to see what a doctor could do for her. The only thing he would do was to suggest antidepressant medication. She thought, I'm not depressed, I'm tired. She heard about a master herbalist and took classes from him and learned what was wrong with her body. She discovered she had low blood sugar. She learned to manage her diet, relieve stress, and learned which herbs were needed to support her adrenals and pancreas. She studied and read a lot of books, and what a change came over her! She took formulas #1 and #2, along with chromium, licorice, pantothenic acid, food enzymes, and others. The more she learned, the more she realized how wrong the doctors were.

- Licorice root acts in the body like the cortin hormone and protects the adrenal glands—helping them to cope with stress. It stabilizes blood sugar levels and provides a feeling of well-being.
- Turmeric, a Mideastern spice, has shown potential in helping regulate blood sugar.
- Fenugreek is another herb that can aid in controlling blood sugar levels.
- Chromium is essential for the proper metabolism of sugar. A deficiency is seen in elevated blood sugar and insulin levels.
- Vitamin A assists in maintaining normal glandular function. It protects against free-radical damage.
- B-complex vitamins are necessary to control the mood swings associated with hypoglycemia. They build the adrenals and calm the nerves. They also help the liver to detoxify toxins.
- Vitamin C with bioflavonoids helps to prevent low blood sugar attacks. It also protects against free-radical damage.
- Vitamin E protects B vitamins from rapid oxidation and reduces cholesterol. It is necessary for rebuilding the adrenal and pituitary glands. Calcium and magnesium help prevent adrenal instability. They work with vitamins A, C, and E, zinc, and inositol for proper absorption.
- Manganese assists in pancreatic development and in maintenance of healthy nerves.
- Acidophilus is beneficial for improving digestion and providing friendly bacteria to grow.
- Blue-green algae and chlorophyll are cleansing and healing.
- Germanium and CoQ10 help provide oxygen to the blood vessels and cells.
- Essential fatty acids serve as precursors to hormone-like substances that help regulate every body function.

### ORTHODOX PRESCRIBED MEDICATION

Oral hypoglycemic drugs are sulfa drugs (sulfonylureas). They include glipizide (Glucotrol), glyburide (DiaBeta, Micronase), and tolbutamide (Orinase). These drugs are not very effective and lose their effectiveness over time. Side effects are abnormally low blood sugar, mental confusion, incoherent speech, bizarre behavior, convulsions, depression, irritability, and other psychological disturbances.

# HYPOTHYROIDISM

Thyroid disease is increasing and is one of the silent epidemics of our time. In most cases, thyroid problems are considered autoimmune diseases, where the body begins attacking itself. Lynne McTaggart, in her article titled "Thyroid: Passing the Salt," writes, "In the case of chronic autoimmune thyroiditis, the highest prevalence occurs in countries with the highest intake of iodine, such as the U.S. and Japan. Even in areas where iodine is deficient, iodine supplementation triples the incidence of conditions that prefigure Graves' disease; the prevalence of thyroid antibodies rises to more than 30 percent within five years" (*What Doctors Don't Tell You*, November 1996).

Dr. Broda O. Barnes, author of *Hypothyroidism: The Unsuspected Illness*, states, "Of all the sly, subtle problems that can affect physical or mental health, none is more common than thyroid gland disturbances." People are walking around with this disease without even knowing it. In one survey, Lynne McTaggart mentions that up to a sixth of people older than fifty-five have what is referred to as hypothyroidism without obvious symptoms. She also says that nearly half of all women and a quarter of all men in the United States and Great Britain will die with an inflamed thyroid. It is understandable why it is considered the silent epidemic.

Hyperthyroidism—Graves' disease—occurs when the thyroid gland produces too much thyroxine hormone, resulting in an overactive metabolism. Some symptoms of hyperthyroidism are irritability, weakness, intolerance, rapid heartbeat, fatigue, insomnia, and sweating.

When the thyroid gland produces too little thyroxine hormone, the condition is known as hypothyroidism. Symptoms of hypothyroidism are frequently missed because they can be associated with other diseases. Some symptoms include anemia, headaches, high blood pressure, insomnia, weight gain and difficulty in losing weight, constipation, hair loss, heart problems, skin problems, muscle cramps, lower back pain, easy bruising, fatigue, PMS, muscle weakness, recurrent infections, depression, and a cold feeling.

The following is a self-test developed by Dr. Barnes: Shake down a thermometer and leave it next to the bed stand. Immediately upon awakening in the morning, place the thermometer in the armpit for ten minutes. A reading below the normal range of 97.8 to 98.2 degrees Fahrenheit strongly suggests low thyroid function. If the reading is above the normal range, it may be an infection or an overactive thyroid gland.

Iodine is not only found in salt but is contained in antiseptics, drugs, cough syrups, and even radiographic contrast agents. Excess iodine can cause either hypothyroidism or hyperthyroidism. Thyroid function may become imbalanced when the body is encumbered with toxins; iodine can collect in the body if it isn't natural. The need for iodine increases when infection invades the body. Using natural herbs like kelp or dulse will help to regulate the gland, whether it is underactive or overactive.

Cooked food kills enzymes and causes the endocrine glands to overwork, leading to body toxicity and disturbance in glandular function. Cooked food overstimulates the thyroid gland and causes the body to retain excess weight. When the glands do not receive the nutrients necessary to satisfy the body's needs, they overstimulate the digestive organs and demand more food because the body is not satisfied. This produces an oversecretion of hormones and an unhealthy appetite, which finally results in exhaustion of hormone-producing glands. The enzymes from live food help the body to maintain proper metabolism. Besides an inadequate or junk-food diet, hypothyroidism can also be caused by chemicals found in the food and water supply, poor absorption of nutrients in the body, and systemic candidiasis—yeast infection throughout the body.

The thyroid gland is the master metabolic regulator. There are three things the body needs to make life possible: oxygen, nutrients, and the thyroid hormone, thyroxine, which increases protein usage throughout the body, increases oxygen use in all the body tissues, and regulates how much sugar is absorbed from the gastrointestinal tract. Low thyroid function is linked to high cholesterol.

## HERBAL COMBINATIONS

The following formulas help to regulate thyroid function by supplying nutrients to balance hormonal deficiencies. They help the body use energy more efficiently.

### Herbal Combination #1

Irish moss purifies and strengthens the cellular structure and vital fluids of the system and is rich in amino acids, chlorine, iodine, iron, magnesium, manganese, calcium, and potassium.

- Kelp promotes glandular health, is the highest natural source of iodine, is rich in minerals, and strengthens tissues in the brain and heart. The thyroid hormone thyroxine is important in regulating blood cholesterol levels.
- Parsley is rich in chlorophyll, potassium, and other minerals. It is a tonic for the urinary system.
- Capsicum increases circulation of blood, ensuring that nutrients are delivered to inflamed and infected areas. It acts upon the heart and then the capillaries to give tone to circulation.
- Hops is calming and soothing to the nervous system, an effective sedative, and relaxing to the entire body. Healing only takes place in a relaxed body.

### Herbal Combination #2

- Irish moss is soothing and relaxing for healing and strengthens the cells and vital fluids of the system.
- Kelp promotes glandular health, is the highest natural source of iodine, is rich in minerals, and strengthens tissues in the brain and heart.
- Parsley is rich in minerals and vitamins, rich in chlorophyll to provide cleansing properties, and contains diuretic properties.
- Sarsaparilla purifies the blood, stimulates the metabolic rate, and is valuable for glandular balance.
- Black walnut is a natural source of iodine, burns up excess toxins, helps to balance sugar levels, expels parasites, and helps to lower blood pressure.
- Watercress acts as a tonic for regulating metabolism and cleans and purifies the blood.

### Other Uses

Energy, epilepsy, fatigue, glands, goiter, hormones, weight loss.

### HEALTHFUL SUGGESTIONS

1. Rule out thyroid problems by taking the basal metabolism test. It is very accurate and can help define the problem. A normal reading should be between 97.6 and 98.2 degrees Fahrenheit. A possible low thyroid reading is around 97.2, and a possible high thyroid reading is around 98.6.

2. A fasting diet would be beneficial using herbal cleansers such as blood, colon, liver, and lymphatic formulas. A change of diet using natural foods will help balance the thyroid function. Use green drinks, vegetable broths, and vegetable juices using carrot, celery, parsley, and garlic diluted with water. Wheatgrass juice is very cleansing. Start with small amounts; it has very strong cleansing properties.

3. Rule out allergies. The foods that cause the most problems are milk, dairy products, chocolate, wheat, caffeine, sugar, and white flour products. Mercury dental fillings may be suspected.

4. Exercise is important to help increase thyroid secretion of hormones and boost cellular response to hormones. Include walking, bicycling, or jumping on a mini trampoline.

5. Eat live foods such as sprouts, salads, raw fruits, and vegetables. Thermos-cooked grains and rice help retain nutrients. Raw, unsalted seeds and nuts (sesame seeds, pumpkin seeds, sunflower seeds, almonds, pecans, and cashews) are nutritious. Green drinks using chlorophyll help nourish the thyroid gland.

6. Avoid all junk foods. They overstimulate the glands and cause exhaustion and weakness. Sugar and white flour products are detrimental. Fried foods are hard to digest and cause the formation of free radicals, which destroy the cells. Avoid drugs, especially oral contraceptives, antibiotics, sulfa drugs, and tranquilizers. Prednisone and estrogen worsen an unbalanced thyroid function. Sulfa drugs and antidiabetic drugs suppress the thyroid. They put a burden on the thyroid gland and cause dysfunction. Fluoride in drinking water inhibits thyroid function.

### HERBS AND SUPPLEMENTS

Vitamin A and E deficiencies reduce thyroid hormone secretion. These vitamins protect against damage to the cells and help to balance thyroid hormones. They also protect the B vitamins from rapid oxidation.

- B vitamins are necessary for the metabolism of carbohydrates, fats, and proteins. They supply energy essential for healthy nerves, skin, hair, eyes, liver, and muscle tone in the digestive tract. A B2 deficiency depresses the function of the thyroid gland. B6 is needed to convert iodine into thyroid hormone. B12 is essential for metabolizing nutrients and for nerve tissue health.

- Minerals are necessary for glandular health. Calcium and magnesium support the glands. Manganese, silicon, selenium, and zinc protect the glands. Magnesium, phosphorus, and potassium are all essential for maintenance of glandular health and hormone production.

- Vitamin C supports normal adrenal function and glandular activity and protects against damage to the glands, especially when radiation therapy is used.

- Essential fatty acids are necessary to correct normal glandular function. Evening primrose and flaxseed oils are very effective in treating thyroid disease.

- Lecithin aids in proper digestion of fats and protects cell linings. It nourishes the myelin sheath protecting the nerves. It is needed for brain health.

### ORTHODOX PRESCRIBED MEDICATION

Levothyroxine is the most common drug prescribed for thyroid replacement therapy. It can cause cold feeling, clumsiness, constipation, dry and puffy skin, headaches, unusual tiredness or weakness, muscle aches, weight gain, and a change in appetite. It can produce hazardous adverse effects in older people. It should not be taken unless it has been taken for years. It is an older drug. Always check with your doctor. Deficiencies in vitamins A and E and the minerals copper, iron, selenium, and zinc, along with the amino acid tyrosine, can interfere with proper thyroid function.

# INDIGESTION

The digestive system is our first line of defense against disease. It is the digestion and assimilation of the food we eat that determines how efficiently our entire body works. Digestion is the breakdown of food by the digestive system. This process involves assimilation of nutrients by the blood and lymph vessels, so they can be distributed to all body cells for healing and rebuilding the body. Indigestion is one of the most common health problems people are faced with today. Digestive diseases are becoming a national health problem. More than twenty million

Americans suffer from digestive problems. Half of all types of cancer are found in the digestive system.

Television commercials are a good indication of the number of people who suffer from digestive problems, and the new drugs advertised to prevent heartburn will eventually cause more problems. The stomach needs hydrochloric acid to destroy germs, viruses, bacteria, parasites, and worms. It is usually the lack of hydrochloric acid that causes heartburn. Some of the drugs are Pepcid, Tagamet, and Zantac. These drugs will destroy any hydrochloric acid left. They used to be prescribed for ulcers and now can be bought over the counter.

A lack of hydrochloric acid and enzymes is the main cause of indigestion. Lack of these can cause bad breath, heartburn, belching, and flatulence. Other symptoms associated with incomplete digestion are skin problems, recurring headaches, muscle wasting, low immunity, delayed wound healing, anemia, poor bowel function, depression, and allergies. If the food stays longer in the digestive tract than it should, constipation, diarrhea, and autointoxication may develop. Poor digestion is the beginning of many chronic diseases.

Digestive disorders include constipation, diarrhea, acidosis and alkalosis, gastric catarrh, chronic gastritis, dilation of the stomach, ulcers, liver disorders, gallstones, enteritis, appendicitis, colitis, diverticulosis, and hemorrhoids.

The main causes of indigestion are overeating, constipation, wrong combinations of food, too much caffeine, alcohol, tobacco, sweets, white flour products, and overcooked food. Meat and dairy products are both high in fat, which is hard on digestion. A lack of hydrochloric acid and enzymes can also contribute to digestive problems, as well as a candida overgrowth. Colon and liver congestion can lead to ulcers, indigestion, and stomach inflammation. Other causes may be allergies, hiatal hernia, gallbladder problems, stress, ulcers, or heart problems.

Indigestion may be one of the main causes of autoimmune diseases. In the 1930s, a Russian scientist named Paul Kouchakoff found that after cooked food is eaten, the number of white blood cells increases in the intestines. The white blood cells are part of the immune system and always increase in number when there is a need to eliminate hostile invaders. This would indicate that a diet comprised primarily of cooked food could initiate the beginnings of inflammation or disease. Cooked food places an added burden on the immune system as well as contributing to digestive disturbances. Eating raw food does not increase white blood cell response.

## EMOTIONAL NEEDS

Stress, tension, and anxiety can burden the digestive system and impair the digestive process. Consequently, symptoms such as heartburn, bloating, and cramping can result after periods of high emotion. We know that the sympathetic nervous system may become overstimulated by emotional stress, which can result in disorders like indigestion. For this reason, eating under the best of circumstances is recommended. De-stress before meals and try to stay away from mealtime conversation that can cause intense emotional responses.

## HERBAL COMBINATIONS
### Herbal Combination #1

This formula is more than a digestive aid; it works with the liver, gallbladder, and spleen to promote normal function of the digestive system. It is healing and nourishing and will benefit the lymphatic and urinary systems. It helps in the production of bile, which digests fat and prevents constipation. It helps with gas, bloating, fluid retention, digestion, and in the assimilation of nutrients.

- Rose hips have a high vitamin content, help in infections, and benefit stomach ailments caused by bacteria.
- Barberry contains antiseptic properties that help when there is inflammation. It increases the flow of bile, is beneficial for all liver problems, and helps eliminate toxins from the stomach and bowels.
- Dandelion helps the liver detoxify poisons and is rich in nutrients to heal liver and stomach problems. It promotes healthy circulation, strengthens weak arteries, and restores gastric balance.
- Fennel helps improve digestion and acts as a diuretic, as well as relaxing the digestive tract nervous system.
- Red beet root is rich in iron and other minerals and is nourishing and healing for the digestive tract.
- Horseradish contains antibiotic properties, stimulates digestion, and helps to eliminate catarrh.

- Parsley is healing for the digestive tract and is rich in vitamins and minerals. It helps to increase the iron content in the blood and is good for liver and spleen problems.

## Herbal Combination #2

This formula will strengthen and heal the digestive and intestinal systems. It contains papaya, ginger, cramp bark, fennel, peppermint, wild yam, and catnip.

## Herbal Combination #3

This Chinese formula helps to nourish and clean the digestive system. It is useful for gas, belching, bloating, and indigestion. It functions as a detoxifying and digestive aid. It benefits the entire body in circulation and constipation. The digestive system is important for nourishing the cells and body systems. The formula contains agastache herb, crataegus fruit, hoelen plant, magnolia bark, oryza seed, shen-qu tea, citrus peel, gastrodia rhizome, *Panax ginseng* root, typhonium rhizome, atractylodes rhizome, cardamom fruit, platycodon root, ginger rhizome, and licorice root.

## Other Uses

Nausea, stomach upset, colon, intestinal mucus.

## HEALTHFUL SUGGESTIONS

1. Use herbs that will help heal the digestive tract, such as fenugreek, licorice, chamomile, ginger, slippery elm, aloe vera, and goldenseal. Herbal teas are very beneficial and will assimilate quickly into the digestive system.

2. Fasting on fresh vegetable juice is very healing. Use cabbage, carrot, celery, and fresh ginger. Fresh pineapple juice and papaya are also healing.

3. Eat smaller meals and chew the food very well so the digestive enzymes in the saliva can be stimulated. Predigested amino acids will help stimulate enzyme activity and heal the stomach. Vegetable broths are rich in minerals. Cook vegetables, strain, and drink the broth. They are healing and rich in potassium.

4. A high-fiber diet is necessary to restore health to the digestive tract. Cook grains in the thermos overnight. They contain live enzymes and are rich in minerals and vitamins as well as high in fiber.

5. Watch food combining—don't mix proteins and starches at the same meal. A protein works well with vegetables. Starch meals work well with vegetables. Whole grains, fresh fruits, and vegetables will help nourish and heal the digestive tract.

## HERBS AND SUPPLEMENTS

Single herbs that are beneficial for indigestion include the bitters, such as gentian and Oregon grape. For a nervous stomach, take chamomile tea with ginger. For acid stomach or heartburn, take raspberry tea or one tablespoon of slippery elm and a capsule of ginger in warm water. For nausea, mix together cinnamon, cardamom, nutmeg, cloves, and a pinch of ginger in a warm cup of herbal tea.

- Aloe is healing and soothing on the digestive tract.
- Buchu and capsicum promote circulation.
- Comfrey is healing and will rebuild tissue.
- Fennel is soothing, and garlic, goldenseal, and gentian are great healers of the intestinal tract.
- Nervine herbs help for nervous indigestion. They include hops, passion flower, skullcap, valerian, and St. John's wort.
- A hydrochloric acid supplement with meals will aid digestion.
- Digestive enzymes are also beneficial for digesting food properly. They are essential for healing the digestive tract, organs, and cells of the body. They help break up and eliminate congested protein in the blood, cells, and organs.
- Deglycyrrhizinated licorice is a natural treatment for heartburn. Papaya and mint are also beneficial.
- Acidophilus protects against overgrowth of bad bacteria and also helps in the digestion of food.
- Chlorophyll and blue-green algae help in the digestion of food while supplying essential vitamins and minerals. They also clean and heal the digestive tract.
- Antioxidants help in preventing free-radical damage. Examples are vitamins A, C with bioflavonoids, E, selenium, zinc, and grapeseed extract.
- B-complex vitamins are essential for a healthy digestive tract. They are involved in eliminating toxins from the liver.
- Amino acids (predigested) are healing for the digestive tract and stimulate enzyme activity.
- Minerals are essential for relieving indigestion, especially calcium, magnesium, and zinc. Potassium is also excellent for healing.

## ORTHODOX PRESCRIBED MEDICATION

Axid (nizatidine), Pepcid (famotidine), and Zantac (ranitidine) are all drugs that were originally prescribed to block the release of stomach acid and were used for treating ulcers. Now they can be bought freely over the counter, as antiheartburn agents. Most people with heartburn actually produce too little acid. These drugs can cause even more problems. Hydrochloric acid is essential for proper digestion to prevent viruses, germs, toxins, parasites, and worms from invading the body. These drugs may cause an imbalance in the body. Many of the B-complex vitamins are produced in the stomach, and these drugs may interfere with the absorption of essential nutrients. Side effects, especially in the elderly, can be poor digestion, slow elimination from the liver, headaches, insomnia, fatigue, diarrhea, stomach pain, and itching. There can also be serious interactions with other drugs.

# INFECTIONS

Infections develop when the immune system is low. It is a condition in which the body or part of it is invaded by a bacteria, virus, or fungus. The immune system becomes weakened when there is inadequate nutrition, an individual is under stress, there is a chronic or long-lasting illness, the body is exhausted, or when there is exposure to toxic material in the food, air, and water. Exposure to toxic metals can weaken the immune system. The symptoms of infection include swollen glands, inflammation, swelling, and soreness in the body.

Infections are the body's warning signal. The body is trying to cleanse itself of built-up toxins. To keep infections from remaining in the system, encourage perspiration, activate the kidneys, and open the bowels, because fevers tend to dry up the bowels and cause constipation. When the body is cleansed naturally, it strengthens the immune system, and eventually infections will occur less and less. Pure water, citrus juices, and vegetable juices are beneficial while a fever lasts. If hunger is experienced during an infection, eat vegetable broths.

## HERBAL COMBINATIONS

### Herbal Combination #1

The following formulas are designed to strengthen the immune system, reduce inflammation, clear the blood of infections, work as natural antibiotics, kill poisons, reduce swelling, and allow the body to heal itself.

- Cat's claw strengthens the immune system, treats viral infections, reduces inflammation, and heals the stomach and bowels.
- Astragalus increases the production of interferon to protect the immune system and contains tonic properties to strengthen the body.
- Echinacea contains strong antibiotic properties and can be used for long periods of time without side effects. It helps clean toxins from the body.

### Herbal Combination #2

- Parthenium is a blood cleanser, excellent for infections, and cleans the liver and kidneys.
- Myrrh is a powerful antiseptic. Like echinacea, it is a valuable cleansing and healing agent. It works on the stomach and colon to soothe and heal inflammation. It stimulates the flow of blood to the capillaries and speeds healing throughout the body.
- Yarrow is a blood cleanser, opens pores to permit perspiration, eliminates impurities, and reduces fevers.
- Capsicum reduces dilated blood vessels in chronic congestion, is a stimulant, and works as a disinfectant.

### Herbal Combination #3

- Goldenseal acts as a natural antibiotic, reduces swelling, heals mucous membranes, and helps to regulate blood sugar levels.
- Black walnut burns up excess toxins, kills infections, and tones the system.
- Althea removes difficult phlegm from the system and heals, soothes, and neutralizes acid in the body.
- Parthenium is an infection fighter, resembles echinacea in its healing properties, and cleans the blood, liver, and kidneys.
- Plantain neutralizes poisons, acts as a laxative, and is soothing to the whole system.
- Bugleweed helps reduce fluid discharges, relieves pain, and relaxes the body.
- Echinacea is useful as a blood purifier and helps in strep and staph infections. It fights chemical toxic

poisoning and helps treat candida and other fungal infections. It is useful for blood poisoning, ulcers, tuberculosis, pyorrhea, childhood diseases, spinal meningitis, and gangrene.

### Other Uses
Infections, colds, contagious diseases, earaches, fevers, flu, gangrene, glandular infections, inflammation, lungs, measles, mumps, sinus infection, sore throat, tonsillitis, typhoid fever.

## HEALTHFUL SUGGESTIONS

1. Fasting will help clean the body and restore health to the immune system. Use pure water and herbal teas such as peppermint, red raspberry, and red clover. Drink citrus juices such as lemon and lime in warm water to stimulate liver and kidney function.

2. A change of diet will help strengthen the immune system and prevent infections. Meat, white flour, and white sugar products have a depressant effect on the immune system. Instead of using meat for protein, use tofu and soy products. Soymilk is also beneficial. Eat more vegetables, brown rice, millet (an alkaline cereal), sprouts, green salads, and fruit. Vegetable broths are high in potassium and help to heal the body.

3. Eat foods that can improve resistance to infections. Live yogurt contains a friendly bacterium, *Lactobacillus acidophilus*, which will protect against harmful bacteria. Use garlic often, because it contains antibacterial and antifungal activity to help prevent infections. Raw vegetable juices are rich in minerals and vitamins that protect the immune system.

4. Check for allergies, for they can be manifested in an individual who suffers from frequent colds, sinus infections, sore throats, or ear infections. Foods eaten frequently can irritate the intestinal lining and cause allergic reactions.

## HERBS AND SUPPLEMENTS

Single herbs to help with infections include alfalfa and mint tea, aloe vera, capsicum, comfrey, dandelion, fenugreek, garlic, ginger (settles stomach), goldenseal, kelp (provides minerals and heals), licorice (provides energy), lobelia (breaks up mucus), marshmallow, mullein, passion flower, red raspberry, rose hips, and slippery elm (for coughs and to heal the throat).

- Vitamin A in large doses for short periods of time promotes healing and fights infections.
- B-complex vitamins are needed with infections because illness can cause a depletion of them. They are necessary to repair and help maintain energy. B6 acts as a natural antihistamine and defends the body against infections.
- Vitamin C with bioflavonoids in large doses at the first sign of infection can help heal. The combination also helps with allergy-related infections. Bioflavonoids strengthen capillaries to help heal infections.
- Vitamin E works with vitamins to promote healing, heal infections, and remove scar tissue.
- Zinc speeds up the healing of external and internal wounds.

## ORTHODOX PRESCRIBED MEDICATION
Antibiotics such as penicillin, tetracycline, or erythromycin are among the most commonly prescribed. When used too often, they lose their effectiveness. Side effects include cramps, burning of stomach, blood in the urine, diarrhea, hives, sensitivity to sunlight, itching, itching of rectal/genital area, nausea, sore mouth or tongue, swelling of face and ankles, and vomiting. Some people are severely allergic to penicillin and could have a fatal reaction if given it without this knowledge.

# INFLAMMATION

The word on the tip of every medical researcher's tongues these days is *inflammation*. A survey of the health section of your local bookstore will reveal a slew of new titles on the subject, and there are more and more news stories on the topic all the time. There is growing awareness of the role of inappropriate inflammation in many conditions, including cardiovascular diseases, autoimmune ailments, Alzheimer's and Parkinson's diseases, obesity, diabetes, and even cancer. The field of inflammation research is experiencing unprecedented growth.

What is it about inflammation, a supposedly healing process, that has doctors and scientists feverishly exploring its role in a variety of diseases? First, let's look at what happens in the inflammatory process.

When the body experiences a traumatic event or injury, such as a laceration to the skin, a complex biological process is triggered. Specialized cells located throughout the body alert the immune system to the presence of bacteria that might enter the wound. A number of those cells release a chemical called histamine that makes nearby capillaries more porous, allowing some plasma to leak out. This slows down the unwanted bacteria and makes it possible for other immune agents to attack. Another group of cells called macrophages also begins fighting the invaders, and these macrophages release more chemicals, called cytokines, which call for reinforcements. Soon, the area is flooded with immune cells that destroy invading pathogens as well as damaged tissue. The visible external result is the familiar pain, swelling, heat, and redness of inflamed tissue.

The problem begins when this inflammatory response goes awry. Sometimes the body fails to shut down the invader-fighting reaction due to a genetic predisposition, high blood pressure, or an environmental factor such as smoking. It is also thought that chronic inflammation is caused by an imbalance in the hormones that control inflammation. These hormones are called prostaglandins, which the body synthesizes from fatty acids. Many Americans eat a diet too rich in omega-6 fatty acids, which the body uses to create prostaglandins that promote inflammation. Omega-3 fatty acids, on the other hand, are used by the body to make prostaglandins that are anti-inflammatory, and the standard American diet tends to be deficient in these fatty acids.

Whatever the reason, when the inflammatory response becomes chronic, it can be the instigator of many degenerative illnesses.

Researchers believe inflammation plays a role in the development of cancer when macrophages and other inflammatory cells produce free radicals, molecules that kill just about anything they come across—including DNA. A cell that is undestroyed but still damaged by free radicals could mutate into a form that allows it to keep growing and dividing. This abnormal growth is not technically a tumor, but to the immune system, it still looks like a wound that needs to be healed.

Inflammation is also suspected as one of the causes of heart disease. The plaques that obstruct arteries were traditionally thought to be caused by too much "bad cholesterol," or low-density lipoprotein (LDL), clogging blood vessels. Now researchers think that when LDL particles remain in blood vessels long enough, they oxidize and make the artery walls sticky. The sticky walls draw specialized white blood cells and envelop them in the inner wall of the artery. A complex chain of chemical events ensues, and it's the immune system's inflammatory response that helps cause strokes and heart attacks.

A postmortem look at the brains of patients who had Alzheimer's disease shows the accumulation of a protein called amyloid peptide. Specialists have long debated whether this plaque is a cause or result of dementia. Some researchers suggest the loss of cognitive ability may in fact be due to the body's inflammatory response to the protein, which destroys brain cells.

Where diabetes is concerned, scientists have discovered a connection between inflammation, insulin, and fat. Fat cells, like immune cells, produce inflammatory chemicals, especially as you gain weight. It's still unclear whether inflammation is a cause or an effect, but it does seem to play a pivotal role. Some researchers have bred mice whose fat cells produce huge amounts of inflammation. These mice become less efficient at using insulin and eventually develop diabetes.

Many of the elements of the Western lifestyle, such as a diet rich in refined carbohydrates and saturated fat, combined with a lack of exercise, also make it easier for chronic inflammation to take hold.

## HERBAL COMBINATIONS
### Herbal Combination #1
This combination contains glucosamine, chondroitin, MSM, and devil's claw.

- Glucosamine helps maintain joint integrity, lubrication, and mobility.
- Chondroitin encourages cartilage tissue generation and draws fluid into the cartilage, making it more resilient.
- MSM is a type of biologically active sulfur found in food. Sulfur is vital to joint health.
- Devil's claw helps relieve joint pain and has been shown to have anti-inflammatory benefits.

### Herbal Combination #2

This combination provides protease enzymes that break down proteins into smaller proteins and amino acids, enhancing digestion. When the body is deficient in protease, undigested proteins can pass through the intestinal tract and remain undigested, inhibiting overall health and vitality. This formula also contains a full spectrum of plant-derived trace minerals, which help activate enzymes.

### Herbal Combination #3

This combination is a blend of fruit juices and nutritional supplements. It contains bioflavonoids, antioxidants, and xanthones.

- Bioflavonoids give fruits and vegetables their vivid colors. Bioflavonoids aid vitamin C absorption and help maintain collagen and capillary walls. They also boost immunity.
- Antioxidants destroy the free radicals that the body accumulates through energy production, pollution, tobacco smoke, ultraviolet light, and radiation. Antioxidants assist virtually every part of the body.
- Mangosteen is a tropical fruit rich in xanthones. Xanthones provide powerful immune and cardiovascular benefits.
- Other ingredients include wolfberry, sea buckthorn, red grapes, grape seeds, grape skins, raspberries, blueberries, apple extract, and green tea.

### HEALTHFUL SUGGESTIONS

1. Eliminate polyunsaturated vegetable oils, margarine, vegetable shortening, partially hydrogenated oils, and all foods (such as deep-fried foods) that contain trans-fatty acids.

2. Use extra-virgin olive oil as your main fat. Canola oil is also a good choice.

3. Increase your consumption of omega-3 fatty acids by eating walnuts, flax seeds, hemp seeds, soy products, sea vegetables, black cod, herring, mackerel, salmon, and sardines.

4. Carbohydrates can influence inflammation. You can limit this by keeping your blood sugar low and stable. To do this, eat fewer processed foods; avoid fast food and products containing high-fructose corn syrup; eat more whole grains, beans, sweet potatoes, winter squashes, other vegetables, and temperate fruits such as berries, cherries, apples, and pears.

5. Eat more fruits and vegetables. They contain vital antioxidants.

6. Eat less meat and poultry as protein sources, as they both contain pro-inflammatory fats. Instead, consume more soy foods, beans, lentils, whole grains, seeds, and nuts.

7. Eat ginger and turmeric regularly.

8. Get regular exercise, thirty to sixty minutes a day most days of the week.

9. Floss your teeth regularly. This fights gum disease, another source of chronic inflammation.

### HERBS AND SUPPLEMENTS

- Turmeric gives curry and American mustard its yellow hue. Turmeric is useful for all inflammatory conditions, such as arthritis, tendonitis, and autoimmune disorders. Turmeric extracts are available in tablets or capsules; 400 to 600 mg three times per day is a standard regimen. Whole turmeric is more beneficial than isolated curcumin, its major component. Seek out products standardized for 95 percent curcuminoids. It takes two months to start seeing results. Turmeric is not recommended for those with gallstones or bile duct dysfunction. Pregnant women should check with their doctors before using it.
- Powdered, dry ginger is an excellent anti-inflammatory herb. One to two capsules (500 to 1,000 mg) twice a day at meals is recommended. As with turmeric, you won't see the full benefits for two months.
- Boswellin is the extract of the herb boswellia. It is used in Ayurvedic medicine and is available in capsule form. It has been used for generalized inflammatory conditions such as fibromyalgia. Unless the product label directs differently, take two capsules twice a day.
- MSM is a natural source of organic, dietary sulfur. The body requires organic sulfur to function properly. A deficiency of dietary MSM impedes the body's ability to promote cell growth and development. If adequate amounts of MSM are not available, poor-quality cells may be developed.
- Noni juice can stimulate the immune function, inhibit the growth of some tumors, normalize cellular function, and boost tissue regeneration.
- Yucca is a precursor to synthetic cortisone and is excellent in controlling inflammation.

- Flaxseed oil helps produce prostaglandins for inflammation control.
- Colloidal minerals provide active enzymes, maintain chemical balance of all body systems, and aid the body's many metabolic regulators.
- Vitamin C with bioflavonoids is a powerful antioxidant, protecting against free-radical damage.
- Colostrum strengthens the immune system to fight infections and diseases.

# INSOMNIA

Insomnia is a growing problem in our society. Many have trouble falling asleep, or they suddenly wake up in the middle of the night and cannot go back to sleep. There are many reasons for insomnia—it could be a symptom of a disease, but it is not a disease itself. Anxiety and pain are the most frequent causes of insomnia. Some people with ailments such as asthma or heart disease may be unable to sleep for fear of suffocation. It could be caused by anxiety, stress, lack of nutrients (especially minerals), hypoglycemia, nervous tension, physical aches and pains, eating heavy meals late at night, or stimulation from soft drinks, coffee, tea, and chocolate.

Insomnia is a nervous disorder, and almost all nervous disorders are affected by autointoxication—self-poisoning by chronic constipation. The brain and nervous system are very sensitive to toxins, and when the bloodstream isn't clean and pure, it has a negative effect on sleep.

## EMOTIONAL NEEDS
Daily tensions and feelings of apprehension can disrupt normal sleep patterns, resulting in insomnia. Learning to diffuse these feelings before bedtime can help prevent impaired sleep.

## HERBAL COMBINATIONS
These formulas are beneficial for an overstressed nervous system. They help relax the body naturally and help with insomnia. They strengthen the nervous system and help relieve anxiety and tense muscles, contributing to a natural sleep. They will gradually build a strong nervous system.

### Herbal Combination #1
- Valerian is a relaxant, sedative, tonic, and tranquilizer.
- Passion flower is soothing for the nervous system and for conditions such as insomnia, hysteria, anxiety, and hyperactivity. It contains calcium and magnesium that help relax the body, lowering blood pressure.
- Hops helps relieve restlessness and acts as a nervine for insomnia.

### Herbal Combination #2
- Black cohosh tonic is an excellent and safe sedative, as well as being beneficial for the central nervous system and helping to prevent spasms.
- Valerian calms the nerves and is a natural tranquilizer.
- Capsicum is a stimulant, cleanses the nervous system, and increases the effectiveness of other herbs.
- Passion flower is excellent for nervous disorders and irritability and is relaxing and soothing.
- Catnip is useful to induce sweating without increasing body heat. It helps in colds, flu, fevers, and childhood diseases, relaxing the body for healing. It helps stimulate appetite and is calming to the nerves.
- Hops has a sedative effect on the nerves, relieves pain, reduces fevers, is good for insomnia, and settles a nervous stomach.
- Wood betony is good for headaches and nervous disorders. It helps to calm the nervous system, works as a pain reliever, and cleans impurities from the blood and liver.

### Other Uses
Convulsions, headaches, hyperactivity, nervous disorders, palsy, and relaxant.

### HEALTHFUL SUGGESTIONS
1. Avoid caffeine drinks, especially in the evening. Many soft drinks have caffeine in them, as well as chocolate, teas, and pain relievers. Avoid alcohol. If you use painkillers, check and make sure they do not contain caffeine. Avoid stimulants in the evening—meat is considered a stimulant. It is best not to eat heavy meals in the evening.

2. Diabetes or hypoglycemia could be a cause of insomnia. When refined carbohydrates are eaten, they can cause a drop in the blood glucose levels and

stimulate the brain, which is a signal that the body needs food. Changing the diet to complex carbohydrates will help keep blood sugar levels normal. Whole grains help the body produce serotonin and melatonin in the brain.

3. Exercise in the late afternoon or evening increases normal sleep patterns. Walking in the evenings if the weather is nice or jumping on a mini trampoline are both beneficial. However, avoid exercising too close to bedtime, for this will stimulate the brain, making it hard to fall asleep. Colon and blood cleansers will help clean toxins from the blood. When toxins are in the blood, it puts stress on the nervous system. Sleep in cotton garments if possible; the skin is eliminating toxins constantly, and this will help skin detoxification.

5. Healing foods include whole grains, oats, millet (high in magnesium), buckwheat, wheat, and barley, which contain B-complex vitamins. Nuts, seeds (sesame, sunflower, pumpkin), almonds (high in calcium and magnesium) are beneficial. Green vegetables are high in calcium for the nervous system. Sprouts, alfalfa, mung beans, radishes, fenugreek, kale leaves, turnip greens, mustard, and spinach are also beneficial.

## HERBS AND SUPPLEMENTS

Single herbs to help insomnia include catnip, chamomile tea, hops (settles the brain), lady's slipper (use extract), lobelia (relaxant), passion flower (settles nerves), skullcap (feeds the nerves), valerian (helps in insomnia), St. John's wort (great relaxant), and wood betony.

- Melatonin is a hormone secreted by the pineal gland at the base of the brain. It is an important hormone in order to get a good night's sleep. It will help the body get back into a pattern of deep, natural sleep. It should be used in small doses.
- B-complex vitamins are very important for insomnia and healthy nerves. Extra B6 is important. A deficiency can cause insomnia. Extra B12 is needed for nervous disorders.
- Antioxidants are needed. Vitamins A, C, E, selenium, and zinc help to prevent free-radical damage to brain cells.
- Calcium and magnesium are an important supplement for the nervous system. Calcium is needed for restlessness and to help prevent waking up

> ### RELAXING COMBINATIONS
> Mary had trouble sleeping for as long as she could remember. Even as a small child, she didn't sleep well. Any noise was a problem. Finally, as an adult, she discovered the above formulas and now uses them about an hour before going to bed. She also has worked on building her nervous system with calcium, magnesium, B vitamins, and nervine herbs. She also takes 1 mg of melatonin occasionally. The combinations help her to relax and calm down before going to bed.

in the night. Magnesium is the relaxant to promote a natural sleep.
- Chromium is needed for blood sugar problems.
- Amino acids are necessary for building the nervous system. Choline and inositol assist in transmission of nerve impulses.

## ORTHODOX PRESCRIBED MEDICATION

Zolpidem tartrate (Ambien) is a drug that is prescribed for sleep. It is a muscle relaxant, sedative, and has a hypnotic effect. It achieves sleep by altering neurotransmitter channels in the brain. It is used for short-term relief of insomnia. Side effects are difficulty breathing, irregular heartbeat, unsteadiness, swelling of face, confusion, dizziness, depression, unusual excitement or nervousness, hallucinations, insomnia, memory loss, and vision changes.

# LEAKY GUT SYNDROME

The gastrointestinal tract performs many important and essential functions. It digests and assimilates nutrients for use by the body. Vitamins and minerals attach to proteins to cross the gut lining and enter the bloodstream. The gastrointestinal tract also works to detoxify chemicals and harmful substances that enter the body, and it fights infection. If the gastrointestinal tract is compromised for various reasons, the body can suffer serious consequences.

Leaky gut syndrome should be considered as an implication in any autoimmune disease, and is believed to be an underlying cause. A healthy gut is damaged by leaky gut syndrome, which damages the protective coating of antibodies normally present in a healthy gut. These antibodies protect us from infections, viruses, bacteria, parasites, and candida. Some of the common diseases suspected of starting with a leaky gut are colitis, diabetes, lupus, scleroderma, rheumatoid arthritis, and multiple sclerosis.

Dr. Sherry A. Rogers, MD, explains leaky gut syndrome. "The leaky gut syndrome is a poorly recognized but extremely common problem that is seldom tested for. It represents a hyperpermeable intestinal lining. In other words, large spaces develop between the cells of the gut wall and bacteria, toxins, and food leak in" (*Let's Live*, April 1995).

A syndrome is a group of signs and symptoms that collectively characterize or indicate a particular disease or abnormal condition. One disease may have many different symptoms to distinguish it from other conditions. Some syndromes are closely related, and an individual may suffer from more than one at a time. Leaky gut syndrome is one condition that can lead to and may be associated with other serious disorders.

If the lining of the intestinal tract becomes more permeable than normal, it can lead to serious health concerns. The large spaces that develop between the cells of the gut wall allow toxic material to enter the bloodstream. Under normal conditions, these toxic substances would be eliminated, but when leaky gut syndrome occurs, parasites, bacteria, fungi, toxins, fats, undigested protein and other foreign matter not normally absorbed enter the bloodstream. These microbes can put an enormous strain on the liver and lessen its ability to detoxify.

The enlarged spaces in the gut wall also allow for the entrance of larger-than-normal protein molecules. These proteins are not completely broken down so the immune system recognizes them as foreign matter and makes antibodies to fight them. When these antibodies are produced, the body begins to recognize relatively common foods or other substances as detrimental, and this leads to allergic reactions. An inflammatory response may occur the next time the food or substance is consumed. If the inflammation occurs in a joint,

rheumatoid arthritis may result. If the antibodies attack the gut lining, various gastrointestinal problems can develop, such as Crohn's disease or colitis. Some cases of asthma are thought to be related to leaky gut syndrome because the inflammatory condition that arises after ingesting a certain food triggers the asthma. Other associated problems include migraines, eczema, and immune problems. It is easy to see how this antibody response can produce symptoms in just about any organ or area of the body. Parasites, candida, diabetes, lupus, multiple sclerosis, and chronic fatigue syndrome are also linked to leaky gut syndrome.

Leaky gut syndrome is a common health condition primarily due to today's lifestyle, but the problem is often overlooked by medical professionals. The symptoms may be masked for a time but the underlying cause remains. Leaky gut is caused by inflammation of the gut lining. This inflammation is usually caused by the following: prescription drugs such as antibiotics, prednisone, also aspirin, ibuprofen, and an unhealthy diet, such as one that includes red meats, white flour, white sugar products, and high consumption of alcohol. Mold and fungi are found in some foods. Chemicals found in many processed foods cause irritation to the intestinal tract. Lack of enzymes and hydrochloric acid are also causes.

Symptoms could include muscle or joint pain, fatigue, food intolerances, abdominal pain, diarrhea, toxic feelings, memory problems, and shortness of breath.

## EMOTIONAL NEEDS

The stomach is very sensitive to stress as well as poor nutritional health. Negative feelings impact the gut. Worrying excessively, feelings of defeat or oppression can cause stomach problems. Anxiety or feelings of anger and not being able to express them in a healthy way can create gastrointestinal problems. Feeling like a martyr can create irritation of the gut. Creating positive feelings is essential.

## HERBAL COMBINATIONS
### Herbal Combination #1

This formula is designed to heal and rebuild the intestinal tract. It is soothing and beneficial for repairing and nourishing the stomach and bowels for better digestion and assimilation.

- Chamomile contains properties that aid digestion and relieve indigestion. It contains anti-ulcer and antibacterial properties. It is a safe and mild sedative to induce sleep.
- Marshmallow is soothing and healing to the digestive tract. It's nourishing, and contains vitamin A, zinc, and high amounts of calcium, which all support the healing process.
- Plantain helps neutralize stomach acids and normalize stomach secretions. It helps to neutralize poisons and clear the gut of unwanted germs, bacteria, and viruses.
- Rose hips help prevent infections and are rich in vitamin C and rutin, which are needed to heal the mucous membranes of the stomach.
- Slippery elm helps neutralize stomach acidity. It is beneficial for those with difficulty digesting food and nutrients.
- Bugleweed is healing and soothing to the tissues of the mucous membranes. It is mild and soothing to the nervous system, and helps increase appetite, and helps in painful areas of the body.

### Herbal Combination #2

This formula is designed specifically to support stomach health. It has been formulated to nourish and support the stomach, and eliminate discomfort and stress, which affect the stomach and entire digestive system. This formula also protects the liver, which is necessary for digestive health.

Herbal Combination #2 contains pau d'arco, cloves, *Inula racemosa*, licorice (deglycyrrhizinated), capsicum, and lecithin.

### HEALTHFUL SUGGESTIONS

1. Colon cleansing is essential to rid the body of intestinal bacteria. Congested colon is the cause of 90 percent of disease. We can poison ourselves with a diseased intestinal tract. Eating the wrong kinds and amounts of food helps perpetuate bacteria that live on and produce toxins that can be absorbed into the bloodstream. The following combination will clean, nourish, and rebuild the colon: Cascara sagrada, buckthorn, licorice, ginger, Oregon grape, capsicum, turkey rhubarb, couch grass, and red clover.

2. Mineral deficiencies are created by leaky gut syndrome. The inflammation process damages the stomach and prevents mineral absorption. Add mineral supplements to prevent depletion. Goat's whey powder will help heal the digestive system, and it's rich in minerals. The stomach and joints need sodium, and goat's whey is rich in sodium and other essential minerals.

3. L-glutamine protects against leaky gut, helps in the healing process, and stimulates glutathione production, which is an important antioxidant.

4. Eliminate meat and dairy products that contain antibiotics, white flour, sugar products, and alcohol. Cola drinks can irritate the stomach.

5. Fasting can be very healing. Use carrot, celery, ginger, and parsley juices. Use a mild food diet, such as salads, steamed vegetables, avocados, squash. Soups using millet are healing and easy to digest. Millet has the ability to sustain human life in the absence of all other foods.

6. Raw cabbage juice contains high amounts of glutamine, an essential amino acid, which is healing for the stomach.

7. Avoid aspirin, which causes the stomach to bleed and has been known to cause bleeding ulcers. Candida can be a problem. It can lead to irritation to the digestive system. The fungus produces toxins that irritate the stomach and colon. Eliminate foods upon which the fungi thrive. They are sugar, white flour products, yeast breads, wine, beer, fruit juices, cheeses, mushrooms, and vinegar products.

8. Allergies can be caused by leaky gut. Watch for foods that irritate and cause problems such as eczema, asthma, and many irritations. Seek a doctor who is interested in treating your whole body and can test for allergies.

### HERBS AND SUPPLEMENTS

- *Ginkgo biloba* is healing and protects the intestines by reducing the damage from oxidation.
- Licorice is well known for healing ulcers, as well as the gastrointestinal system.
- Slippery elm is healing and soothing to the gastrointestinal system.
- Fenugreek is rich in mucilin and is soothing and healing to the intestines.
- Essential fatty acids are found in fish oil, borage oil, evening primrose oil, black currant oil, and especially flaxseed oil, and have strong healing and antifungal properties.

- Acidophilus is very important to provide friendly bacteria for the digestive process.
- Antioxidants help prevent tissue damage that can cause permanent dysfunction. Vitamin A, bioflavonoids like quercetin, grapeseed extract, pine bark extract, bilberry are excellent antioxidants.
- Caprylic acid, olive leaf extract, and garlic are natural antifungal supplements. They are also healing and nourishing for the intestines.
- Colloidal silver has antibiotic properties.
- Bee pollen is nourishing and healing and gives the body stamina and strength.
- Coenzyme Q10 and germanium are rich antioxidants that prevent cell damage.
- Glutamine is an amino acid is beneficial for repairing and rebuilding damage in the intestines.

## ORTHODOX MEDICATIONS

Cimetidine (Tagamet) and ranitidine (Zantac) are both used to block the stomach's response to acid stimulators. They were once sold as anti-ulcer drugs, and are now sold as anti-heartburn drugs.

Cimetidine is prescribed for gastroesophageal reflux disease (GERD), as well as ulcers, heartburn, acid indigestion, sour stomach, and erosive esophagitis. It has also been prescribed for chronic viral warts in children, herpes infections, and many other symptoms.

Possible side effects are sleepiness, dizziness, fatigue, headache, confusion, diarrhea, breast development in males, and impotence. Serious side effects could cause inflammation of the pancreas, skin problems, liver problems, and even cardiac arrhythmias or arrest, and joint pain.

# LUPUS

Lupus is an autoimmune disease where the body begins to attack itself, causing tissue damage anywhere in the body. Lupus can be a very serious condition because it attacks and destroys the body's connective tissues, the skin, and eventually the vital organs. It affects the blood vessels. Raynaud's disease is common with lupus. Lupus is considered a chronic inflammatory disorder of the connective tissues and appears in two forms: discoid lupus erythematosus (DLE), which affects only the skin, and systemic lupus erythematosus (SLE), which generally affects other organs as well as the skin. It can be fatal and is characterized by remissions and flare-ups, like its cousin disease, rheumatoid arthritis.

There are three theories as to the cause of SLE. First, SLE is an abnormal reaction of the body to its own tissues caused by a breakdown in the autoimmune system; second, certain factors may make a person more susceptible to SLE, such as stress, streptococcal or viral infections, parasites, exposure to sunlight, immunization, pregnancy, or genetic predisposition; third, SLE may be aggravated by certain drugs, such as anticonvulsants, penicillin, sulfa drugs, and oral contraceptives. There are more than eighty different drugs that may cause lupus.

Symptoms include nondeforming arthritis (joint pain and stiffness), a butterfly rash, and sensitivity to light. General body symptoms of SLE may include aching, malaise, fatigue, low-grade fevers, chills, anorexia, and arid weight loss. Lymph node enlargements, abdominal pain, nausea, vomiting, diarrhea, and constipation may also occur. Heart and kidney problems may occur, and headaches, irritability, and depression are also common.

Lupus is a complex disease. Natural methods of treatment have been known to decrease or eliminate the use of cortisone and other drugs within six months to a year. Lupus, as well as rheumatoid arthritis, is a condition difficult to move out of the body. Some medical doctors and researchers believe that the degenerative diseases that are increasing in number are side effects from the many immunizations people have been given over the past few decades. These immunizations have the effect of making it impossible for your immune system to know whether a substance in the body is its own or whether it comes from outside the body.

Herbs, diet, and other therapies that would help move out toxic waste matter and mucus with other ailments do not help SLE. The waste simply stirs around in the bloodstream, unable to be removed from the body. This is because the body's ability to remove accumulated waste is hindered and retarded by a constant buildup of parasites. When the parasites are killed, nature has a better chance to cleanse. Another factor may be that protein molecules from dairy products (pasteurized and homogenized) can readily pass through the intestinal wall and form antigen antibody complexes that can cause arthritis and form the complexes of SLE.

## EMOTIONAL NEEDS

Autoimmune diseases have been linked to long-term unexpressed or unresolved emotional factors. While we need more clinical data on the connection, I believe that certain people are vulnerable to emotionally stimulated physical diseases. Successful treatment of lupus should include emotional counseling and support, in combination with other therapies.

## HERBAL COMBINATIONS
### Herbal Combination #1
This formula is beneficial for repairing connective tissues and pain control. It helps eliminate inflammation and stiffness, the cause of pain in autoimmune diseases. It helps boost the immune system to help the body heal itself.

- Glucosamine is very effective in repairing connective tissues, joints, ligament, tendons, and cartilage. Glucosamine supplies the body with building blocks needed to rebuild joint connective tissue naturally. It is very effective in reducing pain and inflammation.
- Cat's claw (uña de gato) is effective in arthritis, rheumatism, and chronic inflammation. It eliminates harmful microorganisms and other harmful substances. It strengthens the immune system.

### Herbal Combination #2
This formula is designed to help rebuild the structural system, strengthening the whole body. It contains anti-inflammatory and detoxifying properties. It helps in building bones, connective tissue, and muscles. It contains glucosamine, MSM, chondroitin, and devil's claw.

### Other Uses
Bones, flesh, cartilage, joint health, arthritis, autoimmune diseases, calcification, bursitis, gout, neuritis, rheumatism.

## HEALTHFUL SUGGESTIONS
1. Parasites are involved more often than a person realizes. A cleanse to help with this contains black walnut, which is very effective in killing parasites, along with other important herbs to help kill as well as expel the invaders. A lower-bowel formula is important to help gradually clean and nourish the colon. A toxic colon is involved if parasites, viruses, and toxins have entered the body. Colonics will help to clean the colon and expel parasites and worms. Use colonics along with oxygen therapy; the oxygen kills parasites and worms.

2. Juice fasting is beneficial to clean the blood and cells. Juices provide minerals and vitamins in their natural state and in a concentrated form to feed, nourish, and clean a sick body. Fasting is one of the oldest methods in cleaning toxins from the body and healing; however, a water fast is not recommended. It releases toxins and heavy metals without supplying nutrients to fortify the system. If you are sick or very weak, wait to fast until after you build and fortify the body. Use lower-bowel, blood, and liver cleansers first; then fasting will be easier. Juices that are beneficial include carrots, celery, endive, or parsley, with ginger (settles the stomach) and garlic (kills parasites). Apple can be added to juices, and it works well with vegetable juices.

3. Allergies are often involved with autoimmune diseases. The environment is full of toxins, in the air, food, and water. The body can only take so much abuse, and then it attempts to fight back. Fluoride in the drinking water is very toxic. Fluoride disrupts the synthesis of collagen and leads to the breakdown of collagen in the skin, muscles, tendons, ligaments, bones, lungs, kidneys, trachea, and cartilage. Use pure water. Distilled water will help eliminate toxins from the body. Dilute juices with distilled water by half. It would be wise to eliminate foods and find if there is an allergy. The foods most involved in allergies are wheat, dairy products, meat, the nightshade family, and eggs. Eggs, dairy products, chicken, and meat all contain antibiotics and hormones, which cause the body to store more toxins.

4. Leaky gut syndrome may also be implicated. If the lining of the intestinal tract becomes more permeable than normal, it can lead to serious health concerns. The large spaces that develop between the cells of the gut wall allow toxic material to enter the bloodstream. Under normal conditions, these toxic substances would be eliminated, but when leaky gut syndrome occurs, parasites, bacteria, fungi, toxins,

fats, and other foreign matter not normally absorbed enter the bloodstream. These microbes can put an enormous strain on the liver and lessen its ability to detoxify. The enlarged spaces in the gut will also allow for the entrance of larger-than-normal protein molecules. These proteins are not completely broken down, so the immune system recognizes them as foreign matter and makes antibodies to fight them. Using digestive enzymes and hydrochloric acid will help to break up the undigested proteins in the bloodstream and cells so they can be eliminated from the body.

5. A candida diet program will help clean and nourish the body, so it can heal and restore the friendly bacteria into the system, which is often part of a lupus problem. Use natural foods such as a lot of vegetables like asparagus, broccoli, cabbage, greens of all kinds, cucumbers, lettuce, okra, beans, turnips, rutabagas, squash, yams, and potatoes. Onions, garlic, Brussels sprouts, and kohlrabi are also good. Millet, brown rice, buckwheat, quinoa, and amaranth are excellent grains. Try to eat organically grown food if possible. If you use eggs and chicken, try to find the ones free of antibiotics and hormones. Antibiotics are one main cause of candida and autoimmune diseases. Use cold-processed oils like olive, soy, and safflower. Fiber is important for cleansing the intestinal tract as well as absorbing toxins. Make grain soups using a lot of vegetables. They supply minerals for healing.

6. Avoid antibiotic therapy, birth control pills, cortisone, progesterone suppositories, altered acid/alkaline balance, meat, high mercury levels, aspirin, chlorine in water, chocolate, fluoride, sleeping pills, nitrates/nitrites, white sugar, white flour products, and stress.

## HERBS AND SUPPLEMENTS

Single herbs that help with lupus include nervine herbs such as hops, lobelia, passion flower, skullcap, St. John's wort, and valerian. Black walnut and goldenseal will kill parasites and worms. Garlic, chaparral, aloe vera, burdock, devil's claw (cleans deep in the cells), cat's claw, red clover, and yucca are also good.

- Acidophilus is a natural way to put the friendly bacteria into the body and help rid it of candida. Use on an empty stomach; the hydrochloric acid needed for digestion can destroy acidophilus.

- Antioxidants such as vitamins A, C, E, grapeseed extract, selenium, and zinc are beneficial to strengthen the immune system and protect from free-radical damage.
- Digestive enzymes are necessary to break up undigested proteins in the blood and cells. Parasites, worms, viruses, germs, and bacteria all have protein coatings. The digestive enzymes also have anti-inflammatory and antiviral properties.
- Glucosamine sulfate is natural and safe to use. It improves symptoms and boosts tissue regeneration. It also helps eliminate pain.
- Cat's claw contains anti-inflammatory properties to eliminate inflammation and pain in the joints. It is a powerful immune system booster.
- Essential fatty acids include flaxseed, borage, black currant, evening primrose, and salmon oil. They improve joint health, strengthen the glands, and boost the immune system.
- B-complex vitamins are necessary for liver health, help to assimilate carbohydrates, and feed the nervous system. Extra B6 and B12 are important.
- Magnesium is very beneficial for joints, bones, and muscles. It also protects the heart.
- Chlorophyll and blue-green algae, also containing chlorophyll, have an indirect action on bacteria, break down poisons, and provide nutrients to the bloodstream.
- Taheebo tea has helped many people eliminate joint pain and inflammation. It cleans the blood and strengthens the body.
- Whey powder is rich in sodium, purifies the blood, and prevents calcium from depositing in the walls of the arteries.

## ORTHODOX PRESCRIBED MEDICATION

Corticosteroids are typically prescribed as the main medical protocol for systemic lupus. These steroid drugs work to reduce inflammation; however, their long-term use can cause bone loss, glaucoma, cataracts, or even diabetes. They can also deplete the body of vitamins and minerals such as B-complex, calcium, and vitamin D. Using these drugs can also cause indigestion, nausea, vomiting, diarrhea, constipation, headache, and dizziness.

# MENOPAUSE

Menopause is a naturally occurring transition period in a woman's life when she stops menstruating. Hormone function gradually decreases for about ten years before menopause is actually reached. It is a physical and emotional transition. It takes approximately five years but can take longer if a woman is in poor mental and physical health.

Some women start menopause early, some later. Some fertility pills can throw women into menopause way before their time. Some drugs can even cause menopausal symptoms. The following drugs can cause cessation of menstruation for varying periods of time, sometimes permanently: oral contraceptives, busulfan, chlorambucil, mechlorethamine, vincristine, and cyclophosphamide.

Some symptoms relating to menopause are hot flashes, night sweats, depression, dizziness, headache, difficulty breathing, and heart palpitations. These have been connected with a decrease in estrogen production. However, if a woman is in good health, has good digestion and elimination, and maintains a positive outlook, these symptoms will hardly be noticed.

With good health habits, the ovaries produce a reduced amount of estrogen following menopause while other glands take over. The adrenals begin to form a type of female hormone that is used along with the small amount of ovarian estrogen. With the right herbs, the body can continue producing the correct amount of hormones needed by the system—even the correct amount of progesterone is produced by other glands.

## EMOTIONAL NEEDS

Depression and anxiety can be associated with menopause. Keeping physically and mentally active is crucial to ward off the emotional ups and downs linked to menopause. Exercise can be a lifesaver in helping to manage mood swings and keep the physical body fit. Knowing that menopause does not signal the end of productivity is also crucial. Remember that for many women it can be the best of times.

## HERBAL COMBINATIONS
### Herbal Combination #1
This formula helps with hot flashes, uterine disorders, headaches, depression, and balancing hormones. It helps in insomnia, irritability, and instability.

- Black cohosh helps the body produce and balance estrogen and progesterone. It strengthens the uterus, is calming, and relaxes the muscles.
- Licorice stimulates the adrenal glands and the natural production of estrogen. It restores energy to the body, stimulates natural interferon in the body, and strengthens the immune system.
- False unicorn stimulates the reproductive organs, helps in uterine disorders, and relieves headaches and depression. It also helps strengthen a weak stomach and improves digestion.
- Siberian ginseng stimulates the entire body, nourishes the blood, and corrects hormonal imbalance. It provides energy to the body.
- Sarsaparilla contains properties to help the body produce progesterone and balance the hormones. It strengthens the female organs and purifies the blood.
- Squaw vine is a uterine tonic and helps the kidneys to eliminate urine. It also relieves congestion in the uterus and ovaries. It is a natural sedative for the nerves.
- Blessed thistle is useful for menopausal problems and helps with cramps and hormone balance. It helps with headaches and supplies oxygen to the brain.

### Herbal Combination #2
This formula helps balance hormones for women. It contains wild yam, false unicorn, and chaste tree. It contains DHEA to strengthen the adrenal glands and reproductive organs. It is an excellent formula for balancing hormones and relieving symptoms in menopause.

### Other Uses
Hormone imbalance, hot flashes, gland malfunctioning, menstrual problems, morning sickness, sexual impotence, uterine problems.

## HEALTHFUL SUGGESTIONS
1. Decrease calories—fewer calories are needed at this time of life. Excess weight can easily accumulate

if the diet is not changed. If complex carbohydrates are added to the diet—with a lot of vegetables and green salads—plus increased exercise, the body can compensate for the weight gain.

2. Exercise regularly. Walking briskly, at least three times a week, in fresh air when possible, will help in the prevention of osteoporosis. Weight lifting is very useful to strengthen the heart and other muscles. A mini trampoline and a rowing machine are also very useful. There are many ways to exercise; pick the ones that you enjoy and vary them.

3. Add soy products to your diet. Phytoestrogens found in soybeans have been shown to relieve some side effects of menopause and even slow down osteoporosis. They may cut the risk of many forms of cancer. Use tofu in mashed potatoes, stir-fry, cream dishes, rice, and millet dishes. Soymilk is useful with cereals or just to drink.

4. Eliminate tea, coffee, cocoa, and chocolate. They contain caffeine, which can interfere with hormonal balance. Caffeine can also prevent the liver from breaking down the bad estrogen that most women have. Coffee can increase the tendency for fibrocystic breast disease as well as other menopausal problems. Caffeine increases the stress effect by increasing the adrenaline output. Tea and coffee interfere with the absorption of minerals such as iron, calcium, and zinc. Sugar and alcohol increase the body's need for B vitamins, calcium, magnesium, zinc, and antioxidants. Smoking can increase the incidence of hormonal problems, as well as the body's need for vitamin C.

5. Allergies and chemical or food sensitivity can create a hormone imbalance. Candida may also be a problem. Eliminate foods that candida feeds on, such as sugar. If allergies are present, eliminate foods that are eaten every day, or at least three days a week. Then reintroduce them gradually to see if they cause irritations.

6. Stress has a negative effect on the endocrine glands, which control mood changes, circulation, digestion, bone structure, emotions, sleep, and weight. When under stress, menopausal changes can result in problems with the areas controlled by the endocrine glands. The hypothalamus is sensitive to stress and can upset the normal hormonal output.

## "MY LIFE IS NOW BALANCED AGAIN"

Patricia began experiencing numerous female problems at the age of eighteen. She went from doctor to doctor and was given antibiotics, over-the-counter medications, or a prescription drug, which for some reason never seemed to work for very long. This went on for about eight years. By age twenty-six her monthly cycles were so debilitating that she spent much of one week out of every month in bed with severe pain. When she moved to Gadsden, Alabama, Patricia was referred by a friend to a caring and concerned gynecologist in Birmingham. After a pelvic exam and other testing, he diagnosed her with what he said was the second most severe case of endometriosis he had ever seen. After two to three laparoscopies, her problems persisted due to major scar tissue and adhesions. Finally she woke up one day with almost unbearable abdominal pains. Her husband called the doctor, who said to get her immediately to his office.

She wound up back in the hospital, where she underwent major surgery for a near-total bowel obstruction that the doctor told her could require a colostomy. She said, "Thank the Lord, I didn't need the colostomy, but a total hysterectomy was necessary at that time." After the hysterectomy, she was placed on an estrogen supplement called Premarin. The side effects she experienced for the next three years were not far from being as bad as the symptoms of her original disease. She developed panic attacks, hot flashes, and chronic headaches, which were things she never had been plagued with before. The emotional changes she was experiencing were becoming unbearable. She was getting so bent out of shape over everything her husband did or said that he dreaded coming home from work every evening.

One day while she was at a neighbor's house, she was given an article on black cohosh and its ability to help produce a natural female estrogen and help with female problems. She realized she had to do something, so she went to an iridologist and nutritional counselor who examined her eyes and began exposing hidden areas of her health. Patricia started on a regimen of black cohosh, herbal combination #1, and other herbs. These have become a mainstay in her life. She has no more hot flashes, headaches, or panic attacks. She says, "My life is now balanced again, and I haven't taken estrogen or any other pharmaceutical medication for over a year." She now has an herb shop where many people come searching, just as she once searched and found.

## HERBS AND SUPPLEMENTS

Single herbs to help with menopause include black cohosh, damiana, dong quai, suma, wild yam, false unicorn, blue cohosh, burdock, cat's claw, cramp bark, horsetail, licorice, milk thistle, red raspberry, St. John's wort, and vitex.

- Dong quai (Angelica sinensis) is very helpful for menopausal symptoms. It helps to balance hormones and acts as a tonic on the uterus. It is beneficial for the female glandular system. It also helps alleviate nervousness, headaches, and hot flashes.
- Natural progesterone is found in wild yam. It is useful for menopausal symptoms such as mood swings, depression, irritability, headaches, and weight gain. Progesterone is needed, not more estrogen.
- Black cohosh helps balance the hormones estrogen and progesterone. It strengthens the uterus and contains calming and muscle relaxant properties.
- A psyllium combination will help alter and eliminate the excess estrogen that most women have. A high-fiber diet, using grains, beans, and vegetables, is very beneficial. A high-fiber diet will help normalize estrogen hormone levels.
- Soy products contain phytoestrogens such as genistein and daidzein, which will help to normalize hormone levels. They will also protect against cancer.
- Antioxidants found in vitamins A, C, E, selenium, zinc, and grapeseed extracts are beneficial. They help prevent free-radical damage. Vitamin E is effective in reducing hot flashes. Vitamin C with bioflavonoids also helps to reduce hot flashes.
- Essential fatty acids, such as evening primrose oil, flaxseed oil, borage, and black currant oil, help nourish and feed the glandular system, which helps hormone levels, as well as other glandular health problems.
- B-complex vitamins are important for eliminating excess estrogen from the liver. They supply energy and help produce a feeling of well-being. Extra B6 and B12 are helpful for symptoms of menopause.
- Calcium, magnesium, silica, and boron are minerals that will help build strong bones and will enhance the body's utilization and absorption of plant estrogens to prevent osteoporosis. Boron is a trace mineral recently spotlighted by scientists who have found that it may be helpful in the prevention of postmenopausal osteoporosis.

## ORTHODOX PRESCRIBED MEDICATION

Estrogen medications such as Estrace, Femogex, Estradiol, and Premarin are prescribed for symptoms such as menopausal hot flashes, night sweats, to prevent postmenopausal heart disease, and osteoporosis; they may even help to prevent Alzheimer's. These are also prescribed as a mental tonic. Possible side effects are increases in the risk of cancer of the uterus and breast. They may increase the risk of gallstones, accelerate the growth of preexisting fibroid tumors of the uterus, increase fluid retention, raise blood pressure, and decrease sugar tolerance. Ray Peat, in his book Nutrition for Women, says, "Millions of women with already high estrogen levels are being sold estrogen pills or injections, often prescribed as treatment for symptoms known to result from excess estrogen. When this treatment fails, and symptoms get worse, a tranquilizer is often added to the treatment. Surgery frequently follows."

# MULTIPLE SCLEROSIS

Multiple sclerosis (MS) is a disease that affects the brain and spinal cord (the central nervous system). It is considered an autoimmune disease, a breakdown of the immune system. In MS, the immune system considers the myelin sheath as foreign material and attacks it. Scar tissue is formed, preventing nerve impulses from flowing along the nerve tissue. Some doctors believe this is caused from a virus attacking the myelin sheath protecting the nerves. Recent studies are linking human herpes virus 6 to MS. In these studies, researchers are trying to decide whether this virus or some other virus actually triggers MS, or if the presence of the virus in tissues is a secondary result of the disease process.

MS is a degenerative state of the nervous system due to starvation of nerves and cerebrospinal cells. MS is one of the most common diseases of the nervous system in the United States—a fact not generally known by the public, because MS is not a sudden killer and does not usually strike dramatically.

The inflammation that occurs in MS also causes hardened patches to develop at random throughout the brain and spinal cord, interfering with nerves in these areas. The damage is first noticed on the myelin coating around the nerve fibers. Myelin is the fatty material that acts as insulation around each nerve fiber. Damage to the myelin leaves the nerves exposed, and the impulses from the brain center run into interference as they move along. The body attempts to repair itself and deposits hard material known as connective tissues (scars), which cannot conduct nerve impulses. The word *multiple* is used to describe the disease because of the many areas it affects, and *sclerosis* is a word that means "scars."

Some causes besides viruses could be metal poisoning, such as lead and mercury. There is a high lead content in the air, and mercury fillings are very common. Breathing toxins causes them to be absorbed much faster than ingesting them. Mercury vapor can leak out of fillings when chewing food, and breathing it is one possibility. Both metals interfere with the nervous system. These metals collect easily when the diet is deficient in essential nutrients such as selenium, zinc, calcium, vitamin E, lecithin, and essential fatty acids.

Candida is often seen with autoimmune diseases. The toxic by-products of candida can tax the immune system and prevent it from destroying invading bacteria, viruses, or other harmful substances.

Symptoms include weakness, loss of bladder or bowel control, slurring of speech, tremors, and blurred or double vision. Emotional disturbances such as mood swings, irritability, euphoria, or depression also occur. Symptoms may be so mild that the patient may be unaware of them or so bizarre that the person appears hysterical.

MS is common in Canada, the United States, and northern Europe, suggesting that a diet heavy in meat, sugar, and refined grains may be a factor in multiple sclerosis. Animal fats, especially those found in dairy products, are linked with MS. The brain tissue of individuals with MS has a higher saturated fat content than those without MS. Another theory is that infants fed cow's milk may experience nervous system disorders later in life. Breast milk has a fifth more linoleic acid—an acid that is essential for nervous tissues—than cow's milk.

## HERBAL COMBINATIONS
### Herbal Combination #1
This formula strengthens and provides nutritional support to the immune system. It helps to detoxify and restore natural functions of the body. It provides protection from infections and toxins. If viruses are one cause of MS, this helps to protect and eliminate them.

- Bupleurum helps protect the adrenal glands from atrophy induced by steroids and has sedative and antipyretic properties. It is an effective pain reliever and antidepressant. It works as an anti-inflammatory and antiseptic.
- *Panax ginseng* is a natural tonic with antifatigue properties. It has an antisenility effect, adjusts metabolism, and improves brain function. It is beneficial for digestion and a stimulant for the adrenals, pancreas, and pituitary glands.
- *Pinellia ternata* is useful in inflammatory conditions, works as a natural sedative, and prevents bleeding. It relieves muscle spasms and absorbs toxins.
- Licorice strengthens the adrenal glands, is soothing to the intestinal tract, contains anti-inflammatory properties, and enhances immune function.
- Cinnamon is used for abdominal and heart pain, kidney troubles, hypertension, and contains antimicrobial properties. It increases blood circulation and improves digestion.
- Dandelion is a natural diuretic, protects the liver, soothes indigestion, and has laxative properties.
- Scute contains antibacterial properties, helps in viral hepatitis, nephritis, and jaundice, and acts as a natural sedative. It relieves muscle spasms and reduces capillary permeability and inflammation.
- Purslane is useful for inflammation, indigestion, parasites, headaches, and dysentery and contains dietary fiber, omega-3 fatty acids, and minerals such as magnesium. It is used for high blood pressure, candida, and digestive tract infections.

- *Thlaspi arvense* is a Chinese herb with antidote, diuretic, and expectorant properties. It is useful for candida, staph, and strep infections. It is high in protein and vitamin C. It helps with inflammatory conditions and eliminates toxins from the blood.
- *Indigofera tinctoria* reduces inflammation, pain, and fever. It relaxes and heals the nervous system. It cleans and detoxifies the liver and blood. It is high in potassium.

### Other Uses

Arthritis, autoimmune diseases, blood cleanser, calcification, gout, rheumatism, lupus.

### HEALTHFUL SUGGESTIONS

1. Rule out allergies. Common foods that may be connected to MS are milk and gluten products. Other possibilities include sugar products, cocoa products, and members of the nightshade family, such as potatoes, tomatoes, eggplants, peppers, and tobacco.

2. Eliminate hydrogenated oils found in margarine, shortening, and packaged products on the grocery shelf, such as pancake mixes, cookies, and crackers, because they become rancid and cause free-radical damage.

3. Strengthen the immune system. Emotional stress, overwork, fatigue, pregnancy, and acute respiratory infections are known to precede the onset of multiple sclerosis. This could very well indicate an impaired immune system.

4. Change to a healthful diet. Fasting and eating less food will help heal the body. There is strong evidence that a diet heavy in meat, sugar, refined grains, and rancid oils may be the main cause of MS. Sugar has a negative effect on the nerves. It leaches out essential minerals such as calcium, magnesium, and the important B-complex vitamins. Eat a diet high in vegetables and fruit. Raw and steamed vegetables supply minerals for a healthy immune system. Use grain soups with lots of vegetables, using onions, shallots, and garlic. Use millet, buckwheat, and brown rice. Thermos cooking is beneficial to supply enzymes along with B-complex vitamins to feed the nerves. Add soybean products such as soymilk, tofu, and tempeh, which are rich in lecithin. Use a lot of leafy green vegetables and seaweed.

5. Exercise is very important for those with MS. It provides more oxygen, which is essential for a healthy immune system. Walking, using a mini trampoline, or any other low-stress exercise will slowly rebuild and strengthen the body. Weight lifting is important to build up the muscles, including the heart, and will help in providing more oxygen to the brain.

### HERBS AND SUPPLEMENTS

Single herbs to help with MS include ginkgo (feeds the brain), hawthorn (strengthens the veins), hops, skullcap, valerian, St. John's wort, horsetail, lobelia, psyllium, licorice, Oregon grape, slippery elm, suma, and yucca.

- Pancreatin enzymes are beneficial for protein digestion. They also help in inflammatory conditions.
- Bromelain, found in pineapple, exhibits inflammatory properties and is beneficial for inflammatory conditions.
- Turmeric acts like natural cortisone without side effects. It contains curcumin, which is shown to lower cholesterol levels and is high in vitamin C.
- Glucosamine sulfate helps to control pain and inflammation. It heals and repairs joints that have deteriorated. It aids in morning stiffness, swelling, and tenderness in one or more joints. It absorbs easily and is nontoxic.
- Essential fatty acids, such as evening primrose oil, flaxseed, borage, and black currant oil, are beneficial. Damaged joints and nerve tissues occur when EFAs are missing. They help prevent inflammation and damage to the nervous system and free-radical damage.
- Grapeseed extract is a powerful antioxidant to prevent nerve damage. It boosts the immune system, reduces inflammation, and promotes healing.
- B-complex vitamins are essential for healthy nerves, especially vitamin B12 and folic acid. They nourish the nervous system, enhance the immune system, and provide energy.
- Cat's claw contains anti-inflammatory properties to eliminate inflammation and pain. It is a powerful immune system booster.
- Digestive enzymes are essential to assure proper digestion and assimilation of nutrients. They will also help digest toxins, protein, viruses, and bacteria in the body to be eliminated.

## "WHY NOT TRY HERBAL THERAPY?"

Anna found out in January 1989 that her daughter Nancy in Minnesota had been diagnosed with MS. She was unable to walk without a walker and was bedridden and without bowel or bladder function. They were told to place her in a nursing home, which they refused. They decided to move her to her parents' home in Kansas. She had taken the conventional treatment, using steroids, and it had the reverse effect. She became weakened to the point she was unable to do anything for herself. Six months later, she lost use of her right arm, and as a professional pianist, it was devastating. The last MRI revealed a lesion over her optic nerve, and if it progressed, she would lose her sight. She spent another two months in the hospital receiving the same treatment; again, the results left her in a wheelchair. Unable to stand or use her right arm, she used her left arm to give herself therapy at the piano. Through much love, prayer, and proper nutrition, she was able to stand with extensions on her walker but was still unable to walk.

At Christmas, she asked to play the piano for the local community to thank them for their support. A lady who had seen her being transferred from her wheelchair to the piano bench asked if she had been injured in an auto accident. She was told that Nancy had MS, and the lady said, "Why not try herbal therapy?" Nancy agreed. When she started using herbal products, she was on fourteen medications, and six of them were painkillers. She took the herbal products and therapeutic massage to build the muscles in her legs. After three weeks on the natural products, she was able to walk without a walker and had normal body functions. After her recovery, she took training for therapeutic massage. She is now doing massage from her own home and selling herbal products. The herbal products she took were combination #l, a lower-bowel formula, formulas to rebuild the nervous system containing nervine herbs, lecithin, and B-complex vitamins, to name a few.

- Antioxidants, such as vitamins A, C, E, selenium, and zinc, help boost the immune system and nourish the central nervous system. They prevent free-radical damage to the nervous system.
- A psyllium formula is very beneficial for the colon to clean and eliminate toxins.
- Lecithin nourishes the myelin sheath surrounding the nerves.
- Chlorophyll and blue-green algae nourish and clean the bloodstream, provide nutrients to build up the immune system, and improve nerve function.
- Aloe vera juice can help to dissolve fatty deposits on the nerves. It can also heal and dissolve scar tissue.
- Germanium and CoQ10 will provide oxygen to the cells and speed healing.

### ORTHODOX PRESCRIBED MEDICATION

Many different drugs, such as muscle relaxants, antidepressants, painkillers, antispasmodics, anti-inflammatories, immunosuppressants, and immuno-modulators, are used. Corticosteroids are the most common ones prescribed, and prednisone is high on the list. When used short-term, it manages inflammatory disease, but long-term use suppresses the natural production of corticosteroids by the adrenal glands. Sudden withdrawal of drugs can cause coma or death. These drugs can cause depression, emotional disturbances, high blood pressure, diabetes, peptic ulcers, insomnia, and muscle cramps.

# OBESITY AND WEIGHT CONTROL

Weight loss is an obsession in the United States. Pick up any magazine and it will have a solution on how to lose weight. These solutions work for some people. But if they only work for some people, then one diet alone cannot fit everyone's needs. Almost half the women in the United States are trying to lose weight. Many have tried weight-loss programs and have had success, but when they go back to their old ways of eating, they gain the weight back. The solution may be finding the right eating pattern for the right body type.

The media, fashion, and peer pressure give a false sense of how a person should look. Not everyone needs to be skinny to look good. Women have all types of figures, and many women who are seemingly overweight still look good. There are also many overweight children in the United States, which will mean more obesity among the adult population if the trend continues. The problem arises when the excess weight affects health.

Being overweight, along with a sedentary lifestyle, most often leads to circulatory problems. It can lead to diabetes and heart disease. High blood pressure is common with obesity and can lead to varicose veins, pressure on the bone structure, respiratory problems, and gallbladder disorders. It can also lead to breast and endometrial cancer in women and colon and rectal cancer in men. It decreases life spans for both men and women. What will this mean for our children of the future?

What causes the body to accumulate excess weight? The tendency to gain weight can be genetic, along with the wrong eating habits for individuals. A lack of exercise and stored-up toxins in the body can create obesity. Eating the wrong diet for your body type can lead to a toxic buildup. A sluggish metabolism, thermogenesis impairment, and thyroid problems can also be factors in obesity.

Dieting is not the answer. Rapid weight loss is dangerous and can lead to heart disease. When the body is deprived of food, it decreases the metabolic rate to ensure survival and to compensate for a smaller calorie intake. When there are food restrictions, one tends to eat excess amounts of the foods that have been limited. Another cause of obesity is when there is a buildup of toxins in the cells, and the body is deficient in vitamins, minerals, and essential nutrients; it will cause you to eat more. The body will be satisfied when it is cleansed properly and fed the proper nutrients.

We need to understand the process of digestion, assimilation, and elimination that prepares nutrients to be assimilated through the wall of the small intestine into the bloodstream. When we learn more about our bodies, we will become convinced that going on a diet is not the answer. The answer is to change our habits, whether it is food, exercise, or how we feel about ourselves. Obesity is a chronic condition, and it may take patience and time.

However, you will feel so much better, and your whole body will feel clean and healthy. You will need less food when you learn to balance your body type. A healthy body produces a healthy mind.

## EMOTIONAL NEEDS

We are beginning to understand that some people eat due to emotional triggers such as depression, rejection, etc. Which comes first, obesity or dysfunctional emotions that initiate overeating, is hard to determine. Overweight individuals often deal with self-esteem issues. Moreover, they may be eating to compensate for other emotional needs that are not addressed. Obesity can sometimes be a form of self-rejection that can stem from the inability to confront emotional issues. Foods can provide a form of emotional comfort.

## HERBAL COMBINATIONS
### Herbal Combination #1

This formula nourishes, increases energy, and stimulates the burning of stored fat. It improves digestion, nourishes the glands, and increases natural weight loss.

- Cordyceps, chromium, and eleuthero protect the body from stress and increase energy.
- Bee pollen, spirulina, and vitamin E provide food and nourishment to strengthen the entire body.
- Kelp is rich in minerals to balance the glands, especially the thyroid.
- Lotus leaf, green tea extract (decaffeinated), and garcinia suppress appetite and increase energy.

### Herbal Combination #2

This formula also increases metabolism and circulation and has a relaxing effect on the nervous system. It contains white willow, wild lettuce, valerian, and capsicum.

### Herbal Combination #3

This formula has a cleansing effect on the body—it acts as a diuretic, a laxative, and helps in digestion and the production of enzymes. It is cleansing, which is vital when promoting weight loss. It contains chickweed, cascara sagrada, licorice, safflower, papaya fruit, gotu kola, hawthorn berries, fennel, dandelion, parthenium, and black walnut.

### Herbal Combination #4

This formula nourishes and protects the glandular system. It is rich in iodine, which is essential for the body to burn fat through exercise. It is well known to be beneficial for improving thyroid function and obesity. These herbs help hormonal balance. The formula contains Irish moss, kelp, black walnut hulls, parsley, watercress, and sarsaparilla.

### Herbal Combination #5

This formula helps to regulate blood sugar, suppress appetite, and reduce obesity. It is rich in minerals and cleans the intestines. It contains gymnema, garcinia, marshmallow, and psyllium hulls.

### Herbal Combination #6

This formula helps balance cortisol levels in the body and helps the body release fat cells. Cortisol is a hormone that is released by the adrenal gland in response to stress. With increased cortisol levels, the body begins to accumulate extra fat around the abdomen. The formula contains Relora (magnolia bark), holy basil, green tea (decaffeinated), L-theanine, phellodendron bark, banaba leaf, DHEA (a hormone precursor that interacts with the adrenal glands, helping lower cortisol levels), vanadium, vitamin C, and chromium.

### Herbal Combination #7

This combination is designed to help support a healthful appetite. The ingredients help maintain blood glucose levels and help protect the digestive system. They are: dry apple cider vinegar, garcinia, L-carnitine, gymnema, chromium, marshmallow, and psyllium hulls.

## HEALTHFUL SUGGESTIONS

1. Allergies and food addictions are one cause of obesity. The most frequently eaten foods are the ones that cause addictions. The foods that are eaten more than three times a week can be the ones that cause allergies. Allergies cause cravings. When one feels better after eating a certain food, it is a pretty good indication that it is affecting the body negatively. If a craving for sweets follows a meal, it could indicate hypoglycemia, which can be due to a food eaten at the meal. Some have lost weight merely by eliminating the foods they are allergic to.

A lack of lipase (the enzyme needed to digest fat) is seen in obese persons.

2. Discover what your personal metabolic type is. Are you a fast burner or a slow burner? Metabolism is the rate the body burns food for energy. Overweight persons can be either fast burners or slow burners. Fast burners have overactive thyroid and adrenal glands; slow burners have underactive adrenal and thyroid glands. If the wrong foods are eaten for your metabolic type, it can cause obesity. If you're a slow burner, you need to eat approximately 65 percent complex carbohydrates, 25 percent protein, and 10 percent fat. If you're a fast burner, you need to eat approximately 40 percent complex carbohydrates, 40 percent protein, and 20 percent fat. The goal is to balance your body type so you can burn calories more efficiently. No matter what your type is, if you go on a cleanse, use nutrients to curb the appetite and nourish the body with wholesome food and add supplements.

3. Fasting is an excellent way to eliminate toxins from the body. If you are a fast burner, it is very hard to fast, because you burn up calories too fast. Take it very slow if you are a fast burner. Use herbal cleansers such as a lower-bowel, liver, and blood cleanser. You can do this and still eat to keep the energy levels up. Slow burners can fast longer; take one day at a time. Use fresh vegetable juices such as carrot, celery, parsley, garlic, and ginger, always diluted. Slow burners should also use herbal cleansers and lower-bowel, liver, and blood formulas. Use digestive enzymes to help digest proteins in the blood. Fast burners can use juices, first a small amount at a time, then, as the body becomes balanced, a little more. Always dilute juices, no matter what body type you are.

4. Parasites may be involved. There is increasing evidence that parasites and other organisms may play a part in overeating. The body is constantly being robbed of essential nutrients when it harbors these unwelcome visitors. As a result, the body craves more food to compensate for the nutrients lost, and overeating becomes a vicious cycle. There are herbs (such as black walnut) that will kill parasites and remove them from the body. Herbal combinations work better and are found under Parasites and Worms. Candida yeast infections can produce toxins that inhibit the conversions of sugars and fats to energy. Candida is very common in obesity.

5. Exercise is very important. Exercise promotes circulation, which is an important factor in how we feel. It improves the quality of our blood. Glandular function is improved with exercise, which releases hormones necessary for health and appetite control. Regular exercise is very beneficial. Calories are burned during exercise, but the body's metabolism increases, so more calories are burned throughout the day, even at rest. Increasing metabolism is the only method for permanent weight loss. Building muscle mass is seen as an excellent way to burn fat. You need to increase heart rate with aerobic exercise but also by using weights. Working the muscles (the heart is also a muscle) using slow, heavy weight lifting builds or maintains muscles. This will increase metabolism.

6. A lack of enzymes may be a problem. Enzymes are found in raw food or in supplements. Eating a diet high in cooked foods, versus eating one consisting mainly of raw foods, can contribute to weight gain. Cooked food overstimulates the glands, causing them to overwork, and they are depleted of natural enzymes. Overstimulating the glands tends to lead to obesity. Raw food is nonstimulating to the glands and tends to stabilize weight. High-fiber foods are essential. They add bulk to help decrease appetite and also clean the intestinal tract for better digestion, assimilation, and elimination. Nutritious foods to consider include green leafy vegetables, carrots, broccoli, celery, tomatoes, apples, cantaloupe, berries, melons, plums, almonds, sesame seeds, asparagus, avocados, and cabbage. Whole grains cooked slowly overnight in a thermos retain enzymes, which help the body with digestion and assimilation. Tofu and soymilk are high in protein and contain phytochemicals to prevent cancer. Eat more beans, peas, lentils, brown rice, millet, amaranth, yellow cornmeal, quinoa, spelt, and teff. Use them in soups and stews; they provide protein, carbohydrates, minerals, and vitamins. Learn and study as much as you can about nutrition. Learn about vitamins, minerals, etc., and what they do for your body. Excessive sugar and starch create an abnormal appetite. This dangerous combination affects the body chemically like alcohol. The more it is used, the more the cravings increase. Sugar hastens decay or fermentation, and acid is rapidly produced. Eight to ten glasses of pure water daily are important. Try drinking two to three glasses at a time, which can jolt the body's metabolism into a higher gear. Any other liquids (juices, pop, coffee, or tea) do not count. It has to be plain, purified water. This will also expedite the body's release of the toxins, which keep fat in the cells.

## HERBS AND SUPPLEMENTS

Single herbs that help with obesity include Chinese ephedra (boosts metabolism), burdock (cleans blood), echinacea (cleans the body of toxins), sarsaparilla (balances the glands), black walnut (increases oxygen in the blood), goldenseal (balances the hormones), chickweed (appetite suppressant), and kelp (regulates metabolism).

- Thermogenic herbs help to increase metabolism and burn fat. Ephedra is very effective but should not be used by anyone with high blood pressure or heart disease. Slow burners seem to do well with ephedra. Fast burners can do well on kola nut, psyllium formulas, and garcinia cambogia.
- Psyllium formulas will increase fiber and assist effectively in losing weight. They produce a full feeling while helping to eliminate toxins.
- B-complex vitamins will help nourish the body and eliminate cravings. B12 and B6 will help relax and boost the body for easier weight loss.
- Lecithin helps nourish the nerves and dissolves the bad fat.
- Essential fatty acids help balance body chemistry and are found in salmon oil, evening primrose oil, borage oil, and flaxseed. All help regulate and eliminate bad fat.
- CoQ10 helps provide oxygen to the cells, improves memory, and helps prevent depression.
- Chromium helps synthesize cholesterol, fats, and protein. It helps stabilize blood sugar levels through insulin. It protects against heart problems.
- L-glutamine and L-tryptophan are supplements that help in cravings.
- Chlorophyll and blue-green algae supply nutrients while cleansing the blood.
- Vitamins A, C, and E improve metabolism.
- Iron helps the thyroid.
- Hoodia has the ability to stimulate the body to control the appetite. It is very promising in eliminating fat cells.

## "I FEEL GOOD ABOUT MYSELF"

Kim says that overeating and dieting have been a big part of her life. At the age of twelve, she began experimenting with different diets, even though she wasn't really overweight. She just thought she was. Her mother and sister were always on a diet, and she wanted to be included. She even once went on a spinach and boiled egg diet, took it to school, and was made fun of. She continued dieting throughout her high school years, mostly using diet pills and starving herself. She would get so weak at times she could hardly stand up. She would lose weight, but only for short periods, because she would then binge until she gained it all back, plus more.

She got married at age nineteen and had her son a year and a half later. Three months after giving birth, she had lost all her weight that she had gained from pregnancy, plus more. She was so pleased, she thought she had finally done it. Her weight was only down for two weeks, and then she began to binge. She says that she loved food, especially sweets, and she didn't like depriving herself of them. So on the weight came.

She finally reached the point, she thought, of no return. She was up to 173 pounds and was wearing a very uncomfortable size sixteen. Tying her shoes was a great task, and she could hardly breathe when she bent over. She really felt at this point that losing weight was hopeless.

As a last resort, she agreed to take the above formulas. She started seeing results immediately. The first week she lost seven pounds with very little effort. She started walking five days a week for about twenty minutes. By the end of her second week, she had lost eleven pounds total. Her whole attitude began changing immediately. She felt great and had a lot of energy. In about two months she had lost a total of twenty-five pounds. The greatest part was that she didn't have to deprive herself of food that she loved so much. She just had to eat the right foods. Candy bars, she discovered, were definitely not the right food! She says, "To date I've lost a total of thirty-nine pounds and am now wearing a size eight in clothes. I can't even begin to express my appreciation for these products. It changed my life. I feel good about myself, and I enjoy going places and being with people, things I didn't enjoy before."

## ORTHODOX PRESCRIBED MEDICATION

Amphetamine-like substances, such as phenylpropanolamine (PPA), are used to promote weight loss by reducing the appetite. This is seen as ineffective as an appetite suppressant and can cause side effects such as nervousness, restlessness, insomnia, nausea, and a rise in blood pressure. They should not be taken by people with high blood pressure, diabetes, thyroid disease, and depression. Fenfluramine cuts the craving for food by increasing the amount of serotonin in the brain. Side effects can be an increased risk of pulmonary hypertension, where the blood vessels that feed the lungs tighten up. Studies done on rats and monkeys suggest that fenfluramine and dexfenfluramine can cause brain damage. The drugs burn out the neurons in the brain that release serotonin. There is also an increased risk of dangerous heart conditions, which have caused this drug to be taken off the market.

# OSTEOPOROSIS

Osteoporosis is a metabolic bone disorder that slows the rate of bone formation and accelerates the rate of bone resorption, causing loss of bone mass. The bones affected by this disease lose essential calcium and phosphate salts and become porous like a honeycomb. As a result they are brittle and vulnerable to fractures, even without serious falls or injuries. In fact, the presence of osteoporosis is usually discovered by the occurrence of spontaneous fractures of the hip, spine, or long bones. Osteoporosis cannot be detected with X-rays until 50 percent of the bone mass has been lost.

Osteoporosis is most common in women due to long-term calcium losses during pregnancies and menstruation. They also have thinner bones than men. The disease is not common in men, and because men have heavier bones they are more resistant to osteoporosis, at least until their later years.

As women age, and the production of estrogen diminishes, calcium, which needs estrogen to be metabolized, is not taken into the bones, and gradual loss of bone tissue through the process of demineralization occurs. However, even young women who don't menstruate because of stress or anorexia are more susceptible to osteoporosis because of diminished estrogen production.

Studies done by Dr. Kervran, a European scientist, found that fractures do not knit when there are high amounts of calcium present in bones but little or no silica. However, he noted that bones knit extremely well when there is an abundance of silica present but little calcium. Kervran found that silica is the first most important supplement in bone health, manganese the second, and potassium the third. Kervran feels that a significant percentage of bone breaks and fractures could be avoided altogether if sufficient silica is present. Horsetail and oatstraw have high amounts of silica, manganese, copper, and other nutrients.

Osteoporosis itself is not painful, but the effects can cause suffering and pain. Vertebrae in the back can collapse and break, which can pinch the nerves and cause intense lower back or sciatic pain. Advanced osteoporosis can cause severe fractures, which occur because of brittle bones. The hips and vertebrae are especially vulnerable.

The incidence of osteoporosis is growing and causes over a million fractures per year. It is the most common bone disorder in the United States, and is directly related to thousands of injuries and deaths per year. Periodontal disease is a type of osteoporosis of the mouth, and is estimated that many of those over sixty years of age have lost their teeth due to this condition.

## Herbal Combination #1

This Chinese formula is designed to strengthen and support the bones as well as kidney health. It is a tonic for the kidneys. It will help strengthen the muscles and spinal disks and is an excellent formula for the entire skeletal system. This formula will keep the bones and entire body healthy and running.

- Chinese therapy actually treats kidney weakness to help build bone structure. Traditional Chinese medicine teaches that the kidneys rule the bones and produce the marrow. Bone health and nourishment depend on kidney health. Insufficient kidney health results in unhealthy bones. There is also a relationship between the kidneys and the ears. This will not only help osteoporosis but will help in weak knees and ankles, arthritis, and related dis-

eases. It will also help in bladder infections, infertility, and impotence. This formula will be beneficial in preventing as well as healing osteoporosis.
- Astragalus helps in arthritic pains and numbness, as well as might sweats, muscle numbness, boils, diarrhea, asthma, and nervousness.
- Cornus is a tonic for the entire body. It expels intestinal worms, treats back pain, dizziness, backache, fever, excessive discharge of urine and excessive menstruation.
- Dioscorea is used for general weakness, diarrhea, coughs, premature ejaculation, excessive urine, and yellowish vaginal discharge.
- Epimedium stimulates hormone secretion and treats impotence and forgetfulness.
- Ligustrum treats swelling, dizziness, headaches, fever, and acts as a painkiller.
- Lycium treats backache, dizziness, general weakness, fever, diabetes, rheumatism, and arthritis.
- *Panax ginseng* acts as a general tonic, sedative, stimulant, aphrodisiac, and is useful for anemia, general weakness, nervous disorders, shortness of breath, and forgetfulness.
- Eucommia acts as a tonic for entire body, treats backache and high blood pressure.
- Drynaria is a tonic for the kidneys, improves blood circulation, treats arthritis, rheumatism, painful joints, fractures, gangrene, ulcers, and wounds.
- Noni strengthens the kidneys, increases menstrual flow, treats bone and tendon ailments, impotence, female infertility, lumbago, hernia, and excessive discharge of urine.
- Rehmannia stops bleeding, treats fevers, ulcers in the mouth, anemia, weak liver, kidneys, back pain, sore throat, irregular menstruation, premature ejaculation, and dizziness.

This formula also contains the following herbs to help with overall health: eucommia, drynaria, *Morinda citrifolia*, cornus, dioscorea, epimedium, ligustrum, lycium, and atractylodes.

## Herbal Combination #2

This formula is designed to nourish the bones and help in the assimilation of minerals, especially calcium, which cannot be absorbed without silica. This will even help protect the myelin sheath surrounding the nerves. This will help the body have a feeling of overall wellness. This formula contains alfalfa, horsetail, oatstraw, plantain, marshmallow, wheatgrass, and hops.

## Other Uses

Arthritis, back pain, ears, muscles, lumbago, overacidity, sciatica, dizziness, disks, calcium deposits, bladder and kidney infections, fatigue, impotency, incontinence, and infertility; helps repair joint damage, and relieve pain. It will also help with tinnitus, uric acid buildup, and is a beneficial formula for overall health.

## HEALTHFUL SUGGESTIONS

1. Exercise: Regular exercise improves calcium absorption and stimulates bone formation. Lack of exercise causes weak muscles, lack of circulation, and oxygen for tissue renewal. The best exercise is weight-bearing exercise, which strengthens the bones. You should exercise at least three times a week. It will not only help your physical health but will improve your mental health as well.

2. Foods to heal: Whole grains such as buckwheat, brown rice, and whole oats are high in magnesium and silica. Whole grains such as millet, amaranth, yellow cornmeal, kamut, quinoa, spelt, and teff. Green leafy vegetables, salads, and lightly steamed vegetables are nutritious. Almonds, soybeans, sesame seeds, lima beans, red, white, and pinto beans are high in magnesium. Sprouts will help in digestion and the assimilation of essential minerals. Foods high in calcium and low in phosphorus are almonds, sesame seeds, kale, leafy greens, kelp, dulse, Irish moss, and parsley.

3. Soy products and fermented foods: Soy is rich in calcium, and helps balance hormones. You can get sour cream products made from soy as well as a soy cream cheese. Soymilk is better than dairy and doesn't cause buildup of mucus. Miso soup is healthy and rich in B vitamins and friendly bacteria that aid in digestion and assimilation. It helps keep the intestinal tract healthy.

4. Lack of hydrochloric acid or low stomach acidity can prevent the body from properly assimilating calcium. Hydrochloric acid prevents germs, viruses, worms, and parasites and many toxins from invading the bloodstream and causing illness.

5. Other factors that are detrimental to bone health include milk consumption (because of the imbalanced calcium-to-phosphorus ratio), antibiotics, steroid medications, and many prescription drugs.

## HERBS AND SUPPLEMENTS

Single herbs to help in osteoporosis: Alfalfa, black walnut (helps balance minerals), horsetail and oatstraw (rich in silicon, which helps in calcium absorption), kelp and Irish moss (rich in needed minerals for bone health). Other herbs important for bone health are red clover, slippery elm, dandelion, echinacea, garlic, ginger, ginseng, goldenseal (heals the digestive tract), hawthorn, licorice, lobelia, marshmallow, papaya, plantain, and sarsaparilla.

- Vitamins and minerals: Vitamins C and D increase the absorption of calcium and other vital minerals. Fluorine, found naturally in herbs, prevents bone loss. Phosphorus is vital to calcium absorption, and the ratio between the two is important. We get too much phosphoric acid in meals, cola drinks, and processed foods. Magnesium helps prevent calcification by making calcium more available so it can be absorbed. Half the amount of magnesium to that of calcium is needed to aid in proper calcium absorption. Silica is essential along with all minerals. A good vitamin and mineral supplement with B vitamins will keep the body strong and healthy.

- Natural progesterone cream made from wild yam will help prevent and reverse bone loss. It should be rubbed on the soft tissues of the body, the inner wrists, breasts, underarms, or the abdomen.

- Soft drinks contain phosphoric acid, which provides excess phosphorus. This upsets mineral balance in the body and prevents calcium and other important minerals from being assimilated. A study in the *Journal of Nutrition* demonstrated that female athletes who consumed carbonated drinks experienced 2.3 more fractures than those who didn't.

- Caffeine: Consumption over a period of time may cause loss of bone mass because it causes the body to eliminate excessive amounts of calcium through the urinary tract.

- Sugar products: Avoid all sugar products, such as soda pop, alcohol, all refined grains—especially refined white sugar and products made with white flour. Urinary secretions of calcium, sodium, zinc, and other minerals increase when the diet is high in sugar. This causes severe mineral imbalances.

Also, when calcium is taken at the same time as sugar, the body will not absorb the calcium. It has been discovered that when healthy subjects ingested large amounts of sugar, their fasting serum cortisol levels increase. Cortisol is a cortisone-like steroid produced by the adrenal glands, normally in small amounts. Cortisol has been liked to stomach fat, which is very hard to lose.

- Salt (sodium chloride), especially in excessive amounts, can significantly increase urinary secretion of calcium. In one study, 200 mg of salt per day was fine, but 2,000 mg caused a high rate of calcium excretion, which is linked to high blood pressure. You can purchase a mineral salt that that's healthier.
- Aluminum can be absorbed and accumulate in the bones. This can reduce the creation of new bone cells and hasten the bone breakdown, which increases the chances of osteoporosis. Dietary sources of aluminum include fluoride-containing products, aluminum beverage cans, antacids, baking powder, aluminum cookware, and processed cheeses and pickles.
- Eating foods containing citric acid at the same time as aluminum-containing substances greatly enhances the body's absorption of aluminum.
- Protein: Excessive animal protein requires the removal of calcium from the bones in order to counteract the acidic by-products of protein breakdown, and then the calcium is excreted from the body via the urinary tract.
- The following supplements help to maintain healthy bone mass: glucosamine, green food supplements such as green barley grass, and essential fatty acids, such as fish oils, evening primrose oil, flaxseed oil, and borage oil.

## ORTHODOX PRESCRIBED MEDICATIONS

Fosamax and Didronel are both prescribed for osteoporosis. They slow bone loss by inhibiting the mechanism by which old bone is reabsorbed. Unfortunately, the old bone that is saved is structurally unsound, and after three to six years tends to increase the rate of bone loss.

Side effects are diarrhea, low calcium, vitamin D deficiency, magnesium deficiency, rash, headache, and muscular pain. Rats given high doses of these drugs developed adrenal and thyroid tumors.

# PAIN

Pain, whether acute or chronic, is a signal alerting the conscious mind that there is an underlying problem. Painkillers don't cure the underlying cause of the pain and can produce a number of side effects. Acute or sudden pain is useful to protect us from further damage, such as when we touch a hot stove and the pain causes us to pull away quickly. It causes increased heart rate, raises blood pressure, and causes heavy breathing or sweating.

Chronic pain is a continual pain lasting longer than six months. Chronic pain has served its warning signal, but if left unchecked, may cause more serious problems. Pain that becomes chronic could be cancer, arthritis, back pain, migraines, or a number of conditions, and should be checked by a professional. Chronic pain could be caused by allergies, which affect the nervous system. It could also be caused by candida, parasites, bacteria, viruses, and autoimmune diseases such as arthritis, chronic fatigue, low thyroid, or adrenal dysfunction, to name a few.

## HERBAL COMBINATIONS
### Herbal Combination #1
This formula is very effective for pain by nourishing and strengthening the nervous system. It contains vitamins and minerals necessary for brain, nerves, and muscles.

- Chamomile is effective and soothing for relaxing the stomach and muscles. It helps to induce a relaxing sleep.
- Passion flower helps soothe and quiet the nervous system and is good for agitation, unrest, and exhaustion. It is very helpful for those who want to wean away from synthetic painkillers, sleeping pills, and tranquilizers.
- Hops is considered one of the best nervine herbs for overcoming insomnia, helping to alleviate nervous tension and promoting a restful sleep.
- Fennel helps digestion, is a natural diuretic, helps to stabilize the nerves, and is used as a sedative for small children. It also acts as an anticonvulsive and pain reliever.
- Marshmallow is relaxing on the bronchial tubes and soothing and healing for lung ailments. It con-

tains anti-inflammatory and anti-irritant properties. It is excellent for gastrointestinal problems.
- Feverfew is a natural remedy for pain relief and is considered excellent for severe headaches and migraines. It works gradually and with a gentle action that allows the body to heal itself.

### Other Uses
Anxiety, convulsions, headaches, hyperactivity, hysteria, insomnia, nervous disorders, and nervous breakdown.

### Herbal Combination #2
This formula helps relax the nervous system, acts as a natural pain reliever, and contains antiseptic properties.
- White willow is a natural pain reliever, contains antiseptic properties, and is cleansing and healing.
- Valerian is a nerve tonic and relieves headache pain.
- Wild lettuce helps after-birth pains and works as a general pain reliever.
- Capsicum is a stimulant, increases blood flow to the pain area, and is also a relaxant. It increases the efficiency of other herbs.

### Other Uses
After-birth pain, cramps, headache, relaxant, and toothache.

### HEALTHFUL SUGGESTIONS
1. Instead of suppressing the symptoms of pain, look into the cause of the pain. When the body is healed both physically and emotionally, the pain can be eliminated. Using pain therapy is only masking the real problem. Learn about natural ways to relieve pain. Many methods can help, such as acupuncture, biofeedback, chiropractic adjustments, and magnetic field therapy. There are many ways to control pain.

2. Allergies can cause irritations to parts of the body that are the weakest and that can bring on pain. Change to a diet high in fiber from brown rice, millet, kamut, organic grains (pesticides and herbicides cause allergies), beans, peas, and lentils. Eliminate red meat, dairy products, saturated fats, alcohol, and caffeine. And avoid refined sugars, including concentrated fruit juices, sodas, pastries, candy, and ice cream. (See the section on allergies.)

## DAVE WAS WELL ON HIS WAY TO RECOVERY

In August 1990, Dave received an electrical shock on the job that should have taken his life. His wife said, "It was only by the grace of God that he survived." Initially Dave's injuries appeared to be minimal, considering the magnitude of the shock, but it was soon obvious that his health was declining instead of improving. He had pain from head to toe that increased as the days went by. Dave was sent from doctor to doctor and was periodically hospitalized while his condition continued to worsen. It was now apparent that his nervous system was deteriorating, and he was diagnosed with reflex sympathetic dystrophy.

By November of 1991, Dave was in a wheelchair and on a host of painkillers. The doctors continued to experiment with various ways to help control the pain, but their efforts were fruitless. By November 1992, the overseeing specialist told Dave that he was deteriorating so rapidly that it was only a matter of time until he would be an invalid. The doctor then suggested he go to California for a very specialized brain surgery that would help control his pain level and possibly slow down the deterioration process. It was apparent the doctors had lost hope. However, the family's hope was not in man but in the Lord, and they knew Dave would be healed. It was at this point that they dismissed the idea of surgery, and they said that God led them to herbs through some concerned friends.

It was Christmas of 1992, and Dave had been on a variety of herbs and vitamins, such as barley juice caps, gotu kola, B-complex vitamins, vitamin E, lecithin, essential fatty acids, lobelia, valerian root, feverfew, and capsicum. He was on the above combination #1, ADHD #1, a formula to feed the structural system, and a Chinese formula to strengthen the immune system and stimulate circulation. Dave took these supplements for six weeks, and already he could see a significant improvement.

Five months later, much to the doctors' surprise, the wheelchair was put up, and Dave was well on his way to recovery, and by October, he was off all prescription drugs. Today Dave works forty to fifty hours a week, driving, walking, measuring commercial parking lots, and sitting for long periods of time to calculate the bids and draw plans, all of which were impossible tasks before. Dave quotes Ezekiel 47:12, "And the fruit thereof shall be for meat, and their leaves will be used for healing."

3. Exercise can reduce pain. The brain releases endorphins during exercise. These are natural pain relievers. Use low-stress exercise in the beginning.

4. Add nutritional supplements. A lack of essential nutrients can cause a heightened sensitivity to pain. Good nutrition is a must for a healthy body, both mentally and physically. Add herbal remedies to feed and nourish the nervous system, which causes the pain.

## HERBS AND SUPPLEMENTS

Single herbs that are beneficial include skullcap (rebuilds nerves), hops (has sedative properties), passion flower (soothing to nerves), willow bark, St. John's wort, lady's slipper, ginkgo, and suma.

- White willow bark has been used as a pain reliever for many years. It has been found to be a very effective pain reliever for arthritis and headaches.
- Feverfew has been proven very effective for headache pain, especially migraine, without side effects. It has been used for arthritis as well as other pain.
- B-complex vitamins are calming for the nerves. B6 and thiamine work together for pain relief. B1 is calming for the nerves, and B12 also calms the nervous system.
- Vitamin C with bioflavonoids is cleansing and healing and protects against pain.
- Amino acids help to rebuild all cells. DL phenylalanine increases blood level of endorphins and reduces inflammation.
- Essential fatty acids such as flaxseed oil and evening primrose oil are needed for healthy brain and nerve function.
- Glucosamine sulfate relieves pain by regenerating new connective tissues. It rebuilds bones, flesh, and cartilage.

- Vitamin K has analgesic properties and is found in chlorophyll and blue-green algae.
- Vitamin E and other antioxidants, such as vitamins A, C, and grapeseed extract, activate endorphins in the system and help to reduce pain.
- Germanium and CoQ10 increase circulation and contain analgesic properties.
- Lecithin is needed by the myelin sheath protecting the nervous system and brain.
- Digestive enzymes are needed to make sure food is being digested properly and to help eliminate undigested protein in the bloodstream, which is one cause of allergies.

## ORTHODOX PRESCRIBED MEDICATION

Painkillers are very popular in the United States, with sales of up to thirty billion dollars a year. Acetaminophen (Tylenol) relieves pain and reduces fever but can cause kidney and liver damage when used too often. It can cause rashes, dizziness, exhaustion, and nausea. Tylenol with codeine (a narcotic) can cause physical and psychological addiction, with side effects such as depressed feelings, allergic reactions, and decreased breathing. Oxycodone and acetaminophen are prescribed for moderate to severe pain and can cause liver or kidney damage with prolonged or excessive use. They can also cause impaired thinking and concentration, confusion, depression, blurred or double vision, anemia, abnormal bleeding, and bruising. They can be habit-forming.

# PARASITES AND WORMS

Parasites and worms are becoming a real problem in the United States. The World Health Organization estimates that nearly half the world's population is infected with parasites. Ann Louise Gittleman, MS, says, "If you think parasites are a problem only in developing countries or the tropics, then you are in for some shocking news. The rate of parasitic-related disorders in the United States is skyrocketing. An astounding one out of six people will test positive for parasites."

One current problem that is sweeping across the country is a parasite that causes intestinal infections. It is called *Giardia lamblia* and has now become the number one cause of waterborne disease in the United States. Tapeworm infection is also increasing by leaps and bounds. It has been linked with Americans' increasing fondness for raw and rare beef.

*Balantidium coli* parasites come from pigs and cause intestinal infections in humans. The painful and serious disease called amoebic dysentery results from amoebas that destroy the intestinal lining. This can cause the body to become dehydrated and eventually lead to bleeding and ulcerations in the bowel.

Flatworms and roundworms are other parasites that cause serious damage and can often kill their hosts. There is one type of flatworm called a fluke that lives and grows quite large in the intestines, liver, lungs, or blood of animals and humans. Another common worm, the tapeworm, absorbs digested foods from its host. The hookworm is the most harmful type. It lives in the intestines and feeds on the blood of the host.

Trichinosis is a disease that comes from eating pork. The trichina is a tiny worm that infects pigs. The larvae, after burrowing into the intestinal wall of the pig, then enter its blood vessels. The blood carries the larvae to the muscle fiber, where they live. Then when humans eat the pork, the cycle begins again in the human body. Symptoms of trichinosis are headaches, fever, sore muscles, swollen eyes, and even painful breathing. These symptoms are similar to other diseases, so people often do not realize that they could have internal worms.

It has been theorized that cancer may also be caused by a parasite. In *The Conquest of Cancers*, Virginia Livingston Wheeler, MD, explains that a parasite called the *Progenitor cryptocids* begins as the lepra or tubercular bacilli and changes form to become a cancer parasite. She says that this microbe is present in all of our cells, and it is only our immune systems that keep it suppressed.

Symptoms of parasites could be diarrhea, constipation, indigestion, hives, gas, fatigue, and food allergies. They can also lead to arthritis or other autoimmune diseases. Other symptoms could be nausea, vomiting, anorexia, cramping, night sweats, and fever. Malnutrition can also develop.

## HERBAL COMBINATIONS

The following three formulas are designed to destroy and eliminate parasites and worms from the body. These are designed to work for a period of ten days. They are also designed to calm and heal the intestinal tract.

### Herbal Combination #1

This formula is designed to kill and expel parasites while healing the intestines.

- Pumpkin seeds expel tapeworms efficiently and are very nutritious.
- Black walnut oxygenates the blood to kill parasites and worms, burns up toxins, and clears fatty deposits.
- Cascara sagrada promotes peristaltic action in the intestinal canal to help expel parasites and worms. It tones and regulates the bowels.
- Chamomile is soothing and relaxing and heals, cleans, and nourishes the intestinal tract.
- Mullein has a calming effect on all inflamed and irritated nerves and is good for bleeding bowels.
- Marshmallow is soothing and healing for the mucous membranes, is rich in vitamin A, and contains a high content of calcium and zinc.
- Slippery elm soothes and disperses inflammation, draws out impurities, and heals and nourishes all parts of the body.
- Violet leaves contain properties that will reach places only the blood and lymphatic fluids penetrate. They are healing for internal irritations.

### Herbal Combination #2

This formula is designed to strengthen the body against yeast infestations and other microorganisms that invade when the immune system is weak. This provides nutrients to strengthen and protect the immune system.

- Black walnut contains astringent and vermifuge properties to expel worms and parasites.
- Caprylic acid is a natural antifungal agent against *Candida albicans* and other invaders in the intestinal tract. It has been found very effective.
- Elecampane is an antiparasitic herb to combat intestinal worms and reduce water retention.
- Red raspberry leaves are soothing and healing to the digestive system and are rich in vitamins and minerals.

### Herbal Combination #3
This herbal formula helps support the intestinal system to eliminate parasites, worms, and toxins. A clean intestinal system will improve digestion, assimilation, and elimination for a better-functioning body. The formula contains pawpaw, pumpkin seeds, black walnut hulls, cascara sagrada bark, violet leaves, chamomile flowers, mullein leaves, marshmallow root, slippery elm bark, oregano, caprylic acid, propionic acid, sorbic acid, echinacea root, garlic, pau d'arco, selenium, zinc, artemisia, wormwood, mugwort, elecampane root, clove, garlic bulb, ginger root, spearmint herb, and turmeric root.

### Other Uses
Blood cleanser, cancer, bowel cleanser, prostate, tumors, and any condition where the body is toxic.

### HEALTHFUL SUGGESTIONS
1. The first step is to do a cleanse. Parasites and worms do not invade a clean body. They live off the waste material that accumulates in the body. A lower-bowel cleanse, blood cleanser, and a parasite cleanse will help rid the body of parasites and worms.

2. Eat a high-fiber diet full of raw vegetables, fruits, and whole grains. Wash vegetables and fruit, especially leafy vegetables for salads. Wash in vinegar water, salted water, or add a little Clorox in water to destroy larvae and parasites. Juices made from celery, carrot, parsley, fresh ginger, and garlic are excellent for destroying worms and parasites. Always dilute the juices.

3. Pumpkin seeds, pomegranate seeds, sesame seeds, and figs can help rid the body of parasites and worms. Garlic, onions, cabbage, and carrots contain sulfur, which aids in expelling parasites from the body. Drink a lot of purified water. Avoid drinking water from rivers and streams. The ground water in the United States has been infested with giardia.

4. Limit or avoid entirely meat products, especially pork. If meat is eaten, make sure it is fully cooked.

5. Avoid sugar, refined foods, white flour products, chocolate, dairy products, alcohol, tobacco, and caffeine.

### HERBS AND SUPPLEMENTS
Single herbs to help rid the body of parasites include aloe vera, black walnut and burdock (equal parts for purging out parasites), chaparral, echinacea, garlic, goldenseal, horsetail, papaya (kills worms), senna (kills parasites), and wormwood (kills worms).

- Black walnut is rich in iodine, which oxygenates the blood to destroy parasites and worms.
- Goldenseal root contains alkaloids that destroy parasites and worms. It helps protect against diarrhea and gastroenteritis.
- Garlic is called Russian penicillin and kills parasites and worms. It is good for destroying toxins in the body.
- Bovine colostrum (transfer factor) helps to boost the immune system and eliminate viruses, worms, parasites, and germs. It helps with diarrhea from giardia and other pathogens.
- Cat's claw cleanses the intestinal tract, assists the body's elimination of parasites, and helps restore immune function.
- Acidophilus is essential to help maintain and encourage normal intestinal flora.
- A multivitamin/mineral supplement is essential to increase the immune function and help the body to recover from parasites.
- Antioxidants help to prevent free-radical damage. Some include vitamins A, C, E, selenium, zinc, grapeseed extract, and CoQ10.
- B-complex vitamins help to prevent anemia, aid in digestion, detoxify the liver, and help support the nervous system.
- Hydrochloric acid helps kill parasites in the body. A deficiency is common. People who take antacids may be even more prone to infestations of parasites, worms, viruses, and germs.
- Digestive enzymes are also missing from most people. Supplements will help break up the protein coating on the worms and parasites and clean the bloodstream.
- Psyllium is high in fiber. It helps clean out the pathogens.
- Grapefruit seed extract is good for getting rid of any pathogens in the bowels.

### ORTHODOX PRESCRIBED MEDICATION
Metronidazole is prescribed to treat trichomonas infections, amoebic dysentery, and giardiasis. Brand names are Flagyl, Metizol, Metryl, and Protostat. It is in the family of antibiotics. Possible side effects include a "superinfection" with yeast organisms,

## THE DOCTORS TOLD HIM THEY HAD NO IDEA HOW TO HELP HIM

Tommy was in his mid-thirties and had been afflicted with horrible health conditions for about eight years. He had a terrible scab that covered most of the top of his head. It was red, scaly, and oozing most of the time. He also had boils over much of his body and terrible allergies. His energy level was so low he went to bed early most nights. Tommy went to several doctors for eight years. The doctors finally told him that they had no idea what the cause of his condition was or how to help him, and they told him he would just have to live with it.

When Barbara met Tommy, she suspected right away that he had parasites. His eating habits were conducive to parasite infestation. Barbara started Tommy on the above three formulas. She advised him to take them continuously for a month to six weeks because he seemed to have such a severe case of parasites.

The boils and the large scab on Tommy's head were his body's way of trying to eliminate all the toxins in his body. Tommy took large doses of blood purifiers to clean his bloodstream. He gradually built up to larger doses, so he would not feel sick with the toxins cleaning out too fast. He also took pau d'arco tea, which cleans the blood and the liver. He began to feel better right away by building up his immune system.

Tommy had a yeast infection (it usually goes along with parasites), so he took caprylic acid. He took acidophilus to restore the friendly bacteria in the intestines. When taking the blood purifiers, he would start developing boils, but then they would go away without fully developing. After a few weeks, Tommy was able to comb his hair without gobs of scab coming out. He used black walnut extract applied externally to his scalp and also took it internally. He also took bee pollen for his allergies.

Tommy continued to get better week by week, but it took about three months before there was a really big change in his condition. It has been about four months now since Tommy began his herbal program. His scalp is still pink from the scab he had on it, but it continues to get better and better. His energy level is way up. He is also eating a much more healthful diet now.

peripheral neuropathy, abnormally low white blood cell count, and aggravation of epilepsy. Other side effects include a sharp metallic taste, yeast infection, allergic reactions, headache, dizziness, unsteadiness, loss of appetite, nausea, stomach cramps, diarrhea, confusion, and depression.

# PARKINSON'S DISEASE

Parkinson's is a degenerative disease of the nervous system that is characterized by tremors and muscle stiffness. As the disease increases it causes stiffness, weakness, trembling of the muscles, stiff shuffling, trouble walking, depression, permanent rigid stoop, and eventually eating, washing, and dressing become difficult. Although the cause of Parkinson's disease is not known, there is an imbalance of two chemicals, dopamine and acetylcholine, seen in patients. Dopamine carries messages from one nerve cell to another, and when the body cannot produce it, the symptoms appear. Chemicals in the brain can be restored with proper nutrients if there is no permanent damage. Because the brain and nervous system are very sensitive to toxins and a lack of nutrients, many health practitioners believe that malnutrition is the cause of this disease. Autointoxication is seen to be the main cause, along with nutritional deficiencies, especially the lack of antioxidants.

Heavy metal poisoning can also be a cause. Mercury and aluminum can accumulate in the brain over the years and causes brain and nerve damage. Some drugs can cause this disease by blocking dopamine and causing a form of secondary Parkinsonism. Over sixty thousand older adults develop drug-induced Parkinson's each year. Drugs are prescribed in excessive amounts to the elderly, especially for chronic anxiety and gastrointestinal complaints. Stelazine, a powerful antipsychotic tranquilizer that is prescribed to calm the intestinal tract, can induce Parkinson's. The irony is that yet another drug is given to control the disease, when a prescription drug is what caused it in the first place. Other drugs that can induce symptoms of Parkinson's include Droperidol, Chlorprothixene, Thiothixene, and lithium, to name a few. Drugs destroy the nervous system and prevent the assimilation of essential nutrients for brain and nerve function.

## HERBAL COMBINATIONS
### Herbal Combination #1
This formula contains natural supplements to strengthen the immune system and rebuild cells. It helps enhance digestion and assimilation. Increases enzyme flora and heals and nourishes the intestinal system. It gives strength to a weakened body, helps the liver to detoxify, and improves immune function for proper healing and rebuilding from diseases.

- Nucleotides are building blocks of DNA and RNA. Dietary supplement of nucleotides enhance the immune system. This will help the immune system to function properly and strengthen the body under stressful situations, and in diseases such as Parkinson's.
- Fructooligosaccharides (FOS) help promote the growth of friendly bacteria in the intestinal system. These are naturally occurring compounds found in fruits and vegetables. They will not break down during digestion, but pass through and inhibit the growth of bad bacteria and enhance the growth of good bacteria.
- Astragalus acts as a tonic to restore energy to a weakened body, enhances the immune system, and increases the production of interferon, which can help immune system function. It contains antiviral properties, both preventive and defensive.
- Milk thistle helps to clean and rebuild liver cells for proper cleansing. It can help reverse both acute and chronic liver problems. It has antioxidant properties. The liver is the most important organ to remove toxins, as well as heavy metals, from the body, in order for the body to heal and rebuild itself.

### Herbal Combination #2
This formula contains vitamins, minerals, supplements, and herbs to help rebuild a worn-out nervous system. The nervous system and immune system are connected; when one fails, the other follows. Rebuilding the nervous system will improve immune function.

This combination contains vitamins C, B1, B2, B6, B12, folic acid, biotin, niacin, pantothenic acid, schizandra fruit, choline bitartrate, wheat germ, inositol, PABA, bee pollen, lemon bioflavonoids, hops, passion flower, valerian root, and di-calcium phosphate.

### Herbal Combination #3
This formula contains nutrients to nourish and protect the body from toxins, heavy metals, and strengthen the immune and nervous systems. It is combination #2 under Alzheimer's Disease.

## HEALTHFUL SUGGESTIONS.
1. Look for the cause. It could be heavy metal poisoning, medications, bad diet, or nutritional deficiencies. A hair analysis would help determine metal poisoning. Blood purification is also therapeutic and improves digestion so the nutrients can circulate to the brain. Using a natural chelation program to dissolve toxins on the artery walls. Exercise is important and a positive attitude is vital for improvement.

2. Healing Diet: a diet that has the ability to purify the bloodstream while nourishing the body. Fruits are cleansers and vegetables are builders. They contain fluorine, chlorine, sulfur, and other mineral substances that will cleanse and heal the body. In-season fruit is best.

3. Vegetable juices that heal and clean are wheatgrass juice, barley grass juice or in capsule form. Blend the following in a juicer: celery, carrots, handful parsley, garlic, and ginger. This is a good spring tonic.

4. Raw vegetables and salads should be eaten at the beginning of a meal to supply enzymes for proper digestion and assimilation. Raw onions and garlic clean the blood and mucus membranes.

5. Use olive oil and lemon juice for salad dressing.

6. Grain-based diet: Whole grains used in thermos cooking help digestion and retain B-complex vitamins and enzymes. Best grains are wheat, whole oats, millet, buckwheat, kamut, quinoa, amaranth, yellow cornmeal, spelt, and teff. Nuts, such as almonds, pecans, and seeds like sesame and sunflower.

7. Avoid cooking in aluminum pots and pans, eliminate antacids, baking powder, pickles, relishes, and some cheeses that contain aluminum. Avoid all drugs and stimulants; they destroy the nervous system and brain cells. Caffeine, tobacco, tea, cola drinks, high-meat diet, alcohol, sugar and white flour products. They contain no nutrients and leach

nutrients that are essential for the brain and nervous system, such as calcium and B-complex vitamins.

8. A low-protein diet has been found to reduce symptoms of Parkinson's disease. Avoid all meats, egg whites, gelatin, dairy products, white flour products, and all sugar products. Those in the experiments improved daytime mobility, thus permitting near-normal function and independence on their job.

## HERBS AND SUPPLEMENTS

Herbs to help cleanse and nourish the body include alfalfa, burdock, dandelion, comfrey, garlic, kelp, echinacea, lobelia, sarsaparilla, mullein, watercress, cayenne, eyebright, nettle, and fennel.

- Essential fatty acids are necessary for normal nervous system and brain function. Evening primrose oil is an excellent source of gamma linolenic acid. Choline is a vital building block for acetylcholine. Salmon and borage are helpful. Soy lecithin is rich in phosphatidylcholine.
- Vitamin E is rich in antioxidants and protects the body from free-radical damage. Coenzyme Q10 supplies oxygen to the brain. Colloidal silver boosts the immune system. DHEA, flaxseed oil, germanium, lutein, MSM, and niacin all will strengthen the immune system.
- Chlorophyll and blue-green algae are high in calcium, magnesium, and potassium to nourish the blood and help in the assimilation of nutrients.
- Sea vegetables have the ability to eliminate radioactive substances from the body. They are rich in minerals that counteract the effects of air pollution. Experiments have found the alginate prepared from kelp, kombu, and other brown seaweeds helps prevent radioactive material from invading the body. Miso has been found effective in removing radioactive elements from the body.
- Acidophilus protects the body from harmful bacteria. Taking it on an empty stomach will assure its effectiveness. It will heal the digestive tract.
- Digestive enzymes are important to break down food for proper digestion and assimilation. They will help also clean the blood and cells of undigested protein.
- Hydrochloric acid is necessary to break down protein into amino acids for proper digestion and assimilation. It destroys bacteria, germs, viruses, parasites, and worms. It is essential for life and the only acid our body produces.

## ORTHODOX PRESCRIBED MEDICATIONS

Two anti-Parkinsonian's drugs, Artane (Lederle) and Cogentin (Merck), showed severe side effects: memory impairment, confusion, hallucinations, and retention of urine. Comtan is used for Parkinson's disease; it is prescribed when doses of the combination drug levodopa/carbidopa (Sinemet) begin to wear off too soon. Side effects could be abdominal pain, back pain, constipation, diarrhea, discoloration of urine, dizziness, nausea, onset of new movement disorders, fatigue, and nausea.

# PERIODONTAL DISEASE

According to the U.S. Public Health Service, 98 percent of all Americans get dental disease at some point. The American Dental Association reveals that by retirement, the average senior citizen has only five teeth left, and 40 percent are wearing dentures. In an advanced modern society, with the latest technology and sophisticated knowledge, why do we have such poor dental health?

The definition of periodontal disease is "of the tissues surrounding and supporting the teeth." One of the first signs of periodontal disease is bleeding gums. When gums are inflamed, this condition is known as gingivitis. Poor diet is the major culprit in gingivitis. Lack of vitamin C can cause scurvy-like symptoms, which include bleeding gums and loose teeth.

This disease needs to be treated by a dental expert. But we want to focus on prevention through nutrition and healthy lifestyle. Good oral hygiene is also necessary. Flossing daily and brushing from the base of the teeth toward the crown can do much to clean away plaque. Plaque, a film on the teeth where bacteria flourish, can harden into a rocklike substance known as tartar. Tartar accumulates at the base of the tooth where the gum line meets. If the plaque isn't brushed off daily, the tartar irritates the gums further and causes more bleeding. The bacteria loosen the teeth from the gums and migrate lower, where they form pus pockets. This extremely dangerous condition is known as pyorrhea. Pus discharges into the mouth and the teeth will actually loosen from the sockets. The roots are destroyed and the teeth are extracted, hence the need for dentures. This entire collection of symptoms is known as periodontal disease. It is essential that you have your teeth checked and cleaned every six months at least. Oral hygiene is very important, but is not sufficient in many cases. The body's immune system must be strengthened, along with a diet free from food that weakens the teeth and body. Dental experts feel that loss of bone mass beneath the teeth is the major contributor to dental problems. It is called osteoporosis of the jaws. A strong bone mass is important beneath the teeth. If not, it will be easier for bacteria to get in and cause further damage.

## HERBAL COMBINATIONS
### Herbal Combination #1
This formula is rich in vitamins, minerals, and herbs designed to strengthen the skeletal system and improve allover health. When the bones are not healthy it affects the entire body and could cause back, knee, and hip problems, and even necessary surgery.

- Vitamin A (beta-carotene) is necessary for healing and strengthening the gums.
- Vitamin C is necessary for protecting against gum problems.
- Vitamin D is necessary for calcium absorption.
- B vitamins help detoxify the liver. Especially B6 and B12 will help protect the immune system and nervous system.
- Calcium is essential for healthy bones. Iron, along with vitamin D, helps calcium absorption.
- Minerals, including phosphorus, magnesium, zinc, copper, manganese, and potassium, are all essential to balance minerals and help keep calcium in solution, and prevent calcium deposits in joints.
- Boron helps calcium absorption and strengthens the bones.

The following herbs are especially beneficial for a healthy skeletal system:
- Horsetail: Bones heal faster when silica is present, which is abundant in horsetail. It is also used in urinary tract disorders, especially lower urinary tract infections. The Chinese feel that a healthy urinary tract is important to bone health.

- Betaine HCl is necessary for the body to absorb calcium and all minerals.
- Papaya contains papain, an enzyme that breaks down protein and other food.
- Parsley is so nutritious that it increases resistance to infections and diseases and is rich in chlorophyll, B vitamins, vitamins A and C, and helps increase iron content in the blood.
- Pineapple helps in the digestion of nutrients and food.
- Valerian is a strong nervine, and healthy nerves are essential for healing. It is rich in magnesium, potassium, copper.
- Licorice works as an adrenal gland stimulant. Helps in inflammation, and strengthens the body.

### Herbal Combination #2
The Chinese herbal combination #1, under Osteoporosis, is an excellent herbal combination to strengthen bone health of the jaws and prevent bone loss.

### Herbal Combination #3
Herbal combination #2 under Osteoporosis contains nutrients that will rebuild and prevent bone loss. It will also help build bone mass.

## HEALTHFUL SUGGESTIONS
1. Natural therapy: Use herbal blood and colon cleansers, which should contain burdock, pau d'arco, red clover, sarsaparilla, yellow dock, dandelion, buckthorn, cascara sagrada, peach, yarrow, Oregon grape, and prickly ash. The bloodstream can carry toxins that can settle in the gums. A clean colon is necessary for a healthy body.

2. Change of diet and lifestyle: Eliminate tobacco, caffeine, and alcohol products. Tobacco constricts the blood vessels and causes weakness. Avoid drugs, when necessary, since they increase the risk of side effects. Eliminate harmful fats; they raise cholesterol levels, thicken the blood, and interfere with the metabolism of essential fatty acids.

3. Foods to heal: Foods high in bone-and-teeth-strengthening fluorine are goat's milk, avocados, cheese, cabbage, garlic, oats, brown rice, and seafood. Foods high in silicon are oats, barley, nuts, seeds, grains, rice polishings. Silicon is also concentrated in the outer skin of fresh fruits and vegetables. Foods

rich in calcium are green leafy vegetables, goat's milk, almonds, avocados, sesame seeds, millet, buckwheat, blackstrap molasses, soymilk, sunflower seeds, beans, dried figs, and whole grains.

4. Apply the following to protect the gums: tea tree oil and vitamin E. Aloe vera will help when rubbed on the gums when they are sore and inflamed. Lobelia extract is beneficial for inflamed and infected gums. Aloe can soothe sore gum tissues.

5. Goldenseal extract (alcohol-free) can be used on a toothbrush or swish in the mouth to help with bacteria and help with sores in the mouth.

## HERBS AND SUPPLEMENTS

Vitamin A is very important for gum health. It heals and strengthens the gum as well as protects from germs.

- Vitamin B-complex is necessary for gum health, for proper digestion, helps the liver to detoxify.
- Vitamin C and bioflavonoids strengthen the gums, prevent infections, help to retard plaque accumulation, and are healing for the gums.
- Vitamin D is necessary, along with calcium, for strong bones. Sunlight is rich in vitamin D.
- Vitamin E protects by enhancing oxygen transport to cells. It also heals gums and tissues.
- Calcium: Herbal calcium formula has been found to build bone mass.
- Black walnut strengthens teeth (add capsule to toothpaste).
- Horsetail contains silica and other minerals to grow bone mass.
- Kelp contains minerals for healthy bones and teeth.
- White oak bark heals and strengthens gums.
- Oatstraw, pau d'arco, slippery elm, yellow dock, and goldenseal will destroy bacteria.
- Chlorophyll found in green plants nourishes the blood and body.
- Coenzyme Q10 helps in circulation and gets oxygen to the head area. Helps in periodontal disease. Strengthens the gums and grows new gum tissues.
- Germanium increases oxygen to the tissues, helps in infections.
- Quercetin and bromelain are excellent to reduce gum inflammation.
- Grapeseed extract contains flavonoids that help heal and rebuild tissues in the gums.

### SHE WAS DELIGHTED AND HAS TOLD MANY PEOPLE

Sara was plagued with all kinds of infections. No matter what she did to heal, it just didn't seem to help. She studied how toxins can accumulate in the body, and mercury tooth fillings could be a definite cause. She had a mouth full of mercury fillings. She found a dentist who agreed to replace all her fillings with a natural substance.

When he started working on Sara, she told him she wanted to use an herbal supplement to see if she could build bone mass and improve her teeth. It was formula #2 under Osteoporosis. It took the dentist two and one-half years to remove and fill the old cavities. Sara had a cleansing crisis and was very sick after the last of the teeth were done. But with all the herbs and vitamins and minerals she took, she felt much better. She used lower-bowel formulas, blood cleansers, and liver cleansers. The good part is, when the dentist finished with the new fillings, he X-rayed her teeth and told her that she had indeed grown new bone mass. She was delighted and has told many people, which has also improved their bone health.

# POST-POLIO SYNDROME

In 1990, there were an estimated 650,000 paralytic polio survivors in the United States, many of whom experienced polio's late effects. There are more than 125,000 who are estimated to have post-polio syndrome (PPS). It is a condition that results in progressive muscle weakness. Swallowing problems are a common sign of the syndrome. Many are often unaware of this condition, which could increase the risk of choking, called dysphagia. The most frequent symptom with PPS is unaccustomed fatigue. It seems to be closely related to chronic fatigue syndrome or fibromyalgia. It affects the muscular, nervous, and immune systems.

Many people suffer silently, and some not so silently, with pain and weakness in their muscles.

Most people have new muscle or joint pain or new muscle weakness or atrophy. Some even have muscle twitching, or fasciculation. Low-stress exercise and low-stress weight lifting have been very beneficial.

Symptoms include chronic pain, decreased stamina, fatigue, fibrositis, debilitation, joint pain, muscle twitching, muscle weakness, respiratory problems, sciatica, scoliosis, and swallowing problems. The major complaints of PPS victims are pain (neck and back), weakness, and fatigue.

## HERBAL COMBINATIONS
Use combinations #1 and #2 under Fibromyalgia Syndrome.

### Other Uses
Ankylosing spondylitis, arthritis, joint pain, rheumatism, calcification deposits, bursitis, gout, neuritis, chronic fatigue syndrome, fibromyalgia.

## HEALTHFUL SUGGESTIONS
1. Low-stress exercise and low-maintenance weight lifting are very beneficial. Starting out slowly and gradually increasing the amount of exercise will help build stamina. Exercise, along with the right supplements, will help restore health in the muscles and joints. Foot reflexology is very beneficial to strengthen the muscles. It may take a lot of patience and time to get the muscles strong again, but it is well worth the time invested.

2. Water is very important. Drink plenty of pure distilled water, which helps to dissolve mineral deposits in the joints. Celery juice is beneficial, along with carrot, parsley, ginger, and garlic. Always dilute the juices. Eat plenty of green leafy vegetables and lightly steamed vegetables. Use brown rice, millet, whole grains, and soy products, such as tofu and soymilk. Add more fiber to the diet, such as psyllium herbal formulas.

3. Avoid alcohol, white sugar, white flour products, meat, fatty foods, and fried foods. Eliminate caffeine, sugar, and chocolate, which can cause imbalances in the body, as well as rob the body of essential nutrients.

4. Allergies can be involved, which irritate the intestinal tract. Proper digestion is essential for good health. Allergies can be from food (eating the same foods constantly), environmental pollutants, or chemicals such as molds, dust, or pollens. There can be a connection between allergies and leaky gut syndrome, which is further aggravated by drugs. The spaces widen between the cells in the intestinal lining and cause material to invade the body, such as viruses, germs, parasites, or undigested protein. These particles of food or other irritants pass through the intestinal tract into the bloodstream and cause allergic reactions and weaken the immune system.

## HERBS AND SUPPLEMENTS
Single herbs to help strengthen the muscles and joints include alfalfa, aloe vera, buckthorn, echinacea, horsetail, oatstraw, pau d'arco, red clover, garlic, and goldenseal.
- White willow bark has been used as a pain reliever for many years. It has no side effects, such as bleeding or ringing in the ears, which aspirin can cause.
- Feverfew has been used for more than two thousand years and is very effective for migraine headaches and arthritis.
- Glucosamine is very effective in treating inflammation, which helps alleviate pain. It also acts as a free-radical scavenger—preventing more damage to the cells. It helps to rebuild and restore new tissue to repair joints.
- Magnesium and malic acid work together to reduce the severity of symptoms associated with inflammation for the joints. Improvement is seen in symptoms when using these together.
- Essential fatty acids help reduce inflammation in the joints. Use cold-pressed flaxseed oil, evening primrose oil, borage oil, and salmon oil. They inhibit prostaglandins that cause pain and swelling. Use vitamin E, along with EFAs; they should be taken after a meal.
- Digestive enzymes help in proper assimilation of nutrients.
- Antioxidants found in vitamins A, C, E, selenium, zinc, and grapeseed extract are beneficial. They help inhibit inflammatory response and scavenge for free radicals that cause muscle pain or damage.
- B-complex vitamins are very important to protect the nervous system, prevent fatigue, and increase resistance to disease. Take extra B6 and B12 to prevent anemia and increase energy. They also help in preventing depression.

## THIS MADE HER A BELIEVER IN HERBS

Hazelle was used to being in pain, and she had long since set aside hope that any doctor could help relieve it. Through the years, she had learned to live with her polio. She was in and out of hospitals trying to find out what the problem was. She was told that maybe she was developing osteoporosis, arthritis, or bone softening. She was sent home with medication. Her daughter had told her about Ron, a reflexologist, iridologist, and herbalist. She wasn't too sure about it, but she decided she would give this "quack" a try. She went to her first examination and would not tell him anything about her medical history. He started by looking at her eyes. He told Hazelle what she had paid seven thousand dollars to find out. He was telling her all that she knew and describing the condition and pain that she lived with.

Hazelle finally decided to cooperate and talk to him about her history. He started to tell her how much her body would be strengthened with a change of diet and the use of herbs, vitamins, and minerals. Hazelle said, "You can save your breath and my time; all I came here for is reflexology."

Ron set her down and began to work on her right toe. He worked on the zone corresponding to the part of the brain that had suffered the most atrophy. He rolled his finger over it, and Hazelle nearly hit the ceiling with pain. Ron said that her toe had such hard crystals that it needed breaking up in order to get the flow of energy in the nervous system moving. He worked harder than he should have at first. Again he said that her diet was producing too much acid. Her high-acid diet was leaching the sodium from her body and causing hardening from the calcium settling out of solution in the joints.

Hazelle continued getting a treatment every week. It was very painful. It was worse than anything she had endured, but she felt it was her only chance—it was better than ending up in a wheelchair. After a month of weekly treatments, she could see an improvement and could do things with her left side that she had never done before. He also did deep massage therapy on her. He encouraged her to exercise in between treatments. Her toe started to become more pliable. The left foot and leg, which had become smaller and had poor circulation from the collapsing effect of polio, were starting to get stronger. She noticed that the periods of pain were less.

Hazelle finally consented to change her diet. She had been on a lot of different medications. She started taking an herbal calcium supplement to help rebuild her joints. She had been using a drug, Premarin (taken from pregnant mare's urine), and was able to eventually substitute the following herbal combination: goldenseal, red raspberry, black cohosh, queen of the meadow, marshmallow, blessed thistle, dong quai, capsicum, and ginger. She eventually stopped taking thyroxin and used an herbal iodine formula containing kelp. As her health increased, her need for estrogen and allergy medications decreased. She finally started to develop a respect for herbs and diet. Hazelle eventually opened her own health food store and now helps others with their health problems.

## ORTHODOX PRESCRIBED MEDICATION

Ibuprofen, like painkillers, is an over-the-counter medication that can be very potent and may cause serious side effects. The most common side effects include digestive system problems such as nausea, vomiting, cramps, gas, bleeding, and ulcers.

# PREMENSTRUAL SYNDROME

Premenstrual syndrome (PMS) is not a disease or a mental disorder, but is often treated as such. More than 150 symptoms have been linked to this disorder, the most common being depression, irritability, faintness, restlessness, sluggishness, impatience, lethargy, delusions, dizziness, nervousness, anxiety, swelling of breasts, feet swelling, constipation, hemorrhoids, skin eruptions, migraines, backaches, and puffiness. This imbalance in the hormonal system could stem from a genetic predisposition, an organic malfunction, a vitamin or mineral deficiency, stress, drugs, chemicals, or a combination of these factors. Many of these symptoms can be linked to nutritional deficiencies.

The liver is responsible for regulating hormonal balance. It has the job of breaking down estrogen and other hormones, and symptoms occur when the liver has trouble breaking down the excess. The liver is responsible for filtering blood levels of estradiol, the unfavorable type of estrogen, but sometimes it can build up in the body. When this excess estrogen is allowed to enter the bloodstream, it travels in the blood to the brain and nervous system and causes depression and bizarre mental manifestations. Excess estrogen acts as a stimulant to the central nervous system and contributes to many women's ailments associated with the menstrual cycle. Women's livers are known to be more sluggish than men's in removing toxins from the body—estrogen accumulates in the body, and estrogen pills and tranquilizers add to the liver's burden.

The problems with PMS are widespread, but they are not normal. Problems are so common that many see them as a normal function of a woman's life. The reproductive organs play an important role in the entire life of every woman. Their functions should not cause pain and discomfort. Menstruation is a form of body cleansing and preparing for a potential pregnancy. In addition, each month many toxins are eliminated with the flow, which acts to purify the blood.

Many scientists believe the culprit for decreased fertility, PMS problems, excess estrogen, and other female disorders may be a group of chemicals that mimic the actions of hormones in the body. One of the most potent, toxic, and carcinogenic chemicals is dioxin. Exposure to dioxins is linked to birth defects, reproductive system diseases, declining fertility (male and female), and cancer. Dioxin is released into the atmosphere as a by-product of manufacturing or disposal processes that use organic chlorine.

## EMOTIONAL NEEDS

We know that stress can intensify the symptoms of PMS. In addition, imbalances between estrogen and progesterone can trigger all sorts of emotional symptoms. Feelings of rage, unprovoked anger, depression, sorrow, etc. may be linked to the way that estrogen chemically manipulates certain neurotransmitters in the brain. Knowing this can help us understand the intense emotions that some women feel prior to their periods.

## HERBAL COMBINATIONS

The following herbal formulas help balance hormones. They help clean, nourish, and heal female organs. They help relax the nerves, feed the glandular system, regulate uterine contractions, and act as a relaxant in cases of hysteria.

### Herbal Combination #1

- Goldenseal kills infection, works as an internal antiseptic, and reduces swelling.
- Red raspberry is high in iron, cleanses the breast for pure milk, and regulates muscles in uterine contractions.
- Black cohosh is a natural estrogen, good relaxant in hysteria, and neutralizes uric acid buildup.
- Queen of the meadow contains diuretic properties, soothes the nerves, and helps relieve uterine pain.
- Ginger distributes herbs and is good for suppressed menstruation.
- Marshmallow is high in calcium, heals the mucous membranes, and is beneficial for menstrual problems.
- Blessed thistle helps lactation, is good for headaches, reduces menstrual pains, and stops excessive bleeding.
- Capsicum stimulates other herbs to do their job and cleans the veins.
- Dong quai relaxes the nervous system, relieves menstrual problems, feeds the female glands, and cleanses and purifies the blood and liver of bad estrogen.
- Lobelia is valuable for helping remove obstructions. It is a powerful relaxant and has a positive effect on the whole system.

### Herbal Combination #2

- Goldenseal reduces swelling, kills infections, and eliminates toxins.
- Capsicum equalizes blood circulation and helps distribute herbs where they are needed.
- False unicorn is useful for uterine disorders, promotes delayed menstruation, and relieves depression.

- Ginger binds herbs together, stimulates the system, and relieves intestinal gas.
- Uva ursi increases the flow of urine and is good for bladder and kidney infections.
- Cramp bark is helpful for severe menstrual or labor pains, regulates pulse, and is soothing to the nerves.
- Squaw vine is an antiseptic for vaginal infections, helps morning sickness, and eliminates toxins.
- Blessed thistle is useful for painful menstruation and helps in headaches due to female problems.
- Red raspberry helps reduce hot flashes, morning sickness, and cramps, and strengthens the uterus.

### Other Uses

Breast problems, cramps, hormone balance, hot flashes, hysterectomy, menopause, menstrual problems, morning sickness, sterility, uterine infections, and vaginal problems.

### HEALTHFUL SUGGESTIONS

1. A cleansing fast using blood, liver, and lower-bowel cleansers will help the liver eliminate toxins that cause PMS symptoms. The body will heal itself when given the natural nutrients. Nervine therapy using herbs to strengthen the nervous system is one of the best methods to help with PMS.

2. Exercise stimulates circulation, and deep breathing improves the supply of nutrients throughout the system. Walking in the fresh air is very stimulating.

3. Caffeine in tea, coffee, soft drinks, cocoa, and chocolate can interfere with hormonal balance. This prevents the liver from eliminating the bad estrogen that women produce. Tea interferes with absorption of iron and zinc. Caffeine in coffee has been shown to increase the tendency for breast problems, including fibrocystic breast disease, painful and lumpy breasts, as well as PMS problems. Sugar depletes nutrients such as B-complex vitamins, which reduces hormone supply to the organs. Smoking contributes to hormonal problems by increasing the need for vitamins and minerals. Alcohol damages the liver and increases the body's need for vitamins and minerals such as calcium, magnesium, zinc, and B-complex vitamins.

4. Eliminate foods that are laced with hormones, such as dairy products, beef, chicken, and eggs. Use soy foods such as tofu and soymilk, which contain phytoe-strogens to help balance hormones. Also, increase foods high in fiber such as grains, nuts, seeds, fruits, and vegetables. Brown rice and millet are versatile and nourishing. Use oats, whole wheat, yellow cornmeal, and buckwheat. Yellow vegetables help keep the bowels clean. Eat salads daily, using leaf lettuce, cabbage, carrots, and other vegetables. Grind and use seeds such as chia, flax, sunflower, and sesame, which are very high in calcium. Foods rich in magnesium are beans, grains, and dark green vegetables.

### HERBS AND SUPPLEMENTS

Single key herbs are black cohosh, false unicorn, blessed thistle, dong quai, vitex (helps in all menstrual problems), hops, kelp, lobelia, red clover (cleans blood and liver), red raspberry (the greatest herb for all female problems), sarsaparilla (helps balance hormones), and skullcap (calms nerves).

- Black cohosh and dong quai help to regulate menstrual flows.
- Wild yam cream is useful to help balance hormones, supply progesterone to balance estrogen, relieve menstrual problems, reduce menopausal symptoms, and alleviate depression. Natural progesterone cream is shown to be very effective in controlling PMS symptoms, as well as many other estrogen-related problems, including irregular cycles, infertility, and weight-related problems, among others.
- St. John's wort helps increase serotonin levels in the brain and aids in depression.
- Soy isoflavones, including genistein and daidzein, are beneficial in controlling the activity of estrogen in women and testosterone in men.
- Magnesium acts as a natural tranquilizer, to relax the muscles and soothe the nerves. Low levels are seen in PMS sufferers. Use along with natural calcium.
- B-complex vitamins, especially pantothenic acid, B6, and PABA, help relieve nervous irritability and are useful for eliminating excess estrogen from the liver.
- Vitamin E helps to alleviate breast tenderness, hormone imbalance, fatigue, depression, and insomnia. It helps to reduce night sweating and is relaxing when taken with unsaturated fatty acids.
- Essential fatty acids found in evening primrose oil, flaxseed, and black currant oil help promote prostaglandin, which helps in fluid retention and in preventing cravings.

## THIS MADE HER A BELIEVER IN HERBS

Laverne became excited about herbs several years ago while she was at work and complaining about her cramps. Someone introduced her to dong quai. She took the herb, and within two hours it began to work. She was amazed that something natural could work that quickly. This made her a believer in herbs, and she went into the business of helping others find herbs as a way of healing.

- Milk thistle repairs liver damage and balances hormone levels regulated by the liver.
- Acidophilus is necessary to provide natural bacteria and helps in the digestion and assimilation of food.
- Vitamin C with bioflavonoids helps prevent heart attacks, assists in removing cholesterol from the body, strengthens the blood vessels, helps absorb iron, and aids in the formation of red blood cells.
- Cat's claw is an herb that has been shown to help with irregularities of the female cycle. It also detoxifies the intestinal tract.
- *Vitex agnus castus* helps normalize the menstrual cycle and flow. It assists the body's elimination of excess estrogen and alleviates PMS symptoms. Vitex balances all the female hormones. It is believed to work by regulating the actions of the pituitary gland—the master gland of the body.
- Chlorophyll and blue-green algae are rich in minerals, especially iron, which can be low in individuals with PMS symptoms.

### ORTHODOX PRESCRIBED MEDICATION

Drugs such as tranquilizers, sedatives, and painkillers are usually prescribed. Oral contraceptives are usually prescribed to regulate menses. They are biphasic (Nelova) or monophasic (Levora or Ovcon). They can cause excess bleeding and spotting. They also increase the risk of blood clots, stroke, heart attacks, and liver, cancer, and gallbladder disease. Oral contraceptives in particular can aggravate PMS symptoms in estrogen-dominant women, and many recent studies state that the pill can increase the risk of breast cancer and other hormonally linked disorders.

# PROSTATE PROBLEMS

Prostate enlargement is common in about one-third of men between the ages of forty and sixty. It is known as benign prostatic hyperplasia (BPH). The prostate becomes enlarged and presses against the urethral canal. This backs up in the kidneys and can obstruct the bladder outlet, causing retention of urine. Prostatitis is an inflammation of the prostate gland. It can block the urine flow. It can cause pain, frequent urination with burning sensation, and blood or pus in the urine.

Prostate cancer is common among men over sixty. It is not easily detected in the early stages. Low levels of zinc, vitamin C, bioflavonoids, and vitamin E have been seen in those with cancer of the prostate. Prostate cancer is a devastating disease that medical doctors treat with surgery and hormone therapy. This disease is also linked to a deficient diet. Prostate cancer, along with some other diseases, first appeared in the twentieth century.

A sometimes related issue, impotence, affects almost ten million American men. Doctors used to believe the cause was psychological, but today they feel most cases of impotence are physiological. A poor diet and a lack of exercise may be responsible.

Many men eat a diet high in fat and low in fiber. Men often eat a lot of animal products, and this can lead to long-term putrefaction and autointoxication that gradually build up in the body. The prostate is especially vulnerable to bacteria that seep in from toxic waste emanating from the colon. Overly processed food has depleted vitamins and minerals in the diet.

### HERBAL COMBINATIONS
#### Herbal Combination #1

These formulas are designed especially for men to support glandular health, particularly of the prostate gland. They also help the urinary tract to heal and prevent infections.

- Pygeum has been used successfully in Europe and Africa for prostate problems. It reduces swelling and inflammation and dissolves deposits that can block urination.

- Saw palmetto cleans and feeds the glands and contains natural antibiotic properties to help infections and an enlarged prostate.
- Stinging nettle is rich in minerals that help when acids are irritating the body. It heals, eliminates excess water, and nourishes the glands.
- Gotu kola works as a blood cleanser, stimulates mental and physical energy, increases mental alertness, and is considered a brain and nervous system nutrient.
- Zinc is necessary for prostate health, essential for cell division, repair, and growth, and healing for wounds and infections.
- Pumpkin seeds strengthen the prostate gland and promote male hormone function. They have been used to treat an enlarged prostate. Myosin, an amino acid found in pumpkin seeds, is known to be essential for muscular contractions.
- Lycopene is a powerful antioxidant found in tomatoes. It has been found to lower the risk of prostate cancer. It helps strengthen the immune system.

### Other Uses
Bladder, kidneys, spleen, hormone regulator, liver.

## HEALTHFUL SUGGESTIONS
1. Cleansing and purifying the blood, colon, and liver is essential to help eliminate the toxins involved with prostate problems. Sit in a tub of hot water with horsetail infusion (put in a cloth packet to avoid a mess). This can be done twenty to thirty minutes twice a day.

2. A change of diet would be very beneficial in eliminating toxins from the body. Eat less meat and more vegetables, fruit, nuts, seeds, brown rice, millet, whole grains, and soy products. Pumpkin seeds, sesame seeds, chia seeds, and flaxseeds are beneficial for the prostate. Eat nuts such as almonds, pine nuts, cashews, pistachios, and pecans. Green salads containing sprouts, parsley, and watercress are beneficial. Steamed vegetables such as winter squash, carrots, asparagus, broccoli, and cabbage are rich in minerals. Dried beans, endives, and dried peas are beneficial. Water is very important—drink about eight glasses a day. This dilutes the urine to help

avoid bacterial growth in the bladder and helps flush the prostate urethra. Cranberry extract is very beneficial for the bladder.

3. Exercise, along with good nutrition, is very beneficial for male health. Aerobic and strength-building exercises help keep the heart rate up and increase muscle mass. Exercise will help improve circulation, lower blood pressure, and reduce toxins to prevent cancer.

4. Relaxation is hard for men. They spend so much time working and building a future that they seldom take time to relax. Unwinding is very important to living a long and healthy life. Getting enough sleep is also very important. Men need to take care of themselves, which they are seldom apt to do.

5. Avoid beer. Researchers have found that a combination of ingredients found in beer stimulates the pituitary gland to release more prolactin, which stimulates the overgrowth of BPH (prostate swelling).

## HERBS AND SUPPLEMENTS
Single herbs to help the prostate include alfalfa, cornsilk, damiana, ginseng, horsetail, kelp, parsley, red clover, and saw palmetto.

- Saw palmetto berries have been found in numerous studies to reduce prostate enlargement. They have shown no side effect and are more effective than some medications.
- Antioxidants are very important. Vitamins A, C, D, E, selenium, zinc, and grapeseed extract are very potent antioxidants. They protect against free-radical damage to the prostate. Vitamin E works with iodine that is found in kelp.
- Essential fatty acids are found in flaxseed, evening primrose, borage, black currant, and salmon oils, and they work with vitamin E to reduce the amount of urine retention in the bladder after urinating. EFAs are the building blocks from which prostaglandins are made to help regulate every organ, tissue, and cell in the human body. They help dissolve brown body fat—the kind that lies deep in the body and surrounds the heart, kidneys, and adrenal glands.
- Minerals are vital for prostate health, especially zinc. Selenium is believed necessary for sperm production. It works with vitamin E, as an antioxidant, to protect against toxins.

- Calcium works with magnesium, sulfur, and zinc, along with B12, C, and inositol, for healthy sexual organs. All vitamins work together to maintain a healthy body.
- Bee pollen contains concentrations of vital nutrients and is rich in vitamins, minerals, and amino acids. It is good for healthy sex glands. It is rich in magnesium, zinc, and essential fatty acids to stimulate sex hormones.
- Lecithin helps eliminate fatty deposits and protect the nerves. It is essential for healthy nerves.
- Germanium and CoQ10 provide oxygen to the cells and improve circulation. They help keep the capillaries and veins in the prostate healthy.
- Acidophilus helps keep the bad bacteria under control. It improves digestion and assimilation of all nutrients.
- Chlorophyll and blue-green algae contain cleansing properties to prevent prostate problems. They protect against infections as well as heal inflammation in the prostate.
- Digestive enzymes are essential to improve proper function of hormones, vitamins, and minerals.

---

### "PRAISE THE LORD FOR HERBS"

Lynn had several operations—one for a tumor partly removed from his brain. It was embedded so deep in his brain that the doctor wasn't able to get it all. At that time he had to have a second surgery on his prostate. In 1990, he had gone back to the doctor for a regular diabetic check-up. The doctor did a prostate check and said that Lynn needed to make an appointment for a third prostate surgery. Lynn told the doctor that he was going to take herbs instead. The doctor laughed and told him good luck.

Lynn started to take combination #1 under Parasites and Worms, zinc and black walnut. Three months later he went back to the doctor for another checkup. The doctor checked his prostate and said that his prostate was smaller and that he didn't need surgery. Lynn said, "Praise the Lord for herbs."

---

Hydrochloric acid is lacking in the elderly, especially when too much cooked food is eaten and not enough raw.

## ORTHODOX PRESCRIBED MEDICATION

Proscar is widely prescribed for prostate enlargement. It is supposed to shrink prostatic tissue and increase urine flow. Adverse sexual effects may resolve in more than 60 percent of patients who continue the medication. It could cause impotence, decreased libido, or decreases in volume of ejaculate. It could cause liver and kidney damage.

# SHINGLES

Shingles is an infection caused by the herpes zoster virus of the nerve endings in the skin. It is the same virus that causes chicken pox, and it can occur in adults who had chicken pox as children. Some medical scientists feel that after a person is exposed to the chicken pox virus, it lies dormant in the body until it may be reactivated decades later in the form of shingles. Shingles affects more than eight thousand Americans annually and usually resolves itself within a few weeks.

Blister and crust formations and severe pain along the involved nerve characterize shingles. The disease usually occurs on the chest and abdomen but may occur on the face, around the eyes, and on the forehead, neck, limbs, and hands. The blisters will become crusty scabs and drop off. The elderly may suffer from attacks of shingles even after healing takes place. The pain may also continue for months after the symptoms disappear.

This is a virus that can lie dormant in the nerve ganglia and spinal cord for years until the immune system breaks down. This can be caused by vaccinations or from drugs used to suppress diseases. Shingles is an acute disease and is a healing and cleansing of the body. When this disease is suppressed, it is pushed deeper into the system to cause even more serious problems later on. If this disease is treated naturally, it will only clean and heal the body.

## HERBAL COMBINATIONS
### Herbal Combination #1

This is an excellent formula to use in cleansing the body of toxins.

- Gentian gives strength to the system, tones the stomach, and cleans the blood.
- Irish moss is high in minerals, gives strength to the body, and soothes the tissues of the lungs and kidneys.
- Goldenseal is cleansing on the system, kills poisons and parasites, and cleans the digestive system.
- Fenugreek dissolves hardened mucus, kills infections, is rich in vitamins and minerals, and is soothing and healing.
- Safflower eliminates gastric disorders, supports adrenal glands, and helps cholesterol buildup.
- Myrrh heals the colon and stomach, speeds the healing action, and stimulates blood flow.
- Yellow dock purifies the blood, stimulates the digestive system, improves liver function, and is rich in iron.
- Black walnut burns up excess toxins and is healing for skin problems.
- Barberry works on the liver to help bile flow freely and removes morbid matter from the stomach and bowels.
- Dandelion gives nutrition to the body, destroys acids in blood, and eliminates toxins.
- Chickweed helps curb the appetite, dissolves plaque in the blood vessels, and strengthens the stomach and bowels.
- Catnip relieves fatigue, is a sedative to the nerves, and rids the body of bacteria.
- Cyani is a stimulating tonic for the body and antiseptic to the blood.
- Parthenium contains blood- and lymphatic-cleansing properties similar to echinacea, is a natural diuretic, and is cleansing for the bladder and kidneys.
- Cascara sagrada cleans and restores bowel function and helps eliminate the built-up glue-like material on the colon walls.
- Slippery elm contains nourishing and healing properties. It soothes and heals while cleansing and restoring the intestinal tract.
- Uva ursi heals and strengthens the urinary tract. It also contains antiseptic properties to help heal infections.

### Other Uses

Arthritis, cancer, colon, constipation, pain, parasites, skin problems, toxic wastes, tumors, worms.

## HEALTHFUL SUGGESTIONS

1. Start with a colon-cleansing formula, enemas, or colonics to open up the bowels. When the bowels and kidneys are not functioning properly, the skin takes over. The skin is called the third kidney. Use blood purifiers and liver cleansers at the same time. This will help nature to assist the body in healing itself.

2. Fasting is the first law of nature to use with an acute disease. When eating during an acute disease, the body has to stop and use its energy to digest the food rather than eliminate toxins. Use pure water with citrus juices. Add ginger and lemon or lime juice. Herbal teas will also help nature do its job, including chamomile (calms the nerves), alfalfa, mint (will help the stomach), red clover blend tea (will help clean the blood), and pau d'arco (will clean the blood and protect the liver). When healing has taken place with juices and herbal teas, add vegetable broths, vegetables (steamed at first), and then raw salads and vegetables.

3. Make a paste with aloe vera juice, black walnut, comfrey, and powdered vitamin C to help the itching and speed healing. Use olive oil with a few drops of tea tree oil and vitamin E on the rash. Vitamin E will also help prevent scarring. These applied to the skin will help stop the pain and rash as well as dry up the blisters.

## HERBS AND SUPPLEMENTS

Single herbs to help with shingles include aloe vera (internally and externally), black walnut (heals skin eruptions), blue vervain, comfrey, dandelion (helps the liver eliminate toxins), echinacea, garlic, kelp, lady's slipper (excellent for the nerve endings), red clover, skullcap, hops, and passion flower.

- Vitamin E has helped some people relieve pain and stop the rash from spreading.
- Vitamin C has also helped stop the pain and dry up the blisters.
- B-complex vitamins are essential for the nerves. Some health providers will give injections of B12 to help speed the healing. All the B vitamins help in healing.

## REAPING THE REWARDS OF GOOD HEALTH

Matt was thirty-three and had been a police officer for twelve years. He was a member of his department's SWAT team and had fitness standards that he had to maintain. He thought he was in pretty good shape until one morning in March of 1994. He woke up with a sharp pain in his right shoulder. Because he had recently completed some training, he thought he had pulled a muscle. However, within two days he broke out into a rash that extended from the left side of his chest around to the left side of his back. He thought it was hives. He visited his father, a chiropractor, who took one look at him and said, "Matt, you have shingles." Matt was shocked, to say the least. He then visited a nurse practitioner who confirmed his father's diagnosis. The nurse practitioner told him that he was young to have shingles and that he had double the lesions that people normally get. She also told him he would be in a great deal of pain to begin with, then after a week or so intense itching would start. He was prescribed an antiviral and a narcotic pain drug and told to buy an over-the-counter antihistamine for the itching. The nurse practitioner gave him a refill prescription for the pain pills because of the amount of pain she felt he would experience. He was also told that he would experience flu symptoms and would become weak. Needless to say, he wasn't very enthused at his prospects for the next two weeks.

The day after his painful awakening, he visited Mary at her health food store. He was a bit skeptical, but having been raised in a chiropractic family, he was open to alternative treatments. He told Mary nothing of his shingles, but after a short while she told him that his nervous system was in an uproar. Mary recommended an herbal program that was not only for the shingles, but also for the entire body. He learned from Mary that his shingles were probably caused by a buildup of toxins and improper functioning of his digestive and intestinal systems. He went home and immediately began the program, using blood cleansers, digestive system strengtheners, intestinal cleansers, combination #1 under Parasites and Worms, and combination #1 under ADHD (for the nervous system). That night he didn't take any pain pills and slept through the night. His health steadily improved as the days went by. Within a week, the lesions were almost completely healed. He had only taken one pain pill that first night. He never experienced the itching, and his skin never turned the dark purple he was told probably would occur.

Ten days after his visit to the nurse practitioner, he returned for a follow-up appointment. The nurse practitioner was amazed at the condition. She told him that she had never seen anyone recover so fast from shingles. He then told her that he had started an herbal program the day after his first visit. She told him to keep up with it, because it was obviously working. He left the office and went fly-fishing! Since that experience, he has continued taking herbs and has changed his eating habits. His wife has also been using herbs and has been reaping the rewards of improved health.

- L-lysine along with vitamin C and cystine will help detoxify toxins and heal eruptions.
- Free-form amino acids are beneficial for healing the body. They are necessary for every cell of the body.
- Chlorophyll and blue-green algae will help clean the blood and provide nutrients to the body.
- Nutrients to stimulate the immune system include licorice, astragalus, chlorophyll, vitamin C with bioflavonoids, kelp, dulse, blue-green algae, ginkgo, milk thistle, pau d'arco, schizandra, Siberian ginseng, suma, wheatgrass juice, dong quai, echinacea, red raspberry, ho-shou-wu, and germanium.
- Essential fatty acids will help heal and nourish the glands. Flaxseed oil, evening primrose oil, borage oil, black currant oil, and salmon oil are beneficial.
- Minerals are essential for healing. Calcium and magnesium are relaxing and soothing for the nerves. Potassium promotes healing and builds resistance to infection. Sodium helps dissolve poisons in the body. Zinc aids healing.
- Antioxidants will help keep shingles under control. They help prevent free-radical damage to the

cells. Vitamin A is very healing for the skin. Vitamins A, C, E, and the minerals selenium and zinc are all beneficial antioxidants. Grapeseed extract is a powerful antioxidant as well.

## ORTHODOX PRESCRIBED MEDICATION

Zovirax is used to treat chicken pox and sudden (acute) shingles (herpes zoster). This is supposed to stop viral multiplication and spread of the acute disease. Side effects can be headache, dizziness, nervousness, confusion, insomnia, depression, fatigue, nausea, vomiting, and diarrhea. Drugs only suppress the acute disease that may manifest itself in the form of a chronic disease later.

# STRESS

We simply can't avoid some stress in life, and all stress isn't bad, especially if we have the physical and emotional resources to deal with it. Stress can be beneficial and can challenge and motivate us to accomplish seemingly impossible tasks. The way we choose to deal with stress is the key to coping with it. If not controlled properly, stress can become distress, and stressful situations can build up in time and take a toll on our physical and emotional health. Symptoms of stress are irritability, change of appetite (some people eat more, and some eat less), memory loss, fatigue, chronic headaches, and even high blood pressure. Overeating, excessive alcohol, drugs, and smoking are usually ways of trying to cope with stress, which creates further stress.

The nervous system is the body's most fragile and delicate system. It is easily affected by physical, emotional, and chemical factors. With all the toxins we deal with daily, it is no wonder our bodies are under constant attack.

Stress can accumulate in the body and eventually cause a breakdown of the adrenal glands. This will cause exhaustion and a complete weakening of the emotional and physical body. It may take twenty years to accomplish this, but it will happen if long-term stress is allowed to continue. It could be a high-pressure job, a bad marriage, unresolved financial problems, loneliness, or a death in the family.

We need to strengthen our bodies so we can withstand the stress we face. It's important to learn to avoid stress we cannot handle and to handle stress we cannot avoid. Some ways to do this are nutritionally building our nerves, fortifying our immune system, and learning to relax and to create an exercise program.

When the body is completely burned out from a lack of nutrients, this puts further stress on the nervous and immune systems. The body, especially the nerves, has to be nourished. Sugar is one of the worst things you can put in your body, and it will wear you down and cause exhaustion. Sugar depletes nutrients from the system—especially B vitamins and minerals, such as calcium. Yet we use sugar to give us a lift, only to have the adrenals eventually burn out. Symptoms of adrenal exhaustion are chronic fatigue, irritability, health problems, anxiety, depression, low stress tolerance, the feeling of being unable to cope or stay in touch with reality, nervous exhaustion, insomnia, difficulty relaxing, and panic attacks.

Free-radical damage can occur when the body is under stress. When free radicals form and become oxidized they can damage body tissues and cell membranes. This puts stress on the body and weakens the immune system, especially with long-term stress. All disease is caused by some type of stress. Chemical stressors can be poisons, bacteria, germs, viruses, drugs, pollution, cigarettes, alcohol, and junk food. Toxic metals, air pollution, and toxic chemicals all put stress on the physical body.

## HERBAL COMBINATIONS
### Herbal Combination #1

This formula helps the body cope with stress. It contains excellent nutrients to fortify the nervous system and boost the immune system. It is to strengthen the body in a ten-day program. It contains three herbal combinations, labeled A, B, and C.

A. Contains chamomile, passion flowers, hops, fennel, marshmallow, and feverfew.

B. Contains suma, astragalus, eleuthero, ginkgo, and gotu kola.

C. Rich in B vitamins B1, B2, B6, B12, folic acid, biotin, niacinamide and pantothenic acid. Also contains schizandra, choline, PABA, wheat germ, bee pollen, valerian, passion flower, inositol, hops, and citrus bioflavonoids. It also contains hops concentrate plus hops herb.

### Herbal Combination #2

This formula is designed with powerful nutrients rich in supporting the immune and nervous systems for energizing the body. It will help energize the body to protect against stressful situations.

- *Rhodiola rosea* stimulates the production of norephinephrine, dopamine, serotonin, and nicotinic cholinergic, which has a positive effect on the central nervous system. It stimulates brain chemistry and fights depression and stress-related disorders.
- Siberian and Korean ginseng help to normalize and adjust the body by restoring and regulating natural immune response. They help protect the body from chemical pollutants, radiation, some poisons, temperature changes, poor diet, and emotional stress.
- Ashwagandha is called Indian ginseng and is strengthening and calming to the nervous system. It relieves nervous exhaustion, fatigue, and memory loss. It acts as a mild sedative and promotes calm rest and sleep. It helps in slowing the aging process.
- Schizandra helps increase energy, replenish and nourish the internal abdominal organs, improves vision, boosts muscular activity, and helps the body heal itself. It stimulates the immune system and protects against free radicals, radiation, the effects of sugar, boosts stamina, normalizes blood sugar and blood pressure, and protects against infections. It has a tonic action on the immune system.
- This formula also contains *Gynostemma pentaphyllum*, rosemary, astragalus, reishi mushroom, suma, and ginkgo. It also contains the following nutrients: alfalfa, kelp, chromium in a fruits and vegetable base to nourish and fortify the body.

### Herbal Combination #3

This is a Chinese formula to strengthen the body against fatigue and stressful situations. It helps strengthen digestion, promote restful sleep, and create a positive feeling.

It contains schizandra, biota, cistanche, cuscuta, dang gui, lycium, ophiopogon, succinum, astragalus, dioscorea, hoelen, lotus, *Panax ginseng*, polygala, polygonum, pizyphus, and rehmannia.

## HEALTHFUL SUGGESTIONS

1. Relaxation therapy: Find a quiet place to practice relaxation and rhythmic breathing, which should be slowly and deeply. Rest on your back or sit in a reclining position, close your eyes, and relax. Count to six as you inhale, and exhale through the nose. Think of pleasant thoughts.

2. When the body tenses up, breathing can become shallow, which decreases the amount of oxygen that reaches the brain.

3. Fasting is beneficial: Vegetable juice is cleansing and healing. Use an herbal blood purifier and a lower-bowel cleanser. This will keep the blood clean so that toxins cannot travel to the brain and nerves and cause stress. A liver cleanser is very beneficial.

4. Congested liver: When the liver is congested and stagnant it can cause depression, stress, and an all-over tired feeling. Whole wheat is cleansing, also sour foods, such as lemon, limes, grapefruit, and sauerkraut; it has a medicinal effect as well. Green leafy vegetables have an energetic effect. Vegetables helpful for liver are broccoli, parsley, collards, and a variety of leaf lettuces. Dark lettuces, such as romaine, are richer in nutrients. Carrots and carrot juice are effective as liver tonics. Use an herbal liver formula that contains milk thistle.

5. Change of diet is the first step in conquering stress. A vegetarian diet is healing. Red meat is hard on the body. It causes uric acid buildup to cause acid in the body. A healthy diet is one that is rich in fruit, vegetables, nuts, seeds, and grains; they are potent foods and contain the germ, the spark of life. They are rich in protein, minerals, B vitamins and are a rich source of unsaturated fatty acids and lecithin.

6. Avoid a high-fat and high-meat diet. Eliminate alcohol, tobacco, and caffeine. Reduce sugar and white flour products; sugar turns to fat in the liver. They all have a negative effect on the brain and nervous system and put stress on the entire body.

## HERBS AND SUPPLEMENTS

Single herbs: Key herbs for stress are alfalfa, chamomile, ginkgo (strengthens the brain), gotu kola (nourishes the brains), hops (builds nerves), kelp (supplies minerals), lady's slipper, licorice (nourishes the adrenals), lobelia, mistletoe, mullein, passion flower, pau d'arco, rose hips, skullcap (improves nerves), suma (builds immunity), valerian, and wood betony.

- Vitamin C is called a wonder vitamin. Helps in coping with stress by inducing the formation of stress-reducing hormones in the body. Emotional and physical stress can deplete vitamin C levels.
- 5-HTP is a boost for those who benefited from L-tryptophan, a supplement that was taken off the market that had benefited many people. It is a brain chemical that supplies serotonin, an important brain chemical, associated with insomnia, depression, fibromyalgia. It helps the body cope with stress. It will help regulate appetite and mood swings.
- Bee pollen is considered to be a perfect food. It is rich in protein, and over twenty-two amino acids, B vitamins, and enzymes. Contains vitamin C and essential fatty acids. It is useful for combating fatigue, depression, and it strengthens the immune system to protect against disease.
- Evening primrose oil is rich in significant quantities of GLA (gamma linolenic acid), and is the richest source, with 9 percent GLA. Regular use will help in the following: chronic fatigue syndrome, schizophrenia, manic depression, weight loss, inhibiting clot formation in the arteries, and it may help kill cancer cells.
- Lecithin made from soy contains phosphatidyl-choline (PC), and when consumed is broken down into the nutrient choline. Choline is used to make acetylcholine, to protect the myelin sheath around the nerves. It can protect the liver from damage, help in brain function, in high cholesterol, and in nerve damage such as in multiple sclerosis.
- SAM-e is known for its ability to enhance dopamine and serotonin function in the brain. It also helps repair the myelin sheath that protects nerve cells. It helps in stress and depression.

### ORTHODOX PRESCRIBED MEDICATION

Benzodiazepines are drugs used to treat stress, nervousness, anxiety, and to ease tension. In the 1970s many women became hooked on the drug Valium, Roche's trademark name for benzodiazepine. All drugs of this type have the potential for abuse and addiction. Side effects can include anxiety, drowsiness, fatigue, light-headedness, and loss of muscle coordination.

# STROKE

A stroke is a clot inside an artery that blocks the flow of blood to the brain, also called thrombus. Embolism is a wandering clot, carried in the bloodstream until it wedges in one of the arteries leading to the brain, Aneurysms are blood-filled pouches that balloon out from weak spots in the artery wall and burst. A hemorrhage is a defective artery in the brain that bursts, flooding the surrounding tissue with blood.

A mild attack can cause temporary confusion and light-headedness, difficulty in speaking clearly, weakness on one side of the body, visual dimness and confusion, severe speech difficulties, and/or sudden or gradual loss or blurring of consciousness. Amnesia can also occur, but is often not permanent. A coma can result for short or long periods.

Watch for early warnings of stroke—which may only last for a few moments—including one or more of the following: fainting, stumbling, numbness or paralysis of the fingers of one hand, blurring of vision, seeing bright lights, loss of speech or memory. It is much wiser and less expensive to start improving health in order to prevent this disease. Some doctors who have treated thousands of people suffering from stroke feel that most strokes can be prevented.

The Chinese see strokes as being caused by "blood stasis" and "stagnation of liver-qi." Chinese medical practitioners prevent strokes and also treat them by treating constipation. Constipation causes a poisoned bloodstream, which sets the stage for a possible stroke. Poisoned blood flows through thousands of miles of arteries, veins, and capillaries. The walls of the arteries consist of cells, which are subject to the same injury from toxins as the cells in the kidneys. The kidneys degenerate at the same time the arteries do and from the same causes. When the walls thicken and harden, this causes degeneration. As they harden they become more brittle and more easily burst under pressure. Pressure increases as the hole through the arteries grows smaller. As the walls become more brittle, extra pressure causes a blood vessel to rupture, which causes a stroke. The brain cells rely on oxygen-rich blood for nourishment. If they don't receive this nourishment, the brain cells die.

Other causes are poor diet, lack of exercise, obesity, and smoking.

## EMOTIONAL NEEDS

Emotional health is important in any healing. Strokes may be associated with resistance to change, giving up on life, getting tired of doing all the same things over and over. We need to learn to accept changes, and go with the flow. Life can be exciting, and changes give us a new perspective on living.

## HERBAL COMBINATIONS
### Herbal Combination #1

This formula is designed to nourish and strengthen the veins. This will help strengthen the blood flow to the heart, brain, and legs. It may help to minimize the appearance of spider and varicose veins in the legs. It may also help with hemorrhoids. This formula is beneficial because it contains many bioflavonoids. It contains the following:

- Horse chestnut strengthens the walls of the veins. Reduces inflammation and pain. Strengthens fragile capillaries to prevent bruising. Tones the muscles to prevent bruising.
- Butcher's broom has been used to treat thrombosis or blood clots, arteriosclerosis, hemorrhoids, peripheral circulation problems, and to lower cholesterol, because of its ability to strengthen the walls of blood vessels. Contains anti-inflammatory properties.
- Rutin is an essential bioflavonoid to strengthen the veins and capillaries. Helps in the assimilation of vitamin C. Help keeps the arteries clean.
- Hesperidin, lemon bioflavonoids, and ascorbic acid all help strengthen the capillaries, veins, and arteries. This helps prevent blood clots and cholesterol buildup.

### Herbal Combination #2

This formula is a must for healthy veins. It will clean, strengthen, and rebuild the circulatory system, as well as nourish and detoxify the body. It acts as an antioxidant to prevent free-radical damage. Free radicals attack blood vessels, causing platelets to clump together, resulting in heart and artery diseases. This formula is found as number #1 under Cardiovascular Disorders.

### Herbal Combination #3

This formula is rich in antioxidants. It is in a liquid form for easily assimilation. It is found as #2 under Aging.

## HEALTHFUL SUGGESTIONS

1. Eliminate saturated fat from the diet. Fat seems to be the primary cause of strokes. It is found in meat and processed food. Margarine and cooking oils are high in fat. These are fats that the body does not know how to handle. These fats plug arteries, which restricts circulation and kills brain cells because of lack of oxygen. Use olive oil, flaxseed oil, and essential fatty acids.

2. Cleanse and purify the blood, colon, and liver. Use a lower-bowel formula as well as blood and liver formulas. Over 90 percent of our health problems are caused by constipation. Dr. Arbuthnot Lane, a well-respected English physician and colon specialist, made the dramatic statement that "constipation was the cause of all ill of civilization."

3. Fasting: Short fasting and a change of diet will help cleanse the arteries. High blood pressure severely strains the arteries, and if the arteries have cholesterol plaque, the risk of having a stroke or heart attack increases.

4. Stress is a big contributor to strokes. Stress is hard to determine, yet a person who is angry and hateful has an extra excretion of hormones and acids, raising blood pressure and contributing to strokes and heart disease. Learn to manage stress by thinking good thoughts and meditating and practicing relaxation therapy.

5. Chelation: Oral chelation will cleanse the entire system and help the blood flow freely; it will improve circulation so that proper nutrition and oxygen can reach the brain. The herbal formula #2 under Stress is a natural form of oral chelation. It contains natural nutrients to nourish and clean the veins and blood.

6. High-fiber foods, such as whole grains (oats, wheat, barley, millet, buckwheat), contain rutin, which strengthens the veins. Whole grains also keep the colon cleaned and nourished. Brown rice, wild rice, beans, nuts, and seeds contain nutrients for capillary health.

7. Vegetables are rich in minerals and low in calories. Potatoes, carrots, celery, cauliflower, broccoli,

cabbage, beets, onions, garlic, cucumbers, and green peppers are nutritious. Use leaf lettuce, tomatoes, green leafy vegetables, string beans, snow peas, and sweet potatoes. Onions, garlic, shallots, scallions, ginger, and cayenne pepper have anticlotting properties.

## HERBS AND SUPPLEMENTS

Key herbs are capsicum (cleans veins, strengthens the walls of the arteries), bugleweed (alleviates pain in heart), burdock, butcher's broom (improves circulation), ephedra, garlic, ginkgo (improves mental clarity), gotu kola (feeds the brain), hawthorn, hops, horsetail, kelp, passion flower, parsley, pau d'arco, psyllium, rose hips, saffron, skullcap, and valerian. Other important herbs are alfalfa (rich in minerals), black cohosh (for slow pulse rate), blessed thistle, dandelion, ginseng, lily of the valley, lobelia, and yellow dock.

- Vitamin E protects the blood vessels, lowers cholesterol levels while increasing the "good" HDL cholesterol. It improves circulation and fights free-radical damage to protect the cells.
- It helps increase energy and a feeling of well-being. It has been found that a deficiency in vitamin E can cause heart disease, cancer, senility, and premature aging.
- Vitamin C is known as the wonder vitamin. It is found to be beneficial in lowering blood cholesterol and triglycerides and helps prevent clots in the blood vessels. It helps in increasing the good cholesterol and lowering the bad. This vitamin will help prevent strokes and heart attacks.
- Coenzyme Q10 is a potent antioxidant, protects against free-radical damage. Like vitamin E, it helps protect the heart from failure by boosting its energy levels. It helps increase energy and protect against disease.
- Garlic is not only a natural antibiotic, but can lower blood pressure and serum cholesterol levels. It will help strengthen the veins and arteries. It helps protect against colon and stomach cancer. It helps protect against heart disease and hardening of the arteries.
- Evening primrose oil, along with borage oil and blackcurrant oil, is rich in gamma-linolenic acid (GLA). These oils improve cellular function. They also help protect the heart and veins.

- Lecithin helps build and strengthen the cells and protects the myelin sheath that covers the nerves. Improves vein health and prevents blood clots, therefore protect against strokes.
- Chlorophyll and blue-green algae protect the immune system by stimulating the body to produce interferon.
- Flaxseed oil and salmon oil are essential for healthy arteries. They help eliminate toxins from the blood.
- Germanium improves the supply of oxygen to the tissues and organs. Helps rebuild heart damage and prevent strokes.

## ORTHODOX PRESCRIBED MEDICATIONS

Coumarins are drugs given to prevent stroke and blood clots. It can be dangerous if you have bleeding ulcer, adrenal insufficiency, heavy bleeding during menstruation, or liver or kidney problems. Side effects are easy bruising, nosebleeds, dark urine, and tarry or red stools.

# ULCERS

It is estimated that forty million people suffer from ulcers in the United States. Ulcers can be very devastating. An ulcer is an erosion in the stomach lining or anywhere in the digestive tract. The erosion can extend deep into the wall of the intestines, damaging blood vessels and causing bleeding.

Ulcers were thought to be stress-related, but evidence has identified a mop-shaped bug in the stomach tissue that bores deep into the stomach's mucous lining, causing damage. H. pylori has been implicated in up to 90 percent of patients with ulcers. It is no wonder that viruses and bacteria form in the intestinal tract when antacids are widely prescribed. When hydrochloric acid is decreased, viruses, parasites, and worms thrive in the stomach and other parts of the intestinal system. H. pylori is found in a large number of patients suffering from stomach and duodenal ulcers.

The germs thrive when toxins are already in the body. Then when drugs are prescribed to neutralize or suppress stomach acid, the germs, parasites, worms, and viruses thrive even more. Zantac and

Tagamet are prescribed and are very popular. They control the ulcers, but when the drugs are stopped, the ulcers often recur. As many as 60 to 90 percent of ulcer sufferers have a relapse. With an increase in the use of antacids, there may be higher incidence of autoimmune diseases, stomach problems, bacteria, worms, and parasites invading the body. The most common ulcers are found in the duodenum and in the lower part of the stomach.

Symptoms are gnawing pain in the abdomen, mostly when the stomach is empty, heartburn, nausea, bleeding, and vomiting. Stress can play a major role in ulcers, but there are probably other considerations for the stomach forming sores, including autointoxication and constipation. When the lower colon is clogged and delays the passage of food from the stomach, fermentation and acid conditions will irritate the stomach wall. The glands are continually producing enzymes to help in the digestion process and can become overworked. The pancreas swells when we eat too much cooked food. Mucus is formed every time we eat cooked food, and this leaves our stomachs vulnerable to all kinds of germs, viruses, and toxins.

## EMOTIONAL NEEDS

In spite of the fact that ulcers may have a bacterial cause, there is some speculation that highly stressed people may experience more severe cases of ulcers. Worry, anxiety, and tension can certainly make ulcers worse. Internalizing feelings of tension or being out of control may also contribute to this disease.

## HERBAL COMBINATIONS
### Herbal Combination #1

This formula will help heal, strengthen, and nourish the intestinal system. This will help the body digest and assimilate nutrients.

- Slippery elm is useful for inflammation and ulcerations of the digestive tract. It helps in colitis, gastric and duodenal ulcers, and diarrhea.
- Marshmallow is soothing and healing on the mucous membranes and stimulates healing.
- Goldenseal heals infections, stops bleeding, and eliminates toxins from the digestive system.
- Fenugreek has the ability to dissolve hardened mucus. It helps expel toxic waste through the lym-

phatic system. It contains lecithin, which dissolves cholesterol, as well as lipotropic (fat-dissolving) substances.

### Herbal Combination #2

This formula helps soothe, heal, and nourish the digestive system. It helps improve digestion and acts as a natural diuretic. It helps in inflammation and ulcerations of the gastrointestinal tract and helps control bleeding.

- Chamomile is relaxing for anxiety and insomnia and soothing for the digestive system; it also reduces swelling and inhibits development of gastric ulcers.
- Marshmallow contains mucilage that is soothing on the mucous membranes and encourages healing.
- Rose hips contain natural vitamin C for healing and pectin for healing the digestive tract.
- Slippery elm bark is useful for inflammation and ulcerations of the digestive tract, as well as colitis, gastric and duodenal ulcers, and diarrhea.
- Plantain heals wounds, soothes the mucous membranes, and is nourishing.
- Bugleweed heals and controls bleeding, helps in digestion, and is useful for nervous indigestion.

### Other Uses

Bad breath, canker sores, colitis, colon, diverticulitis, dysentery, heartburn, indigestion, stomach ulcers.

## HEALTHFUL SUGGESTIONS

1. Eat only when hungry and not while under stress. When the body is under stress, it secretes stomach acid. This depletes the acid that is really needed to digest food. Learn to treat acute diseases naturally. Drink cabbage, celery, and carrot juice often. Cabbage juice has been proven to heal ulcers. Ginger can be added to other juices. Millet is easy to digest and nourishing. It is rich in calcium, magnesium, and protein. Eat more fruit, steamed vegetables, and whole grains. Potato peel broth is healing. Make grain and vegetable soups. Barley helps rebuild the stomach lining. It is rich in B1, B2, and bioflavonoids. Cook slowly in a thermos to retain the enzymes and B vitamins.

2. Eliminate foods that cause distress to give the stomach a chance to heal. Meat and dairy products can make an ulcer worse. Stay away from coffee,

alcohol, soft drinks, sugar, and white flour products. A high-fiber diet will help clean and eliminate toxins. Eliminate aspirin and all drugs that suppress the symptoms.

3. Go on a colon, blood, and liver cleanse. This will help the body heal itself. Fasting using juices will help repair and heal the stomach lining. Resting the stomach and digestive juices will speed the healing. Cabbage, celery, carrots, and parsley are excellent juices. Add ginger and garlic to help the healing.

4. Papaya fruit contains enzymes that promote good digestion and heal the stomach lining. Okra powder acts as a demulcent to stop inflammation. Almond milk is beneficial for its acid-neutralizing properties. Persimmon helps to facilitate healing of the stomach lining, and whey powder contains compounds that help heal ulcerated tissue. Flaxseeds soaked overnight in pure water are very healing. Drink the water and chew the seeds. Avocados, bananas, yams, and cooked carrots are also healing.

## HERBS AND SUPPLEMENTS

Single herbs that help with ulcers include aloe vera (healing), capsicum, comfrey, fenugreek, garlic, goldenseal (healing for the digestive system), hops (for the nerves), psyllium, pau d'arco, slippery elm, white oak, and licorice extract.

- Aloe vera juice is healing and will soothe and help in pain.
- Raspberry and chamomile teas are relaxing and healing for the intestines.
- Licorice (*Glycyrrhiza glabra*) has been shown to have anti-ulcer properties without side effects. It seems to stimulate growth and regenerate stomach and intestinal cells.
- Essential fatty acids, including flaxseed, borage, evening primrose, salmon, and black currant oils, will help coat and heal the ulcers. They also feed and nourish the glands.
- Capsicum stops bleeding and heals ulcers.
- Free-form amino acids are essential for healing and repairing tissue.
- Food enzymes are essential to clean and repair the stomach. Take them with meals and between meals for healing.

- Fiber supplements will help prevent ulcers and aid in healing the lining of the intestines. High-fiber foods can increase bulk in the intestines and eliminate invading bacteria, worms, parasites, and germs that accumulate in the intestines. Guar gum and psyllium have mild laxative effects and create bulk to help the body eliminate waste without straining.

## ORTHODOX PRESCRIBED MEDICATION

Cimetidine (Tagamet) and famotidine (Pepcid) are H2 blockers and are prescribed to block acid production in the stomach. They were once prescribed as anti-ulcer drugs and are now being sold over the counter. H2 blockers can cause mineral imbalances. The minerals calcium, phosphorus, and magnesium are affected. They could also deplete vitamin B12. Side effects could be headaches, insomnia, fatigue, confusion, diarrhea, kidney or liver impairment, impotence, ringing in the ears, and heart palpitations.

### SHE COULD EVEN ENJOY SPICY FOODS AGAIN

Lorina had an ulcer and didn't like being on her medication, Tagamet. She knew there were side effects, and it was expensive. She was willing to try something natural. A friend gave her a list of ailments that chlorophyll was good for, and she noticed one of them was an ulcer. She purchased some and faithfully drank it daily. The ulcer pain began to dwindle. She started learning what else was good for ulcers and started combining the chlorophyll with aloe vera juice. A week later, she noticed the morning pain and discomfort were no longer there. She could even enjoy spicy foods again.

# PART 4

# Nutrition, Herbs, and the Human Body

# NUTRITIONAL THERAPIES

## CLEANSING AND FASTING

A cleansing diet is good during colds, flu, or illness. The body has the ability to rid itself of toxins if it is given the chance. Toxins are expelled through the skin, which needs to be kept clean and scrubbed, and through the nose, mouth, colon, and stomach. The purpose of cleansing the body is to eliminate excessive mucus and toxins. The first step is to stay away from white sugar products, white flour products, animal protein, and salt.

The benefits of a cleansing fast are many. It dissolves toxins and mucus in the body, cleanses the kidneys and the digestive system, purifies the glands and the cells, and eliminates built-up waste and hardened material in the joints and muscles. It relieves pressure and irritation in the nerves, arteries, and blood vessels and builds a healthy bloodstream. In summary, it provides an overall boost to one's health.

Fasting is one of the oldest ways of healing and cleansing the body of diseases and buildup of mucus and toxins. Juice fasting helps restore the body to health as well as rejuvenating the system. It eliminates dead cells and toxic waste products that cause sickness and sluggish feelings. This method of fasting is safer than a water fast because poisons in the body are released into the blood-stream more slowly. Some people fast anywhere from three to ten days.

Taking enemas is suggested during juice fasting by some nutritionists, for it helps the body in its cleansing and detoxifying effort by washing out all the toxic wastes from the alimentary canal. The following is a good example of what is commonly taken during a juice fast:

2 Tbsp. fresh lemon or lime juice
2 Tbsp. pure maple syrup
1/10 tsp. cayenne pepper
Pure water: combine in 10 oz. hot or cold water
Use 6 to 12 glasses daily

The lemon used in this diet is a loosening and cleansing agent with many important building factors. The elements in the lemon and the maple syrup, along with the cayenne pepper, work together for maximum benefit.

The natural iron, copper, calcium, carbon, and hydrogen found in the sweetening supply more building and cleansing material. The cayenne pepper is necessary, as it breaks up mucus and increases warmth by building the blood for an additional lift. It also adds many of the B vitamins and vitamin C. The following is a great example of a cleansing diet (there are various types). You can find many outstanding reference books that provide other effective cleansing diets.

If you become constipated, taking an herb laxative in the morning and evening is helpful. Also use lemon skin or pulp with the cleansing drink. Use mint tea to neutralize odors from the mouth.

Fasting is very beneficial, but it must be remembered that during a prolonged fast, the body is cleansing itself without any opportunity to replenish or regenerate the cells and tissues. (Read *Discover Your Fountain of Health* by Norman W. Walker, DSc, PhD.) The system is depleted of some of its most vital essential elements. Dr. Walker says that the immediate result of prolonged fasting is a feeling of well-being, but the damage to the system may not show up for one or two years longer. Therefore, the safest way to fast would be to go on fruit juices for three to four days at a time, or no longer than six days, and then break the fast by drinking vegetable juices to build the body and also by eating raw vegetables and fruits for two or three days. This procedure can be repeated as long as it is felt necessary, but be sure not to fast more than six days. A mild food diet should follow a fast. This way you don't overload the system with hard-to-digest food.

A green drink is another excellent cleansing method and can be used to prepare for a fast. It is nourishing and very high in chlorophyll. I use this drink when I feel a cold coming on or when I feel that my body is full of toxins. In my favorite green drink, I use pineapple juice or fresh unfiltered apple juice, blended with alfalfa sprouts, spearmint, parsley, and comfrey.

# MILD FOOD DIET

A mild food diet is used in chronic sickness and for periodic cleansing. The following foods are recommended:

Fruits, raw
Vegetables, raw
Half fruit juice, half water
Vegetable juices
Raw, cold-pressed oils
Raw nuts
Honey, raw
Pure maple syrup
Seeds (sunflower, sesame)
Sprouts
Bake all starch vegetables

Note: The following foods should be avoided during illness: grains, sugar, dairy products, butter, eggs, dried legumes, meats, peanuts, chips, soft drinks (including diet drinks).

# "GOOD-FOR-YOU" FOODS

- Fresh, raw fruits: Especially good when eaten in season; contain many vitamins and minerals.
- Fresh, raw vegetables: Eat as many raw or lightly steamed vegetables as possible.
- Fresh, raw fruit juices: Wonderful when used in a fast; full of enzymes, vitamins, and minerals.
- Fresh, raw vegetable juices: Considered living food; full of enzymes, vitamins, and minerals.
- Yogurt, kefir, cottage cheese products: Made with certified raw milk when possible.
- Kelp: Contains iodine; use instead of salt.
- Cheeses: Made naturally without artificial coloring and synthetic processing.
- Seeds: Eat ground or sprouted seeds; important to have sprouts on hand, as they are living foods.
- Nuts: Eat raw and fresh; keep in freezer to keep from going rancid.
- Whole grains: Freshly ground when ready to use or sprouted for live enzymes.
- Honey: Use pure and natural (raw) honey; full of vitamins and minerals and easily assimilated.
- Pure maple syrup: Contains vitamins and minerals.
- Cold-pressed oils: Contain vitamin E; use with lemon juice or apple cider vinegar; use on salads.
- Fertile eggs: Contain protein and vitamins.
- Herbs: Use garlic, capsicum, parsley, watercress, and paprika often.
- Dried fruits: Must be dried naturally in the sun with no chemicals added; should be soaked in water before eating to be more effective.
- Natural sauerkraut: Made at home fresh without added chemicals or salt; very rich in calcium and has great curative value.
- Herbal teas: Drink chamomile, licorice, spearmint, and red raspberry.

# NATURAL FOODS

The following are specific food items that are "natural," untainted by processing or manufacturing:

- Almonds: High in protein, vitamin E, calcium.
- Apples: Contain high levels of protein, enzymes, and minerals; useful for whatever ails you.
- Apricots: Are rich in minerals, especially iron; detoxify the liver and pancreas; high in vitamin A; good for blood, skin, and destroying worms.
- Avocados: High in protein and fat; good for the diabetic and hypoglycemic.
- Blackberries: Good for the colon and diarrhea.
- Blueberries: Nourish the pancreas.
- Strawberries: Good for the skin; clean the body and remove metallic poisons, such as arsenic.
- Carob powder: Alkaline; contains minerals and is a natural sweetener.
- Cherries: Cleanse intestines and provide minerals; eat in season for one cleansing food diet; also drink cherry juice.
- Citrus fruits: Provide vitamin C; use lemons, limes, and pure water on occasional fasts; act as a cleanser, eliminating toxins; juice of three lemons or limes in quart of warm water is good to drink during a fast; help eliminate the flu.
- Coconuts: Supply roughage.
- Dates: High in protein, iron, mineral content, calcium, and potassium.
- Figs: Contain iron and minerals; food for constipation.
- Fruits: All fruits are very nourishing, especially when eaten in season; clean and build the body.
- Grains: Concentrated food; buckwheat, barley, millet, oats, rye, and wheat are high in protein; food for the vegetarian.
- Grapes: Blood builder; good for anemia; antitumor food.
- Honey: High in vitamins and minerals; use as substitute for white sugar; use pure honey.
- Mustard seeds: Good for digestion and gas.
- Nut butter: More nourishing than dairy butter; grind fresh when ready to use.
- Nuts: Best raw; contain protein, unsaturated fats, minerals. Almonds, cashews, pecans, pistachios, and walnuts.
- Oils: Cold-pressed are needed to assimilate the proteins from vegetables. Considered a kidney food.
- Papaya: Good for digestion, especially for protein foods.
- Seeds: Contain the germ and embryo. Rich in oil, vitamin E.
- Vitamin B-complex: Minerals and proteins.
- Sprouted seeds: Very healthful, the freshest food you can eat. Rich in enzymes, B vitamins, and hormones. Alfalfa, wheat, mung beans, radish, fenugreek, sunflower, and chickpeas are the most common and the best sprouted seeds.
- Sunflower seeds: Contain protein, vitamins, and minerals. Feed the eyes, sinuses, and glands.
- Vegetables: High in enzymes, vitamins, and minerals; carrot juice diluted is very good.
- Watercress: Natural immune properties. High in vitamins A and C.
- Yogurt: Beneficial for intestinal health.

# HERBS FOR MOTHERS AND CHILDREN

THE BEST THING AN EXPECTANT MOTHER can do for her child is to obtain proper nutrition, exercise, fresh air, lots of pure water, sunshine, adequate sleep, and relaxation. About 80 percent of the diet should be raw, natural food. Some of the best foods a pregnant woman can eat include grains (buckwheat, brown rice, whole wheat), nuts (almonds, pecans, piñons), seeds (sunflower, flax, pumpkin), and all types of vegetables and fruits.

## HERBS FOR MOTHERS

Herbs are also very helpful for dealing with some of the physical traumas of pregnancy. One herb that is especially known for its uses during pregnancy is red raspberry. It can be used as a tea or in capsule. It is safe and effective, strengthens the uterus for easier delivery, and lessens bleeding during and after delivery. It is high in iron and helps relieve "after-pain." Women who take red raspberry usually have shorter labors. The following subsections outline some of the ailments common to pregnancy and give their herbal and nutritional therapies.

### ANEMIA

Anemia is characterized by a lack of red blood cells, which are mainly responsible for transporting oxygen and nutrients to the body cells. Iron assists in this process and is essential for improving one's anemic condition. Pregnant women need extra iron for this purpose. Yellow dock contains a high level of iron, as does red raspberry. This easy and tasty "green drink" recipe provides a large amount of natural iron. Combine raw apple juice or pineapple juice with either comfrey, alfalfa sprouts, and spearmint or peppermint leaves, parsley, and wheatgrass. Blend in blender until smooth. Add about 500 mg of vitamin C, which helps iron absorb into the bloodstream. Adding vitamin E can also help improve an anemic condition because it strengthens the blood cells.

### CONSTIPATION

For anyone who suffers from constipation, eating raw vegetables and fruits daily will inevitably help. Brewer's yeast and yogurt are useful for improving the growth of flora needed for proper digestion. Daily bran intake is especially effective for preventing constipation (remember to always drink large amounts of water when taking a bran supplement, as otherwise it can cause further constipation). Psyllium supplements or a lower-bowel herbal formula can also be very helpful.

### FALSE LABOR

Drinking catnip as a tea in small amounts will help relieve false contractions. Also, blue cohosh is known to help relax the uterus, thereby preventing the false contractions.

### HEARTBURN

Papaya tablets can help relieve the sometimes severe heartburn that accompanies pregnancy. A combination of comfrey and pepsin can also help.

### INSOMNIA

Extra calcium can help improve sleep. The following herbal combination can also help decrease a tendency toward insomnia: comfrey, alfalfa, oatstraw, Irish moss, horsetail, lobelia, and chamomile tea.

### MISCARRIAGE

Taking red raspberry tea throughout the pregnancy can help prevent miscarriage. The following is a common uterine herbal combination used to prevent miscarriage: wild yam, squaw vine, false unicorn, and cramp bark. Lobelia and capsicum will help relax the uterus. Bayberry and catnip can help prevent miscarriage.

### MORNING SICKNESS

Teas made of red raspberry, catnip, peppermint, or spearmint can help relieve nausea and morning sickness. Digestive enzymes can be helpful. Ginger is widely known as an aid to nausea. Essential oils have also been useful.

### TOXEMIA

A green drink is helpful in cleansing the circulatory system. Alfalfa, raspberry, and comfrey tea is also cleansing and nourishing to the body. The following combinations are useful: (a) kelp, dandelion, and alfalfa; (b) red beet, yellow dock, strawberry, lobelia, burdock, nettle, and mullein. Stay away from red meat, white sugar products, and white flour products. Add more vitamins A and C to your diet.

### OTHER

The following formulas will make the delivery and labor easier; it is suggested to start administering the formulas approximately six weeks before one's due date: (a) black cohosh, squaw vine, lobelia, pennyroyal, and red raspberry; (b) black cohosh, false unicorn, squaw vine, blessed thistle, lobelia, and red raspberry.

# NURSING MOTHERS

There are several herbs known to assist with the various ailments that a nursing mother can encounter. Refer to the following list.

Nursing: Blessed thistle is known to increase mother's milk. Brewer's yeast taken daily will increase milk as well as give the mother necessary energy. Red raspberry and marshmallow tea is good. Alfalfa is excellent for rich milk and strength for the mother. Fennel seed boiled in barley water helps increase mother's milk.

Breasts: At the first signs of a breast becoming infected, take 1,000 mg of vitamin C every hour. Take extra vitamin A and E and garlic capsules. A green drink can also be very helpful for infections. For cracked, sore, or dry nipples, apply thin honey or almond oil.

# HERBS FOR CHILDREN

First year of life: Fruit and vegetable juices or nut milks, always diluted. Raw apple juice and fresh carrot juice are very nourishing. Vitamin C must be given, which is needed daily to build up resistance to germs. Babies need the amino acid taurine, and mother's milk has a good supply, but synthetic formulas don't. A deficiency of this amino acid in experiments has induced epileptic seizures. Taurine and B6 is a good combination for seizure problems.

- Colic: Catnip tea has been used for years for colic in babies. Fennel and peppermint tea are good. Tincture of lobelia may be added to the tea.
- Constipation: A small amount of mullein added to warm water or weak licorice tea is good for babies. A nursing mother should watch her diet.
- Cradle cap: Vitamin E or almond oil rubbed into scalp.
- Digestion: For difficulty in digesting cow's milk in children, add powdered apple or papaya to milk.
- Diaper rash: Take ground comfrey and goldenseal and make a paste with aloe vera juice. Vitamins E and A are good.
- Diarrhea: Carob flour in pure water every few hours. Carob in boiled milk is good. Herb teas

like those made of red raspberry, slippery elm, ginger, strawberry, sage, yarrow, and oak bark are recommended.

- Dry skin: Olive oil, vitamins A and E and almond oil. Aloe vera is good.
- Ear infection: Garlic oil in ear. Garlic capsule in the rectum. Mullein oil and lobelia extract.
- Fever: Catnip, red raspberry, or spearmint tea. Enemas help to bring fevers down.
- Hyperactivity: Keep children away from sweets, artificial coloring and flavoring, and preservatives. B-complex in water or juice, calcium herbal formula, vitamin D, and multiple vitamin and mineral tablets are excellent for hyperactivity.
- Pinworms: Raisins soaked in senna tea for older children is an old-time remedy. Chamomile and mint tea helps. Garlic in child's rectum will discard worms.
- Restlessness: Chamomile tea; lobelia extract on the tongue will help relax the body.
- Teething: Restless, crying babies who are teething need more calcium and vitamin D. Weak, warm tea of catnip, chamomile, peppermint, or fennel will help. Licorice root to chew on can dull the pain and irritation that teething causes.
- Sore gums: Rub the gums with thick honey to which a pinch of salt has been added. Honey with oil of chamomile, lobelia extract rubbed on gums, and peppermint oil rubbed on gums will help.
- Urination problems: For infants who cannot urinate, administer crushed watermelon seeds in a tea. Give small amounts often.

# THE BODY SYSTEMS

HERBAL MEDICINES HAVE BEEN USED with success for centuries. They are one of the oldest forms of therapy practiced by humans. Millions of people have testified to the benefits of herbal medicine. Approximately 80 percent of the world's population today depends on medicinal plants to heal and prevent disease. The world's population, as well as its numerous physicians, are turning more and more to herbal medicines because they are considered safer than drugs. The side effects associated with the use of drugs are too numerous to mention. Drug companies are being sued constantly and settle out of court to prevent publicity.

Americans are becoming educated and more involved in their own health. We as individuals realize we have to take responsibility for our own health. Drugs will not heal the body—they just cause more problems and suppress the disease further in the system. Good health comes through learning more about diet, herbs, vitamins, minerals, and supplements that protect as well as help the body heal itself.

Currently, and in the past, doctors have said that herbs are unscientific, primitive, unproven, ineffective, possibly dangerous, and do not have a place in our society today. This can no longer be said. There is now evidence of the validity of herbal medicine. Science can now prove why herbs work to help the body heal itself. They are natural and do not cause side effects. When used with knowledge and guid-

ance, herbs strengthen, clean, nourish, and stimulate body functions, and even prevent disease. We now know why herbs work to heal the body. The following subsections give a brief overview of each of the body's systems, along with the various disorders that commonly affect these systems, as well as herbal and nutritional supplements used to treat these disorders.

## THE CIRCULATORY SYSTEM

Heart disease is the number one killer of adults in the United States. Nearly one million people die each year of heart disease and related cardiovascular illness. Heart disease is striking people at younger ages each year, without warning and often fatally. It hits, in many cases, without chest pains, shortness of breath, or other symptoms common in heart disease. Cholesterol collects around the heart first, then accumulates in the veins and arteries. This is why the heart can suffer damage first without symptoms. These illnesses are related to bad diet, alcohol, smoking, and lack of exercise. Lifestyle and diet change should be considered in order to protect the circulatory system. A typical American diet of meat and potatoes, sugar, and white flour products is paving the way for heart disease. A proper diet of whole grains (high in fiber), fresh vegetables, and fruits and herbs will clean and nourish the arteries.

Poor bowel function is another important cause of accumulation of fats and other toxins on the artery walls. It creates stagnation in the bowels, which fosters anaerobic bacteria that produce toxic waste. If the bowels are not properly eliminated after each meal, these toxins circulate in the bloodstream and are deposited in the organs and other parts of the body.

## ORAL CHELATION FORMULA

An oral chelation formula that cleans the entire system and helps the blood flow more freely will improve circulation so that proper nutrition and oxidation can function in the body. The natural chelating elements work in a bonding reaction and surround the plaque, much as a magnet attracts metals. The chelation elements remove the built-up deposits on the arterial wall.

The natural chelation formula contains vitamins, minerals, glandular extracts, amino acids, and herbs. It contains chelated minerals, a process that makes them better absorbed by the body. It contains L-cystine, HCL, choline, PABA, L-methionine, fish lipids, citrus bioflavonoids, rutin, adrenal substance, spleen extract, thymus substance, and inositol. Hawthorn berries and *Ginkgo biloba* are two herbs beneficial for circulation. This formula contains vitamins A, D, E, C, B1, B2, B6, B12, niacin, pantothenic acid, folic acid, biotin, magnesium, iron, iodine, copper, and zinc. It also contains chromium, selenium, potassium, manganese, and calcium.

## BLOOD PURIFYING FORMULAS

Impurities in the blood affect the heart. The toxins are collected by both the blood and the lymph fluid that pass through the heart continually. It is important to purify the blood. The following formulas will help purify the bloodstream.

1. Red clover, burdock, pau d'arco, sage leaves.

2. Ganoderma, dang gui, peony, lycium, bupleurum, curcuma, cornus, saliva, ho-shou-wu, atractylodes, achranthes, ligustrum, alisma, astragalus, ligusticum, rehmannia, *Panax ginseng*, cyperus.

3. Pau d'arco, red clover, yellow dock, burdock, sarsaparilla, dandelion, cascara sagrada, buckthorn, peach bark, prickly ash, yarrow, Oregon grape.

## CIRCULATORY SYSTEM ENHANCERS

1. This formula will provide nutrients to the eyes, ears, and nose areas to clean and nourish: goldenseal, bayberry, eyebright, red raspberry.

2. This formula increases resistance to stress with its natural nutrients to enhance the circulatory, glandular, and nervous systems: Siberian ginseng, bee pollen, yellow dock, licorice, gotu kola, kelp, schizandra, barley grass, rose hips, capsicum.

3. This formula feeds and strengthens the heart: hawthorn berries, capsicum, garlic.

4. This Chinese formula is known to nourish the heart and strengthen the circulatory system: schizandra, dang gui (dong quai), cistanche, succinum, ophiopogon, lycium, *Panax ginseng*, polygonum, hoelen, dioscorea, astragalus, lotus, polygala, acorus, zizyphus, rehmannia, dioscorea.

5. This stimulates circulation and elimination, which has a positive effect on the immune system: garlic, capsicum, parsley, goldenseal, ginger, eleuthero.

6. This formula contains ginkgo and hawthorn. The ginkgo protects the cells of the body and especially those of the brain. It increases circulation to deliver oxygen and glucose to the cells. It protects against free-radical damage and protects the nervous system.

7. Capsicum, garlic, and parsley are also beneficial to nourish the heart. Parsley is a natural diuretic and rich in minerals. Garlic helps to dissolve cholesterol plaque on the artery walls. It stimulates the lymphatic system to eliminate toxins and is a natural antibiotic.

8. This formula is rich in iron for healthy blood: red beet root, yellow dock, red raspberry, chickweed, burdock, nettle, mullein.

## OTHER HERBS AND SUPPLEMENTS

The following are single herbal and supplemental products that have shown beneficial qualities for improving cardiovascular health.

• Omega-3 fatty acid: An essential nutrient for the body. It helps the body create a hormone-type substance called prostacyclin. This prevents blood cells from sticking together and decreases the danger of blood clotting and producing strokes and heart attacks.

- Coenzyme Q10 formula: Contains the minerals copper, iron, magnesium, and zinc, and the amino acids leucine, histidine, and glycine, and the herbs capsicum and hawthorn. This formula increases oxygen to the brain and cells, prevents circulatory problems, and strengthens the heart and immune system.
- Liquid chlorophyll: Repairs tissues. Helps to neutralize pollution that we eat and breathe. It helps in the assimilation of calcium and other minerals. Purifies and strengthens the entire body.
- Suma, astragalus, Siberian ginseng, ginkgo, and gotu kola: A powerhouse of herbs to increase circulation and feed and strengthen the brain, eyes, ears, nose, and throat. Improves memory, alertness, and sense of well-being.
- L-carnitine: Energizes the body, lowers cholesterol, cleans the veins and arteries, and strengthens the muscles, especially the heart. It burns fat and reduces built-up fat in the body.

Other single herbs for the circulatory system: Aloe vera, bilberry, bugleweed, butcher's broom, cayenne, cloves, garlic, ginger, ginkgo, hawthorn, horseradish, prickly ash, suma, Virginia snake root.

# THE DIGESTIVE SYSTEM

Digestive disorders are one of the most common health problems that plague people today. Both the old and the young are having increased digestive problems. Improper digestion can cause poor assimilation, especially of essential minerals. Lack of minerals and essential fatty acids can produce unhealthy cells. Digestive upsets are mainly caused by stress, constipation, faulty diet, drugs, alcohol, and tobacco. Eating wholesome, natural food nourishes the digestive system and strengthens the whole body.

## DIGESTIVE FORMULA

This formula is more than a digestive aid; it works with the liver, gallbladder, and spleen to promote normal function of the digestive system. This will also benefit the lymphatic and urinary systems. It helps in the production of bile, which digests fat and prevents constipation. It helps with gas and bloating, fluid retention, digestion, and in the assimilation of nutrients.

1. Rose hips, barberry, dandelion, fennel, red beet root, horseradish, parsley.

2. This formula contains enzymes to supplement the body's production of digestive enzymes. These enzymes are important because food requires them to be processed, especially when we eat too much cooked food and not enough raw food. This formula will help the body digest a minimum of 30 grams of protein, 30 grams of carbohydrates, and 30 grams of fat. It contains alpha-amylase, betaine HCl, bile salt, bromelain, lipase, pancreatin, papain, and pepsin.

3. This formula is in liquid form for easier assimilation and digestion. It contains gentian root, cardamom, orange peel, dandelion, red raspberry, and potassium sorbate.

## DIGESTIVE SYSTEM FORMULAS

These formulas improve digestion, and most ailments are benefited when digestion is strengthened. These herbs help to calm a nervous stomach, aid digestion, and provide enzymes and protein digestive aids.

1. This is a formula that enhances the digestive system and also benefits the urinary system in the elimination of toxins. It will help prevent nausea, gas, bloating, allergies, motion sickness, and cravings for sweets. It includes magnolia, shenqu tea, crataegus, oryza, hoelen, *Panax ginseng*, pinellia, saussurea, gastrodia, citrus, atractylodes, cardamom, platycodon, ginger, licorice, agastache typhonium.

2. Papaya, ginger, peppermint, wild yam, fennel, dong quai, spearmint, catnip, lobelia.

3. Ginger, cramp bark, peppermint, wild yam, fennel, catnip, Oregon grape.

4. Red beet root, dandelion, parsley, horsetail, black cohosh, birch, blessed thistle, angelica, chamomile, gentian, goldenrod, yellow dock.

5. Papaya and mint.

6. Goldenseal, juniper, uva ursi, cedar berries, mullein, yarrow, garlic, slippery elm, capsicum, dandelion, marshmallow, nettle, white oak bark, licorice.

7. This formula benefits the stomach and the intestinal system. It helps prevent indigestion, infections, inflammations, ulcers, and toxic accumulation: slippery elm, marshmallow, dong quai, ginger, wild yam, lobelia.

8. This Chinese formula is very beneficial to the digestive and nervous systems. This will benefit many health problems. When the nerves are strengthened, it fortifies the immune system. This also benefits the urinary and intestinal systems. It includes bupleurum, peony, cinnamon, dang gui (dong quai), fushen, zhishi, scute, atractylodes, *Panax ginseng*, ginger, licorice, typhonium flagelliforme.

9. This is another beneficial Chinese formula that works with the digestive system. This strengthens digestion to prevent indigestion, colitis, poor circulation, and many health problems that go along with an unbalanced center of digestion. It includes *Panax ginseng*, astragalus, atractylodes, hoelen, dioscorea, lotus, galanga, chaenomeles, magnolia, saussurea, dang gui (dong quai), citrus peel, dolichos, licorice, ginger, zanthoxylum, cardamom, typhonium flagelliforme.

10. This combination will strengthen and heal the digestive and intestinal systems. It includes ginger, capsicum, goldenseal, licorice.

## SINGLE HERBS FOR THE DIGESTIVE SYSTEM

Alfalfa provides essential minerals and aids digestion. Aloe vera heals and protects the mucous membranes, will heal ulcers, and will even heal scars from adhesion. Buchu heals the digestive tract, absorbs excessive uric acid, and acts as a tonic. Capsicum heals and stops internal bleeding, acts as a disinfectant, and aids in digestion. Other beneficial herbs include comfrey, fennel, gentian, ginger, papaya, parsley, peppermint, and slippery elm.

# THE GLANDULAR SYSTEM

The glandular or endocrine system consists of the pituitary gland, thyroid gland, parathyroid gland, thymus gland, sex glands (ovaries, testes), pancreas, hypothalamus, and adrenal glands. Along with the nervous system, hormones, which are secreted by the glands, are the major means of controlling the body's activities. The glandular system has a direct effect upon mood, mind, behavior, immune defense, memory, control of metabolic rate, and control of blood sugar, to name a few.

All the glands depend upon one another and work together synergistically. The glandular system is necessary for survival; a healthy system is essential for health. An imbalance in any gland of the glandular system will cause enormous problems for the entire body. There are many problems that can happen because of glandular imbalance. Vitamins, minerals, and herbs nourish and restore glandular health.

## GLANDULAR FORMULA

This was formulated to nourish and strengthen the entire glandular system. The nutrients of vitamins, minerals, and herbs are combined with necessary essential ingredients to stimulate proper hormone production and metabolism.

Vitamin A nourishes the thymus gland, as well as all the glands, to increase its size and antibody production. Zinc protects the immune system and supports the T cells. Low zinc intake decreases thymus growth. Lecithin breaks down fatty deposits, especially effective on the liver. Vitamin C nourishes and cleans all the glands and, with the lemon bioflavonoids, helps protect the immune system. The minerals, especially the trace minerals in the herbs, are vital for glandular health. Kelp is rich in iodine and contains all essential minerals. Alfalfa is rich in minerals and eliminates uric acid from the body. Parsley is a natural diuretic and eliminates toxins such as uric acid. Dandelion stimulates bile production and benefits the spleen and pancreas. Licorice root strengthens the adrenals, pancreas, and spleen.

## HERBAL FORMULAS FOR THE GLANDULAR SYSTEM

1. This formula enhances the glandular system. It is especially beneficial for the pancreas in the production of pancreatin and bile from the gallbladder. It also helps improve liver function and is beneficial for the urinary system. This formula includes cedar berries, burdock, goldenseal, eleuthero, horseradish.

2. This formula strengthens the digestive system. Lack of proper digestion can cause malfunction of the glands. The formula includes Oregon grape, ginger, cramp bark, fennel, peppermint, wild yam, and catnip.

3. This formula nourishes the pancreas, liver, adrenals, and the digestive system. It includes licorice, safflower, dandelion, horseradish, sesquiterpene lactones.

4. This formula provides nutrition, especially for the thyroid, but is beneficial for all the glands because of the complete mineral content. The minerals help eliminate toxic metal and poisons from the body. The formula includes Irish moss, kelp, black walnut, parsley, watercress, and sarsaparilla.

5. This formula helps bile production to digest fat and prevent constipation. It nourishes the liver, gallbladder, digestive system, spleen, and immune system, as well as the glandular system: rose hips, barberry, dandelion, fennel, red beet root, horseradish, and parsley.

6. This formula is designed to feed the liver. The liver is vital to detoxify the system. A healthy liver is important to the glandular system. The formula includes red beet root, dandelion, parsley, horsetail, yellow dock root, black cohosh root, birch leaves, blessed thistle herb, angelica root, chamomile flowers, gentian root, goldenrod herb.

7. This formula nourishes the glandular system, especially the pancreas and prostate. It includes goldenseal, juniper, uva ursi, cedar berries, mullein, yarrow, garlic, slippery elm, capsicum, dandelion, marshmallow, nettle, white oak bark, and licorice.

8. This formula is rich in minerals to support the glandular system, especially the hypothalamus and thyroid glands. This contains chelated minerals for easy absorption to benefit specific body systems. It includes zinc, manganese, kelp, Irish moss, parsley, hops, and capsicum.

9. This formula helps balance the glandular system. It is rich in iodine, iron, calcium, and magnesium. It includes kelp, dandelion, and alfalfa.

10. This is a formula to benefit the glandular system, especially the thyroid, the master gland. The hops are added to control the stress of the system. Stress depletes nutrients, and this will add extra nutrients to protect the glands. It includes kelp, Irish moss, parsley, hops, and capsicum.

11. This formula is designed to nourish the glandular, nervous, and circulatory systems. This is a natural way to provide the body with nutrients that help it adapt to stress. The formula includes Siberian ginseng, bee pollen, yellow dock, licorice, gotu kola, kelp, schizandra, barley grass, rose hips, and capsicum.

12. This formula is to support the glandular system when the body is undergoing fasting or cleansing programs. It will help nourish, strengthen, and fortify the glands when under stress. It includes chickweed, cascara sagrada, licorice, safflower, parthenium, black walnut, gotu kola, hawthorn, papaya, fennel, and dandelion.

13. This formula is excellent for athletes. It provides the body with nutrients for anyone who is physically active. It could also help parents who are active with children. It includes Siberian ginseng, ho-shou-wu, black walnut, licorice, gentian, fennel, slippery elm, bee pollen, bayberry, myrrh, peppermint, safflower, eucalyptus, lemongrass, and capsicum.

14. This formula is to help the body maintain a balance in weight control. Along with a high-fiber diet, using whole grains, fruits, vegetables, and natural supplements, this formula will help in weight control. It includes licorice, red beet root, hawthorn, and fennel.

15. This formula is for an overstressed body, where the glands become weakened and put stress on the entire body. This will give the body nutrients essential for the energy it needs to function properly. The formula includes suma, astragalus, Siberian ginseng, ginkgo, and gotu kola.

16. This formula is designed to support the nutritional needs of the pancreas: chromium, zinc, goldenseal, juniper, uva ursi, huckleberry, mullein, yarrow, garlic, slippery elm, capsicum, dandelion, marshmallow, nettle, white oak, and licorice.

17. This is a Chinese formula that is very beneficial to strengthen the glandular system. When the glands are out of balance, it can cause a number of health problems. It includes dendrobium, eucommia, rehmannia, ophiopogon, trichosanthes, pueraria, anemarrhena, achyranthes, hoelen, asparagus, moutan, alisma, phellondendron, cornus, licorice, and schizandra.

## FEMALE GLANDS

This female glandular formula contains vitamins, minerals, and herbs to provide nutritional support and prevent deficiencies that cause emotional and physical symptoms and problems common to women. This nutritional support will help prevent physical and mental stress, which causes fatigue, depression, irritability, and chemical imbalances that can lead to a dependency on antidepressant drugs.

It contains vitamins A, C, B1, B2, niacinamide, vitamins D, E, B6, folic acid, B12, biotin, pantothenic acid, calcium, iron, iodine, magnesium, zinc, copper, manganese, chromium, selenium, and potassium. It also contains choline, inositol, bioflavonoids, and PABA. It contains the following Chinese herbs: dong quai, peony, bupleurum, hoelen, atractylodes, codonopsis, alisma, licorice, magnolia, ginger, peppermint, moutan, gardenia, and cyperus.

## FEMALE FORMULAS

1. This is designed to help maintain the female glands as well as other glands. This will nourish and strengthen the reproductive glands and prevent menstrual pain, premenstrual tension, insomnia, menopausal symptoms, sexual disinterest, and other problems that are caused by chemical imbalance. It includes black cohosh, licorice, Siberian ginseng, sarsaparilla, squaw vine, blessed thistle, and false unicorn.

2. This formula is designed to help prepare a woman for giving birth by strengthening the glands and reproductive system. This supplies nutrients to build a weakened body and prevent menstrual disorders, morning sickness, miscarriage, and menopausal symptoms. It includes black cohosh, squaw vine, dong quai, butcher's broom, and red raspberry.

3. This is formulated especially for the female reproductive organs and also benefits the glandular system. This is rich in herbs that contain vitamins and minerals that feed and strengthen the female glands. The formula includes red raspberry, dong quai, ginger, licorice, black cohosh, queen of the meadow, blessed thistle, and marshmallow.

4. This is designed to strengthen the female reproductive system and the urinary system. This helps to prevent cramps, bloating, morning sickness, and menstrual disorders. It includes goldenseal, red raspberry, black cohosh, queen of the meadow, althea, blessed thistle, dong quai, capsicum, and ginger.

5. This is a nutritional herbal supplement to help balance hormones, prevent bad estrogen from accumulating, reduce bloating, avoid postpartum problems, help with weakness in the veins, prevent

hemorrhaging, alleviate anemia, and strengthen the urinary system. It includes goldenseal, capsicum, ginger, uva ursi, cramp bark, squaw vine, blessed thistle, red raspberry, and false unicorn.

6. A liquid formula for easy digestion and assimilation. It enhances nutritional support for the digestive and glandular systems. It includes peppermint, rose hips, hibiscus, and red raspberry.

## MALE FORMULAS

1. A special formula for the prostate gland as well as for the glandular system. This will help balance hormones in the body. It helps to supply nutrients for inflammation and pain in the prostate gland. It includes saw palmetto, pumpkin seeds, sarsaparilla, damiana, *Panax ginseng*, DHEA.

2. A special formula for the male reproductive system as well as the urinary system. It contains nutrients to help prevent kidney stones, inflammation, infections, impotence, edema, joint pain, and prostatitis. The formula includes capsicum, goldenseal, ginger, parsley, uva ursi, marshmallow, juniper berries, eleuthero root, queen of the meadow leaves.

3. This is especially formulated for the male reproductive system. It provides nutrients to nourish and strengthen the prostate. It helps prevent swelling, inflammation, and pain. This is important for older men, who need nutrients for proper function of the male glands. It includes muira puama, yohimbe bark, epimedium extract powder, L-arginine, damiana leaves, oatstraw leaves, saw palmetto berries, DHEA.

4. This formula is designed to help strengthen the glandular system, especially the pancreas and prostate. It helps in infections and water retention and supplies circulation to prevent toxins from accumulating in the glands. The formula includes black walnut, damiana, ho-shou-wu, sarsaparilla, saw palmetto, Siberian ginseng, American ginseng, suma, pumpkin seed, licorice root, black cohosh root, gotu kola, capsicum fruit, goldenseal root, ginger, dong quai root, lobelia, kelp.

## SINGLE HERBS FOR MALES

Black walnut, damiana, ho-shou-wu, sarsparilla, saw palmetto, Siberian ginseng, American ginseng, suma.

# THE IMMUNE SYSTEM

The immune system is a network of mechanisms and processes that keeps us safe from bacteria, viruses, fungal infections, and any other toxins that may invade our tissues. The immune system accumulates damage and gradually becomes defective over many years and is implicated in the autoimmune diseases that are prevalent now. Diet and lifestyle have a profound effect on the immune system. Evidence has been produced that shows stress and how we cope with it is the main cause of illness.

Stress affects the body by depleting the adrenal glands. This causes a suppressed immune system. This happens because the immune system requires enormous amounts of nutrients. The body also requires large amounts of nutrients, and the average American diet does not supply the body's needs. Our food is processed, with added chemicals, food coloring, preservatives, and taste enhancers. The natural food is depleted of vital vitamins, such as B vitamins and minerals, that are essential for a healthy immune system.

Viruses are composed of living and nonliving material. They can be dormant for years and, if the immune system is weak, come to life. The virus inserts its genetic material through the cell wall. It then dissolves the wall and fuses with the contents of the cell, and thus multiplies and begins to do its damage.

## IMMUNE FORMULA

This formula contains nutrients to protect and strengthen the immune system. It contains the necessary ingredients for a healthy immune system to fight toxins, germs, and viruses that constantly invade our bodies. The formula includes the following: vitamin A from fish oils and beta-carotene, vitamin C, vitamin E, zinc, selenium, barley grass juice powder, wheatgrass juice powder, asparagus powder, astragalus, broccoli powder, cabbage powder, ganoderma, parthenium, schizandra, eleuthero, myrrh gum, and pau d'arco.

## SPECIAL IMMUNE FORMULAS

1. This formula is beneficial for the immune and circulatory systems. This helps protect against germs and viruses that cause illness. It includes rose hips, chamomile, slippery elm, yarrow, capsicum, goldenseal, myrrh gum, peppermint, sage, and lemongrass.

2. This not only strengthens the immune system but aids digestion and the lymph system. It helps in fever, vomiting, motion sickness, chills, abdominal pain, and water retention. It includes ginger, capsicum, goldenseal, and licorice.

3. Germanium is an antioxidant that neutralizes free radicals to prevent them from damaging tissues in the body. Echinacea helps neutralize toxins and rid them from the body. This formula includes germanium and echinacea.

4. This formula protects the body from stress that weakens the immune system. It also is beneficial for the lymphatic and respiratory systems. It includes parthenium, yarrow, myrrh gum, and capsicum.

5. This formula strengthens the eliminative system, which can cause a weakened immune system. A weak immune system will open the door to all kinds of illness. This formula includes goldenseal, black walnut, althea (marshmallow), parthenium, plantain, bugleweed, echinacea.

6. This formula helps purify and eliminate toxins, germs, and viruses from the body. It is also useful in liquid form for easy assimilation for those who have faulty digestion. The formula includes spice, red clover blossoms, burdock, pau d'arco bark, sage leaves.

7. This formula contains organic chelated minerals along with amino acids, for better absorption and assimilation by the body. It contains arginine, leucine, glycine, vitamins C, B6, B12, pantothenic acid, folic acid, niacin, calcium, phosphorus, iodine, zinc, copper, potassium, bee pollen, eleuthero root, gotu kola herb, capsicum fruit, licorice root, glutamine, and choline.

8. This formula is designed to fortify the body to protect against yeast infestations and other microorganisms that invade when the immune system is weak. This provides nutrients to strengthen and protect the immune system. The formula includes caprylic acid, vitamins A, E, C, pantothenic acid, biotin, zinc, selenium, calcium, phosphorus, pau d'arco, garlic bulb, goldenseal root, yucca root, lemongrass herb, rose hips concentrate, hesperidin, citrus bioflavonoids.

9. This formula is designed to protect and build up the immune system. It contains nutrients that are vital for the protection of the immune system. It contains beta-glucans, which stimulates the immune system and increases natural killer T cells; arbinogalactan, which stimulates natural killer cells and increases the intestinal flora; colostrum, which is rich in immune-stimulating transfer factors; reishi and maitake mushrooms, to boost the immune system; and cordyceps, which protects the genes and increases T-cell and B-cell activity that is vital to immune response.

10. A combination of goldenseal and parthenium in an extract form is designed to heal and strengthen the immune system and protect against diseases. Goldenseal is the greatest healer in the herbal kingdom. It will heal and repair the entire digestive tract. Parthenium will help the lymphatic system to keep the body clean.

11. This Chinese formula is carefully designed to strengthen the immune system. It protects against viral infections and germs. The formula includes dandelion, purslane, indigo, thlaspi, bupleurum, scute, pinella, ginseng, cinnamon, licorice.

12. This formula is in an extract for quicker assimilation and quicker action. It strengthens the immune and nervous systems. This is useful to help fight infections, especially for all kinds of ear problems, such as ear infections, accumulation of wax in the ears, and itching ears. It has been used for some types of hearing loss. It can also be used for throat infections. The formula includes black cohosh, chickweed, goldenseal, desert tea, licorice, valerian, skullcap.

## SINGLE HERBS FOR THE IMMUNE SYSTEM

Single herbs that are known to assist in building and maintaining a healthy immune system include the following: barley juice powder, blue vervain, burdock, chaparral, echinacea, ginkgo, goldenseal, parthenium, pau d'arco, rose hips, and suma.

# THE INTESTINAL SYSTEM

The colon is the body's sewer system, and if not treated properly, it can accumulate toxic poisons that are absorbed into the bloodstream. This will then cause many diseases. Lack of fiber in the diet is the main cause of intestinal diseases. Years of poor diet cause bowel problems.

The small intestine is where most nutrition is absorbed. Stress can affect nutrient absorption and cause irritation of the small intestine. The large intestine absorbs minerals and water. When the membrane of the large colon is unhealthy, it cannot assimilate and absorb the minerals, and this creates deficiency diseases. The health of the entire body is maintained when the intestinal system is working properly.

## BOWEL FORMULA

This formula benefits the entire gastrointestinal tract. It supplies nutrients for a healthy colon. It strengthens and heals the stomach, nourishes and cleans the intestines, and stimulates bile function and liver health. It dissolves and eliminates mucus from the intestinal tract. It contains nutrients for proper digestion and assimilation.

It contains betaine HCl, bile salts, pancreatin, pepsin, psyllium hulls, algin, cascara sagrada bark, bentonite clay, apple pectin, marshmallow root, parthenium root, charcoal, ginger root, and sodium copper chlorophyll.

## GYMNEMA FORMULA

Excellent for the digestive and glandular systems. Research on gymnema shows good results on nourishing the pancreas and helping with problems such as diabetes, obesity, and glandular problems. The formula includes gymnema leaves, marshmallow, psyllium hulls, garcinia, herbal pumpkin.

## PUMPKIN SEED FORMULA

This formula is good for parasites, colon cleansing, skin problems, removing toxins from the system, constipation, prostate, tumors, and worms. The formula includes pumpkin seeds, culver's root, cascara sagrada, violet, chamomile, mullein, marshmallow, and slippery elm.

## LOWER-BOWEL FORMULAS

The herbs in these formulas tone, rebuild, and strengthen the bowels. They will gradually clean and restore bowel function. Constipation causes poisons to accumulate in the blood and prevents food from being assimilated.

1. This formula is designed to help the entire intestinal tract. This will enhance normal liver function. It strengthens the gall bladder and the urinary and lymphatic systems. The formula includes rose hips, barberry, dandelion, fennel, red beet root, horseradish, parsley.

2. This formula will help heal and restore normal lower-bowel function. It will also help purify the blood. The formula includes cascara sagrada, buckthorn, licorice, capsicum, ginger, Oregon grape, turkey rhubarb, couch grass, red clover.

3. This formula is rich in fiber and minerals for the lower bowels. It helps restore normal function to weakened bowels. The formula includes dong quai, cascara sagrada, turkey rhubarb, goldenseal, capsicum, ginger, Oregon grape, lobelia, fennel, red raspberry.

4. This formula contains natural fibers. It will absorb toxins and rid them from the body. It will help lower cholesterol. It is a natural way to restore normal bowel function. The formula includes psyllium, apple fiber, oat fiber, lobelia.

5. This formula is an excellent way to clean the bowels. The ginger helps prevent any cramps that might be caused by the senna. The catnip helps relax the bowels, and the formula is rich in minerals, which are absorbed in the lower bowels. The formula includes senna leaves, fennel, ginger, catnip.

6. This formula works on the lower bowels to promote the friendly bacteria, essential for a healthy colon. This is soothing and healing to the entire intestinal system. The formula includes slippery elm, marshmallow, plantain, chamomile, rose hips, bugleweed.

7. This Chinese formula supports the digestive and detoxifying functions of the body. It has a cleansing and strengthening effect on the urinary system. The Chinese use these herbs to move energy to the head and support the natural elimination of excess moisture and toxins. The formula contains agastache herb, crataegus fruit, hoelen plant, magnolia bark, oryza seed, shenqu tea, citrus peel, gastrodia rhizome, *Panax ginseng* root, typhonium rhizome, atractylodes rhizome, cardamom fruit, platycodon root, ginger rhizome, licorice root.

## GENERAL CLEANSING FORMULA

This formula benefits the colon, blood, and cells of the body. It is an excellent formula to use on a weight-loss program. It is an excellent blood cleanser to use for any disease.

This formula includes gentian, Irish moss, cascara sagrada, goldenseal, slippery elm, fenugreek, safflower, myrrh, yellow dock, parthenium, black walnut, barberry, dandelion, uva ursi, chickweed, catnip, cyani.

## SUPPLEMENTS AND SINGLE HERBS

Acidophilus, aloe vera, hydrated bentonite, liquid chlorophyll, magnesium, black walnut, buckthorn, cascara sagrada, chaparral, dandelion, fennel, fenugreek, flax, ginger, goldenseal, licorice, marshmallow, Oregon grape, peppermint, psyllium, safflower, sarsaparilla, senna, vervain, slippery elm.

# THE NERVOUS SYSTEM

The nervous system is a very delicate and important part of the body and needs to be treated properly. The nervous system and the immune system are closely connected. When one system fails, the other is affected. The brain has the job of transmitting information back and forth from the immune system. It is vital to nourish and strengthen the nervous system in order to protect the immune system.

## STRESS FORMULA

Stressful situations leach nutrients from the body. Nutritionists regard inadequate nutrients as the most stressful on the immune and nervous systems. This formula is designed to fortify the body against depleted essential nutrients and protect the body under stress. It contains vitamins C, B1, B2, B6, B12, folic acid, biotin, niacinamide, pantothenic acid, schizandra, choline bitartrate, PABA, wheat germ, bee pollen, valerian root, passion flower, inositol, hops, citrus bioflavonoids.

## HERBAL FORMULAS FOR THE NERVES

1. This formula is designed to relax the nerves and nourish and strengthen the nervous system. It is especially good for spastic colon and muscle spasms. It helps prevent migraine headaches. It is

rich in calcium and B-complex vitamins, which provide nutritional support for the nervous system. The formula includes chamomile, passion flower, hops, fennel, marshmallow, feverfew.

2. This formula is designed to strengthen weakened nerves and help in nervous tension, cramps, headaches, hysteria, pain, and insomnia. This will build the nerves to help in coughs, vertigo, colds, flu, and fevers. The formula includes white willow, valerian, lettuce leaves, and capsicum.

3. This is a formula to strengthen the nervous system as well as a cleansing power to clean the muscles and tissues. The devil's claw is similar to chaparral and enhances this formula. The formula includes white willow, black cohosh, capsicum, valerian, ginger, hops, wood betony, devil's claw.

4. This formula not only strengthens the nervous system but benefits peripheral blood circulation. It helps relieve anxiety and tense muscles. It will gradually build a strong nervous system, which protects the immune system. Valerian is rich in calcium, and passion flower is beneficial for the eyes. The formula includes black cohosh, valerian, capsicum, passion flower, skullcap, hops, wood betony, catnip herb.

5. This Chinese formula is beneficial for the nervous system. It helps to prevent depression, insomnia, fatigue, anxiety, and menopause symptoms. It also strengthens the urinary, respiratory, and female reproductive systems. The formula includes perilla, saussurea, gambir, bamboo sap, bupleurum, aurantium, zhishi, ophiopogon, cyperus, platycodon, liqusticum, dang gui, *Panax ginseng*, hoelen, coptis, ginger, licorice.

6. Valerian root herb supports the central nervous system. It aids in relaxing the body and helps with sleeping disorders. When the body is relaxed, it heals faster. This formula contains valerian root.

7. This combination supplies nutrients that strengthen the nervous system. It also benefits the respiratory and muscle systems. The formula includes blessed thistle, pleurisy, catnip herb, yerba santa.

## SINGLE HERBS FOR THE NERVES

Bilberry, black currant oil, catnip, chaparral, feverfew, hops, lady's slipper, passion flower, skullcap, valerian, wood betony.

# THE RESPIRATORY SYSTEM

Respiratory infections are the most frequent single cause of illness. One-third to one-half of industrial absenteeism from sickness is caused by acute respiratory illness. The lungs have the responsibility of supplying oxygen necessary for body energy. Toxins present in the atmosphere, such as nitrogen and ozone dioxide, are increasing as a major cause of respiratory problems. Pollutants can attack the body repeatedly over a long period before symptoms appear. The respiratory system consists of the lungs, nose, throat, and trachea.

Herbs, vitamins, minerals, and proper diet will help keep the respiratory system strong and healthy. A colon cleanse is essential for a healthy respiratory system.

## RESPIRATORY FORMULA

This formula was developed for severe lung congestion, allergies, lungs filling with fluid, mucus, pneumonia, coughs, and toxic buildup in the lungs. It also helps in digestion. The herbs in this formula will help protect the lungs from all the pollutants in the air. The formula helps loosen hard mucus from the sinuses, throat, and lungs. It will help in asthma, bronchitis, coughs, hay fever, nasal drainage, earache, sinus swelling, and swollen glands. The formula includes boneset, fenugreek, horseradish, mullein, fennel.

## SPECIAL RESPIRATORY FORMULAS

1. This Chinese formula is beneficial for the respiratory system. It also helps with the circulatory and lymphatic systems. It increases circulation and eliminates toxins from the system. The formula includes astragalus root, aster root, qinjiao root, platycodon root, anemarrhena rhizome, bupleurum root, dang gui root, lycium bark, ophiopogon root, *Panax ginseng* root, atractylodes rhizome, blue citrus peel, citrus peel, typhonium rhizome, schizandra fruit, and licorice root.

2. These two combinations are very beneficial for the respiratory system. Fenugreek and thyme are especially beneficial for the sinuses and head area. They both help prevent and eliminate mucus from

the respiratory system. The formula helps keep the lungs and the nasal passages clean to prevent germs and viruses from multiplying. The formula includes fenugreek, thyme.

3. This formula is designed for the nervous and muscle system as well as the respiratory. This supplies nutrients to heal and strengthen the respiratory system. The formula includes blessed thistle, pleurisy, catnip, yerba santa.

4. This formula is excellent for the lungs. It supplies nutrition for the respiratory system. This helps in asthma, allergies, coughs, sinus headache, and sinus irritation that causes drainage in the throat. The formula includes rose hips, chamomile flowers, mullein leaves, yarrow flowers, yerba santa leaves, goldenseal root, myrrh gum, peppermint leaves, sage flowers, astragalus root, slippery elm bark, lemongrass herb, capsicum fruit.

5. This formula is designed for the entire respiratory system and is especially effective for the sinuses. It helps clean and strengthen the mucous membranes of the nose, throat, and lungs to prevent allergies and other respiratory problems. It helps with hay fever, sinus irritations, itching eyes, irritating coughs, asthma, bronchitis, and respiratory infections. The formula includes burdock root, orange peel, capsicum fruit, goldenseal root, parsley herb, horehound herb, althea root, yerba santa herb.

## SINGLE HERBS FOR THE RESPIRATORY SYSTEM

Angelica, boneset, comfrey, ephedra, fenugreek, flaxseed, goldenseal, licorice, lobelia, marshmallow, mullein, yerba santa.

# THE STRUCTURAL SYSTEM

The structural system consists of bones, muscles, and connective tissue. Poor nutrition and the inability to assimilate minerals contribute to bone loss. Diets high in protein and sugar, smoking, alcohol, caffeine drinks, and lack of exercise all contribute to bone loss and pave the way for other diseases.

Bone loss in women after menopause is a special concern. This happens when decreased secretion of the hormone estrogen is greatest. This isn't necessary if a balanced diet is followed with ample supply of minerals. The ability to assimilate minerals is a concern in the young as well as the elderly.

## STRUCTURAL FORMULA

This formula is designed to provide nutrition for the bones, flesh, and cartilage of the structural system. There are many nutrients that contribute to a healthy structural system, and the following have been beneficial. The formula includes vitamin A (beta-carotene), vitamin C, calcium (chelated for easier assimilation), iron, vitamins D, B6, B12, phosphorus, magnesium, manganese, potassium, boron, betaine HCI (necessary for the assimilation of calcium and other minerals), papaya, parsley, pineapple, valerian, horsetail, licorice.

## SPECIAL STRUCTURAL FORMULAS

1. This formula contains nutrients to nourish, lubricate, and help maintain mobility of the joints. It will help relieve joint pain and contains anti-inflammatory properties. It nourishes the joints, promotes cartilage tissue regeneration, and maintains fluid in the cartilage. The formula includes glucosamine, chondroitin, MSM, and devil's claw.

2. This is especially beneficial for increasing bone mass as well as strengthening the nervous system. It is rich in calcium and minerals to help in the assimilation of calcium. The formula includes alfalfa, marshmallow, plantain, horsetail, oatstraw, wheatgrass, hops.

3. This is formulated to nourish the hair, skin, and nails. It is a benefit to the structural system. It is rich in silicon, which has been shown to be beneficial in calcium assimilation. The formula includes dulse, horsetail, sage, rosemary.

4. This is a formula to use internally and externally. It will heal and rebuild tissues. It will help in cases of adhesion, which cause a lot of pain and misery. The formula includes slippery elm, marshmallow, goldenseal, fenugreek.

5. This Chinese formula is designed to strengthen the bones. It also helps enhance the urinary system. It helps in backaches, fatigue, arthritis, osteoporosis, and tones up the structural system. The formula

includes eucommia, cistanche, rehmannia, morinda, drynaria, achyranthes, hoelen, dipsacus, lycium, dioscorea, ligustrum, cornus, dang gui (dong quai), *Panax ginseng*, astragalus, epimedium, liquidambar, atractylodes.

## SINGLE HERBS FOR THE STRUCTURAL SYSTEM

Aloe vera, bayberry, comfrey, horsetail, oatstraw, red raspberry, white oak bark, yucca.

# THE URINARY SYSTEM

The urinary system consists of the kidneys, bladder, ureter, and urethra. Keeping this system in good working condition will help prevent the body from poisoning itself. The proper function of this system is vital to our inner health. The kidneys help maintain a balance of body fluids. The kidneys have the ability to filter out harmful toxic material while retaining the vital vitamins, proteins, sugars, fats, and minerals. But if this system is overloaded with more toxins than it can eliminate, diseases will invade the body. It will cause protein in the blood to be lost in the urine. Potassium, calcium, magnesium, and zinc can also be lost. This causes nutritional depletion and illness. Diseases associated with kidney failure are high blood pressure, stroke, heart attack, or heart disease. It is important to protect the urinary system and nourish it with the proper food, vitamins, minerals, herbs, and supplements that strengthen these vital organs.

## URINARY FORMULA

This formula will help clean, nourish, and heal the urinary system. It contains juniper berries, goldenseal root, capsicum fruit, parsley herb, ginger root, eleuthero root, uva ursi leaves, queen of the meadow leaves, and marshmallow root.

## SPECIAL URINARY FORMULAS

1. This formula is designed especially for the urinary system. It strengthens the kidneys to release toxins, and it nourishes and cleans the urinary system. It contains herbs and nutrients that are rich in vitamins and minerals. The formula includes uva ursi, hydrangea, hops, eleuthero, schizandra, asparagus stem, dandelion leaf, parsley leaves, cornsilk, watermelon seed, dong quai root, horsetail stems, strobilus.

2. This formula strengthens the urinary, reproductive, and digestive systems. The formula includes dong quai, goldenseal, juniper, uva ursi, parsley, ginger, marshmallow.

3. This formula provides nutrition for the urinary system. It will help protect the urinary organs from kidney stones, infections, and water retention. The formula includes juniper berries, parsley, uva ursi, dandelion, chamomile.

4. This formula strengthens the urinary system as well as the lymph system. This Chinese formula contains the following: stephania, hoelen, morus, chaenomeles, astragalus, atractylodes, alisma, magnolia, polyporus, areca, cinnamon, typhonium, ginger, citrus peel, licorice.

## SINGLE HERBS FOR THE URINARY SYSTEM

Cornsilk, garlic, grapevine, horsetail, hydrangea, juniper berries, marshmallow, parsley, peach bark, slippery elm, uva ursi.

# APPENDIX

In this section I have put together some specific extract formulas and what they are good for. The advantage of extracts is that they either go directly into the bloodstream or are absorbed within minutes in the walls of the stomach. In an extract, the more active elements of medicinal herbs are liberated from insoluble, pulpy material. This is beneficial when digestion is poor, which is usually the problem when one is ill.

There are herbs that extract better in alcohol because it draws out more medicinal properties than vinegar. But vinegar and glycerin are also beneficial ways of extracting herbs. Vegetable glycerin has a sweet taste and is useful for children's remedies. It is a preservative and draws out medicinal properties better than water, but not as well as alcohol. Extracts are excellent to use internally and externally. If using alcohol extracts is a problem, place the amount of extract you will use in a cup of boiling water, allow the alcohol to evaporate, then drink the water.

## BONESET, FENUGREEK, HORSERADISH, MULLEIN, AND FENNEL EXTRACT

This extract formula is excellent for the lungs. It is soothing, cleansing, and healing for the mucous membranes. It helps with allergies, asthma, bron-chitis, emphysema, coughs, congestion, lung ailments, mucus congestion, pneumonia, the immune system, and is excellent to help heal and clean the stomach and aid in digestive problems.

## BLACK WALNUT EXTRACT

Black walnut is rich in organic iodine and tannins, both of which contain antiseptic properties. This extract is useful for skin problems, parasites, worms, bruises, itching skin, ringworm, syphilis, and athlete's foot. It can help regulate blood sugar levels and eliminate toxins and fatty material.

## BLUE VERVAIN EXTRACT

This extract is used as a natural tranquilizer because it relaxes the body. It is good for fevers, upset stomach, colds, respiratory problems, and spleen and liver conditions. It helps to stimulate suppressed menstruation. This extract is also effective for hysteria, epilepsy, palsy, nervous exhaustion, hallucinations, coughs, earaches, headaches, diarrhea, insomnia, and dysentery.

## CAPSICUM EXTRACT

Capsicum is one of the best stimulants in the herbal kingdom. It is healing for the arteries, veins, and capillaries. It can help stop bleeding internally and externally. It has been used to stop heart attacks, strokes, colds, flu, low vitality, headaches, indigestion, depression, arthritis, and ulcers. This is a good extract to have on hand for emergencies.

### CATNIP AND FENNEL EXTRACT

This is an excellent extract for infants and children. It is relaxing for fevers and restlessness. It can help relieve colic, ease stomach cramps, soothe an upset stomach, reduce acid indigestion, and relieve gas. It can be taken internally or simply rubbed on the stomach.

### GARLIC OIL EXTRACT

Garlic is nature's antibiotic. This extract is useful for high blood pressure, infections, and earaches. It works well with mullein oil for ear infections.

### ECHINACEA AND GOLDENSEAL EXTRACT

An excellent extract for fighting infections. It acts as a natural antibiotic and is good for viral and bacterial infections. It helps with colds, flu, bronchitis, sinus infections, throat problems, and coughs. It is effective for cleaning the lymphatic and glandular systems of toxins and mucus.

### GOLDENSEAL AND PARTHENIUM EXTRACT

This extract is useful for infections of all kinds. It can kill parasites and worms and is good to take when traveling to prevent diarrhea. It can help the body heal lymphatic congestion, contagious diseases, childhood diseases, colds, flu, and sore throats.

### HAWTHORN BERRY EXTRACT

This extract is beneficial for the circulatory system. It nourishes the heart and can help prevent arteriosclerosis, weak heart action, and angina pectoris. It can heal heart valve defects, an enlarged heart, and breathing problems due to weak heart action and lack of oxygen.

### LICORICE ROOT EXTRACT

Licorice is considered food for the adrenal glands. It stimulates the body to produce interferon, which is an immune substance that counteracts cancer and viruses. It stimulates the body to produce its own natural estrogen and cortisone, an action which

helps balance female hormones. This extract is useful for lung conditions, hypoglycemia, diabetes, and to help counteract stress. It can also help with hoarseness and throat damage.

### LOBELIA EXTRACT

Lobelia is one of the best relaxants in the herbal kingdom. It is excellent for strengthening the nervous system and cleaning obstruction from the stomach. It helps remove congestion from any part of the body. Lobelia extract is helpful for bronchial spasms, the clearing of allergies, asthma, bronchitis, childhood diseases, convulsions, croup, headaches, and spasms. It can be rubbed on a child's spine to promote relaxation and healing.

### GINKGO, KOREAN GINSENG, AND GOTU KOLA EXTRACT

This herbal extract is excellent for the brain. It can help improve concentration and memory and reduce the symptoms of Alzheimer's and ADHD. It helps improve blood circulation and works to feed, nourish, and clean the brain.

### OREGON GRAPE EXTRACT

This extract works on the liver, blood, stomach, and intestines. It helps the body in chronic diseases such as blood poisoning, skin problems, liver congestion, and staph infections. It helps the body heal itself.

### PAU D'ARCO EXTRACT

Pau d'arco is a natural blood cleanser and builder, and it helps protect the liver from damage. This extract has antibiotic properties which can help destroy viral infections. It has helped in many kinds of cancers. It has been used for healing arthritis, asthma, diabetes, gonorrhea, hernia, infections, liver ailments, lupus, Parkinson's disease, tumors, Epstein-Barr, pyorrhea, skin problems, spleen ailments, ulcers, and varicose veins.

### RED CLOVER, BURDOCK, AND SPICE EXTRACT

This is an excellent and proven formula for cleansing the blood and eliminating toxins from the bloodstream. It helps with infections, cancers, skin problems, and chronic diseases. It is a tonic for nerves and is useful for colds, flu, and childhood diseases.

## RED RASPBERRY, PEPPERMINT, ROSE HIPS, AND HIBISCUS EXTRACT

This is an excellent extract formula for all female problems. It can help reduce nausea during pregnancy and also feeds and strengthens the uterus. It can help in balancing hormones, preventing hemorrhage, reducing pain, and curing diarrhea. It is also helpful for children with fevers, colds, colic, and vomiting.

## CHAMOMILE, PASSION FLOWER, FENNEL, MARSHMALLOW, HOPS, AND FEVERFEW EXTRACT

This extract is useful for nervous disorders. It can help the body handle stressful situations by calming the nerves, relaxing the body, and promoting sleep. It is a good remedy for insomnia, irritability, and nervous fatigue.

## MA HUANG, WHITE WILLOW, DANDELION, AND STINGING NETTLE EXTRACT

This extract formula increases thermogenesis. It helps to decrease appetite and increase energy levels, so it is a good stimulant for weight loss.

## VALERIAN, ANISE, BLACK WALNUT, DESERT TEA, GINGER, AND LICORICE EXTRACT

This extract formula contains antispasmodic properties to strengthen the nervous system. It helps repair and rebuild the nervous system. It helps with spastic conditions, convulsions, asthma attacks, nervous disorders, insomnia, and fevers. It is an excellent formula for acute and chronic diseases.

## DANDELION, INDIGO, THLASPI, SCUTE, BUPLEURUM, PINELLIA, GINSENG, CINNAMON, AND LICORICE EXTRACT

This extract is formulated to strengthen and provide nutritional support to the immune system. It can help improve the digestive system and the liver. This formula can help in healing the many autoimmune diseases that are plaguing mankind.

## COMMON POULTICES

- Bayberry: Can be applied to skin for cancerous and ulcerated sores. It is a strong cleanser and healer.
- Catnip: Reduces swelling; especially good for under the eyes. The English herbalist Nicholas Culpeper wrote about catnip for hemorrhoids, applied topically.
- Clay: Excellent healing agent. Good for skin problems such as eczema. Swollen liver can be helped with clay packs. It is suggested that clay should be taken internally a few days before using it as a pack on the body. It can be used for boils, carbuncles, and tumors.
- Comfrey: Excellent for healing wounds and broken bones. It can be applied externally for burns, sprains, and wounds, and has been used as a hot poultice to help ease pain caused by bursitis.
- Ginger: Add powdered ginger to boiling water. Soak a cloth in ginger water and apply to affected areas to help relieve pain, or to bring blood to the surface of congested areas. Ginger baths and soaking the feet will help reduce pain.
- Hops: A poultice made of hops soothes inflammations and boils and helps reduce the pain of toothache. Its lupulon and humulon properties help to prevent infections.
- Mullein: Used for swollen lymph glands and lymph congestion. Use one part lobelia and three parts mullein.
- Onion: Used for boils, ears, infections, sore throats, and sores. When using as a poultice, chop and heat the onions.
- Plantain: This is a valuable first-aid remedy. Apply mashed or crushed herb on a cut or a swollen or running sore and secure with a clean bandage. Discard pulp and replace as needed.
- Potato: Good for infections, tumors, and warts. Use by grating raw potato and add ginger (to stimulate the action of the potato).
- Slippery elm: Excellent for abscesses, bites, blood poison, boils, and stings. (Note: Slippery elm is used as a jelling agent for poultices. It is excellent mixed with other herbs.)
- White oak bark: Use for hemorrhoids and varicose veins.
- Yarrow: This is a good poultice for wounds and inflammations. It has been used to reduce swellings and ease earaches. The poultice will also soothe bruises and abrasions. For nosebleeds, the leaves are steeped in water and then placed in the nostrils. It is also useful for nicks and cuts. Yarrow has anti-inflammatory properties and can be applied as a tea to sore nipples in nursing mothers.

It can be used as a wash for eczema, rashes, and poison ivy.

## NATURAL ANTISEPTICS

- Black walnut: External and internal antiseptic, good for internal parasites, infection, and tonsillitis.
- Cabbage leaves: Contain rapine, an antibiotic. The warm leaves placed on the ulcerated sore will draw out the pus on sores.
- Carrots: Mashed and boiled and applied to a sore, they have helped in drawing out pus and healing the area. They are said to be a strong antiseptic.
- Clove: The oil is a strong germicide. It is used for toothaches, pains, nausea, and vomiting.
- Cornflowers: Contain important glycosides that have strong antiseptic properties. This herb has been used in eyewashes. Its germicidal and anti-bacterial properties have been used as an effective antidote for snake venom and scorpion poisons.
- False unicorn: Contains chamaelirin, a strong antiseptic. Helps ease evacuation of tapeworms and worms in the intestinal tract. It creates a pure environment in the body.
- Garlic: Is a powerful antibacterial agent. It contains allicin. The powder on wounds is good for the healing process. Garlic oil is useful for ear infections.
- Goldenseal: Contains the antibiotic berberine, which is used for mouth and gum problems. It is also used for worms and infection.
- Lemon: A natural antiseptic. Helps fade freckles.
- Myrrh: Has sensational antiseptic properties; contains gums, essential oils, resins, and other bitter compounds. Good for uterus, vaginal infections, and dysentery. It is also used for serious periodontal diseases. Laboratory tests have proven this to be one of the finest antibacterial and antiviral agents.
- Queen of the meadow: Used as an antiseptic to treat diseases of the uterus and cancer of the womb.
- Tea tree oil: Contains antifungal properties; aids in athlete's foot, acne, boils, burns, warts, vaginal infections, tonsillitis, sinus infections, ringworm, skin rashes, impetigo, herpes, corns, head lice, cold sores, canker sores, insect bites. It is a remarkable oil with valuable properties for healing.
- Thyme: Contains an antiseptic called thymol. Use small amounts for dressing wounds. Thyme

should be crushed and added to boiling water, then steeped and strained. It can be used for sprains and bruises.

## EMERGENCY AIDS

### Alcoholism

- Hops: Good for delirium.
- Cayenne: Reduces dilated blood vessels.
- Goldenseal: Natural antibiotic.
- Chaparral: Helps clean the residue of alcohol.
- Bee pollen: Gives nourishment and strength to the body.
- Glutamine (amino acid): Has been used in large doses to reduce the craving for alcohol.

### Allergies

The best natural antihistamine is to cut orange peels in small strips and soak in apple cider vinegar for several hours, drain, and cook down in honey until soft (but not the consistency of candy). Keep in refrigerator and use as needed. Relieves stuffiness and clogged passages. Allergies are treated with tyrosine, especially cases of hay fever from grass pollen.

### Arthritis

- Histidine: Is good for tissue growth and repair and is useful for its anti-inflammatory effect. It is used in rheumatoid arthritis.
- Proline (amino acid): Is used in multiple amino acid and vitamin formula for arthritis.

### Asthma

For an acute attack, a few drops of lobelia extract in the mouth will relax and put a stop to the spasms. Pour one cup cold water over one or two teaspoons of shredded elecampane root. Let stand eight to ten hours, then reheat. Take very hot, in small sips. Can sweeten with honey. Use one cup twice a day.

### Bleeding

- Cayenne pepper: A small amount applied in the nose has stopped bleeding immediately; taken internally with water helps internal bleeding; also helps a bleeding cut.

- Plantain: Powdered herb or fresh leaf applied directly on wound; dampen first.

- Marigold: The tincture in boiled water is used to wash wounds; very useful in bleeding conditions.
- Shepherd's purse: Works as a styptic. Use as a tea and apply as a poultice to the wound.

## Blisters

- Methionine: This amino acid helps heal rashes and blisters in babies with high ammonia content in their urine.
- Lysine: This amino acid has helped heal fever blisters when given 500 mg daily, with acidophilus and yogurt.

## Boils

- Figs: Fresh figs applied hot; also used for mouth sores.
- Honey: An antibiotic; apply with a small amount of comfrey powder and it will help bring boils to a head.
- Slippery elm: Use the powder added to water to make a paste; healing as a poultice. Can be used for wounds, boils, and skin problems.

## Bronchitis

- Comfrey, mullein, and lobelia: Are excellent for bronchitis. Bowels must be opened; an enema is helpful.
- Lobelia tincture: For immediate needs if there is shortness of breath or gasping; if the throat needs to be cleared of mucus, a few drops of lobelia tincture will relax the throat and bronchi.
- Irish moss: Good for chronic bronchitis.
- Cystine (amino acid): Builds white cell activity and helps build resistance for respiratory diseases such as chronic bronchitis, emphysema, and tuberculosis.

## Bruises

- Comfrey powder, goldenseal mixed with aloe vera juice: Is very good for bruises.
- Mullein: Oil of mullein flowers with olive oil is good for bruises.
- St. John's wort: The flowers are infused in olive oil and applied to bruises and wounds.
- Shepherd's purse: The whole plant is used as a poultice for wounds.

- Witch hazel: A compress dipped in distilled witch hazel is good for bruises and swellings.

## Burns

- Cool water: Immediately immerse in cool water, apply vitamin E oil, and take vitamin E orally.
- Aloe vera plant: Cut off leaves, slit them open, and squeeze juice onto burn, or lay exposed side of leaf directly on burn.
- Wheat germ oil and honey: Make a paste of wheat germ oil and honey in blender, mixing at low speed, then add comfrey leaves to make a thick paste. Apply to burn and keep remainder in refrigerator.
- Marshmallow compress: Can be used for mild burns.
- Potatoes: Peeled raw potatoes will help burns.
- Vitamin C: Applied topically and taken internally, it reduces pain, eliminating the need for morphine.

## Chapped Hands

- Aloe vera gel: Can be applied to chapped hands and chapped lips.

## Chicken Pox

- External teas: Red raspberry, catnip, and peppermint with vinegar to relieve itching.
- Goldenseal tea: For severe itching.
- Lemonade: With honey and fresh vegetable and fruit juices, if possible.
- L-lysine and immune-supporting herbs and vitamins can help facilitate wound healing.

## Colds and Flu

- Mild teas: Teas made from catnip or peppermint or red raspberry; use boneset, elderberry, and peppermint teas for cases of the flu; give natural vitamin C liquid.
- Chamomile tea: Relaxing and soothing for colds and flu.
- Lemon and honey water: Steeped and used for colds and coughs; refreshing and restorative.
- Honey: Added to herb drinks, it will help destroy bacteria, for the honey is a bactericide.
- Barley water: Wash two ounces of barley and boil in one pint of water for a few minutes. Discard water, then place barley in four pints pure water. Add clean lemon peel and boil down to two pints. Strain and add two ounces of honey. Can be used freely for children.

## Constipation

- Prevention is the best method. The diet for children should include whole-grain cereals, leafy greens, and raw fruits with skins. These are essential in keeping the bowels working normally. Emotional disturbances in the mother affect the baby if nursing.
- Chamomile tea: Weak chamomile tea is good for constipation.
- Cascara sagrada: Small amounts for children.
- Elderflower: Good in cases of constipation.
- Licorice: Added to herbal teas, it has a slight laxative action.

## Convulsions

- Chamomile tea: In small, weak doses several times a day helps. A warm chamomile tea enema is helpful.
- Lobelia tincture: Can also be rubbed well into the neck, chest, and between the shoulders.

## Coughs

- Onion remedy: Peel and chop onions, cover with honey. Simmer. Strain and use as a cough syrup.
- Honey and licorice root: Or honey and horehound herb, or honey and wild cherry bark are useful.
- Mullein: Good for croup cough.
- Marshmallow, mullein, comfrey, lobelia, and chickweed: Combine in equal parts; good for coughs.
- Pitted dates: Crushed and made into a syrup; has been used for coughs, sore throat, and bronchitis.
- Tea of sage and thyme: In equal parts with a pinch of cardamom, ginger, cloves, and nutmeg, is another remedy for coughs.

## Heavy Cough

- Cherry bark and coltsfoot tea: Chew on licorice or candied ginger.
- Almond drink: For cough and fever, grind almonds into powder and steep in one pint cold water.
- Horehound remedy: Use two tablespoons of the fresh leaves with two cups of boiling water; drink in small amounts.

## Croup

- Catnip or chamomile tea: Brings perspiration.
- Lobelia tincture: A few drops in catnip or peppermint tea is helpful.

## Depression

- Tyrosine: Has been found to have a fantastic effect on depression for its management and control, compared to a drug used for depression, with one great difference—no side effects.
- Gotu kola: Helps in mental fatigue, which is common in depression.
- Ginseng: Helps stimulate the entire body energy to overcome depression.
- Kelp: Contains all the minerals for glandular health.
- Herbal combinations: Black cohosh, capsicum, valerian, mistletoe, ginger, St. John's wort, hops, wood betony.
- B-complex and 5-HTP can also be helpful.

## Diarrhea

- Red raspberry tea: Is soothing for diarrhea.
- Carob powder in boiled milk: Usually about one teaspoon to one cup milk.
- Barley water: Given to small babies is good for diarrhea.
- Licorice or ginger: Is good to help colic pains from diarrhea.
- Carrot soup: Is an excellent remedy for infant diarrhea; the cooked soup coats the inflamed small bowel, soothes it, and helps promote healing.
- Slippery elm tea: Nourishing as well as healing.
- Ginger: A weak ginger tea settles the stomach and helps in diarrhea.

## Diphtheria

- Pineapple juice, lemon juice, and honey: Or cider vinegar and honey is useful.
- Cayenne: A pinch can be used for older children.

## Earache

- Oil of garlic: In the ear; hold in with cotton.
- Oil of lobelia: In each ear; hold in with cotton.

## Fever

- High fevers: An enema is used to reduce the fever.
- Barley water: Use for high fever (use linen cloth to tie barley and boil for half an hour).

## Headaches

- Hops: In capsule form with water.
- Wood betony, chamomile tea, tei-fu oil: Rub on temples.

- For severe headaches: Fasting with juice and green drinks.

## Hemorrhoids
- Ginger tea, yarrow extract, white oak bark: Applied externally.

## Herpes Simplex I (fever blisters or cold sores)
- Lysine: Inhibits the virus, together with vitamins C, A, and zinc.
- Yogurt and buttermilk: Will eliminate the pain, halt the spread of the lesions, and promote healing.

## Herpes Simplex II
- Black walnut: Used internally as well as externally.
- Goldenseal: Mixed with aloe vera for external use, internally to speed healing of infection.

## Insect Bites and Bee Stings
- Clay: A clay paste dampened and applied to the bite and sting will help relieve the pain.
- Plantain: Wet plantain leaf with a little olive oil and place on bee or hornet sting after the stinger is removed; will help healing; replace the leaf as it dries.
- Honey: Apply honey after removing the stinger.
- Comfrey: Mixed with aloe vera juice will reduce swelling.

## Insomnia
- Plain, warm milk: It contains generous amounts of the amino acid tryptophan, which quiets the nervous system, and vitamin B6 keeps the tryptophan high in the bloodstream. It is an essential ingredient for the regeneration of the body tissues. This is a natural alternative to tranquilizers.
- Hops: Help relax the body.
- Calcium: Herbal combinations help.
- Passion flower: Excellent for insomnia.
- Valerian: Can be used occasionally; prolonged use can cause depression in some people.

## Kidney Stones
- Apple juice and lemon juice fasts: With olive oil.

## Measles
- Hot catnip tea or chamomile tea: Will break out the rash and check the fever; use three tablespoons

of the herb in a quart of water and boiled down to one pint.

## Memory
- Glutamine: Has been used safely when given to children who can't learn or retain information.
- Gotu kola: Has been used with children to improve their learning ability and concentration.

## Mumps
- Catnip tea: Served hot, relieves pain.

## Ringworm
- Seal location: A fungoid parasite is best stopped by sealing off the air.
- Undiluted lemon juice, white of egg, nail varnish. Apply every few hours.
- Garlic: Used internally is helpful.
- Lobelia and olive oil: Apply tincture.

## Sunburn
- Vinegar and sunflower oil: To avoid sunburn, mix one teaspoon vinegar to one-half cup thin sunflower oil and apply.
- Aloe vera: Gel from aloe vera plant is useful for sunburn.
- Honey and wheat germ oil with powdered comfrey: Combine equal parts of honey and wheat germ oil with powdered comfrey added. Make paste ahead of time and it will keep well in a covered jar.

## Toothache
- Hot poultices: Will reduce the pain of toothache.
- Chamomile and hops tea: Will help relax the body.
- Oil of clove: Can be mixed with zinc oxide powder in a paste; this will protect the cavity from food.

## Tonsillitis
- Catnip tea enema: Pineapple juice.
- Vegetable juices: Are useful in removing waste.
- Red raspberry tea: Comfrey tea.

## Weight Control
- Phenylalanine: Is effective in weight control because of its positive effect on the thyroid.
- Kelp: Helps regulate the thyroid.
- Fasting formula: Licorice, beet root, hawthorn, and fennel.

## Worms

- Apples: Grated raw apples sprinkled with anise seed in a salad will get rid of worms.
- Cold sage tea: Is also good for worms.
- Garlic: Excellent body cleanser.
- Papaya latex: Is used in Asia for children to expel worms (obtain at health food stores).
- Yarrow: Serves as a tonic to the bowels after expelling worms.
- Pomegranate: Good for pinworms, roundworms, and tapeworms.
- Pumpkin seeds: Help eliminate worms.

# HERBAL FIRST-AID KIT

The following list comprises herbs and other medicinal items that could come in handy if regularly kept in a first-aid kit.

- Aloe vera gel: Excellent for burns and skin rashes; also used for insect bites and stings, poison oak and ivy, acne, and itchy skin.
- Antispasmodic extract: Contains valerian, anise, lobelia, black walnut, brigham tea, licorice, and ginger. Used for the nerves and spastic conditions; excellent in emergency conditions such as hysteria, shock, poisonous bites, and stings; used externally for pain and muscular spasms.
- Capsicum: Powder and extract; can be rubbed on toothaches, inflammation, and swellings; in treating arthritis, rub capsicum extract over the inflamed joint and wrap with flannel for the night. Is useful to stop bleeding internally and externally by helping to normalize the circulation. Capsicum and plantain will draw out foreign bodies embedded in the skin.
- Cascara sagrada: Safe tonic, laxative, very important to keep the bowels open in illness and avoid constipation.
- Chamomile: Used as a tea, chamomile is safe for children in colds, indigestion, and behavioral and nervous disorders; relieves menstrual cramps; externally, apply to swellings, sore muscles, and painful joints.
- Charcoal: Used for diarrhea and intestinal gas;

can be used as a poultice. Can be used in some poisoning.

- Chlorophyll: I keep liquid chlorophyll on hand for all kinds of emergencies. It is a good cleanser for the blood. It is good to clean the bowels. Good for children and nursing mothers. It is rich in minerals.
- Comfrey: Can be used for bleeding by using a strong decoction. It can be used internally and externally for healing of fractures, wounds, sores, and ulcers. It is an old-time remedy from the Middle Ages, and is as follows: Place burned area in ice water until pain is gone; mix the following in blender—one-half cup wheat germ oil, one-half cup honey, and add as much dried or fresh comfrey leaves as it will take to make a thick paste, and add a pinch of lobelia.
- Eucalyptus oil: Useful for bronchial spasms, chills, colds, sore throat, rheumatism; good antiseptic and expectorant.
- Fenugreek: Dissolves mucus; good for infections of nose, throat, and lungs. Helps to lower fevers. Excellent for children.
- Flowers and plants, edible and nutritious: Chicory, clover, dandelion, elderberry, squash, borage, nasturtium, lamb's quarters, plaintain, purslane, rose petals, violets, and wild watercress.
- Garlic powder and oil: "Nature's antibiotic," the oil is used for earaches. Garlic taken with capsicum and vitamin C at the beginning of a cold will often help.
- Ginger: Excellent for upset stomach, nausea, colds, and flu.
- Lobelia extract: Can be used internally and externally to relax all spasms; a few drops in the ear will relieve earaches; lobelia used with catnip as an enema is effective for fevers and infections; used externally in baths, compressions, poultices, and liniments for muscle spasms.
- Peppermint oil: Aids nausea, is an excellent stomach aid, assists in digestion, cleanses and gives tone to the entire body; sedative for nervous and restless persons of all ages; promotes relaxation and sleep.
- Red raspberry: Excellent for pregnancy, relieving nausea, preventing hemorrhage and bleeding, reducing pain, and easing childbirth; reliable for

children with stomach problems, fevers, colds, and flu.

- Sarsaparilla: A hot decoction, made with an ounce of root in a pint of water, will promote profuse sweating and will act as a powerful agent to expel gas from the stomach and intestines.

- Tea tree oil: Contains antifungal properties and helps with conditions such as athlete's foot, acne, boils, burns, warts, vaginal infections, tonsillitis, sinus infections, ringworm, skin rashes, impetigo, herpes, corns, head lice, cold sores, canker sores, insect bites, and fungal infections.

# BIBLIOGRAPHY

Abdullaev, F.I., and G.D. Frenkel. "Effect of Saffron on Cell Colony Formation and Cellular Nucleic Acid and Protein Synthesis." *Biofactors* 3 (1992): 201.

Abelin, J., et al. "Fat Binder as a Weight Reducer in Patients With Moderate Obesity." *ARS Medicina* (Aug./Oct. 1994).

Adlercreutz, H., et al. "Plasma Concentrations of Phytoestrogens in Japanese Men." *Lancet* 342 (8881) (Nov. 13, 1993): 1209–1210.

Ageel, A.M., et al. "Experimental Studies on Antirheumatic Crude Drugs Used in Saudi Traditional Medicine." *Drugs Exptl. Clin. Res.* 15 (1989): 296–301.

Airola, Paavo, Ph.D., N.D. *How to Get Well*. Health Plus, 1974.

Anderson, James W., et al. "Meta-Analysis of the Effects of Soy Protein Intake on Serum Lipids." *New England Journal of Medicine* (88) (1993): 3008–29.

Anderson, Nina, and Howard Peiper. *The Secrets of Staying Young (From the Inside Out)*. Sheffield, Massachusetts: Safe Goods Publishing, 1999.

Aonuma, S., et al. "Effects of Coptis, Scutellaria, Rhubarb, and Bupleurum on Serum Cholesterol and Phospholipids in Rabbits." *Takugaku Zasshi* 77 (1957): 1303–7.

"Artemisia Vulgaris." Wikipedia: The Free Encyclopedia. http://en.wikipedia.org

Astrup, A., et al. "The Effect and Safety of an Ephedrine/Caffeine Compared to Ephedrine, Caffeine, and Placebo in Obese Subjects on an Energy-Restricted Diet." *Inter Jour Obes* 16 (1992): 269–77.

Avorn, J., et al. "Reduction of Bacteriuria and Pyruia After Ingestion of Cranberry Juice." *JAMA* 271 (10) (Mar. 9, 1997): 751–4.

"Bacopa Monniera—Monograph." *Alternative Medicine Review* (March 2004).

"Bacopa Monnieri." Wikipedia: The Free Encyclopedia. http://en.wikipedia.org

Balch, James F., M.D., and Phyllis Balch. *Prescription for Nutritional Healing*. Garden City Park, New York: Avery Publishing Group, 1997.

"Banaba Leaf." www.supplementwatch.com

Barney, Paul, M.D. "The Cranberry Cure." *Herbs for Health* (Nov./Dec. 1996): 45.

———. *Doctor's Guide to Natural Medicine*. Pleasant Grove, Utah: Woodland Publishing, 1998.

Bauer, R., and H. Wagner. "Echinacea Species as Potential Immunostimulatory Drugs." *Econ Med Plant Res* 5 (1991): 253–321.

Beattie, Shelley, and John Romano. "The Ten Best Performance Supplements." *Muscular Development and Fitness* (July 1995): 192.

Beguin, M.H. *Natural Foods, Healthy Teeth*. La Chaux-de-Fonds, Switzerland: Edition de 1-Etoile, 1979.

Berkarda, B., et al. "The Effect of Coumarin

Derivatives on the Immunological System of Man." *Agents Actions* 13 (1983): 50–2.

Berwick, Ann. *Holistic Aromatherapy*. St. Paul, Minnesota: Llewellyn Publications, 1994.

"Best of Health World." *Health World Magazine*. 1993.

Bethel, May. *The Healing Power of Herbs*. 1969.

———. *The Healing Power of Natural Foods*. Wilshire Book Co., 1978.

Bianchini, Francesco, and Francesco Corbetta. *Health Plants of the World*. New York: Newsweek Books.

Bircher-Benner Clinic. *The Bircher-Benner Children's Diet Book*. New Canaan, Connecticut: Keats Publishing, 1977.

"Bitter Melon." *The Review of Natural Products* (Nov. 2004).

"Bitter Melon." Wikipedia: The Free Encyclopedia. http://en.wikipedia.org

"Bitter Orange." *The Review of Natural Products* (Oct. 2005).

Bliznakov, Emile G., M.D., and Gerald L. Hunt. *The Miracle Nutrient Coenzyme Q10*. New York: Bantam Books, 1987.

"Boswellia Serrata." www.supplementwatch.com

"Boswellia." Wikipedia: The Free Encyclopedia. http://en.wikipedia.org

"Boswellia." www.wholehealthmd.com

Braly, James, M.D. "A Scientific Herb for the Symptoms of Aging." *Doctor's Best*. Laguna Hills, California.

Braverman, Eric. *The Healing Nutrients Within*. New Canaan, Connecticut: Keats Publishing, 1997.

Breggin, Peter R., M.D. Toxic Psychiatry. St. Martin's Press, 1991.

Broadhurst, C. Leigh. "Turmeric." *Herbs for Health* (Nov./Dec. 1996): 41.

Brown, Donald J., N.D. "Shiitake Mushroom: A Model for the Efficacy of Immunomodulators in Cancer and HIV Infection." *Quarterly Review of Natural Medicine* (Spring 1994): 19.

———. "Herbs for Health." *Let's Live* (August 1994): 47.

———. "Valerian Root: Non-Addictive Alternative for Insomnia and Anxiety." *Quarterly Review of Natural Medicine* (Fall 1994): 222.

———. *Herbal Prescription for Better Health*. Prima Publishing, 1997.

Brown, Norman. "Mushrooms as Medicine." *Delicious!* (Jan. 1997): 54.

Brown, Royden. *Bee Hive Product Bible*. Garden City Park, New York: Avery Publishing, 1993.

Bucco, Gloria. "Wild Yam for Menopause." *Let's Live* (Jan. 1998): 78.

Buchanan, Clive. *Herbal Knowledge*. Pleasant Grove, Utah: Woodland Publishing, 1996.

Bukowiecki, L., et al. "Ephedrine, a Potential Slimming Drug, Directly Stimulates Thermogenesis in Brown Adipocytes via B-adrenoreceptors." *Inter Jour Obes* 6 (1982): 343–50.

Capelli, R., et al. "Extracts of Ruscus Aculeatus in Venous Disease in the Lower Limbs." *Drugs Exp Clin Res* 14 (4) (1988): 277.

"Caralluma Fimbriata: A New Dietary Supplement in Weight Management Strategies." Report to the U.S. Food and Drug Administration.

Carr, Anna, et al. *Rodale's Illustrated Encyclopedia of Herbs*. Emmaus, Pennsylvania: Rodale Press, 1987.

Castleman, Michael. *The Healing Herbs*. Emmaus, Pennsylvania: Rodale Press, 1996.

"Cat's Claw." *Energy Times* (May–June 1995).

Caujolle, F., P. Muriel, and E. Stanislas. *Annales Pharmaceutiques Françaises* (1953): 109–120.

Ceci, F., et al. "The Effects of Oral 5-HTP Administration on Feeding Behavior in Obese Adult Female Subjects." *J Neural Transm* 76 (1989): 109–17.

Center for Nutritional Research. "Most Frequently Asked Questions About Colostrum." CNR Publications: Internet, 1999.

———. "The Colostrum Miracle: Too Good to Be True?" CNR Publications: Internet, 1999.

Challem, Jack, and Renate Lewin-Challem. *What Herbs Are All About*. New Canaan, Connecticut: Keats Publishing, 1980.

Challem, Jack. "Good Bacteria That Fight the Bad." *Let's Live* (Oct. 1995): 55.

———. "Recharge With CoQ10." *Let's Live* (April 1996): 41.

———. "Vitamin E Fights Heart Disease." *Let's Live* (May 1993): 50.

Champault, G., et al. "Medical Treatment of Prostatic Adenoma." *Ann Urol* 18 (1984): 407–10.

Child, S.J. "Dimethysulfone (DMSO2) in the Treatment of Interstitial Cystitis." *Urol Clin North*

Am 21 (1) (Feb. 1994): 85–8.

Chilton, J.S. "The First International Conference on Mushroom Biology and Mushroom Products." *HerbalGram* 31: 57.

Christopher, John R. "Red Raspberry." *Herbalist Magazine* Vol. 1 (4) (1976): 129.

———. *The School of Natural Healing*. Orem, Utah: BiWorld Publishers, 1976.

Cichoke, Anthony J. "Pau d'Arco: Divine Herb from the Rain Forest." *Let's Live* (Dec. 1994): 36.

———. *Enzymes and Enzyme Therapy*. New Canaan, Connecticut: Keats Publishing, 1994.

Claustrat, B., et al. "Melatonin and Jet Lag: Confirmatory Results Using Simplified Protocol." *Bio Psychiatry* 32 (1992): 705–11.

Clymer, R. Swinburne, M.D. *Nature's Healing Agents*. The Humanitarian Society, 1905.

Cohen, M.L. "Epidemiology of Drug Resistance: Implications for a Post-Antimicrobial Era." *Science* 257 (1992): 1050–1055.

Colby, Benjamin. *Guide to Health*. 1846. Reprint. Orem, Utah: BiWorld Publishers.

Coon, Nelson. *Using Plants for Healing*. Rodale Press, 1979.

Cooper, Kenneth H. *Dr. Kenneth Cooper's Antioxidant Revolution*. Nashville: Thomas Nelson Publishers, 1994.

Cooper, Remi. *Antioxidants*. Pleasant Grove, Utah: Woodland Publishing, 1997.

Cowley, Geoffrey. "Melatonin." *Newsweek* (Aug. 7, 1995): 46.

Culpeper, Nicholas. *Culpeper's Herbal Remedies*. Wilshire Book Co., 1971.

———. *Culpeper's Complete Herbal*. England: W. Foulsham and Co.

Cunnane, S.C., et al. "High A-linoleic Flaxseed: Some Nutritional Properties." *Br J Nutr* 69 (1993): 443–53.

Dahlitz, M., et al. "Sleep-Inducing Effects of Low Doses of Melatonin Ingested in the Evening." *Lancet* 337 (1991): 1121–24.

Dawson, Adele G. *Health, Happiness, and the Pursuit of Herbs*. Vermont: The Stephen Greene Press, 1980.

Deihl, H.W. "Cetyl Myristoleate Isolated From Swiss Albino Mice: An Apparent Protective Agent Against Adjuvant Arthritis." *Journal of Pharmaceutical Sciences* 3 (1994): 296.

Della Loggia, R., et al. "Evaluation of Some Pharmacological Properties of a Peppermint Extract." *Fitoterapia* 61 (1990): 215–21.

Destreot, Raymond. *Our Earth, Our Cure*. Swan House Publishing, 1974.

Di Silvero, F., et al. "Evidence That Serenoa Repens Extract With Placebo by Controlled Clinical Trial in Patients Prostatic Hypertrophy." *Eur Urol* 21 (1992): 309–14.

Drovanti, A., et al. "Therapeutic Activity of Oral Glucosamine Sulfate in Osteoarthritis: A Placebo-Controlled Double-Blind Investigation." *Clinical Therapy* 3 (4) (1980): 260–72.

Duffield, P.H., and D. Jamieson. "Development of Tolerance to Kava in Mice." *Clin Exp Pharmacol Physiol* 18 (1991): 495–508.

Duke, James A. *Handbook of Medicinal Herbs*. Boca Raton, Florida: CRC Press, 1985.

Elkins, Rita. *Alpha Lipoic Acid*. Pleasant Grove, Utah: Woodland Publishing, 1998.

———. *Bee Pollen, Royal Jelly, Propolis, and Honey*. Pleasant Grove, Utah: Woodland Publishing, 1996.

———. *Blue-Green Algae, Spirulina, and Chlorella*. Pleasant Grove, Utah: Woodland Publishing, 1995.

———. *CMO*. Pleasant Grove, Utah: Woodland Publishing, 1997.

———. *Depression and Natural Medicine*. Pleasant Grove, Utah: Woodland Publishing, 1996.

———. *Encyclopedia of Fruits, Vegetables, Nuts, and Seeds for Healthful Living*.

———. *Noni*. Pleasant Grove, Utah: Woodland Publishing, 1996.

———. *Pycnogenol, The Miracle Antioxidant*. Pleasant Grove, Utah: Woodland Publishing.

———. *Shark Cartilage*. Pleasant Grove, Utah: Woodland Publishing, 1996.

———. *The Complete Home Health Advisor*. Pleasant Grove, Utah: Woodland Publishing, 1994.

———. *Wild Yam, Nature's Progesterone*. Pleasant Grove, Utah: Woodland Publishing, 1996.

Faber, K. "The Dandelion-Taraxacum Officinale." *Pharmazie* 13 (1958): 423–35.

Farwell, Edith Foster. *A Book of Herbs*. The White Pine Press, 1979.

Fischer-Rasmussen, W., et al. "Ginger Treatment of Hyperemesis Gravidarum." *Eur J Obstet Gynecol*

*Reprod Biol* 1 (1991): 19.

Fluck, Hans. *Medicinal Plants.* J.M. Rowson, trans. England: W. Foulsham & Co., 1973.

Foster, Steven, and James A. Duke. *Medicinal Plants.* Boston: Houghton Mifflin, 1990.

Foster, Steven. "Asian Ginseng." Botanical Series 303 (1991): 5.

———. "Evening Primrose." *Herbs for Health* (March/April 1997): 57.

———. "Milk Thistle." *Nutrition News* Vol. XII (10) (1989).

Fox, Arnold, M.D., and Nadine Taylor. "The Wonders of Shark Cartilage." *Let's Live* (March 1994): 14.

Fox, W. Shaffer. *100 & Healthy: Living Longer With Phytomedicines From the Republic of Georgia.* Orem, Utah: Woodland Publishing, 2004.

Franz, G. "Polysaccharides in Pharmacy, Current Applications and Future Concepts." *Planta Medica* 55 (1989): 493–7.

Gaby, A., M.D. *Preventing and Reversing Osteoporosis.* Rocklin, California: Prima Publishing, 1994.

Gagliardi, Gary. "Shark Cartilage for Achy Joints." *Muscle and Fitness* (Oct. 1995): 52–7.

Gainer, J.L., and J.R. Jones. "The Use of Crocetin in Experimental Atherosclerosis." *Experientia* 31 (1975): 548.

Gerard, John. *The Herbal: The Complete 1633 Edition.* Rev. by Thomas Johnson. New York: Dover Publications, 1975.

Gibbons, Euell. *Stalking the Wild Asparagus.* New York: David McKay Co., 1962.

Gilman, A.G., et al. *The Pharmacologic Basis of Therapeutics.* New York: Macmillan, 1980.

Goldberg, Burton. *Alternative Medicine.* Tiburon, California: Future Medicine Publishing, 1999.

Goleman, Daniel, Ph.D., and Joel Gurin, eds. *Mind, Body Medicine.* Consumer Reports Books, 1993.

Gordon, David, et al. "The Rumored Dope on Beijing's Women." *Newsweek* (Sept. 27, 1997): 63.

Gorman, Christine, et al. "The Fires Within." *Time* (Feb. 23, 2004).

Graedon, Joe. *The People's Pharmacy.* New York: Avon Publishers, 1980.

*The Green Book: A Summary of Scientific Literature on Herbal and Nutritional Supplements.* Orem, Utah: Woodland Publishing, 1999.

Grieve, M. A *Modern Herbal.* 2 vols. Dover Publications.

Griffin, LaDean. *Is Any Sick Among You?* Orem, Utah: BiWorld Publishers, 1974.

Griggs, Barbara. *Green Pharmacy.* Rochester, Vermont: Healing Arts Press, 1981.

Gunther. *The Greek Herbal of Dioscorides.* Cited in Christopher Hobbs, "Feverfew," HerbalGram 6 (1988): 28.

Harmon, N.W. "Herbal Medicine, The Chamomiles." *Can Pharm J* (Nov. 1989): 612.

Harris, Ben Charles. *The Complete Herbal.* New York: Larchmont Books, 1972.

———. *Eat the Weeds.* Keats Publishing, 1961.

Hawken, C.M. *Green Foods.* Pleasant Grove, Utah: Woodland Publishing, 1998.

He, G., et al. "Effect on the Prevention and Treatment of Atherosclerosis of a Mixture of Hawthorn and Motherwort." *Chung Hsi I Choeh Ho Tsa Chih* 10 (1990): 361.

Hennen, William J. *Chitosan.* Pleasant Grove, Utah: Woodland Publishing, 1996.

Herschler, Robert J. "Methylsulfonylmethane and Methods of Use." U.S. patent #4296130, issued Oct. 20, 1981.

———. "Methylsulfonylmethane in Dietary Products." U.S. patent #4616039, issued Oct. 7, 1986.

———. "Use of Methylsulfonylmethane to Relieve Pain and Nocturnal Cramps to Reduce Stress-Induced Deaths in Animals." U.S. patent # 4973605, issued Nov. 27, 1990.

Hikino, H. "Recent Research on Oriental Medicinal Plants." *Economic Medical Plant Research* 1 (1985): 53–85.

Hirazumi, A., et al. "Anticancer Activity of Morianda Citrifolia on Intraperitoneally Implanted Lewis Lung Carcinoma in Syngenic Mice." *Proc West Pharmacol* 37 (1994): 145–46.

Hobbs, Christopher. "A Literature Review." *HerbalGram* 17 (1988): 10–5.

———. "Cayenne, This Popular Herb Is Hot." *Let's Live* (April 1994): 55.

———. "Help Your Heart With Hawthorn." *Let's Live* (Feb. 1996): 78.

———. "Milk Thistle Therapy." *Herbs for Health* (July/August 1997): 49.

———. "St. John's Wort." *HerbalGram* (Fall/Winter 1988): 167.

———. *Foundations of Health, The Liver and Digestive Herbal*. Capitola, California: Botanica Press, 1992.

Hobson, Katherine. "The Body on Fire." *U.S. News and World Report* (Oct. 20, 2003).

Hoffman, David L. "Bugleweed." *Herbal Materia Medica*. Health World Online

Holmes, Peter. *The Energetics of Western Herbs*. Boulder: Artemis Press, 1989.

*Hoodia*. Orem, Utah: Woodland Publishing, 2005.

"Houpu Magnolia." Wikipedia: The Free Encyclopedia. http://en.wikipedia.org

Howell, E., M.D. *Food Enzymes for Health and Longevity*. Woodstock Valley, Connecticut: Omangod Press, 1980.

Hruby, K., et al. "Silybin in the Treatment of Deathcap Fungus Poisoning." *Forum* 6 (1984): 23–26.

Hutchens, Alma R. *Indian Herbology of North America*. Ontario, Canada: Merco, 1969.

Ikumoto, T., et al. "Physiologically Active Compounds in the Extracts From Tochukaso and Cultured Mycelia of Cordyceps and Msaria." *Yakugaku Zasshi* 111 (9) (1991): 504–9.

Inatani, R., et al. "Structure of a New Antioxidative Phenolic Diterpene Isolated From Rosemary." Agric. *Biol Chem* 6 (1982): 1661.

Ingram, Cass. *Killed on Contact*. Cedar Rapids, Iowa: Literary Visions Publishing.

Inouye, S., et al. "Inhibitory Effect of Volatile Constituents of Plants on the Proliferation of Bacteria." *Microbial Biochem* 100 (1984): 232.

Jackson, Deb, and Karen Bergeron. "Wild Quinine." http://altnature.com

Jacob, S., et al. "Enhancement of Glucose Disposal in Patients With Type 2 Diabetes by Alpha-Lipoic Acid." *Arzneim Forsch* 45 (1995): 872–4.

Jacob, Stanley W., M.D. "Pharmacologic Management of Snoring." U.S. patent #5569679, issued Oct. 29, 1996.

Jarrard, Greg. *Ashwagandha: Ayurveda's Miracle Herbal Adaptogen*. Orem, Utah: Woodland Publishing, 2004.

Jensen, Bernard, D.C. *Nature Has a Remedy*. 1978.

Johnson, E.S., et al. "Efficacy of Feverfew as Prophylactic Treatment of Migraines." *British Medical Journal* 291 (1985): 569–73.

Jones, K. "An Ancient Chinese Secret Promotes Longevity and Endurance." *Healthy and Natural Journal* 3 (3) (1997): 90–2.

———. *Cordyceps: Tonic Food of Ancient China*. Seattle: Sylvan Press, 1997.

Jones, Susan Smith, and Brian Bailey. "Tofu Is a Superfood for the 1990s." *Let's Live* (June 1995): 84.

Jones, Susan Smith. "Honeybee Pollen." *Let's Live* (Dec. 1995): 60.

Kadans, Joseph, N.D., Ph.D. *Encyclopedia of Medicinal Herbs*. New York: Arco Publishing, 1970.

Kamen, Betty. "Gymnema Extract." *Let's Live* (Sept. 1989): 40–1.

Kao, P.C., and F.K. P'eng. "How to Reduce the Risk Factors of Osteoporosis in Asia." *Chung Hua I Hsueh Tsa Chih* (Taipei) 3 (55) (March 1995): 209–13.

Keville, Kathi. *Herbs for Health and Healing*. Emmaus, Pennsylvania: Rodale Press, 1996.

Kight, Juli. "Bacopa." http://healthyherbs.about.com
——— . "Banaba Leaf." http://healthyherbs.-about.com

Kinosian, B.P., and J.M. Eisenber. "Cutting Into Cholesterol: Cost-Effective Alternatives for Treating Hypercholesterolemia." *JAMA* 259 (15) (April 15, 1988): 2249–54.

Kirschmann, John D. *Nutrition Almanac*. Rev. ed. McGraw Hill, 1979.

Kloss, Jethro. *Back to Eden*. Loma Linda, California: Back to Eden Books, 1971.

Koch, Carolee Bateson, D.C., N.D. *Allergies: Disease in Disguise*. Alive Books, 1994.

Kordel, Lelord. *Natural Folk Remedies*. Manor Books, 1974.

Krampf, Leslie. "Green Giants: The New Superfoods." *Delicious* (April 1996).

Krinsky, Norman. "Carotenoids and Cancer: Basic Research Studies." *Natural Antioxidants in Human Health and Disease*. Boston: Academic Press, 1994.

Krochmal, Arnold, and Connie Krochmal. *A Guide to the Medicinal Plants of the United States*. The New York Times Book Co., 1973.

Kroeger, Hanna. *Good Health Through Diets*. Boulder, Colorado.

"Kudzu." Wikipedia: The Free Encyclopedia. http://en.wikipedia.org

"Kudzu." www.wholehealthmd.com

Kuroda, K., and K. Takagi. "Pharmacological and Chemical Studies on the Alcohol Extract of Capsella Bursa Pastoris." *Life Sciences* 3 (1969): 151–5.

———. "Physiologically Active Substances in Capsella Bursa Pastoris." *Nature* 5169 (1968): 707–8.

Lane, I. William, and Linda Comac. *Sharks Don't Get Cancer*. Garden City Park, New York: Avery Publishing, 1993.

Lee, Deborah. *Essential Fatty Acids*. Pleasant Grove, Utah: Woodland Publishing, 1997.

Lee, John R., M.D. "Osteoporosis Reversal: The Role of Progesterone." *Int Clin Nutr Rev* 10 (1990): 384–91.

Lee, K.N., et al. "Conjugated Linoleic Acid and Atherosclerosis in Rabbits." *Atherosclerosis* 108: 19–25.

Leicester, R.J., and R.H. Hunt. "Peppermint Oil to Reduce Colonic Spasm During Endoscopy." *Lancet* II (1982): 989.

Leung, A.Y. *Encyclopedia of Common Natural Ingredients Used in Food, Drugs, and Cosmetics*. New York: J. Wiley and Sons, 1980.

Lewis, Walter H., and Memory P.F. Elvin. *Medical Botany: Plants of the United States*. The New York Times Book Co., 1973.

Ley, Beth M. DHEA: *Unlocking the Secrets to the Fountain of Youth*. Newport Beach, California: BL Publications, 1996.

Lieberman, Shari, and Nancy Bruning. *The Real Vitamin and Mineral Book*. Garden City Park, New York: Avery Publishing Group.

Lipsky, H., et al. "Dietary Fiber for Reducing Blood Cholesterol." *Journal of Clinical Pharmacology* 30 (8) (Aug. 1990): 699–703.

Loren, Karl. *The Report of Germanium*. Glendale, California: Life Extension Educational Service, 1987.

"Maca." Wikipedia: The Free Encyclopedia. http://en.wikipedia.org

"Maca." www.supplementwatch.com

"Maca." www.wholehealthmd.com

"Magnolia Bark." www.supplementwatch.com

Maitra, I., et al. "Alpha Lipoic Acid Prevents Buthionine Sulfoximine-Induced Cataract Formation in Newborn Rats." *Free Radical Biology and Medicine* 18 (1995): 823–9.

Malstrom, Stan, N.D., M.T. *Own Your Own Body*. Fresh Mountain Air Publishing, 1977.

———. *Herbal Remedies* II. Rev. ed. Woodland Books, 1975.

"Mangosteen." Wikipedia: The Free Encyclopedia. http://en.wikipedia.org

"Mangosteen." www.supplementwatch.com

Margen, Sheldon, M.D. *The Wellness Encyclopedia of Food and Nutrition*. New York: Rebus, 1992.

Mars, Brigette. "Mullein as Medicine." *Let's Live* (April 1996): 79.

———. "Evening Primrose Oil." *Let's Live* (May 1995): 25.

Marti, James E. *Alternative Health Medicine Encyclopedia*. Detroit: Visible Ink, 1995.

Mascolo, N., et al. "Biological Screening of Italian Medicinal Plants for Anti-Inflammatory Activity." *Phytother Res* 1 (1987): 28–31.

Mautner, H.G., et al. "Antibiotic Activity of Seaweed Extracts." *J Amer Pharm Ass* 5 (1953): 294–6.

McCabe, D., et al. "Polar Solvents in the Chemoprevention of Dimethybenzanthracene-Induced Rat Mammary Cancer." *Arch Surg* 121 (12) (Dec. 1986): 1455–9.

McCaleb, Rob. "Bilberry, Health From Head to Toe." *Better Nutrition for Today's Living* (June 1991).

———. "Garlic, Infection Fighter." *Better Nutrition* (August 1993): 47.

———. "Mental Function and Gotu Kola." *HerbalGram* 28 (1993): 32.

———. "Research Reviews." *HerbalGram* 24 (1991): 21.

McCleod, Dawn. *Herb Handbook*. Wilshire Book Co., 1968.

Mckenzie, L.S., et al. "Osteoarthritis: Uncertain Rationale for Anti-Inflammatory Drug Therapy." *Lancet* 1 (1976): 908.

Menchini-Fabris, G.F., et al. "New Perspectives on Treatment of Prostato-Vesicular Pathologies With Pygeum Africanum." *Arch Int Urol* 60 (1988): 313–22.

*Merck Manual*. 9th ed. Merck and Co.

Messina, Mark, and Virginia Messina. *The Simple Soybean and Your Health*. New York: Avery Publishing Group, 1994.

Meyer, Joseph E. *The Herbalist*. Glenwood, Illinois: Meyer Books, 1918.

Montagna, Joseph F. *The People's Desk Reference.* Lake Oswego, Oregon: Quest for Truth Publishing, 1979.

Moore, Michael. *Medicinal Plants of the Mountain West.* Museum of New Mexico Press, 1980.

Morales, A., et al. "Nonhormonal Pharmacological Treatment of Organic Impotence." *J Urol* 128 (1982): 45.

Moriga, M., et al. "The Activity of N-Acetyl-Glucosamine Kinase in Rat Gastric Mucosa." *Gastroenterol Japonica* 15: 7.

Mowrey, Daniel B. "Chlorella: A Jack of All Trades for Your Health." *Let's Live* (Feb. 1989): 80.

———. *Herbal Tonic Therapies.* New Canaan, Connecticut: Keats Publishing, 1993.

"Mugwort." Natural Medicines Comprehensive Database. Stockton, California: Therapeutic Research Faculty, 2005.

Murphy, J.J., et al. "Randomized Double-Blind, Placebo-Controlled Trial of Feverfew in Migraine Prevention." *Lancet* 2 (1988): 189–92.

Murray, Frank. "Suma Lauded." *Better Nutrition* (June 1987): 17.

Murray, M.J., et al. "Oil Composition of Mentha Aquatica X. M. Spicata F1 Hybrids in Relation to the Origin of M. X. Piperita." *Canad. J. Genet. Cytol.* 14 (1972): 13–29.

Murray, Michael T. "Natural Approaches to Impotence." *Let's Live* (July 1995): 44.

———. "Sexual Vitality for Men and Women." *Let's Live* (May 1994): 16.

———. *Arthritis.* Rocklin, California: Prima Publishing, 1994.

———. *The Healing Power of Foods.* Rocklin, California: Prima Publishing, 1993.

———. *The Healing Power of Herbs.* Rocklin, California: Prima Publishing, 1995.

———. *Natural Alternatives to Over-The-Counter and Prescription Drugs.* Rocklin, California: Prima Publishing.

Murray, Michael T., and Joseph Pizzorno. *Encyclopedia of Natural Medicine.* Rocklin, California: Prima Publishing, 1991.

Nadraszky, Bill. "Caralluma—Appetite Suppressant." www.nadraszky.com (Apr. 20, 2006).

Nagabhushan, M., and S.V. Bhide. "Curcumin as an Inhibitor of Cancer." *J Am Coll Nutr* 11 (1992): 192.

Nair, S.C., et al. "Antitumor Activity of Saffron." *Cancer Lett* 57 (1991): 109.

Nauss, J.L., et al. "The Binding of Micellar Lipids to Chitosan." *Lipids* 10 (1983): 714–9.

O'Dwyer, P.J., et al. "Use of Polar Solvents in Chemoprevention of 1,2-Dimethyldrazine-Induced Colon Cancer." *Cancer* 62 (5) (Sept. 1, 1988): 944–8.

Ody, Penelope. *The Complete Medicinal Herbal.* London: Dorling Kindersley, 1993.

Olsen, Cynthia B. *Australian Tea Tree Oil.* Pagosa Springs, Colorado: Kali Press, 1991.

Orey, Cal. "Chamomile Secrets," *Let's Live* (March 1995).

Osawa, T., et al. "A Novel Antioxidant Isolated From Young Green Barley Leaves." *J Agr Food Chem* 40 (1992): 1135–37.

Packer, Lester, et al. "Alpha Lipoic Acid as a Biological Antioxidant." *Free Radical Biology and Medicine* 19 (1995): 227–50.

Pariza, Michael, et al. "Mammary Cancer Prevention by Conjugated Dienoice Derivative of Linoleic Acid." *Cancer Research* 51 (Nov. 15, 1991): 6118–24.

Passwater, Richard A. *Cancer Prevention and Nutritional Therapies.* New Canaan, Connecticut: Keats Publishing, 1987.

———. "Coenzyme Q10: The Nutrient of the 90s." *Health Connection* (April 1987).

———. *The Antioxidants.* New Canaan, Connecticut: Keats Publishing.

"Pawpaw." *The Review of Natural Products* (July 2004).

"Pawpaw." Wikipedia: The Free Encyclopedia. http://en.wikipedia.org

"Phellodendron." Wikipedia: The Free Encyclopedia. http://en.wikipedia.org

"Phellodendron." www.supplementnews.org

Picozzi, Michele. "Drink Up, Green Tea Offers Bounty of Health Benefits." *Let's Live* (March 1996): 45.

———. "Medicinal Mushrooms." *Let's Live* (Aug. 1995): 80.

Pitchford, Paul. *Healing With Whole Foods.* Berkeley, California: North Atlantic Books, 1993.

Pizzorno, J.E., and Michael T. Murray. *A Textbook of Natural Medicine.* Seattle: JBC Publications, 1985.

"Plants for a Future: Parthenium Integrifolium."

http://www.ibiblio.org

Pohl, P. "Therapy of Radiation-Induced Leukopenia by Esberitox." *Med Klin* 64 (1969): 1546.

*Professional Guide to Diseases*, Medical Desk Reference. Intermed Communications Books.

Rai, V., et al. "Effect of Ocimum Sanctum Leaf Powder on Blood Lipoproteins, Glycated Proteins, and Total Amino Acids in Patients With Non-Insulin-Dependent Diabetes Mellitus." *J Nutr Environ Med* 7 (1997): 113–8.

Ramazanov, Zakir, Ph.D., et al. *Stress and Weight Management: Effective Herbal Therapy Using Rhodiola Rosea and Rhododendron Caucasicum.* Sheffield, Massachusetts: Safe Goods Publishing, 1999.

*Reader's Digest Family Guide to Natural Medicine.* Pleasantville, New York: The Reader's Digest Association, 1993.

Reuben, Carolyn. *Antioxidants, Your Complete Guide.* Rocklin, California: Prima Publishing, 1995.

"Rhodiola." www.wholehealthmd.com

"Rhodiola Rosea." Wikipedia: The Free Encyclopedia. http://en.wikipedia.org

Ritchason, Jack. *The Little Herb Encyclopedia.* Pleasant Grove, Utah: Woodland Publishing, 1994.

———. *The Vitamin and Health Encyclopedia.* Pleasant Grove, Utah: Woodland Publishing, 1996.

Sabir, M., and N. Bhide. "Study of Some Pharmacologic Actions of Berberine." *Ind J Phys Pharm* 15 (1971): 111–32.

Schardt, David. "Grading Vitamin C." *Nutrition Action Newsletter* (Nov. 1994): 10.

Schechter, Steve. "Schizandra." *Let's Live* (Sept. 1994): 76.

Scheer, James F. "Acidophilus, Nature's Antibiotic." *Better Nutrition for Today's Living* (Aug. 1993): 34.

Schlegelmilch, R., and R. Heywood. "Toxicity of Cratageus (Hawthorn) Extract." *J Amer College Toxicol* 13 (1994): 103–11.

Schmidt, Michael A., Lendon H. Smith, and Keith W. Sehnert. *Beyond Antibiotics.* Berkeley, California: North Atlantic Books, 1994.

Schoneberger, D. "The Influence of Immune-Stimulating Effects of Pressed Juice From Echinacea Purpurea on the Course and Severity of Colds." *Forum Immunol* 8 (1992): 2–12.

"Sea Buckthorn." www.supplementwatch.com

"Sea-buckthorn." Wikipedia: The Free Encyclopedia.

http://en.wikipedia.org

Selvam, R., et al. "The Antioxidant Activity of Turmeric." *Journal of Ethnopharmacology* 47 (1995): 59–67.

Sharaf, A., et al. "Glycyrrhetic Acid as an Active Estrogenic Substance Separated From Glycyrrhiza Glabra." *Egyptian J Pharm Sci* 2 (1975): 245–51.

Sharma, R., et al. "Berberine Tannate in Acute Diarrhea." *Indian Pediatr* 7 (1970): 496–501.

Sharp, David. "Six Teas That Promise Much More Than Comforting Warmth on a Chilly Day." *Health* (Nov./Dec. 1996): 102.

Shealy, C. Norman, M.D. *DHEA: The Youth and Health Hormone.* New Canaan, Connecticut: Keats Publishing, 1986.

Shomon, Mary. "What You Need to Know About Caralluma Fimbriata." http://thyroid.about.com

Shook, Edward E. *Advanced Treatise in Herbology.* Lakemont, Georgia: CSA Press, 1978.

Singletary, K.W., and J.M. Nelshoppen. "Inhibition of 7,12-Dimethylbenza Anthracene (DMBA)-Induced Mammary Tumorigenesis and of In Vivo Formation of Mammary DMBA-DNA Adducts by Rosemary Extract." *Cancer Lett* 2 (1991): 169.

Smith, Gary Robert, and Sotiris Missailidis. "Cancer, Inflammation, and the AT1 and AT2 Receptors." *Journal of Inflammation* (Sept. 30, 2004).

Sotolongo, Jose R., M.D., et al. "Successful Treatment of Lupus Erythematosus Cystitis with DMSO." *Urology* 23 (2) (Feb. 1984): 125–7.

Soucek, M., et al. "Constitution of Parthenolide." *Collection of Czechoslovak Chemical Communications* 26 (1959): 803–810.

Spencer, Mike. "Yucca, New Hope for Arthritics." *Let's Live* (Feb. 1975).

Sporn, A., and O. Schobesch. "Toxicity of Nordihydroquaiaretic Acid." *Igiena* (1966): 725–6.

Srivastava, K.C., and T. Mustafa. "Ginger and Rheumatic Disorders." *Med Hypothesis* 29 (1989): 25–8.

Stanko, R.T., et al. "Body Composition, Energy Utilization, and Nitrogen Metabolism With a Severely Restricted Diet Supplemented With Pyruvate." *American Journal of Clinical Nutrition* 55 (1992): 771–5.

———. "Enhancement of Arm Exercise Endurance Capacity With Dihydroxyacetone and Pyruvate." *J Appl Physiol* 68 (1) (Jan. 1990): 119–20.

———. "Pyruvate Inhibits Clofibrate-Induced Hepatic Peroxisomal Proliferation and Free Radical Production in Rats." *Metabolism* 44 (2) (Feb. 1995): 166–71.

———. "Pyruvate Inhibits Growth of Mammary Adenocarcinoma 13762 in Rats." *Cancer Research* 54 (1994): 1004–7.

———. "Pyruvate Supplementation of a Low-Cholesterol, Low-Fat Diet: Effects on Plasma Lipid Concentrations and Body Composition in Hyperlipidemic Patients." *American Journal of Clinical Nutrition* 59 (2) (Feb. 1994): 423–7.

Steenblock, David A. "Chlorella and Detoxification." *Let's Live* (March 1989): 28.

Steinberg, Philip N. "Uncaria Tomentosa (Cat's Claw): A Wondrous Herb From the Peruvian Rainforest." *Townsend Letter* 130 (May 1994): 2.

———. "Uncaria Tomentosa (Cat's Claw): Wonder Herb From the Amazon." *New Editions Health World* (Feb. 1995): 43.

Steinmetz, K.A., et al. "Vegetables, Fruit, and Colon Cancer in the Iowa Women's Health Study." *Am J Epidemiol* 139 (1994): 1–5.

Stoll, B.A. "Eating to Beat Breast Cancer: Potential Role for Soy Supplements." *Ann Oncol* 3 (March 8, 1997): 223–25.

Suzuki, O., et al. "Inhibition of Monoamine Oxidase by Hypericin." *Planta Medica* 50 (1984): 272–74.

Suzuki, Y.J., et al. "Lipoate Prevents Glucose-Induced Protein Modifications." *Free Radical Res Commun* 17 (1992): 211–17.

Szturma, W. "Method for Treating Gastro-Intestinal Ulcers With Extract of Herb Cetair." U.S. Patent 4150123 (April 17, 1979).

Tauchert, M., et al. "Effectiveness of the Hawthorn Extract Li 132 Compared With the ACE Inhibitor Captopril." *Munch Med* 136 (1994): 27–33.

"Tell Me About Phellodendron (Huang Bai)." www.acupuncturetoday.com

Tenney, Louise. *Ginkgo*. Pleasant Grove, Utah: Woodland Publishing, 1996.

———. *The Encyclopedia of Natural Remedies*. Pleasant Grove, Utah: Woodland Publishing, 1995.

*The Lawrence Review of Natural Products*. St. Louis: Facts and Comparisons.

Tkac, Debora. *The Doctor's Book of Home Remedies*. New York: Bantam Books, 1991.

Tsunoo, A., et al. *Science and Cultivation of Edible Fungi*. Rotterdam: Elliott Balkema, 1995.

Tyler, Varro E. *The Honest Herbal*. New York: PPP, 1993.

Udall, Kate Gilbert. *Amino Acids, The Building Blocks of Life*. Pleasant Grove, Utah: Woodland Publishing, 1997.

Vahouny, G., et al. "Comparative Effects of Chitosan and Cholestryramine on Lymphatic Absorption of Lipids in the Rat." *Am J Clin Nutr* 2 (1983): 278–84.

Vennet, B. "Anti-Ulcer Activity of Procyanidin Preparation of Water-Soluble Procyanidin Cimetidine Complexes." *Pharm Acta Helv* 11 (1989): 316–20.

Voaden, D., and M. Jacobson. "Identification and Synthesis of Oncolytic Hydrocarbon From American Coneflower Roots." *J Med Chem* 5 (1972): 619–23.

Vogel, G. Proceedings of the International Bioflavonoid Symposium. Munich, 1981.

Vukovic, Laurel. "Breathe Deeply . . . and Relax." *Natural Health* (Nov/Dec 1995): 64.

Wagner, H., et al. "The Chemistry of Silymarin (Silybin), the Active Principle of the Fruits of Silybum Marianum." *Arzenium-Forsch* 18 (1968): 688–96.

Wang, H., and Y. Wu. "Inhibitory Effect of Chinese Tea on N-Nitrosation In Vitro and In Vivo." *IARC Sci Publ* 105 (1991): 546.

Wardlaw, G.M., et al. "Serum Lipid and Apolipoprotein Concentrations in Healthy Men on Diets Enriched in Either Canola Oil or Safflower Oil." *American Journal of Clinical Nutrition* 54 (1991): 104.

Weil, Andrew, M.D. "A Bitter Route to Long Life?" www.drweil.com (Aug. 1, 2002).

———. "A Magic Route to Health and Wealth?" www.drweil.com (May 20, 2004).

———. "Can Herbs Combat Inflammation?" www.drweil.com (Dec. 3, 2002)

———. "Eating to Ease Inflammation?" www.drweil.com (July 12, 2005)

———. *Eating Well for Optimum Health: The Essential Guide to Food, Diet, and Nutrition*. New York: Alfred A. Knopf, 2000.

———. "Energizing the Elderly?" www.drweil.com

(Mar. 24, 2005).

———. "Influencing Inflammation?" www.drweil.com (Nov. 3, 2005).

———. *Natural Health, Natural Medicine.* Boston: Houghton Mifflin, 1990.

———. "Preventing Breast Cancer With a European Herb?" www.drweil.com (June 24, 2003).

———. "Should You Try Thermogenic Supplements for Weight Loss?" www.drweil.com (Jan. 22, 2002).

———. "Turning Off Cravings for Alcohol?" www.drweil.com (Mar. 3, 2005).

Weiner, Michael A., and Janet A. Weiner. *Herbs That Heal.* Mill Valley, California: Quantum Books, 1994.

Weiss, Rudolf Fritz, M.D. *Herbal Medicine.* Beaconsfield, England: Beaconsfield Publishers, 1988.

Weissman, G. "Aspirin." *Scientific American* (Jan. 1991): 58–64.

Williams, Lane. *CLA.* Pleasant Grove, Utah: Woodland Publishing, 1997.

———. *Griffonia.* Pleasant Grove, Utah: Woodland Publishing, 1998.

Wilson, Roberta. *A Complete Guide to Understanding and Using Aromatherapy.* Garden City Park, New York: Avery Publishing, 1995.

Wright, Jonathan V., M.D. "Safe Uses of DHEA." *Let's Live* (July 1996): 26.

Yaginuma, T., et al. "Effect of Traditional Herbal Medicine on Serum Testosterone Levels and Its Induction of Regular Ovulation in Hyper-Androgenic and Oligomenorrhetic Women." *Nippon Sanka Fujinka Gakkai Zasshii* 7 (1982): 939–44.

Yang, W., et al. "Treatment of Sexual Hypofunction With Cordyceps Sinensis." *Jiangxi Zhongyiyao* 5 (1985): 46–7.

Yaychuk-Arabei, Irene, Ph.D. "Successful Slimming Hastened With Herbs." *Health Naturally* (June/July 1996): 26.

Zinchenko, T.C., and I.M. Fefer. "Investigation of Glicosides from Betonica Officinalis." *Farmatsevt Zhurnal* 3 (1962): 35–8.

Zoltan, Rona P., M.D. "The Joys of Soy." *Health Naturally* (Oct./Nov. 1997): 23.

Zucker, Martin. "Vitamin E." *Let's Live* (Nov. 1997)

# INDEX